Surgical Management
of Congestive Heart Failure

CONTEMPORARY CARDIOLOGY

CHRISTOPHER P. CANNON, MD
SERIES EDITOR

SURGICAL MANAGEMENT OF CONGESTIVE HEART FAILURE

Edited by

JAMES C. FANG, MD

GREGORY S. COUPER, MD

Brigham and Women's Hospital, Harvard Medical School, Boston, MA

Foreword by

LYNNE W. STEVENSON, MD

Brigham and Women's Hospital, Harvard Medical School, Boston, MA

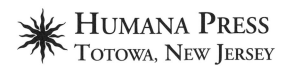

HUMANA PRESS
TOTOWA, NEW JERSEY

© 2005 Humana Press Inc.
999 Riverview Drive, Suite 208
Totowa, New Jersey 07512

humanapress.com

For additional copies, pricing for bulk purchases, and/or information about other Humana titles, contact Humana at the above address or at any of the following numbers: Tel.: 973-256-1699; Fax: 973-256-8341, E-mail: humana@humanapr.com; or visit our Website: www.humanapress.com

Production Editor: Robin B. Weisberg
Cover Illustration: From Fig. 2 in Chapter 4, "Mitral Valve Surgery With Severe Left Ventricular Dysfunction," by Vinay Badhwar and Steven F. Bolling.
Cover design by Patricia F. Cleary

This publication is printed on acid-free paper. ∞
ANSI Z39.48-1984 (American National Standards Institute) Permanence of Paper for Printed Library Materials.

eISBN 1-59259-842-0

Library of Congress Cataloging-in-Publication Data

Surgical management of congestive heart failure / edited by James C. Fang, Gregory S. Couper.
    p. ; cm. -- (Contemporary cardiology)
 Includes bibliographical references and index.
 ISBN 1-58829-034-4 (alk. paper)
 1. Heart--Surgery. 2. Congestive heart failure.
    [DNLM: 1. Cardiac Surgical Procedures--methods. 2. Heart Failure, Congestive--surgery. WG 169 S9615 2005] I. Fang, James C. II. Couper, Gregory S. III. Sereis: Contemporary cardiology (Totowa, N.J. : Unnumbered)
 RD598.S854 2005
 616.1'29--dc22

                                                                              2004004129

FOREWORD

There are 4 to 5 million people with heart failure in the United States alone. Included in this diagnosis are patients who have decreased left ventricular contractility and ejection fraction but no symptoms, and patients who have "preserved" ejection fraction, even supernormal in hypertrophic cardiomyopathy, in whom an impairment of ventricular filling leads to exercise intolerance and elevated venous pressures. However, the majority of patients currently diagnosed have left ventricular ejection fraction 20–40% and mild to moderate symptoms of heart failure.

Medical Therapy for Heart Failure

For these patients, there have been major advances in pharmacologic therapy since the late 1980s, since the demonstration that vasodilator therapy improves outcome in heart failure. Subsequent trials showed that inhibition of the renin-angiotensin system enzyme bestows additional benefit, decreasing recurrent ischemic events and improving outcomes for patients with diabetes, as well as decreasing the left ventricular dilation, or "remodeling" that characterizes heart failure progression. Even more striking for survival benefit has been the addition of β-adrenergic blocking agents. The complexity of initiation and uptitration of β-blocking agents has highlighted the chasm between the recommended therapeutic regimen and the limited experience and resources available to establish and maintain that regimen in the community. The true impact of the therapies proven in clinical trials has not yet been realized, but may be less than anticipated when those therapies are provided without clinical trial-level surveillance to populations on average 10 years older and with more co-morbidities.

Although inhibition of the renin-angiotensin system and β-receptors of the sympathetic nervous system have provided the cornerstones of our pharmacologic therapy, it is not clear whether more benefit can be derived from further neurohormonal modulation. Trials of central sympatholysis, angiotensin receptor blockers, cytokine inhibitors, and endothelin antagonists may even be deleterious on top of the known therapies. Furthermore, as heart failure progresses, an increasing proportion of patients are unable to tolerate reflex inhibition, first showing intolerance to β-blockers, then to angiotensin-converting enzyme (ACE) inhibitors. Symptoms of congestion can be relieved at most stages of heart failure until close to the end stage, when the cardiorenal syndrome often becomes limiting before there is other evidence of refractory low output states. Oral inotropic therapy to improve cardiac output was abandoned owing to a small but significant increase in mortality. Paradoxically, intravenous inotropic therapy is increasingly used to provide palliation at the end stage of heart failure. Expected survival is less than 50% at 6 months for patients who are dependent on chronic inotropic therapy.

Surgery for Heart Failure: Repair, Remodeling, and Replacement

Since medical therapy for heart failure has delayed but not prevented disease progression, there is increasing interest in more definitive therapy. Many previous surgical approaches were tried and subsequently abandoned, whereas transplantation became an accepted therapy without any controlled experiment. More recently, the template of the double-blind randomized clinical trial that has validated drug therapies has been superimposed with some awkwardness on investigation of procedures and devices. After initial feasibility has been shown, systematic performance and documentation of outcomes with a new therapy without randomization can provide conclusive evidence of lack of sufficient efficacy to merit a controlled trial, as with the commendable experience of the Cleveland Clinic with the left ventriculectomy procedure. For cardiomyo-plasty, the limited functional improvement observed was not sufficient to maintain enthusiasm for the courageously planned randomized trial, subsequently plagued with slow enrollment. For benefit, it remains possible that early experience carefully recorded with a new procedure could be sufficiently positive to constitute a "breakthrough" development, after which equipoise could not then be established for a randomized trial. More often, there are encouraging results that warrant further investigation with a prospective control arm. It should be recognized, however, that inability to provide an ethical double blind limits both patient enrollment and the interpretation of results for such trials. These limitations and the inherently greater cost and risk of surgical procedures mandate a higher bar of obvious benefit before acceptance of a new surgical procedure for heart failure.

Inherent in consideration of surgery for heart failure is the recognition that some patients are more likely to benefit than others. In this respect, the surgical approaches are already advanced beyond the medical approaches, which have been hindered by the assumption of homogeneity of the heart failure populations. In *Surgical Management of*

Congestive Heart Failure, multiple different procedures for heart failure are presented, together with careful description of the candidate populations for each. For procedures such as revascularization and valve repair or replacement, the benefit has been well established for some populations. The challenge here is to push the envelope to identify when such procedures may offer meaningful benefit for patients once considered to be "too late" in the stage of their disease. Other procedures under active investigation for advanced stages of disease, such as ventricular reconstruction or external constraint devices, may eventually be introduced earlier in the course of disease to limit disease progression. At the end of the road, the goal of effective cardiac replacement looms large. Cardiac transplantation at this time remains the greatest success story for truly end-stage disease, with more than 50,000 patients now transplanted worldwide. The breadth of its impact far exceeds the actual recipients, however, because the lure of cardiac transplantation called attention to the newly defined population of advanced heart failure, whereas the restricted donor supply inspired the development of better heart failure management and of new strategies for replacement, such as mechanical cardiac devices and xenotransplantation.

The Right Therapy for Each Patient

Heart failure has legitimately moved into a field of its own. After a barren period in the mid-1990s when medical therapy was ACE inhibitors and surgical therapy was transplantation, better understanding of the physiology of heart failure has yielded a cornucopia of potential options. At the same time, survival alone is no longer the only count of success. The implanted defibrillators have decreased the cloud of sudden death, and biventricular pacing has shown larger improvement in symptoms than seen with neurohormonal therapy, but issues of functional capacity and quality of life are increasingly relevant. Heart failure is not one disease, and the heart failure patient is not a composite of averages. The individual patient has developed heart failure uniquely through injury and adaptation, suffers the limitations of heart failure uniquely, and seeks therapy with unique expectations regarding length and quality of survival, tempered by risk-taking preferences that can be honored but not predicted. This book seeks to encompass both the large studies and the vital experiences. Improved outcome in heart failure must be calibrated and tracked for populations, but will ultimately be provided by individual physicians for individual patients.

Lynne W. Stevenson, MD

PREFACE

Congestive heart failure (CHF) is one of the leading causes of hospitalization in the United States and is associated with significant morbidity and mortality. Pharmacologic therapies have had a significant impact on the disease, but have been primarily limited to angiotensin-converting enzyme inhibitors and β-blockers. Inotropic agents and other vasodilators are available and effective for the acute management of heart failure, but are associated with poor long-term outcomes. Until recently, few surgical therapies were available for severe end-stage CHF short of cardiac transplantation. With the advent of better surgical techniques and improved pre- and postoperative medical management, traditional surgeries for severe left ventricular dysfunction can now be performed with reasonable success. Furthermore, the advances in mechanical circulatory support devices have made the concept of bridging to transplant and bridging to recovery a reality. Even permanent mechanical circulatory support is now available. Finally, other novel approaches using various devices are constantly being investigated.

The surgical options for the end-stage heart failure patient are now numerous and effective. The aim of *Surgical Management of Congestive Heart Failure* is to bring together the latest clinical, scientific, and investigational surgical approaches to improve the lives of this challenging group of patients. The book is written by leading authorities in both cardiovascular surgery and cardiology as the management of these patients has necessitated an increasingly multidisciplinary approach. We hope that the readers will get a broad yet in-depth understanding of the options that can be offered to their patients and what the future holds for the surgical and device-oriented treatment of heart failure.

James C. Fang, MD
Gregory S. Couper, MD

CONTENTS

CONTRIBUTORS

MICHAEL A. ACKER, MD, *Division of Cardiothoracic Surgery, University of Pennsylvania School of Medicine, Philadelphia, PA*

FRANCISCO A. ARABIA, MD, *Department of Surgery, Sarver Heart Center, University of Arizona College of Medicine, Tucson, AZ*

VINAY BADHWAR, MD, *Section of Cardiac Surgery, University of Michigan, Ann Arbor, MI*

STEVEN F. BOLLING, MD, *Section of Cardiac Surgery, University of Michigan, Ann Arbor, MI*

JOHN G. BYRNE, MD, *Division of Cardiac Surgery, Department of Surgery, Brigham and Women's Hospital, Harvard Medical School, Boston, MA*

BLASÉ A. CARABELLO, MD, FACC, *Department of Medicine, Baylor College of Medicine, Veterans Affairs Medical Center, Houston, TX*

JACK G. COPELAND, MD, *Section of Cardiovascular and Thoracic Surgery, Department of Surgery, Sarver Heart Center, University of Arizona College of Medicine, Tucson, AZ*

GREGORY A. COUPER, MD, *Division of Cardiac Surgery, Department of Surgery, Brigham and Women's Hospital, Harvard Medical School, Boston, MA*

TERESA DE MARCO, MD, *Division of Cardiology, University of California at San Francisco, San Francisco, CA*

PAUL L. DIGIORGI, MD, *Division of Cardiothoracic Surgery, Department of Surgery, Columbia University College of Physicians and Surgeons, New York, NY*

VINCENT DOR, MD, *Cardio Thoracic Center of Monaco, Monaco*

JAMES C. FANG, MD, *Cardiovascular Division, Brigham and Women's Hospital, Harvard Medical School, Boston, MA*

JAMES P. GREELISH, MD, *Department of Cardiac Surgery, Vanderbilt University Medical Center, Nashville, TN*

RUEDIGER HOERBELT, MD, *Division of Cardiac Surgery and Transplantation Biology Research Center, Department of Surgery, Massachusetts General Hospital, Harvard Medical School, Boston, MA*

KATHERINE J. HOERCHER, RN, *George M. and Linda H. Kaufman Center for Heart Failure, Cleveland Clinic, Cleveland, OH*

JOHN ADAMS JARCHO, MD, *Cardiovascular Division, Department of Medicine, Brigham and Women's Hospital, Harvard Medicine School, Boston; and UpToDate Inc., Wellesley, MA*

UDAY N. KUMAR, MD, *Department of Medicine, University of California, San Francisco, CA*

RICHARD LEE, MD, MBA, *Division of Cardiothoracic Surgery, Department of Surgery, St. Louis University School of Medicine, St. Louis, MO*

PATRICK M. MCCARTHY, MD, *Cardiovascular Institute, Northwestern University Medical School, Chicago, IL*

JOREN C. MADSEN, MD, DPhil, *Division of Cardiac Surgery and Transplantation Biology Research Center, Department of Surgery, Massachusetts General Hospital, Harvard Medical School, Boston, MA*

YOSHIFUMI NAKA, MD, PhD, *Division of Cardiothoracic Surgery, Department of Surgery, Columbia University College of Physicians and Surgeons, New York, NY*

MEHMET C. OZ, MD, *Division of Cardiothoracic Surgery, Department of Surgery, Columbia University College of Physicians and Surgeons, New York, NY*

BRADLEY J. PHILLIPS, MD, *Division of Cardiac Surgery, Brigham and Women's Hospital, Harvard Medical School, Boston, MA*

MOHAMMED A. QUADER, MD, *Division of Cardiothoracic Surgery, Department of Surgery, Nebraska Heart Institute, Lincoln, NE*

HARRY RAKOWSKI, MD, *Division of Cardiovascular Surgery, University of Toronto, Toronto, Ontario, Canada*

ANTHONY C. RALPH-EDWARDS, MD, *Division of Cardiovascular Surgery, University of Toronto, Toronto, Ontario, Canada*

LESLIE A. SAXON, MD, *Division of Cardiovascular Medicine, Department of Medicine, Keck School of Medicine, University of Southern California, Los Angeles, CA*

LEONARD SCHWARTZ, MD, *Division of Cardiovascular Surgery, University of Toronto, Toronto, Ontario, Canada*

RICHARD G. SMITH, MSEE, CEE, *Marshall Foundation Artificial Heart Program, University of Arizona Sarver Heart Center, Tucson, AZ*

LYNNE W. STEVENSON, MD, *Cardiovascular Division, Department of Medicine, Brigham and Women's Hospital, Harvard Medical School, Boston, MA*

JEFFREY J. TEUTEBERG, MD, *Cardiovascular Division, Department of Medicine, Brigham and Women's Hospital, Harvard Medical School, Boston, MA*

E. DOUGLAS WIGLE, MD, *Division of Cardiovascular Surgery, Department of Medicine, University of Toronto, Toronto, Ontario, Canada*

WILLIAM G. WILLIAMS, MD, *Division of Cardiovascular Surgery, Department of Medicine, The Hospital for Sick Children, University of Toronto, Toronto, Ontario, Canada*

1 Recent Advances in Cardiac Allotransplantation

John Adams Jarcho, MD
and James C. Fang, MD

CONTENTS

INTRODUCTION

Heart transplantation has become a routine approach to the management of severe cardiac failure *(1)*. Indeed, given the excellent survival statistics for heart transplant recipients, heart transplant outcomes are now an important standard against which the success of other therapies is routinely measured. There are more than 200 institutions currently performing heart transplants worldwide, two-thirds of them in the United States. In 1995, there were 4049 heart transplants reported to the International Society for Heart and Lung Transplantation (ISHLT);

From: *Contemporary Cardiology: Surgical Management of Congestive Heart Failure*
Edited by: J. C. Fang and G. S. Couper © Humana Press Inc., Totowa, NJ

2359 of these took place in the United States. The same figures for the year 2000 were 3175 and 2197, respectively *(2)*. It is clear that more patients would benefit from heart transplantation if more donor organs were available; in 2000, there were 3452 new registrations on US waiting lists, according to data from the United Network for Organ Sharing (UNOS). In that same year, the median waiting time for a heart transplant in the United States, considering all patients regardless of waiting list priority, was 346 days *(3)*.

Over the last decade, the field of heart transplantation has evolved in response to many changes, including the following:

- Rapid improvements in heart failure management
- Increasing availability of mechanical ventricular assist devices (VADs)
- Better appreciation of the risk factors influencing transplant outcome
- Shortage of suitable donor organs
- Increasingly competitive behavior between transplant centers
- Advances in the science of immunology, with the development of new approaches to immunosuppression
- Improved management of posttransplant complications, including especially posttransplant coronary artery disease (CAD)
- Increasing number of long-lived heart transplant recipients

This chapter focuses on recent developments in cardiac transplantation and relates them to current clinical practice.

THE HEART TRANSPLANT CANDIDATE

Heart transplantation is generally considered the choice of last resort in heart failure management, which means that all other feasible approaches, whether medical or surgical, should have been exhausted. Furthermore, the standard of practice has required the demonstration of a survival advantage—that is, the expectation that a heart transplant recipient will benefit, not only by the resolution of symptoms, but also by an improvement in life expectancy. This strict standard has grown harder to meet as the medical management of congestive heart failure has improved.

Data from the Cooperative North Scandinavian Enalapril Survival Study (CONSENSUS) trial, published in 1987, showed that patients with New York Heart Association class III to IV heart failure had an anticipated 1-year survival of less than 50% without angiotensin-converting enzyme (ACE) inhibitor therapy *(4)*. A decade and a half later, in the COPERNICUS trial, a similar population of patients achieved a 1-year survival of 89% with ACE inhibitors and β-blockade

(5). This prognosis is comparable to that of heart transplant recipients; in a review from Stanford University, patients transplanted between 1987 and 1998 had a 1-year survival of 85% *(6)*.

Thus, it has become progressively more important to define the survival of patients with heart failure precisely. Although many variables influence prognosis, the single variable most frequently used to estimate prognosis in heart transplant candidates is the peak oxygen uptake with exercise. In a study that did much to establish this approach, Mancini et al. *(7)* performed exercise tests on 114 patients with advanced heart failure. Those with a peak oxygen uptake less than or equal to 14 mL/kg/min had a survival rate of 47% at 1 year, suggesting that such patients would derive a survival benefit from heart transplantation. It was on the basis of this and similar studies that the American College of Cardiology's 24th Bethesda Conference recommended the use of a peak oxygen uptake of 14 mL/kg/min as a threshold in selecting transplant candidates *(8)*.

However, the results of a single test are an inadequate indication for heart transplantation because no one measurement can be expected to capture all of the individual variability in prognosis. In practice, a combination of test data and clinician judgment are typically used to evaluate potential recipients. Efforts have been made to derive a multivariate risk score, such as the Heart Failure Survival Score *(9)*, that would permit a more accurate prediction of survival in advanced heart failure and thus improve the accuracy of candidate selection. Some centers have used the Heart Failure Survival Score as a criterion in selecting patients for transplant. An important limitation to such scoring systems is that they were developed and validated in the era before β-blockers were shown to be beneficial in patients with heart failure, and therefore may not reflect the significant impact this medical therapy has had on survival.

Heart transplant candidates must also be free of other medical problems that could be expected to jeopardize the success of the transplant or reduce the likelihood of a satisfactory long-term outcome *(10)*. The contraindications to transplantation, unlike the indications, are based primarily on a combination of empiricism and clinical experience (*see* Table 1). Absolute contraindications are those considered sufficient to exclude transplantation; relative contraindications are evaluated on a case-by-case basis.

The application of these contraindications, and the "unacceptable" values for measurements such as pulmonary vascular resistance and creatinine clearance, vary somewhat from institution to institution. New data have influenced judgment about many of these clinical issues:

Table 1
Contraindications to Heart Transplantation

Absolute contraindications
    Current malignancy other than skin cancer
    Hepatatis B or C infection with active hepatitis
    AIDS (acquired immunodeficiency syndrome)
    Fixed pulmonary hypertension
Relative contraindications
    Age over 65 years
    Diabetes mellitus with end-organ damage
    Significant renal, liver, or lung disease
    Severe peripheral or carotid vascular disease or abdominal aortic
      aneurysm
    HIV infection
    Hepatitis B or C infection
    Previously treated malignancy other than skin cancer
    Reversible pulmonary hypertension
    Recent pulmonary embolus
    Active peptic ulcer disease
    Infiltrative myocardial disease
    Collagen vascular disease
    Major psychiatric disorder
    History of persistent noncompliance with medical care
    Drug, alcohol, or tobacco addiction

- The age limit for heart transplantation, once as low as 55 years, has continued to extend upward. In one report comparing 15 patients aged 70 years and older with 98 younger patients, all undergoing transplantation between 1994 and 1999, there were no significant differences between the two groups in 1-year or 4-year survival (11).
- Although diabetes with end-organ damage is considered a contraindication to transplantation, selected patients may have outcomes as good as those without the disease. In an analysis of 374 cardiac transplant recipients, 76 with diabetes, the 1-year and 3-year survival rates of the two groups were comparable (12).
- Pulmonary hypertension has been demonstrated to be a risk factor for early posttransplant mortality in data from the ISHLT (2) and from the Cardiac Transplant Research Database (CTRD) (13). However, there is a significant difference between reversible pulmonary hypertension (i.e., pulmonary hypertension that can be reduced with acute vasodilator therapy) and fixed or irreversible pulmonary hypertension in this regard. In one study of 293 cardiac transplant candidates, those with a pulmonary vascular resistance (PVR) less than 2.5 Wood units

(200 dynes-s/cm^5) at baseline had a 3-month mortality rate of 6.9% *(14)*. Those who had an elevated PVR at baseline that could be reduced below 2.5 Wood units using nitroprusside had a 3-month mortality of only 3.8%; those with a fixed elevation in PVR had a 3-month mortality of 40.6%.

Although fixed pulmonary hypertension is a contraindication to transplantation, the evolution of newer approaches to reduce PVR has made this criterion somewhat more flexible. Continuous intravenous infusion of a vasodilator such as dobutamine *(15)*, milrinone *(16)*, prostaglandin E1 *(17)*, or prostacyclin *(16)* during the weeks or months prior to transplant may reduce PVR significantly. For transplant candidates with persistent mild-to-moderate pulmonary hypertension, the decision is often made to accept only a heart from a donor who weighs more than the recipient; larger hearts are less likely to develop right ventricular failure in response to elevated PVR *(18)*. The implantation of a VAD to reduce an elevated PVR has been reported *(19,20)*, although this approach is not typically employed in the absence of other indications for VAD support. Additional management strategies for elevated PVR in the posttransplant setting are discussed in another section (*see* The Immediate Posttransplant Course).

- Patients with a history of malignancy may be appropriate candidates for transplantation if they have been successfully treated and if enough time has passed to have a reasonable certainty of cure. In the reported experience of two large transplant centers, 31 of 1388 patients (2%) had a history of malignancy *(21,22)*. Of these 31 patients, 4 had recurrence of the original malignancy after transplantation. The recurrent cancers included a uterine leimyosarcoma that had previously required treatment for distant metastases, a malignant melanoma (which was presumably incurable), an adenocarcinoma of the bladder that was not actually resected until after transplantation, and a renal hypernephroma resected only 3 months before transplantation. These data suggest that recurrent malignancy tends to occur primarily in patients with metastatic or untreatable disease or in those treated within a short time of the transplant.

- The hepatitis B and hepatitis C viruses are of particular concern in cardiac transplantation because they can produce chronic infection, liver disease, and cirrhosis. In a study using data from the Joint ISHLT/UNOS Thoracic Registry, 30 patients were identified who were known to have a positive serologic test for hepatitis B surface antigen (HBsAg) prior to transplant *(23)*. Of these, 11 developed active hepatitis or cirrhosis, and 5 died of hepatitis B. The authors suggested caution in accepting HBsAg-positive heart transplant candidates. However, a study of heart transplant recipients in Taiwan, where hepatitis B is endemic, found that lamivudine was effective in controlling hepatitis B virus reactivation in six of seven patients, suggesting that newer antiviral agents may make heart transplantation in HBsAg-positive patients feasible (24). Similar improvements are evolving in the management of hepatitis C (25).

• Human immunodeficiency virus (HIV) infection has been regarded as an absolute contraindication to organ transplantation because of the expectation that the immunological consequences would be unpredictable and likely fatal. However, limited experience has demonstrated that, in the era of highly active antiretroviral drug therapy, organ transplantation is feasible in HIV-positive patients (26,27). The experience with this approach is still too limited to make any firm statements about the anticipated outcome for such patients, however.

Heart transplant candidates must also be evaluated for evidence of immune sensitization against non-self tissue types. Human leukocyte antigen (HLA) tissue types are determined by cell surface molecules that are highly heterogeneous; exposure to non-self HLA molecules typically produces a vigorous immune response (28). Such exposure can occur as a result of blood product transfusions or, for women, exposure to nonidentical fetal HLA molecules during pregnancy. Anti-HLA sensitization is of concern in transplantation because it can cause an aggressive immune response against the transplanted organ, termed hyperacute rejection, which can destroy the organ and potentially cause the death of the patient (29,30). Evaluation for anti-HLA sensitization typically involves testing of the transplant candidate's serum for the presence of anti-HLA antibodies by any one of several methods, including a complement-dependent cytotoxicity assay, an enzyme-linked immunosorbent assay, or flow cytometry (31). These tests all result in a quantitative measurement called the percent reactive antibody.

If the PRA is elevated, donor-specific crossmatching (testing of the recipient's serum for antibodies against donor tissue) is generally performed. Although crossmatching has typically been performed using a complement-dependent cytotoxicity assay, more sensitive flow cytometric crossmatching has been shown to correlate with clinical outcomes after transplantation (32–34).

The advent of VAD technology has complicated the problem of anti-HLA sensitization. Patients supported with a VAD have a significantly increased likelihood of developing anti-HLA sensitization; some series suggested that this occurs in one-third to two-thirds of VAD recipients (35,36). Women and recipients of multiple blood transfusions are at greater risk of sensitization, just as is seen among transplant candidates without VADs (37). The mechanism for this increase in sensitization in VAD recipients appears to be T-cell activation as a result of contact between circulating blood elements and the material components of the device itself, leading to B-cell stimulation and increased production of immunoglobulins by existing B-cell clones *(38)*. Hence, the device "turns on" latent anti-HLA sensitization.

The increase in elevated PRA results seen in VAD patients has led to the development of a number of approaches to decrease anti-HLA sensitization. Efforts are routinely made to limit blood product use as much as possible and to use leukocyte-depleted blood for transfusion, although these approaches do not prevent sensitization completely *(39)*. More aggressive strategies for decreasing sensitization have included the use of plasmapheresis to remove bulk immunoglobulins *(40,41)*, immunoadsorption columns specifically designed to remove anti-HLA antibodies *(42,43)*, the administration of exogenous intravenous immunoglobulin to inhibit native antibody production and function *(44,45)*, and the use of chemotherapeutic agents (typically cyclophosphamide) *(46)* to inhibit antibody production. Reports of the use of anti-CD20 monoclonal antibody (rituximab) for treatment of "humoral rejection" have suggested that this agent might also be beneficial in decreasing anti-HLA sensitization *(47,48)*.

THE HEART TRANSPLANT WAITING LIST

In the United States, patients who are accepted as suitable candidates for heart transplantation are registered with UNOS and are placed on the candidate waiting list. At the time of listing, each patient is assigned one of three priority status codes based on acuity of illness (*see* Table 2). The rationale for this status system is the expectation that it ranks patients fairly according to urgency; status 1A patients are presumably at a higher risk of death in the near term than status 1B or status 2 patients and are thus entitled to priority for the next available donated heart *(49)*. Additional policies intended to help ensure fair organ allocation include

- The requirement that the transplanting institution provide clinical information to justify all status 1A listings
- A time limit on all status 1A listings (in most cases, 14 days), with automatic downgrading to status 1B unless the transplanting center provides new justification to extend the listing
- A regional review board for each UNOS-defined geographic region of the United States, appointed to review all clinical justification information and approve or deny status 1A listings; the decisions of the regional review board may be appealed to the national Thoracic Organ Committee of UNOS

Table 2
Status Priorities for Heart Transplantation

1A. A patient listed as status 1A is admitted to the listing transplant center hospital and has at least one of the following devices or therapies in place:
  (a) Mechanical circulatory support for acute hemodynamic decompensation that includes at least one of the following:
    (i) Left and/or right VAD implanted for a maximum of 30 days at any point after being implanted
    (ii) Total artificial heart
    (iii) Intraaortic balloon pump
    (iv) Extracorporeal membrane oxygenator
  (b) Mechanical circulatory support with objective medical evidence of significant device-related complications, such as thromboembolism, device infection, mechanical failure, and/or life-threatening ventricular arrhythmias.
  (c) Mechanical ventilation.
  (d) Continuous infusion of a single high-dose intravenous inotrope (e.g., dobutamine ≥ 7.5 µg/kg/min, or milrinone ≥ 0.50 µg/kg/min), or multiple intravenous inotropes, in addition to continuous hemodynamic monitoring of left ventricular filling pressures.
1B. A patient listed as status 1B has at least one of the following devices or therapies in place:
  (a) Left and/or right VAD implanted (beyond the 30 days of status 1A allotted to such patients)
  (b) Continuous infusion of intravenous inotropes
2. A patient who does not meet the criteria for status 1A or 1B is listed as status 2.

- A provision for exceptional cases in which patients with highly urgent need who do not meet formal status criteria may be granted a status 1A or 1B listing on approval of the regional review board

Despite the considerable effort devoted to creating and enforcing these policies, it is evident that unresolved inequities persist in the allocation system for heart transplantation. In a study conducted by UNOS in 1999, data on heart transplants taking place between 1994 and 1996 were analyzed separately for each of the 11 geographical UNOS regions. The number of patients placed on the waiting list during that interval in the different UNOS regions ranged from 11.5 to 33 per million population; the number of transplants varied from 5.3 to 10.7 per million (50). With such disparities from region to region, it is not surprising to find that the wait for a donor organ across the country varies widely. During 2000 and 2001, the median waiting time for status 1A candidates varied from 25 days in Region 1 (New England) to 67 days in Region 7 (the northern Midwest). During the same period, the median waiting time for status 2 candidates varied from 248 days in Region 4 (Texas and Oklahoma) to 945 days in Region 9 (New York) *(51)*.

Disparities encountered from region to region of the country may be explained as arising from differences in organ procurement rates, because most hearts are transplanted locally within the relatively limited geographic area served by a single organ bank or organ procurement organization (OPO). However, inequalities have also been demonstrated among transplanting institutions served by the same OPO. An analysis of heart transplants performed within the Delaware Valley OPO (now called the Gift of Life Donor Program) reviewed 662 transplants that were performed between 1992 and 1995 (before status 1 had been separated into status 1A and 1B). Significant differences in waiting times and mortality rates were found among the four institutions performing heart transplants in the OPO service area (Hahnemann University Hospital, Hershey Medical Center, Temple University Hospital, and Hospital of the University of Pennsylvania) *(52)*. The median waiting time for status 1 patients varied by institution from 18 to 42 days, and the mortality rate on the waiting list for status 1 patients varied from 9 to 25%. The likelihood that a status 1 patient would be transplanted within 30 days varied from 17 to 53%.

These disparities in waiting time and mortality rates within a local organ allocation unit raise the concern that differences in institutional clinical practice may be significant enough to alter a patient's likelihood of undergoing a heart transplant or of dying while waiting. Clinical management variables that could contribute to the observed disparities include

- How long and how vigorously medical alternatives are pursued before the decision is made to list a patient for transplant
- Whether exclusion criteria are applied strictly or loosely
- Which approach to therapy is taken while the patient is waiting, including the choice of medications, the doses, and the clinical follow-up
- How ill the patient must be before the decision is made to make management changes that result in the patient's advancing to a higher status
- How often and how readily the clinicians at an institution resort to the use of mechanical cardiac support

In many cases, these management decisions have no right or wrong answers, and experts may disagree about the best course of action in a given clinical situation. Certainly, such decisions could not be successfully policed or regulated without impeding the flexibility that is critical to good medical care. Unfortunately, such differences in practice do have a direct influence on the likelihood that a patient will survive to undergo a heart transplant. The public availability of institutional statistics (on the UNOS Internet website, for example) makes it likely that patients will take these data into account in making their own decisions about where to seek treatment for advanced heart disease.

An additional strategy to increase donor organ availability is the development of an "alternate" waiting list that matches less-ideal transplant candidates with less-optimal organs. The largest experience with an alternate recipient waiting list is that of the University of California at Los Angeles *(53)*. In a report of 62 patients transplanted from the alternate list, the survival rate at 90 days posttransplant was 82% (compared with 91% for 401 contemporaneous transplants from the standard list). After 90 days, the death rates per 1000 patient-months were 4.3 for the alternate list and 3.6 for the standard list. The authors concluded that the satisfactory long-term survival of patients transplanted from the alternate list supports the use of this approach, although it is not clear whether the data would not also support the use of a single waiting list with broader acceptance criteria for both donors and recipients.

THE CARDIAC DONOR

In the fields of kidney, lung, and even liver transplantation, the shortage of donor organs has to some extent been mitigated by the use of living organ donors. In heart transplantation alone, this approach is not a possibility; all cardiac donors are cadaveric donors who have suffered brain death but maintain cardiopulmonary function. In 2000 and 2001, the cause of brain death for most cadaveric donors was either a cerebrovascular event (43%) or head trauma (42%), with the remainder mostly caused by cerebral anoxia or central nervous system tumors *(54)*.

Organ transplantation from brain-dead donors is complicated by the fact that physiological stability is not maintained after brain death. Initially, the increase in intracranial pressure that often accompanies brain death (because of cerebral edema and herniation) causes an abrupt increase in catecholamine release, with blood levels increasing 10-fold over baseline values. This catecholamine surge is accompanied by a sudden rise in systolic and diastolic blood pressure; in one animal model, the mean systolic blood pressure rose from 125 to 402 mmHg during this phase *(55)*. The heart rate often slows initially (the "Cushing reflex"), but then accelerates; the baseline heart rate may double. The severity of the hemodynamic and neurohormonal changes appears to be influenced by how rapidly intracranial pressure rises *(56)*.

The sudden catecholamine release that occurs with brain death causes ischemic injury to the myocardium. Histologically, contraction band necrosis and focal myocyte necrosis are seen, with neutrophil infiltration and subendocardial hemorrhage. Myocardial lactate production increases, and a significant decrease in adenosine triphosphate has been demonstrated by nuclear magnetic resonance spectroscopy *(57)*. β-Adrenergic receptors are decoupled from adenylyl cyclase, and contractility is impaired *(58)*.

Brain death also causes injury to the coronary vascular endothelium *(59)*. Endothelium-dependent vasodilation is impaired *(60)*, and there is an increase in the cell-surface expression of adhesion molecules and HLA antigens *(61)*. As a result, the allograft is more immunogenic; in animal studies, hearts from brain-dead donors suffered more rapid rejection than hearts obtained without the induction of brain death *(62)*.

These effects of brain death may have clinical consequences for the allograft recipient, depending on how severe the catecholamine surge is. One study compared the outcomes when donors had died of an intracranial bleed, typically associated with an abrupt rise in intracranial pressure (group I) with outcomes when donors had died by other means, possibly associated with less-significant catecholamine release (group II). Compared with group II, group I had a higher mortality rate by discharge posttransplant (14 vs 5%) *(63)*.

Once the catecholamine surge accompanying brain death recedes, the loss of central nervous system function results in progressive physiological instability. Respiration by definition ceases and must be supported by artificial ventilation. Blood pressure, having risen acutely during brain death, now declines progressively as a result of decreasing circulating levels of catecholamines *(64)* and vasopressin *(65)*. Diabetes insipidus occurs in about half of cases, also because of the decrease in vasopressin levels; left untreated, diabetes insipidus results in hypernatremia and volume depletion. Declines in other hormone levels, including adrenocorticotropic hormone, cortisol, thyroxine, triiodothyronine, and glucagon, have also been described *(66)*.

Given these physiological events in the setting of brain death, it is evident that the clinical evaluation of a potential cardiac donor is complex (*see* Table 3) *(67)*.

Table 3
Optimal Assessment of the Organ Donor

- The inciting event, including cause of brain death, any information about possible chest trauma, and cardiac arrest with cardiopulmonary resuscitation.
- Past history, focusing on cardiac disease, hypertension, and other coronary risk factors; high-risk behaviors for hepatitis or HIV infection (intravenous drug use, incarceration, etc.); and history of malignancy.
- Clinical course from the inciting event until the present examination, including sequential data regarding vital signs, central venous pressure, cardiac rhythm, and fluid intake and output, as well as medications (especially inotropes and/or pressors).
- Examination for chest trauma, cardiac rubs, murmurs or gallops, peripheral pulses, and perfusion.
- Laboratory data, including blood gases, electrocytes, blood counts, hepatic and renal function, cardiac enzymes, and bacterial cultures.
- Consideration of pulmonary artery catheterization for more complete hemodynamic monitoring.
- An echocardiogram to evaluate cardiac structure and function, including evidence of left ventricular hypertrophy, valvular abnormalities, and global and regional wall motion.
- Cardiac catheterization in patients with risk factors for coronary artery disease.

The ideal donor is young; has no cardiac history; did not require resuscitation; has had stable hemodynamics since brain death, with an optimal volume status and a minimum of inotropes; and has a normal echocardiogram (and angiogram, if necessary). Unfortunately, such donors are rare, and the pressing need for more organs has led to questions about what departures from the "ideal" are acceptable and can be tolerated without endangering the transplant recipient. As with the selection of the acceptable transplant candidate, the identification of the acceptable cardiac donor has varied from institution to institution. A survey from the Association of Organ Procurement Organizations in 1999 found that the "donor yield" for hearts (i.e., the number of hearts procured and transplanted divided by the total number of potential donors in a given OPO) ranged from 19 to 62% *(68)*.

Such statistics clearly indicate the need for defined criteria for donor acceptability. In 2001, a committee of experts at a conference in Crystal

City, Virginia, suggested that the following donor characteristics were compatible with successful heart transplantation *(69)*:

- Age greater than 55 years (the upper end of the acceptable donor age spectrum is uncertain)
- Small donor size relative to the transplant candidate; an adult male donor weighing 70 kg or more is suitable for most recipients
- Hepatitis B or C seropositivity
- Modest cardiac enzyme elevation without left ventricular dysfunction
- Mild left ventricular hypertrophy (wall thickness less than or equal to 13 mm)
- Minor cardiac structural abnormalities, including mild mitral or tricuspid regurgitation, bicuspid aortic valve, secundum atrial septal defect
- In some cases, the presence of mild coronary disease on angiography

Single-institution studies have demonstrated that donors with such relative contraindications ("marginal" donors) can be used successfully with an acceptable posttransplant outcome *(70)*, although an analysis from the CTRD confirmed that the mortality rate for the recipients of hearts from marginal donors is higher *(71)*. Institutional experience is likely to be a critical factor in determining the success of such efforts to expand the donor pool.

One of the most frequently encountered donor problems is distinguishing acceptable from unacceptable donor hemodynamic instability. The Papworth Hospital in Cambridge, UK, was one of the first institutions to examine this issue systemically. They evaluated 150 organ donors on whom hemodynamic data were collected between 1990 and 1993. Of these, 52 (35%) were found to be unacceptable initially because of hypotension, elevated filling pressures, a low left ventricular stroke work index, or a high inotrope requirement. However, with optimal hemodynamic and hormonal management, including optimization of volume status and the judicious use of vasopressin, triiodothyronine, steroids, insulin, and glucose, 44 of the 52 originally unacceptable donors yielded transplantable organs. At follow-up 13 to 48 months later, 37 of the 44 recipients (84%) were alive and well *(72)*. Based on this experience and the comparable experience of a few other institutions, a consensus conference in Crystal City, Virginia, recommended an approach to optimal donor management to improve organ yield (*see* Table 4) *(71)*. It is anticipated that the widespread use of such a protocol would greatly increase the number of cardiac transplants nationally, but this outcome remains to be demonstrated.

Table 4
Recommended Approach to Optimal Donor Management

Conventional management prior to the initial echocardiogram
  a. Adjust volume status (target central venous pressure 6–10 mmHg).
  b. Correct metabolic perturbations, including
      Acidosis (target pH 7.40 to 7.45)
      Hypoxemia (target pO_2 > 80 mm Hg, O_2 saturation > 95%)
      Hypercarbia (target pCO_2 ≥ 30 to 35 mmHg)
  c. Correct anemia (target hematocrit > 30%, hemoglobin > 10 g/dL)
  d. Adjust inotropes to maintain mean arterial pressure ≥ 60 mmHg.
      Norepinephrine and epinephrine should be tapered off rapidly in
      favor of dopamine or dobutamine.
  e. Target dopamine < 10 g/kg/min or dobutamine < 10 g/kg/min.
Initial echocardiogram
  a. Rule out structural abnormalities (substantial left ventricular
      hypertrophy, valvular dysfunction, congenital lesions).
  b. If left ventricular ejection fraction is ≥ 45%, proceed with
      recovery (consider aggressive management as shown below to
      optimize cardiac function before recovery), with final evaluation
      in the operating room.
  c. If left ventricular ejection fraction is < 45%, aggressive
      management with placement of a pulmonary arterial catheter
      and hormonal resuscitation is strongly recommended.
Hormonal resuscitation
  a. Triiodothyronine: 4 g bolus, then infusion at 3 g/h.
  b. Arginine vasopressin: 1-U bolus, then infusion at 0.5 to 4 U/h,
      titrated to a systemic vascular resistance of 800
      to 1200 dyne/s/cm⁵.
  c. Methylprednisolone: 15-mg/kg bolus.
  d. Insulin: 1 U/h minimum. Titrate to maintain blood sugar 120
      to 180 mg/dL.
Aggressive hemodynamic management
  a. Initiated simultaneously with hormonal resuscitation.
  b. Placement of pulmonary artery catheter.
  c. Duration of therapy ≥ 2 h.
  d. Adjustment of fluids, inotropes, and pressors every 15 min based
      on serial hemodynamic measurements to minimize use of
      α-agonists and meet the following target (Papworth) criteria:
      Mean arterial pressure > 60 mmHg.
      Central venous pressure 4 to 12 mmHg.
      Pulmonary capillary wedge pressure 8 to 12 mmHg.
      Systemic vascular resistance 800 to 1200 dyne/s/cm⁵.
      Cardiac index > 2.4 L/min/m².
      Dopamine < 10 g/kg/min or dobutamine < 10 g/kg/min.
Follow-up echocardiogram may be useful to reassess ventricular
function, although data are currently limited on this issue.

THE TRANSPLANT OPERATION

The cardioplegia solution that is used to perfuse the heart during donor harvest and to transport the heart from donor to recipient is intended to optimize myocardial preservation and minimize the amount of ischemic injury the heart sustains. Myocardial injury during ex vivo ischemia results from several distinct phenomena, including cellular swelling, extracellular edema, intracellular acidosis, depletion of metabolic substrate, calcium overload, endothelial injury, and reperfusion injury *(73)*. Therefore, most cardioplegia solutions include osmotic agents, buffering agents, antioxidants, a metabolic substrate, and magnesium to retard calcium influx.

Unfortunately, the best composition for cardioplegia is unclear. Two broad categories of cardioplegia solutions have been developed: "intracellular" solutions, with a high potassium concentration and a low sodium concentration, such as the University of Wisconsin, Collins, and Stanford solutions; and "extracellular" solutions, with a low potassium concentration and a high sodium concentration, such as Celsior and the St. Thomas solution.

A survey of heart transplant programs in the United States published in 1997 retrospectively evaluated 9401 heart transplants performed between 1987 and 1992 and concluded that intracellular solutions were superior to extracellular solutions in their effect on mortality at 1 month posttransplant (odds ratio 0.85; $p < 0.05$) *(74)*. However, the survey also found that 167 different solutions were in current use—a number equivalent to the number of heart transplant programs—suggesting that experimental proof of superiority has not been a prerequisite for the use of any given formulation.

It has been proposed that continuous perfusion of the donor heart should be a more effective way of preventing ischemic injury than cold storage alone. This has been confirmed in animal studies, in which viable organ function is markedly prolonged by perfusion techniques *(75–77)*. However, the acceptable results for most cardiac transplant recipients with cold ischemic storage, and the cost and logistical difficulties associated with continuous perfusion systems, have thus far precluded clinical adoption of a continuous perfusion approach.

There are two commonly employed approaches to the implantation of the donor heart. In the first, the standard or Shumway technique, the left and right atria of the donor heart are anastomosed to cuffs of left and right atrium created in the recipient *(78)*. With this technique, the left and right atria of the recipient are divided during the excision of the native heart, leaving a cuff of atrial tissue on each side. The donor atria are opened posteriorly to create corresponding left and right atrial cuffs.

In the second, the bicaval or Wythenshawe technique, the superior and inferior vena cavae of the recipient are anastomosed to an intact donor right atrium; the left atrial anastomosis is created in the same way as in the standard technique *(79)*. For the bicaval approach, the recipient right atrium is divided to create superior and inferior vena caval cuffs. No incisions are made in the donor right atrium. A third technique, designated "total" orthotopic heart transplantation, involves the anastomosis of left and right pulmonary vein cuffs to a nearly intact left atrium; this approach is used infrequently *(80)*.

Comparative studies have suggested that there are at least two disadvantages to the standard technique that are overcome by the bicaval technique *(81–83)*:

- Significant tricuspid regurgitation may occur after heart transplantation, in part because of distortion of right atrial geometry with the standard technique; this occurs less often with the bicaval approach.
- Sinus node dysfunction may occur with the standard technique because of injury to the sinus node; this is also less common with bicaval transplantation.

These advantages have led to a progressive increase in the use of the bicaval technique. In a worldwide survey of heart transplant programs reported in 1999, the bicaval technique was preferred by 54% of centers, the standard technique by 23%, and the total technique by 6%; the remaining 17% had no consistent preference *(84)*.

THE IMMEDIATE POSTTRANSPLANT COURSE

The immediate postoperative period after heart transplantation is dominated by concern for hemodynamic stability. Early graft failure accounts for the majority of the operative mortality and for 20 to 25% of deaths in the first posttransplant year, a figure that has not changed in the last decade *(85)*. Optimal hemodynamics require good intrinsic function of the right and left ventricles of the allograft, acceptable systemic and pulmonary vascular resistance, and appropriate cardiac filling pressures.

There is a close correlation between total ischemic time and the function of any allograft organ; however, the time constraints are strictest in heart transplantation, with the optimal ischemic time less than 4 hours. In a study of 911 heart transplant recipients from the CTRD, patients with an ischemic time of less than 4 hours had a 1-month survival of 85%, compared to those with longer ischemic times, who had a 1-month survival of 71% *(86)*. Analyses of data from the ISHLT also demonstrated that ischemic time has a statistically significant, linear relationship to mortality at 1 year posttransplant (odds ratios for ischemic times of 0, 3, 7, and 10 hours are 0.6, 1.0, 2.1, and 3.5, respectively) *(87)*. The impact on survival at 5 years, although still statistically significant, is much less pronounced.

Right ventricular function is possibly of even greater concern than left ventricular function after heart transplantation. Several factors contribute to a significant incidence of right ventricular dysfunction in this setting, including the following:

- Most cardiac transplant recipients have some degree of pulmonary hypertension, as noted in The Heart Transplant Candidate section.
- Pulmonary vascular resistance may be further elevated during cardiopulmonary bypass by several factors. Atelectasis, hypoxic pulmonary vasoconstriction, and microemboli probably all play a role. In addition, cardiopulmonary bypass induces a systemic inflammatory response, with cytokine and protease release and activation of leukocytes and complement *(88,89)*. Direct injury to the pulmonary vascular endothelium, with the loss of endothelium-dependent vasodilation, has also been demonstrated *(90)*.
- The right ventricle appears to be more vulnerable than the left ventricle to the cardiac injury that occurs with brain death, as suggested by animal models *(91)*.

As described regarding the management of pulmonary hypertension in the pretransplant setting, a variety of intravenous agents with vasodilatory and/or inotropic properties have been used postoperatively to reduce pulmonary vascular resistance and support right heart function. Dobutamine *(92)* and milrinone *(93)* are effective in this setting, combining inotropic support for both the left and the right ventricle with pulmonary vasodilation. The utility of nonspecific vasodilators like dobutamine, milrinone, and isoproterenol may be limited by systemic vasodilation and hypotension, especially if the systemic vascular resistance is already low (*see* below). Intravenous prostaglandin E1 *(94)*, intravenous or inhaled prostacyclin *(95,96)*, and inhaled nitric oxide *(97)* all have greater specificity for the pulmonary vascular bed and are effective in reducing pulmonary vascular resistance. Nitric oxide in particular has seen increasing use in the immediate postoperative period, although it can only be administered to an intubated patient.

Severe right ventricular dysfunction with consequent cardiogenic shock occurs in 2 to 3% of patients after heart transplantation. Mechanical support with a right VAD can be life-saving *(98–100)*. Unfortunately, only about 25 to 30% of such patients recover, usually because, by the time mechanical support is instituted, secondary complications such as sepsis, coagulopathy, or renal failure have supervened. Close observation of hemodynamics in the immediate postoperative period and rapid intervention in the event of progressive right heart failure are necessary for right VAD support to be successful.

It has been recognized that as many as 10% of patients undergoing cardiopulmonary bypass experience vasodilatory shock in the postoperative period; in many cases, this vasodilatory state persists despite high levels of endogenous or exogenous catecholamines *(101)*. It is possible that patients receiving high doses of long-lasting vasodilators (such as angiotension-converting enzyme inhibitors) are at increased risk of this complication. In addition, however, an improved understanding of the pathogenesis of shock has led to the recognition that, with prolonged hypotension, neurohypophyseal stores of the vasoconstrictor vasopressin are depleted *(102)*. A lack of vasopressin may underlie many cases of vasodilatory shock in the postbypass setting. In one study of 145 patients undergoing cardiopulmonary bypass, 11 had vasodilatory shock. All of these patients had inappropriately low serum arginine vasopressin concentrations, and all responded to low-dose arginine vasopressin infusions *(103)*.

Finally, the use of mechanical cardiac assistance (if appropriately timed) for catastrophic early graft failure is often preferable to high doses of vasoconstricting catecholamines as the sole means of hemodynamic support and allows for patient stability while issues of urgent relisting for transplantation are considered.

IMMUNOSUPPRESSION

Calcineurin Inhibitors

Most patients receive some form of triple-drug therapy (a calcineurin inhibitor, an antiproliferative agent, and a corticosteroid) for maintenance immunosuppression with or without the addition of antilymphocyte antibody therapy during the initiation of treatment *(104)*. The calcineurin inhibitors cyclosporine and tacrolimus are a mainstay of the triple-drug regimen *(105,106)*. The advent of this class of drugs (cyclosporine was first introduced for clinical use in the United States in 1983) resulted in a rapid improvement in posttransplant survival from approx 50% at 1 year to above 80% at 1 year *(107)*. The inhibition of calcineurin decreases the transcription of interleukin-2 (IL-2), an essential cytokine for the activation and proliferation of T lymphocytes *(108)*.

Several small studies have compared the efficacy and side-effect profile of cyclosporine with that of tacrolimus, but even the largest of these studies included only 243 patients *(109)*. None was able to detect a significant difference in acute rejection or in patient survival; there were reported differences in side-effect profile, but they were not consistent from study to study. As a result, there are no compelling data to support the choice of one of these two agents over the other in most instances. In some cases, switching from cyclosporine to tacrolimus may be effective for a specific patient in improving control of rejection or in ameliorating specific side effects, such as hyperlipidemia, hypertension, and hirsutism. Data from the ISHLT Registry indicate that 72% of patients transplanted between 1999 and 2001 were receiving cyclosporine and 25% were receiving tacrolimus; 3% were not receiving a calcineurin inhibitor *(2)*.

Antiproliferative Agents

The second component of most heart transplant drug regimens is an antiproliferative agent. For many years (since the advent of clinical heart transplantation), azathioprine was virtually the only drug used for this purpose. Mycophenolate mofetil was introduced as an alternative antiproliferative agent in 1992. It is metabolized to mycophenolic acid, which is a noncompetitive inhibitor of the enzyme inosine monophosphate dehydrogenase. This enzyme converts inosine monophosphate to guanosine monophosphate, which is an essential step in *de novo* purine biosynthesis. Proliferating lymphocytes are uniquely dependent on the *de novo* pathway *(110)*.

After initial trials in renal transplant patients suggested that mycophenolate might be more effective than azathioprine for preventing rejection, a randomized trial was undertaken comparing the two drugs in heart transplant recipients *(111)*. A total of 650 patients were enrolled, but 72 of these patients (11%) were withdrawn from the study before receiving the study drug because of inability to take oral medication within a prespecified time limit of 6 days after transplant. When the results of the study were analyzed by intention to treat, there was no beneficial effect of mycophenolate compared with azathioprine. However, by received-treatment analysis, patients receiving mycophenolate had a significant reduction in rejection-requiring treatment (65.7 vs 73.7%) and in mortality at 1 year (6.2 vs 11.4%).

Despite several methodological problems with this study, the results were generally interpreted to suggest that mycophenolate may be superior to azathioprine for the prevention of cardiac allograft rejection. A subsequent report from the ISHLT Registry also compared mycophenolate with azathioprine and found a significant improvement in survival at 1 year (96 vs 93%) and 3 years (91 vs 86%), providing further support for the superiority of mycophenolate in a larger (although retrospective) analysis *(112)*. Data from the ISHLT Registry indicated that 70% of patients transplanted between 1999 and 2001 were receiving mycophenolate, and 15% were receiving azathioprine *(2)*.

Two newer drugs, sirolimus (also called rapamycin) and its derivative everolimus, are also antiproliferative agents; they are collectively referred to as TOR (target of rapamycin) inhibitors. Sirolimus was first identified as an immunosuppressive agent in the 1970s, but was not introduced into clinical organ transplantation until the 1990s. This agent has a structure similar to that of tacrolimus, and like tacrolimus, it binds to FK506-binding protein (FKBP) in the cell. However, rather than inhibiting calcineurin, the complex of sirolimus and FKBP then binds to another intracellular protein, TOR. Although the effects of TOR have not been completely defined, it is known to play a central role in the G1 phase of the cell cycle and IL-2-stimulated cell growth and proliferation *(113)*.

The place of TOR inhibitors in the immunosuppressive regimen is still not clearly established. In studies in renal transplant recipients, sirolimus has been used in place of a calcineurin inhibitor (with mycophenolate or azathioprine) or in place of mycophenolate or azathioprine (with cyclosporine). Sirolimus was an effective immunosuppressant in both settings. However, when sirolimus is substituted for cyclosporine, there is an increase in the incidence of acute rejection, and when sirolimus is combined with cyclosporine, there is an increase in the frequency of significant nephrotoxicity *(114)*.

Only one major randomized trial to date has evaluated the efficacy of TOR inhibitor therapy for preventing rejection in heart transplant recipients *(115)*. In this study, 634 patients were randomly assigned to receive either azathioprine or one of two doses of everolimus in combination with cyclosporine and prednisone. At 6 months, there was a significant reduction in the incidence of rejection with everolimus. In both this study and a single-center trial of sirolimus *(116)*, TOR inhibitor therapy was also found to reduce the severity of allograft vasculopathy *(see* Cardiac Allograft Vasculopathy). Data from the ISHLT Registry indicated that only 3% of patients transplanted between 1999 and 2001 were treated with sirolimus, although this figure is undoubtedly increasing *(2)*.

Corticosteroids

Although corticosteroids form the third cornerstone of the immuno-suppressive regimen, their side effects can be unacceptably morbid. As a result, during the late 1980s and early 1990s several large centers attempted, using a variety of different approaches, to withdraw patients from steroids after transplantation *(117–121)*. These studies demon-strated that rapid steroid tapering (within the first 2 months) results in the greatest reduction in steroid morbidity, but two-thirds of patients have recurrent rejection and require the resumption of steroid therapy. Slower steroid weaning (after the first 6 months) is associated with a higher rate of successful steroid withdrawal, but the reduction in steroid side effects is more modest. Patients who are successfully weaned from steroids appear to have better long-term survival than those who are not. However, it is not clear whether this is a consequence of the reduction in steroid morbidity or whether successful steroid weaning merely iden-tifies a subset of patients with a less severe response to their allograft who would be likely to have a better long-term survival in any case.

Induction Therapy

Antilymphocyte antibody therapy is initiated at the time of trans-plantation at some centers as an adjunct to triple-drug immunosup-pression. The earliest antilymphocyte antibody preparations were crude sera derived from the immunization of animals (horses, rabbits, etc.) with human lymphocytes. Progressive refinement of these sera, with isolation of the globulin fraction and with use of pure T-cell popula-tions for immunization, led to the development of commercial prepara-tions. A monoclonal antibody directed against the T-cell surface molecule CD3 (OKT3) was introduced for clinical use in kidney trans-plantation in 1981 and in heart transplantation in 1987. Numerous small trials have compared these preparations to one another and to initiation of immunosuppression without antilymphocyte antibodies, but there has been no conclusive evidence that one approach is superior to another *(122)*. In the most recent survey of transplant programs, less than 50% use any sort of induction therapy, and this proportion is falling.

There may be certain clinical indications for which such therapy is warranted. For example, in the patient who is at high-risk for rejec-tion, this more potent immunosuppression may be advantageous. Anti-lymphocyte therapy also has sufficient immunosuppressive potency that it may permit postponement of the initiation of calcineurin inhibitor therapy, which may be especially useful in patients who have early postoperative renal dysfunction. However, these indications have not been prospectively studied in cardiac transplantation.

These advantages of antilymphocyte therapy must be balanced against potential disadvantages. The administration of OKT3 is associated with a risk of an acute inflammatory process called the cytokine release syndrome, thought to be caused by release of tumor necrosis factor from the targeted lymphocytes (123). This syndrome is characterized by high fever, headache, elevated blood pressure, and in severe cases, pulmonary edema. The cytokine release syndrome is not seen with other antilymphocyte preparations. Increases in infection rates and decreased effectiveness with repeated use (because of an allogeneic response against these nonhuman antibodies) also occur with antilymphocyte therapy.

The anti-IL-2 receptor antibodies daclizumab and basiliximab are a new class of immunoglobulins introduced in the 1990s (124,125). Unlike earlier antilymphocyte antibodies, these agents specifically target only activated T cells, that is, T cells that have been specifically stimulated in response to foreign antigen. They do so because they are directed against the high-affinity form of the IL-2 receptor, which is expressed only on activated T cells. Initial experience in renal transplantation demonstrated that both daclizumab and basiliximab significantly reduced the incidence of rejection during the first 6 months after transplant compared to placebo without a significant increase in side effects or adverse events.

The success of these agents in renal transplantation led to a cardiac transplant study conducted at Columbia-Presbyterian Medical Center and reported in 2000 (126). Individuals in a group of 55 patients undergoing heart transplantation were randomly assigned to receive five doses of either daclizumab or placebo. All patients also received triple-drug immunosuppression with cyclosporine, mycophenolate mofetil, and prednisone. During the "induction period" (the first 3 months after transplantation, based on the dosing regimen and the half-life of daclizumab), the proportion of patients experiencing acute rejection was significantly greater in the daclizumab group than the placebo group (63 vs 18%). There was no difference between the two groups during the subsequent 3 months (43 vs 37%). The use of daclizumab was not associated with an increased risk of adverse events, and there were no episodes of cytokine release syndrome.

The data from this study and the renal transplant studies suggested that anti-IL-2 receptor antibodies may have efficacy similar to other antilymphocyte antibodies with a more benign side effect profile. There are insufficient data at present to determine whether these antibodies truly reduce rejection frequency over the longer term or merely post-pone rejection, as with other induction agents. There are also no data on other long-term effects, such as malignancy.

THE POSTTRANSPLANT CLINICAL COURSE

Rejection

Rejection is a significant cause of mortality after heart transplanta-tion, accounting for approx 15% of deaths in the first posttransplant year; fortunately, it declines in frequency over time *(127)*. However, the incidence of rejection-related deaths is declining; approx 6% of patients transplanted in 1990, but fewer than 2% of those transplanted in 2000, died of rejection within the first 3 years after transplantation *(128)*. Improvements in immunosuppression (*see* Immunosuppression) are likely responsible for this decline.

The diagnosis of rejection is still based on invasive procurement of myocardial tissue and histological examination. Although noninvasive strategies, such as echocardiographic diastolic abnormalities, biomark-ers such as troponin I and T, and magnetic resonance imaging, have been studied, they have not proven reliable enough to permit confident early diagnosis *(129)*.

The management of cellular rejection (i.e., the presence of lympho-cytic infiltration) is relatively uniform, although there is debate for cer-tain histological pictures. There is some variation from institution to institution in the treatment approach. For example, there is debate about whether an ISHLT biopsy grade 2 requires treatment; studies suggest that a grade 2 biopsy early after transplant may progress to more severe rejection, while late grade 2 episodes (more than 6 months to 1 year after transplant) typically resolve spontaneously *(130)*. Whenever a biopsy finding is thought to require treatment, a follow-up biopsy is obtained within the subsequent few weeks to con-firm resolution of rejection.

In 1989, Hammond et al. described a distinct form of rejection with-out histological evidence of a lymphocyte infiltrate *(131)*. This entity has been called *humoral rejection* or *vascular rejection* and has been the subject of extended debate, including disagreement about its exis-tence, its clinical features, its pathologic characteristics, its etiology, and its management. A general characterization of humoral rejection has evolved gradually; in 2003, a panel of pathologists, cardiologists, cardiac surgeons, and other scientists published a summary description of the current understanding of this entity, although no consensus diag-nostic criteria have yet emerged *(132)*.

Humoral rejection occurs early after transplantation (usually within the first month). As its name indicates, it is thought to be a humorally mediated, rather than cell-mediated, form of rejection. Clinically, it often presents with an abrupt decline in cardiac function; some patients present with cardiogenic shock. Histologically, a cellular infiltrate is not present. However, immunofluorescence studies can detect the deposition of immunoglobulin and complement (such as C4d) within the myocardium, especially in the capillaries and other small vessels. In severe cases, light microscopic changes may be seen, including endothelial cell swelling, interstitial edema and hemorrhage, and a perivascular inflammatory infiltrate (vasculitis). Ischemic damage to the myocardium may be seen, perhaps as a result of vascular inflammation and subsequent occlusion by thrombus.

Treatment of humoral rejection has been unsatisfactory. One moderately successful approach is to use plasmapheresis for removal of immunoglobulin with or without high-dose cyclophosphamide to eliminate B cells responsible for the production of antibodies targeting the allograft *(133)*. The use of rituximab, a monoclonal antibody against the CD20 molecule expressed on B cells, has also been described *(134)*. Despite aggressive treatment, the mortality rate of humoral rejection remains high (13% in one recent series) *(135)*. Those who survive have a significantly increased incidence of cardiac allograft vasculopathy (CAV).

Infection

Infection is the counterpart to rejection in the heart transplant recipient *(136)*. The aggressive immunosuppression necessary to prevent rejection leads to a significant risk of infectious complications. Infection causes 25% of deaths in the first posttransplant year. Unlike rejection, which has become a less frequent cause of posttransplant mortality over the last decade, infection has consistently accounted for approx 4.5% of deaths within the first 3 years after transplantation *(134)*.

One of the most important infectious pathogens in the heart transplant setting is cytomegalovirus (CMV) *(137)*. The CMV virus is latent (as a result of prior, often inapparent, infection) in about two-thirds of adults. Usually, CMV does not cause significant clinical illness except in the immunosuppressed patients. After transplantation, reactivation of the CMV virus, or *de novo* infection, can cause an acute febrile illness as well as gastroenteritis, hepatitis, pneumonia, and even myocarditis.

The incidence of clinical CMV disease after heart transplantation is approx 20 to 25%, but varies depending on whether the transplant recipient and/or the organ donor have previously been infected (as demonstrated by positive or negative CMV serology). Recipients who are CMV negative and receive an organ from a CMV-positive donor are at highest risk (in one report, 85% of such patients developed clinical CMV illness requiring treatment) *(138)*.

In addition to the acute manifestations of CMV disease, CMV infection can have an immunosuppressive effect, increasing the risk of fungal, bacterial, and other superinfection *(139)*. Furthermore, CMV infection increases the incidence of rejection and has been implicated as a risk factor for the development of CAV *(140)*. It has also been suggested that CMV infection contributes to the pathogenesis of posttransplant lymphoproliferative disease (*see* below).

The drug of choice for treating CMV disease is ganciclovir or valganciclovir. Although such antiviral therapy is typically effective in the treatment of active CMV illness, the morbidity associated with CMV infection has led most transplant centers to adopt a strategy of prophylaxis after transplantation with either an antiviral agent or CMV immune globulin *(141)*. Such prophylactic therapy is usually given to CMV-negative recipients of CMV-positive donor hearts. In another approach, referred to as *preemptive therapy*, patients are screened repeatedly for evidence of CMV viremia by polymerase chain reaction and are treated only if active viral replication is detected. Whether CMV prophylaxis will influence the later development of CAV is still under investigation.

Cardiac Allograft Vasculopathy

CAV is a form of CAD unique to heart transplant recipients. CAV differs from typical coronary atherosclerosis in that it is a diffuse process involving the entire coronary arterial tree. The lesions of CAV are concentric rather than eccentric, resulting in a progressive circumferential narrowing of the vessel. Histologically, CAV lacks the lipid accumulation and cholesterol crystal formation seen in native coronary disease; smooth muscle cell proliferation and macrophage infiltration predominate *(142)*.

CAV also develops and progresses much more rapidly than typical coronary disease. Angiographically, CAV is detectable in 40 to 50% of heart transplant recipients by 5 years posttransplant *(143)*. However, angiography underestimates the frequency of CAV because the diffuse, concentric nature of the disease process makes it difficult to be certain of the "normal" luminal diameter. Intravascular ultrasound (IVUS) studies have demonstrated that CAV is detectable in more than 80% of patients as early as 1 year after transplantation *(144)*.

Once CAV is evident by angiography, the prognosis is poor, with progressive vascular narrowing, diffuse myocardial ischemic injury, and cardiac failure. Revascularization, including percutaneous coronary intervention and coronary artery bypass grafting, is usually not feasible in patients with advanced CAV because of the diffuse nature of the disease process, which extends to the arteriolar level. Cardiac retransplantation is an option for some patients, but most heart transplant recipients with CAV die of their disease. Although rejection and infection are the predominant causes of death in the first year after transplantation, CAV is responsible for 20 to 25% of subsequent mortality *(134)*.

Because CAV is very difficult to treat once it is established, efforts to manage this serious condition have focused on prevention. The first breakthrough in reducing the incidence of CAV was described in 1995 by Kobashigawa et al. *(145)* in their report of a randomized trial of pravastatin in 97 heart transplant recipients. Patients taking pravastatin at a dose of 40 mg per day had a significant reduction in the frequency of angiographically detectable coronary disease at 1 year posttransplant when compared to controls not taking the drug (6 vs 20%). In addition, survival at 1 year was significantly better in the pravastatin group (94 vs 78%). Because most of the deaths in the study patients were caused by rejection, it has been suggested that pravastatin may also have an immunological effect on heart transplant recipients, although a mechanism for such an effect has not been established. A similar study of simvastatin also found reductions in both CAV and mortality *(146)*.

The pathogenesis of CAV is multifactorial, but it is clear that the immune response to the allograft is one important variable. As a result, various maintenance immunosuppressive regimens have been studied for their potential ability to reduce the development of graft coronary disease. The first agents for which such a beneficial effect has been clearly demonstrated are the TOR inhibitors sirolimus and everolimus. In the study of everolimus for rejection prophylaxis described in the Immunosuppression section, IVUS studies were also performed at baseline (within 6 weeks after transplantation) and at 1 year. Measurements were made of the maximal intimal thickness from both studies, and CAV was considered to have developed if the maximal intimal thickness had increased by at least 0.5 mm between the baseline and 1-year studies. Patients taking azathioprine had a higher incidence of CAV than those taking either the 1.5 mg or 3.0 mg dose of everolimus (52.8 vs 35.7 and 30.4%) *(147)*. In another trial, sirolimus was substituted for either azathioprine or mycophenolate in patients with established, severe CAV. After 2 years, adverse cardiac events and angiographic worsening of disease were seen less often than in patients who continued previous therapy *(148)*.

Antioxidant vitamins, although they have not been shown to be beneficial in typical CAD, may be effective in the posttransplant setting. This was illustrated in a trial of 40 heart transplant recipients randomly assigned to either vitamin C and E supplementation or placebo. IVUS was performed at baseline and 1 year later, and measurements of average intimal index (plaque area divided by vessel area) were made. Patients treated with antioxidants had no significant change in intimal index; there was an 8% increase in intimal index among the placebo group *(149)*.

The calcium channel blocker diltiazem was also found to reduce the progression of CAV in a randomized trial of 106 heart transplant recipients. Angiography was used to evaluate changes in mean coronary artery diameter. The average coronary diameter decreased in the control group, from 2.41 mm at baseline to 2.19 and 2.22 mm at 1 and 2 years, respectively, but was unchanged in the diltiazem-treated group *(150)*.

Malignancy

The chronic use of immunosuppressive agents in heart transplant recipients increases the risk of malignancy approx 80 to 100 times that in the general population *(151)*. The most common cancers in this setting are skin cancers (primarily squamous cell carcinoma), lymphoma, lung cancer (especially among smokers), and Kaposi's sarcoma *(152,153)*. Malignancy, like CAV, is responsible for 20 to 25% of posttransplant deaths after the first year. Unlike CAV, however, the incidence of malignancy as a cause of death has not fallen over the past decade, but has remained constant *(134)*.

Most posttransplant malignancies are treated in the same way as in nonimmunosuppressed patients, with standard surgical resection, chemotherapy, and radiotherapy. The dose of immunosuppression is usually reduced; a common approach is to discontinue the antiproliferative agent (azathioprine or mycophenolate) and to decrease the calcineurin inhibitor dose substantially. Surgically, resection can cure carcinoma *in situ*, including skin cancer, colon cancer, renal cell carcinoma, and other solid tumors. However, the prognosis is poor in patients with advanced disease, and the clinical course tends to be more aggressive in the immunosuppressed host.

The term *posttransplant lymphoproliferative disorder* (PTLD) is used to encompass three different forms of disease that can occur after transplantation *(154)*:

- Benign polyclonal lymphoproliferation, which is not a true malignancy, but is an acute illness characterized by fever, malaise, fatigue, and rapidly progressive lymphadenopathy; it is responsible for about 55% of cases.
- Polyclonal B-cell proliferation with evidence of early malignant transformation, which is similar to the first disorder, but with the development of clonal cytogenetic abnormalities; it is responsible for about 30% of cases.
- True monoclonal malignant lymphoma, which is usually an extranodal disease that often involves the gastrointestinal tract, lungs, central nervous system, and sometimes the allograft organ; it is responsible for about 15% of cases.

The overall incidence of these disorders in heart transplant recipients is approx 4% (164), although it is much higher (>10%) in patients who have received OKT3 (see Immunosuppression) (156). The pathogenesis of PTLD in most cases is de novo infection or reactivation of Epstein-Barr virus (EBV), with consequent B-cell proliferation and transformation (157). In one study of 381 nonrenal transplant recipients, the risk of PTLD was 24 times higher for EBV-seronegative transplant recipients than for seropositive recipients, suggesting that primary EBV infection carries a much greater risk than reactivation of latent virus from previous infection (158).

Treatment of PTLD depends on the type of disease present, as outlined above. Patients with benign polyclonal lymphoproliferation are often treated with reduction in immunosuppression alone. Although antiviral therapy with acyclovir or ganciclovir has been suggested as an option, there is no solid evidence of the efficacy of this approach (159). In patients who have true malignant lymphoma, standard chemotherapy regimens such as CHOP (cyclophosphamide, doxorubicin, vincristine, and prednisone) or the more aggressive ProMACE-CytaBOM (cyclophosphamide, doxorubicin, etoposide, cytarabine, bleomycin, vincristine, methotrexate, and prednisone) have been used successfully (160). The use of the anti-CD20 monoclonal antibody rituximab has also been described in this setting (161).

CONCLUSION

Because of the complexity of their clinical condition, heart transplant patients require lifelong follow-up care at an institution with expertise in the field. Nonetheless, despite the risks posed by the immune attack on the allograft and the immunosuppression necessary to control it, an increasing number of heart transplant recipients are enjoying extended survival. The patient half-life (time to 50% survival) and 1-year conditional half-life (time to 50% survival for patients who live more than 1 year) for all patients in the ISHLT Registry are 9.3 and 11.8 years, respectively; prognosis tends to be better at institutions that perform a larger number of transplants annually *(2)*. Recipients tend to report excellent functional status, with more than 90% having no activity limitation.

Although heart transplantation is an option for only a small number of patients, it is an effective form of therapy that continues to evolve with new advances in both basic science and clinical medicine. Furthermore, the creation of heart transplantation as a field of expertise, both in medicine and in surgery, has had the consequence of dramatically increasing the understanding of advanced heart failure and has led directly to the development of other approaches (such as ventricular assist) to manage this common and mortal disease.

REFERENCES

1. Hunt SA. Current status of cardiac transplantation. JAMA 1998;280:1692.
2. Hertz MI, Taylor DO, Trulock EP, et al. The Registry of the International Society for Heart and Lung Transplantation: 19th Official Report—2002. J Heart Lung Transplant 2002;21:950.
3. 2001 Annual Report of the US Organ Procurement and Transplantation Network and the Scientific Registry for Transplant Recipients: Transplant Data 1991–2000. Rockville, MD: Department of Health and Human Services, Health Resources and Services Administration, Office of Special Programs, Division of Transplantation; Richmond, VA: United Network for Organ Sharing; Ann Arbor, MI: University Renal Research and Education Association, Ann Arbor, MI.
4. Effects of enalapril on mortality in severe congestive heart failure. Results of the Cooperative North Scandinavian Enalapril Survival Study (CONSENSUS). The CONSENSUS Trial Study Group. N Engl J Med 1987;316:1429.
5. Packer M, Coats AJ, Fowler MB, et al. Effect of carvedilol on survival in severe chronic heart failure. N Engl J Med 2001;344:1651.
6. Robbins RC, Barlow CW, Oyer PE, et al. Thirty years of cardiac transplantation at Stanford University. J Thorac Cardiovasc Surg 1999;117:939.
7. Mancini DM, Eisen H, Kussmaul W, et al. Value of peak exercise oxygen consumption for optimal timing of cardiac transplantation in ambulatory patients with heart failure. Circulation 1991;83:778.
8. Mudge GH, Goldstein S, Addonizio LJ, et al. Twenty-fourth Bethesda conference: cardiac transplantation: Task Force 3: recipient guidelines/prioritization. J Am Coll Cardiol 1993;22:21.
9. Aaronson KD, Schwartz JS, Chen TM, et al. Development and prospective validation of a clinical index to predict survival in ambulatory patients referred for cardiac transplant evaluation. Circulation 1997;95:2660.
10. Cimato TR, Jessup M. Recipient selection in cardiac transplantation: contraindications and risk factors for mortality. J Heart Lung Transplant 2002;21:1161.
11. Blanche C, Blanche DA, Kearney B, et al. Heart transplantation in patients 70 years of age and older: a comparative analysis of outcome. J Thorac Cardiovasc Surg 2001;121:532.

12. Mancini D, Beniaminovitz A, Edwards N, et al. Survival of diabetic patients following cardiac transplant. J Heart Lung Transplant 2001;20:168.
13. Bourge RC, Kirklin JK, Naftel DC, et al. Predicting outcome after cardiac transplantation: lessons from the Cardiac Transplant Research Database. Curr Opin Cardiol 1997;12:136.
14. Costard-Jackle A, Fowler MB. Influence of preoperative pulmonary artery pressure on mortality after heart transplantation: testing of potential reversibility of pulmonary hypertension with nitroprusside is useful in defining a high risk group. J Am Coll Cardiol 1992;19:48.
15. Stanek B, Sturm B, Frey B, et al. Bridging to heart transplantation: prostaglandin E1 vs prostacyclin vs dobutamine. J Heart Lung Transplant 1999;18:358.
16. Canver CC, Chanda J. Milrinone for long-term pharmacologic support of the status 1 heart transplant candidates. Ann Thorac Surg 2000;69:1823.
17. Frey B, Zuckermann A, Koller-Strametz J, et al. Effects of continuous, long-term therapy with prostaglandin E1 preoperatively on outcome after heart transplantation. Transplant Proc 1999;31:80.
18. Yeoh TK, Frist WH, Lagerstrom C, et al. Relationship of cardiac allograft size and pulmonary vascular resistance to long-term cardiopulmonary function. J Heart Lung Transplant 1992;11:1168.
19. Petrofski JA, Hoopes CW, Bashore TM, et al. Mechanical ventricular support lowers pulmonary vascular resistance in a patient with congential heart disease. Ann Thorac Surg 2003;75:1005.
20. Adamson RM, Dembitsky WP, Jaski BE, et al. Left ventricular assist device support of medically unresponsive pulmonary hypertension and aortic insufficiency. ASAIO J 1997;43:365.
21. Koerner MM, Tenderich G, Minami K, et al. Results of heart transplantation in patients with preexisting malignancies. Am J Cardiol 1997;79:988.
22. Goldstein DJ, Seldomridge A, Addonizio L, et al. Orthotopic heart transplantation in patients with treated malignancies. Am J Cardiol 1995;75:968.
23. Hosenpud JD, Pamidi SR, Fiol BS, et al. Outcomes in patients who are hepatitis B surface antigen-positive before transplantation: an analysis and study using the joint ISHLT/UNOS thoracic registry. J Heart Lung Transplant 2000;19:781.
24. Ko WJ, Chou NK, Hsu RB, et al. Hepatitis B virus infection in heart transplant recipients in a hepatitis B endemic area. J Heart Lung Transplant 2001;20:865.
25. Nguyen MH, Wright TL. Therapeutic advances in the management of hepatitis B and hepatitis C. Curr Opin Infect Dis 2001;14:593.
26. Fishman JA, Rubin RH. Solid organ transplantation in HIV-infected individuals: obstacles and opportunities. Transplant Proc 2001;33:1310.
27. Calabrese LH, Albrecht M, Young J, et al. Successful cardiac transplantation in an HIV-1-infected patient with advanced disease. N Engl J Med 2003;348:2323–2328.
28. Abbas AK, Lichtman AH, Pober JS. Immune responses to tissue transplants. In: Abbas AK, Lichtman AH, Pober JS, eds. Cellular and Molecular Immunology, 2nd ed. WB Saunders, Philadelphia, PA: 1994.
29. Smith JD, Danskine AJ, Laylor RM, et al. The effect of panel reactive antibodies and the donor specific crossmatch on graft survival after heart and heart-lung transplantation. Transplant Immunol 1993;1:60.
30. Baid S, Saidman SL, Tolkoff-Rubin M, et al. Managing the highly sensitized transplant recipient and B cell tolerance. Curr Opin Immunol 2001;13:577.
31. Betkowski AS, Graff R, Chen JJ, Hauptman PJ. Panel-reactive antibody screening practices prior to heart transplantation. J Heart Lung Transplant 2002;21:644.

32. Bishay ES, Cook DJ, Starling RC, et al. The clinical significance of flow cytometry crossmatching in heart transplantation. Eur J Cardiothorac Surg 2000;17:362.
33. Przybylowski P, Balogna M, Radovancevic B, et al. The role of flow cytometry-detected IgG and IgM anti-donor antibodies in cardiac allograft recipients. Transplantation 1999;67:258.
34. Aziz S, Hassantash SA, Nelson K, et al. The clinical significance of flow cytometry crossmatching in heart transplantation. J Heart Lung Transplant 1998;17:686.
35. McKenna DH Jr, Eastlund T, Segall M, et al. HLA alloimmunization in patients requiring ventricular assist device support. J Heart Lung Transplant 2002;21:1218.
36. Massad MG, McCarthy PM, Smedira NG, et al. Does successful bridging with the implantable left ventricular assist device affect cardiac transplantation outcome? J Thorac Cardiovasc Surg 1996;112:1275.
37. Massad MG, Cook DJ, Schmitt SK, et al. Factors influencing HLA sensitization in implantable LVAD recipients. Ann Thorac Surg 1997;64:1120.
38. Itescu S, Ankersmit J-H, Kocher AA, Schuster MD. Immunobiology of left ventricular assist devices. Prog Cardiovasc Dis 2000;43:67.
39. Stringham JC, Bull DA, Fuller TC, et al. Avoidance of cellular blood product transfusions in LVAD recipients does not prevent HLA allosensitization. J Heart Lung Transplant 1999;18:160.
40. Ratkovec RM, Hammond EH, O'Connell JB, et al. Outcome of cardiac transplant recipients with a positive donor-specific crossmatch—preliminary results with plasmapheresis. Transplantation 1992;54:651.
41. Pisani BA, Mullen GM, Malinowska K, et al. Plasmapheresis with intravenous immunoglobulin G is effective in patients with elevated panel reactive antibody prior to cardiac transplantation. J Heart Lung Transplant 1999;18:701.
42. Ruiz JC, de Francisco AL, Vazquez de Prada JA, et al. Successful heart transplantation after anti-HLA antibody removal with protein-A immunoadsorption in a hyperimmunized patient. J Thorac Cardiovasc Surg 1994;107:1366.
43. Robinson JA. Apheresis in thoracic organ transplantation. Ther Apher 1999;3:34.
44. Dowling RD, Jones JW, Carroll MS, Gray LA Jr. Use of intravenous immunoglobulin in sensitized LVAD recipients. Transplant Proc 1998;30:1110.
45. John R, Lietz K, Burke E, et al. Intravenous immunoglobulin reduces anti-HLA alloreactivity and shortens waiting time to cardiac transplantation in highly sensitized left ventricular assist device recipients. Circulation 1999;100:II229.
46. Itescu S, Burke E, Lietz K, et al. Intravenous pulse administration of cyclophosphamide is an effective and safe treatment for sensitized cardiac allograft recipients. Circulation 2002;105:1214.
47. Aranda JM Jr, Scornik JC, Normann SJ, et al. Anti-CD20 monoclonal antibody (rituximab) therapy for acute cardiac humoral rejection: a case report. Transplantation 2002;73:907.
48. Garrett HE Jr, Groshart, K, Duvall-Seaman D, et al. Treatment of humoral rejection with rituximab. Ann Thorac Surg 2002;74:1240.
49. Renlund DG, Taylor DO, Kfoury AG, Shaddy RS. New UNOS rules: historical background and implications for transplantation management. United Network for Organ Sharing. J Heart Lung Transplant 1999;18:1065.
50. Kauffman HM, McBride MA, Shield CF, et al. Determinants of waiting time for heart transplants in the United States. J Heart Lung Transplant 1999;18:414.
51. Data from the Organ Procurement and Transplantation Network Web site at http://www.optn.org/latestData/stateData.asp?type=region.

52. Whellan DJ, Tudor G, Denofrio D, et al. Heart transplant center practice patterns affect access to donors and survival of patients classified as status 1 by the United Network of Organ Sharing. Am Heart J 2000;140:443.

53. Laks H, Marelli D, Fonarow GC, et al. Use of two recipient lists for adults requiring heart transplantation. J Thorac Cardiovasc Surg 2003;125:49.

54. Data from the Organ Procurement and Transplantation Network Web site at http://www.optn.org/latestData/step2.asp.

55. Chen EP, Bittner HB, Kendall SW, Van Trigt P. Hormonal and hemodynamic changes in a validated animal model of brain death. Crit Care Med 1996; 24:1352.

56. Shivalkar B, Van Loon J, Wieland W, et al. Variable effects of explosive or gradual increase of intracranial pressure on myocardial structure and function. Circulation 1993;87:230.

57. Pinelli G, Mertes PM, Carteaux JP, et al. Myocardial effects of experimental acute brain death: evaluation by hemodynamic and biological studies. Ann Thorac Surg 1995;60:1729.

58. White M, Wiechmann RJ, Roden RL, et al. Cardiac beta-adrenergic neuroeffector systems in acute myocardial dysfunction related to brain injury. Evidence for catecholamine-mediated myocardial damage. Circulation 1995;92:2183.

59. Stoica SC, Goddard M, Large SR. The endothelium in clinical cardiac transplantation. Ann Thorac Surg 2002;73:1002.

60. Szabo G, Buhmann V, Bahrle S, et al. Brain death impairs coronary endothelial function. Transplantation 2002;73:1846.

61. Koo DD, Welsh KI, McLaren AJ, et al. Cadaver vs living donor kidneys: impact of donor factors on antigen induction before transplantation. Kidney Int 1999; 56:1551.

62. Wilhelm MJ, Pratschke J, Beato F, et al. Activation of the heart by donor brain death accelerates acute rejection after transplantation. Circulation 2000;102: 2426–2433.

63. Tsai FC, Marelli D, Bresson J, et al. Use of hearts transplanted from donors with atraumatic intracranial bleeds. J Heart Lung Transplant 2002;21:623.

64. Schnuelle P, Berger S, de Boer J, et al. Effects of catecholamine application to brain-dead donors on graft survival in solid organ transplantation. Transplantation 2001;72:455.

65. Chen JM, Cullinane S, Spanier TB, et al. Vasopressin deficiency and pressor hypersensitivity in hemodynamically unstable organ donors. Circulation 1999; 100:II244.

66. Chen EP, Bittner HB, Kendall SW, Van Trigt P. Hormonal and hemodynamic changes in a validated animal model of brain death. Crit Care Med 1996;24:1352.

67. Hunt SA, Baldwin J, Baumgartner W, et al. Cardiovascular management of a potential heart donor: a statement from the Transplantation Committee of the American College of Cardiology. Crit Care Med 1996;24:1599.

68. Ozcan YA, Begun JW, McKinney MM. Benchmarking organ procurement organizations: a national study. Health Serv Res 1999;34:855.

69. Zaroff JG, Rosengard BR, Armstrong WF, et al. Consensus conference report: maximizing use of organs recovered from the cadaver donor: cardiac recommendations, March 28–29, 2001, Crystal City, Virginia. Circulation 2002;106:836.

70. Jeevanandam V, Furukawa S, Prendergast TW, et al. Standard criteria for an acceptable donor heart are restricting heart transplantation. Ann Thorac Surg 1996;62:1268.

71. Young JB, Naftel DC, Bourge RC, et al. Matching the heart donor and heart transplant recipient: clues for successful expansion of the donor pool: a multivariable, multiinstitutional report. J Heart Lung Transplant 1994;13:353.

72. Wheeldon DR, Potter CD, Oduro A, et al. Transforming the "unacceptable" donor: outcomes from the adoption of a standardized donor management technique. J Heart Lung Transplant 1995;14:734.

73. Jahania MS, Sanchez JA, Narayan P, et al. Heart preservation for transplantation: principles and strategies. Ann Thorac Surg 1999;68:1983.

74. Demmy TL, Biddle JS, Bennett LE, et al. Organ preservation solutions in heart transplantation—patterns of usage and related survival. Transplantation 1997;63:262.

75. Hassanein WH, Zellos L, Tyrrell TA, et al. Continuous perfusion of donor hearts in the beating state extends preservation time and improves recovery of function. J Thorac Cardiovasc Surg 1998;116:821.

76. Nickless DK, Rabinov M, Richards SM, et al. Continuous perfusion improves preservation of donor rat hearts: importance of the implantation phase. Ann Thorac Surg 1998;65:1265.

77. Jones BU, Serna DL, Beckham G, et al. Recovery of cardiac function after standard hypothermic storage vs preservation with Peg-hemoglobin. ASAIO J 2001: 47:197.

78. Shumway NE, Lower RR, Stouffer RC. Transplantation of the heart. Adv Surg 1966;2:265.

79. Sarsam MA, Campbell CS, Yonan NA, et al. An alternative surgical technique in orthotopic cardiac transplantation. J Cardiac Surg 1993; 8:344.

80. Dreyfus G, Jebara V, Mihaileanu S, et al. Total orthotopic heart transplantation: an alternative to the standard technique. Ann Thorac Surg 1991;52:1181.

81. Blanche C, Nessim S, Quartel, A, et al. Heart transplantation with bicaval and pulmonary venous anastomoses. A hemodynamic analysis of the first 117 patients. J Cardiovasc Surg 1997;38:561.

82. Aziz T, Burgess M, Khafagy R, et al. Bicaval and standard techniques in orthotopic heart transplantation: medium-term experience in cardiac performance and survival. J Thorac Cardiovasc Surg 1999;118:115.

83. Milano CA, Shah AS, Van Trigt P, et al. Evaluation of early postoperative results after bicaval vs standard cardiac transplantation and review of the literature. Am Heart J 2000;140:717.

84. Aziz TM, Burgess MI, El-Gamel A, et al. Orthotopic cardiac transplantation technique: a survey of current practice. Ann Thorac Surg 1999;68:1242.

85. Kirklin JK, Naftel DC, Bourge RC, et al. Evolving trends in risk profiles and causes of death after heart transplantation: a ten-year multi-institutional study. J Thorac Cardiovasc Surg 2003;125:881.

86. Bourge RC, Naftel DC, Costanzo-Nordin MR, et al. Pretransplantation risk factors for death after heart transplantation: a multiinstitutional study. J Heart Lung Transplant 1993;12:549.

87. Hosenpud J, Bennett L, Keck B, et al. The Registry of the International Society for Heart and Lung Transplantation: 17th Official Report—2000. J Heart Lung Transplant 2000;19:909.

88. Asimakopoulos G, Smith PL, Ratnatunga CP et al. Lung injury and acute respiratory distress syndrome after cardiopulmonary bypass. Ann Thorac Surg 1999; 68:1107.

89. Butler J, Rocker GM, Westaby S. Inflammatory response to cardiopulmonary bypass. Ann Thorac Surg 1993;55:552.

90. Wessel D, Adatia I, Giglia T, et al. Use of inhaled nitric oxide and acetylcholine in the evaluation of pulmonary hypertension and endothelial function after cardiopulmonary bypass. Circulation 1993;88:2128–2138.

91. Bittner HB, Chen EP, Kendall SW, et al. Brain death alters cardiopulmonary hemodynamics and impairs right ventricular power reserve against an elevation of pulmonary vascular resistance. Chest 1997;111:706.

92. De Broux E, Lagace G, Dumont L, et al. Efficacy of dobutamine in the failing transplanted heart. J Heart Lung Transplant 1992;11:1133.

93. Levy JH, Bailey JM, Deeb GM. Intravenous milrinone in cardiac surgery. Ann Thorac Surg 2002;73:325.

94. Vincent JL, Carlier E, Pinsky MR, et al. Prostaglandin E1 infusion for right ventricular failure after cardiac transplantation. J Thorac Cardiovasc Surg 1992; 103:33.

95. Kieler-Jensen N, Lundin S, Ricksten SE. Vasodilator therapy after heart transplantation: effects of inhaled nitric oxide and intravenous prostacyclin, prostaglandin E1, and sodium nitroprusside. J Heart Lung Transplant 1995; 14:436.

96. Haraldsson A, Kieler-Jensen N, Ricksten S-E. Inhaled prostacyclin for treatment of pulmonary hypertension after cardiac surgery or heart transplantation: a pharmacodynamic study. J Cardiothorac Vasc Anesth 1996;10:864.

97. Rajek A, Pernerstorfer T, Kastner J, et al. Inhaled nitric oxide reduces pulmonary vascular resistance more than prostaglandin E(1) during heart transplantation. Anesth Analg 2000;90:523.

98. Chen JM, Levin HR, Rose EA, et al. Experience with right ventricular assist devices for perioperative right-sided circulatory failure. Ann Thorac Surg 1996; 61:305.

99. Barnard SP, Hasan A, Forty J, et al. Mechanical ventricular assistance for the failing right ventricle after cardiac transplantation. Eur J Cardiothorac Surg 1995; 9:297.

100. Kaul TK, Fields BL. Postoperative acute refractory right ventricular failure: incidence, pathogenesis, management and prognosis. Cardiovasc Surg 2000;8:1.

101. Albright TN, Zimmerman MA, Selzman CH. Vasopressin in the cardiac surgery intensive care unit. Am J Crit Care 2002;11:326.

102. Landry DW, Oliver JA. The pathogenesis of vasodilatory shock. N Engl J Med 2001;345:588.

103. Argenziano M, Chen JM, Choudhri AF, et al. Management of vasodilatory shock after cardiac surgery: identification of predisposing factors and use of a novel pressor agent. J Thorac Cardiovasc Surg 1998;116:973.

104. Taylor DO. Cardiac transplantation: drug regimens for the 21st century. Ann Thorac Surg 2003;75:S72.

105. Valantine H. Neoral use in the cardiac transplant recipient. Transplant Proc 2000; 32:S27.

106. Taylor DO, Barr ML, Meiser BM, et al. Suggested guidelines for the use of tacrolimus in cardiac transplant recipients. J Heart Lung Transplant 2001; 20:734.

107. Opelz G. Multicenter evaluation of immunosuppressive regimens in heart transplantation. Transplant Proc 1997;29:617.

108. Wiederrecht G, Lam E, Hung S, et al. The mechanism of action of FK-506 and cyclosporin A. Ann NY Acad Sci 1993;696:9.

109. Kobashigawa JA. Controversies in heart and lung transplantation immunosuppression: tacrolimus vs cyclosporine. Transplant Proc 1998;30:1095.

110. Allison AC, Kowalski WJ, Muller CD, et al. Mechanism of action of myco-phenolic acid. Ann NY Acad Sci 1990;696:63.
111. Kobashigawa J, Miller L, Renlund D, et al. A randomized active-controlled trial of mycophenolate mofetil in heart transplant recipients. Transplantation 1998; 66:507–515.
112. Hosenpud JD, Bennett LE. Mycophenolate mofetil vs azathioprine in patients surviving the initial cardiac transplant hospitalization: an analysis of the Joint UNOS/ISHLT Thoracic Registry. Transplantation 2001;72:1662.
113. Schmelzle T, Hall MN. TOR, a central controller of cell growth. Cell 2000; 103:253.
114. Saunders RN, Metcalfe MS, Nicholson ML. Rapamycin in transplantation: a review of the evidence. Kidney Int 2001;59:3.
115. Eisen HJ, Tuzcu EM, Dorent R, et al. Everolimus for the prevention of allograft rejection and vasculopathy in cardiac-transplant recipients. N Engl J Med 2003; 349:847.
116. Mancini D, Pinney S, Burkhoff D, et al. Use of rapamycin slows progression of cardiac transplantation vasculopathy. Circulation 2003;108:48.
117. Prieto M, Lake KD, Pritzker MR, et al. OKT3 induction and steroid-free maintenance immunosuppression for treatment of high-risk heart transplant recipients. J Heart Lung Transplant 1991;10:901.
118. Miller LW, Wolford T, McBride LR, et al. Successful withdrawal of cortico-steroids in heart transplantation. J Heart Lung Transplant 1992;11(2 part 2):431.
119. Olivari MT, Jessen ME, Baldwin BJ, et al. Triple-drug immunosuppression with steroid discontinuation by 6 months after heart transplantation. J Heart Lung Transplant 1995;14(1 part 1):127.
120. Kobashigawa JA, Stevenson LW, Brownfield ED, et al. Corticosteroid weaning late after heart transplantation: relation to HLA-DR mismatching and long-term metabolic benefits. J Heart Lung Transplant 1995;14:963.
121. Taylor DO, Bristow MR, O'Connell JB, et al. Improved long-term survival after heart transplantation predicted by successful early withdrawal from maintenance corticosteroid therapy. J Heart Lung Transplant 1996;15:1039.
122. Taylor DO, Kfoury AG, Pisani B, et al. Antilymphocyte-antibody prophylaxis: review of the adult experience in heart transplantation. Transplant Proc 1997;29 (suppl 8A):13S.
123. Norman DJ, Chatenoud L, Cohen D, et al. Consensus statement regarding OKT3-induced cytokine-release syndrome and human antimouse antibodies. Transplant Proc 1993;25(2 suppl 1):89.
124. Nashan B, Moore R, Amlot P, et al. Randomised trial of basiliximab vs placebo for control of acute cellular rejection in renal allograft recipients. CHIB 201 International Study Group. Lancet 1997;350:1193.
125. Vincenti F, Kirkman R, Light S, et al. Interleukin-2-receptor blockade with daclizumab to prevent acute rejection in renal transplantation. Daclizumab Triple Therapy Study Group. N Engl J Med 1998;338:161.
126. Beniaminovitz A, Itescu S, Lietz K, et al. Prevention of rejection in cardiac transplantation by blockade of the interleukin-2 receptor with a monoclonal antibody. N Engl J Med 2000;342:613.
127. Kirklin JK, Naftel DC, Bourge RC, et al. Rejection after cardiac transplantation: a time-related risk factor analysis. Circulation 1992;86(suppl II):II-236.
128. Kirlin JK, Naftel DC, Bourge RC, et al. Evolving trends in risk profiles and causes of death after heart transplantation: a 10-year multi-institutional study. J Thorac Cardiovasc Surg 2003;125:881.

129. Valantine HA, Yeoh TK, Gibbons R, et al. Sensitivity and specificity of diastolic indexes for rejection surveillance: temporal correlation with endomyocardial biopsy. J Heart Lung Transplant 191;10 (5 part 1):757.

130. Winters GL, Loh E, Schoen FJ. Natural history of focal moderate cardiac allograft rejection: is treatment warranted? Circulation 1995;91:1975.

131. Hammond EH, Yowell RL, Nunoda S, et al. Vascular (humoral) rejection in heart transplantation: pathologic observations and clinical implications. J Heart Lung Transplant 1989;8:430.

132. Rodriguez ER. The pathology of heart transplant biopsy specimens: revisiting the 1990 ISHLT working formulation. J Heart Lung Transplant 2003;22:3.

133. Grauhan O, Knosalla C, Ewert R, et al. Plasmapheresis and cyclophosphamide in the treatment of humoral rejection after heart transplantation. J Heart Lung Transplant 2001;20:316.

134. Garrett HE, Groshart K, Duvall-Seaman D, et al Treatment of humoral rejection with rituximab. Ann Thorac Surg 2002;74:1240.

135. Michaels PJ, Espejo ML, Kobashigawa J, et al. Humoral rejection in cardiac transplantation: risk factors, hemodynamic consequences and relationship to transplant coronary artery disease. J Heart Lung Transplant 2003;22:58.

136. Fishman JA, Rubin RH. Infection in organ-transplant recipients. N Engl J Med 1998;338:1741.

137. Rubin RH. Prevention and treatment of cytomegalovirus disease in heart transplant recipients. J Heart Lung Transplant 2000;19:731.

138. Madden BP, Reynolds L, Tryhorn Y, et al. Is routine post-operative surveillance for cytomegalovirus infection following heart transplantation necessary? Eur J Cardiothorac Surg 1998;14:15.

139. Avery RK. Prevention and treatment of cytomegalovirus infection and disease in heart transplant recipients. Curr Opin Cardiol 1998;13:122.

140. Koskinen PK, Kallio EA, Tikkanen JM. Cytomegalovirus infection and cardiac allograft vasculopathy. Transpl Infect Dis 1999;1:115.

141. Valantine HA, Luikart H, Doyle R, et al. Impact of cytomegalovirus hyperimmune globulin on outcome after cardiothoracic transplantation: a comparative study of combined prophylaxis with CMV hyperimmune globulin plus ganciclovir vs ganciclovir alone. Transplantation 2001;72:1647.

142. Billingham ME. Histopathology of graft coronary disease. J Heart Lung Transplant 1992;11(3 part 2):S38.

143. Costanzo MR, Naftel DC, Pritzker MR, et al. Heart transplant coronary artery disease detected by coronary angiography: a multiinstitutional study of preoperative donor and recipient risk factors. Cardiac Transplant Research Database. J Heart Lung Transplant 1998;17:744.

144. Rickenbacher PR, Pinto FJ, Chenzbraun A, et al. Incidence and severity of transplant coronary artery disease early and up to 15 years after transplantation as detected by intravascular ultrasound. J Am Coll Cardiol 1995;25:171.

145. Kobashigawa JA, Katznelson S, Laks H, et al. Effect of pravastatin on outcomes after cardiac transplantation. N Engl J Med 1995;333:621.

146. Wenke K, Meiser B, Thiery J, et al. Simvastatin reduces graft vessel disease and mortality after heart transplantation: a 4-year randomized trial. Circulation 1997;96:1398.

147. Eisen HJ, Tuzcu EM, Dorent R, et al. Everolimus for the prevention of allograft rejection and vasculopathy in cardiac-transplant recipients. N Engl J Med 2003;349:847.

148. Mancini D, Pinney S, Burkhoff D, et al. Use of rapamycin slows progression of cardiac transplantation vasculopathy. Circulation 2003;108:48.

149. Fang JC, Kinlay S, Beltrame J, et al. Effect of vitamins C and E on progression of transplant-associated atherosclerosis: a randomized trial. Lancet 2002;359:1108.

150. Schroeder JS, Gao SZ, Alderman EL, et al. A preliminary study of diltiazem in the prevention of coronary artery disease in heart-transplant recipients. N Engl J Med 1993;328:164.

151. Penn I. Cancers complicating organ transplantation. N Engl J Med 1990;323:1767.

152. Penn I. Solid tumors in cardiac allograft recipients. Ann Thorac Surg 1995; 60:1559.

153. Rinaldi M, Pellegrini C, D'Armini AM, et al. Neoplastic disease after heart transplantation: single center experience. Eur J Cardiothorac Surg 2001;19:696.

154. Nalesnik MA, Jaffe R, Starzl TE, et al. The pathology of posttransplant lymphoproliferative disorders occurring in the setting of cyclosporine A-prednisone immunosuppression. Am J Pathol 1988;133:173.

155. Armitage JM, Kormos RL, Stuart RS, et al. Posttransplant lymphoproliferative disease in thoracic organ transplant recipients: 10 years of cyclosporine-based immunosuppression. J Heart Lung Transplant 1991;10:877.

156. Swinnen LJ, Costanzo-Nordin MR, Fisher SG, et al. Increased incidence of lymphoproliferative disorder after immunosuppression with the monoclonal antibody OKT3 in cardiac-transplant recipients. N Engl J Med 1990;323:1723.

157. Hanto DW. Classification of Epstein-Barr virus-associated posttransplant lymphoproliferative diseases: implications for understanding their pathogenesis and developing rational treatment strategies. Annu Rev Med 195;46:381.

158. Walker RC, Marshall WF, Strickler JG, et al. Pretransplantation assessment of the risk of lymphoproliferative disorder. Clin Infect Dis 1995;20:1346.

159. Paya CV, Fung JJ, Nalesnik MA, et al. Epstein-Barr virus-induced posttransplant lymphoproliferative disorders. ASTS/ASTP Task Force and the Naymo Clinic Organized International Consensus Development Meeting. Transplantation 1999; 68:1517.

160. Swinnen LJ, Mullen GM, Carr TJ, et al. Aggressive treatment for postcardiac transplant lymphoproliferation. Blood 1995;86:3333.

161. Zilz ND, Olson LJ, McGregor CG. Treatment of post-transplant lymphoproliferative disorder with monoclonal CD20 antibody (rituximab) after heart transplantation. J Heart Lung Transplant 2001;20:770.

2

Surgical Revascularization in the Management of Heart Failure and Ischemic Left Ventricular Dysfunction

Jeffrey J. Teuteberg, MD and James C. Fang, MD

CONTENTS

INTRODUCTION

More than 5 million Americans have congestive heart failure, and 550,000 new cases are diagnosed each year. This condition results in almost 1 million hospital discharges and more than 50,000 deaths a year at a cost of $28.8 billion *(1)*. Coronary artery disease (CAD)

From: *Contemporary Cardiology: Surgical Management of Congestive Heart Failure*
Edited by: J. C. Fang and G. S. Couper © Humana Press Inc., Totowa, NJ

remains a leading cause of heart failure. Since the early trials of surgical vs medical management of coronary artery disease in the late 1970s, there have been substantial changes in the surgical techniques and the medical management of chronic CAD, acute coronary syndromes, and heart failure.

Despite these advances, the optimal role of surgical revascularization in the management of heart failure and ischemic left ventricular (LV) dysfunction remains unclear and primarily anecdotal. There is still no large prospective randomized experience with coronary artery bypass graft (CABG) surgery for patients with heart failure in the current era of mechanical revascularization. Although retrospective surgical series have suggested benefit for this population, these studies have rarely included the most recent advances in medical, surgical, and device therapies for heart failure (2–8). Furthermore, basic questions about bypass surgery and heart failure remain, including the optimal methods for assessing viability, the most appropriate end points (other than mortality) that should be targeted, and whether cost considerations and quality-of-life (QoL) measures should be paramount. Nonetheless, surgical revascularization remains one of the therapeutic cornerstones in the management of advanced heart failure from CAD.

CORONARY BYPASS SURGERY AND HEART FAILURE: THE CLINICAL EXPERIENCE

There are no randomized, controlled trials of patients with multivessel CAD and significant LV dysfunction because most early clinical trials of surgical revascularization excluded patients with advanced heart failure because of their high perioperative mortality. However, the three large randomized trials of bypass surgery vs medical management of the 1970s, the Veterans Administration Cooperative Study (VACS), the European Cooperative Coronary Study (ECSS), and the Coronary Artery Surgery Study (CASS), did include some patients with decreased LV function. Therefore, some insight into the role of CABG in these patients can be gleaned from a review of these trials (Table 1).

Randomized Trials

The VACS was the first large, multicenter, randomized controlled trial of medical therapy vs CABG for patients with stable angina. A total of 686 patients were randomized between 1972 and 1974. LV dysfunction was defined as an ejection fraction (EF) less than 50%. A minority of patients in either group had LV dysfunction, 35% in the medical arm and 31% in the CABG arm. A subgroup of patients with

Table 1
Comparison of Major Characteristics From the Three Large, Randomized Trials of Coronary Bypass Surgery vs Medical Management

	VACS	ECSS	CASS
Number of patients	686	768	780
Inclusion criteria			
Age (years)	≤65	≤65	≤65
Male sex (%)	100	100	90
EF (%)	>35	>50	>30
Significant stenosis (%)	≥50	≥50	≥70
Baseline characteristics (%)			
CHC class I/II angina	42[a]	57	74
β-Blockers	12	75	43
EF < 50%	26 (<45%)	0	21
Three-vessel disease (≥50% stenosis)	50	53[b]	51
Randomized to surgery			
Operative mortality (%)	5.8	3.3	1.4
Grafts/patient in three-vessel disease	2.3	2.4	2.8
Graft patency (%)			
12–18 months	70	75	90
60 months	67	69	82
Randomized to medical therapy (%)			
CABG by 10–12 years	38	36	38

CABG, coronary artery bypass graft surgery; CASS, Coronary Artery Surgery Study; ECSS, European Cooperative Coronary Study; EF, ejection fraction; CHC, Canadian Cardiovascular Association Classification; VACS, Veterans Administration Cooperative Study.

[a]Twenty-six percent were asymptomatic after myocardial infarction or had nonexertional chest pain.

[b]Eight percent of patients had left main coronary artery disease with lumen narrowing of 50% or more. (Adapted from ref. *16.*)

three-vessel disease and impaired LV dysfunction (but without left main CAD) was defined as having high angiographic risk. In this subgroup, the 7-year survival was 52% in the medically treated group vs 76% in the CABG group ($p = 0.002$). The survival advantage of bypass surgery was sustained at 11 years (38% medical vs 50% surgical, $p = 0.026$) *(9,10)*, but not by 18 years (23% medical vs 24% surgical, $p = 0.49$) *(11)*.

The ECSS was the second large, multicenter, randomized controlled trial of medical therapy vs CABG for patients with stable angina. It enrolled 768 patients from 1973 until 1976, but excluded any patient with an EF less than 50% *(12)*.

CASS was the third large, multi-center, randomized controlled trial of bypass surgery for stable angina. Patients in New York Heart Association (NYHA) class III/IV or with an EF less than 35% were specifically excluded. A total of 780 patients were randomly assigned from 1975 to 1979. There were, however, 160 patients with an EF less than 50%; in this subgroup, there was a survival benefit to bypass surgery at 7 years (70% medical vs 84% surgical, $p = 0.01$). Importantly, most of the survival advantage was in those patients with triple-vessel disease, whose survival was 65% with medical therapy and 88% with CABG ($p = 0.009$) *(13)*. A survival benefit was also seen in those with LV dysfunction in combination with more severe angina and left main coronary disease *(14,15)*. Although there was no difference in overall survival for all patients at 10 years, patients with an EF less than 50% had a survival benefit with surgery (61% vs 79% for the medical and CABG groups, respectively) *(16)*.

In summary, the landmark randomized trials of coronary bypass surgery did demonstrate a survival benefit to patients with advanced CAD and decreased LV function, but it is important to note that these studies were primarily trials of angina and not heart failure. Moreover, they were conducted in an era when surgical mortality was much higher than it is today, and medical therapy for both atherosclerosis and heart failure was essentially nonexistent. In fact, some have argued that the trials have no relevance in today's practice.

Contemporary Retrospective Studies

With improvements in surgical techniques and a growing perception that CABG benefits ischemic LV dysfunction, more contemporary experiences have been reported and are arguably more reflective of current practices. Duke University reported 710 patients with an EF of 40% or less, 301 of whom had CABG. After adjusting for differences between those who did and did not receive operations, the 3-year survival was 86% in the surgical group and 68% in the medical group. The benefits were greatest in the subgroup with the worst tertile of LV function *(17)*.

Yale University reported 83 consecutive patients with an EF of 30% or less who underwent CABG, half of whom had heart failure as the indication for surgery. The survival in this cohort at 3 years was 80%, with concomitant improvements in symptoms (by one NYHA functional class) and ventricular function (EF improved from a mean of 24.6 to 36%, $p < 0.001$) *(18)*.

Finally, in a review of 12 retrospective surgical series, bypass surgery improved 3-year survival by 30 to 50% in patients with LV dysfunction *(19)*, but at the cost of a higher surgical mortality. This increase in surgical mortality was, not surprisingly, consistent across studies. In a study of 12,471 patients undergoing bypass surgery, the operative mortalities with an EF above 40%, from 20 to 40%, and less than 20% were 2.3, 4.8, and 9.8%, respectively ($p < 0.001$) *(20)*. In fact, this surgical mortality paradox is often the clinical dilemma of whether to accept the high perioperative mortality for the potential long-term mortality benefit.

ISCHEMIC HEART DISEASE AND HEART FAILURE: PATHOPHYSIOLOGY

Historically, the prevailing perception was that LV dysfunction was the consequence of nonviable scar from myocardial infarction. Yet, early surgical revascularization experience with advanced CAD and concomitant LV dysfunction resulted in improvements in overall ventricular performance, and this improvement was not easily explained by the concept of a scarred hypocontractile ventricle. By the early to mid-1980s, the phenomenon of painless ischemia at rest and myocardial viability began to supplant the previous notion of an irreversibly scarred heart *(21)*. This concept that chronic resting hypoperfusion could result in resting wall motion abnormalities without infarction and was reversible with revascularization was termed *hibernating myocardium (22,23)*.

In a related manner, some areas of myocardium, although well perfused at rest (therefore not hibernating), may easily become ischemic because of a tenuous blood supply from severe epicardial CAD. With repeated bouts of episodic ischemia, the myocardium may become dysfunctional, a process referred to as *stunning*. Although these entities are thought of as clinically distinct (stunning in acute ischemic events and hibernation in chronic stable coronary disease), they often coexist in the same patient and even in the same myocardial territory *(24)*. Most important, both conditions are potentially reversible with revascularization.

Hibernation is an adaptive response of the myocyte to a level of perfusion sufficient for the preservation of the low-energy demands of maintaining cellular integrity, but inadequate for the high-energy demands of contractile function *(25)*. Although the myocyte can maintain cellular integrity when blood flow is reduced by 40–60%, greater reductions in blood flow usually result in membrane dysfunction *(26)*. In the setting of hypoxia, the myocyte shifts to glucose utilization to meet its metabolic demands. However, glycolysis can only be maintained if there is enough blood flow to ensure the supply of glucose and the removal of inhibitory metabolites, such as lactate *(27,28)*. Thus, hibernating myocardium exists in a delicate balance between blood flow adequate enough to avert cellular death, but insufficient for contractile function.

Although cellular integrity may be maintained, intracellular functions may be altered. Hibernating myocardium at the time of bypass surgery demonstrates characteristics of dedifferentiation with loss of contractile elements and an increase in the interstitial space *(29)*. Subsequent investigations have shown cytoskeletal disorganization, interstitial fibrosis, and markers of apoptosis, but not signs of ischemic cell death. Therefore, the hibernating myocyte is not merely a normal cell with reduced metabolic activity *(30)*. It eventually undergoes a process of architectural disorganization and extracellular fibrosis that may lead to apoptotic signaling. Hence, the time from restoration of flow to clinically detectable improvement in contractile function depends on the severity of the intracellular alterations that have occurred. If hypoperfusion is allowed to persist long enough, there may be myocyte loss, irreversible cell damage, or an unfavorable extracellular matrix that may diminish the magnitude of any potential improvement in contractile function *(31)*. However, if hibernation (and/or stunning) can be identified before irreversible cell damage or death, restoring adequate blood flow by revascularization should improve myocardial function. This concept of recoverable myocardial function in the setting of compromised blood flow is known as *myocardial viability.*

ASSESSMENT OF MYOCARDIAL VIABILITY

Early techniques to assess myocardial viability were primitive but important because perioperative morbidity and mortality could be prohibitive if clinical improvement was not likely. Early strategies included the use of ventriculography or echocardiography to assess improvements in regional ventricular contractility after nitrate administration *(32–34)* or after provoked extrasystoles *(35,36)*. Other provocative methods have used inotropic agents *(37)* and exercise *(38)*. In contemporary practice, detection of myocardial viability employs one of three strategies: (1) identifying metabolically active myocardium (i.e., radionuclide perfusion imaging), (2) assessing contractile reserve (i.e., dobutamine echo), or (3) quantifying myocardial scar (i.e., cardiac magnetic resonance imaging [MRI]).

Positron Emission Tomography

The determination of viability with positron emission tomography (PET) scanning involves the independent assessments of myocardial blood flow and cell viability. Blood flow to the myocardium is most commonly measured with ^{13}N-ammonium, but ^{15}O-water, ^{82}Rb, and other single-photon emission computed tomography (SPECT) perfusion tracers have been employed *(39)*. Metabolically active myocytes, especially hypoperfused myocytes that rely more heavily on glycolysis, will transport glucose intracellularly; thus, myocardial cell viability is inferred by uptake of ^{18}F-deoxyglucose (FDG) *(40)*. The perfusion scan is then matched with the metabolism scan. Normal myocardium will have normal perfusion and metabolism. Scar will have both decreased perfusion and decreased metabolism. Hibernating and viable myocardium will have decreased perfusion, but normal metabolism *(41)*. For these reasons, PET is often considered the gold standard for the noninvasive assessment of viability. Unfortunately, the lack of wide availability of this technology has limited its clinical utility.

A landmark study by Tillisch et al. in 1986 first applied PET to the assessment of myocardial viability and found an accuracy of 92% for the prediction of postoperative improvements in LV wall motion *(42)*. Their observations have been confirmed in numerous subsequent studies of PET in the prediction of viability. A meta-analysis of 17 such studies (including 462 patients) demonstrated an overall positive predictive accuracy of 76% and a negative predictive accuracy of 82% for improvement of wall motion after revascularization *(41)*. Furthermore, in a multivariate model for predicting improvement in LV function, PET viability was a strong independent predictor of recovery *(43)*.

Thallium Perfusion Imaging

There are two basic protocols for assessing viability with thallium 201 (Tl 201), rest–redistribution and stress–redistribution–reinjection. Thallium 201, a potassium analogue, is actively transported into the myocardium by a sodium–potassium pump. After injection, the tracer initially distributes into viable cells based on the distribution of blood flow. After several hours, thallium can be redistributed into myocardium independent of blood flow and thus is a marker of preserved cellular metabolism and hence viability *(44)*. During a rest–redistribution scan, Tl 201 is injected at rest, and baseline images are obtained. Hypoperfusion is manifested by a defect on the resting scan. The redistribution images are obtained 3 or 4 hours later. The resting scan is then compared to the redistribution scan. Viability is inferred by defects in Tl 201 uptake at rest that "fill in" on the redistribution scan.

However, this technique may incorrectly identify scar as viable myocardium. Both hibernating myocardium and nontransmural scar

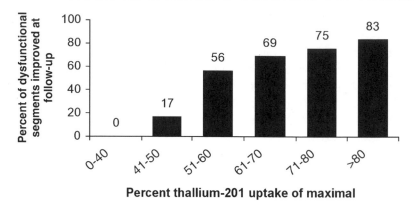

Fig. 1. Improvement in dysfunctional segments after revascularization based on the level of Tl 201 uptake after 4 hours of redistribution. (Adapted with permission from ref. *53*.)

can produce an area of decreased perfusion that redistributes (fills in) and is associated with a resting wall motion abnormality *(45)*. Conversely, the lack of uptake after redistribution does not necessarily equate with scar *(26,46,47)*. When the redistribution phase is lengthened from several hours to as long as 8–48 hours, there is greater distinction between scar and hibernating myocardium *(48)*. Unfortunately, longer intervals between rest and redistribution scans lead to poor image quality because of tracer decay or washout *(49)*. A second injection of Tl 201 has been used to overcome this loss of tracer intensity and substantially improves viability detection *(50–52)*. As many as half of fixed defects in a redistribution scan can show enhancement after reinjection *(51)*.

Because Tl 201 activity in the myocardium is present across a continuum of values, a minimum value is often arbitrarily used as a cutoff to determine clinical viability. Myocardial defects with counts below this cutoff are therefore labeled "irreversible." Although there is no ideal single value, 50% of the maximal tracer uptake is commonly used as this cutoff. However, viability is not binary at a prespecified cutoff value, although the chance of functional recovery decreases progressively as thallium counts fall (Fig. 1) *(53)*. Moreover, the ability of thallium techniques to predict functional recovery at a particular activity value for viability is worse in areas of akinesis than hypokinesis *(53)*. Therefore, it is possible that irreversible defects by Tl 201 may still be viable, especially when assessed by PET. Only the most severe perfusion defects correlate well with PET nonviability *(54)*. These cutoff values are important to note and may account for the variable diagnostic accuracy of this technique in the literature.

The diagnostic accuracy of Tl 201 scintigraphy can be improved with exercise. In areas with equivocal viability by tracer uptake, the finding of reversible ischemia on stress imaging predicts recovery of function *(55)*. Exercise stress imaging also provides the additional prognostic information of exercise capacity. Finally, combining various features of Tl 201 scintigraphy, such as stress-induced ischemia, wall motion abnormalities, late redistribution activity, and the use of absolute of tracer counts, can refine the interpretation of viability.

Despite these technical issues, Tl 201 scintigraphy is sensitive. Pooled data from several studies showed that the use of Tl 201 for viability has a sensitivity of 86–90% and specificity of 47–54% for predicting improvement in postrevascularization wall motion *(40)* and compares favorably to PET *(56)*.

Technetium-99 Perfusion Imaging

The technetium-based tracers ^{99m}Tc-sestamibi and ^{99m}Tc-tetrofosmin have also been used for the assessment of myocardial viability. Technetium-based agents cross cell membranes passively and then bind to mitochondria. These tracers distribute according to perfusion and viability of the myocardium *(44,57)*, but do not redistribute as extensively as Tl 201. However, they are similar to Tl 201 in their ability to demonstrate viability and predict recovery of function *(58–61)*. Pooled data from seven studies of ^{99m}Tc-sestamibi showed a sensitivity of 81% and specificity of 60% for the detection of functional recovery after revascularization and can be improved with the administration of nitrates *(40)*. Finally, in one series, ^{99m}Tc-tetrofosmin had a sensitivity of 96% and specificity of 30% for predicting viability *(58)*.

In summary, the primary advantages to the use of thallium- or technetium-based scintigraphy are their widespread availability and high sensitivity. The tracers are generally similar in their ability to predict improvement in LV function. Drawbacks to the technology include motion artifacts, attenuation of counts from other organs, and the time to obtain, process, and interpret the data. Continuous technological improvements are helping to minimize these disadvantages.

Dobutamine Echocardiography

In early studies of myocardial viability, inotropic agents often improved the function of hypokinetic or akinetic myocardial segments. Although the hibernating myocyte may have a perturbed cytoskeletal structure and a decreased quantity of contractile fibers, it is often still capable of responding to inotropic agents through β-receptor stimulation.

Low-dose dobutamine stress echocardiography (LDSE) can demonstrate this contractile reserve and imply viability. During infusion of low-dose dobutamine (<5 μg/kg/min), hypocontractile viable myocardium is stimulated to contract (via adrenergic β-1-receptors), but not to a level at which the increased oxygen demand outstrips its supply. The sensitivity, specificity, and diagnostic accuracies of LDSE to predict postoperative improvements in LV function are variable and range from 71 to 97%, 63 to 96%, and 70 to 91%, respectively (62). When compared to Tl 201, LDSE generally shows a higher specificity and lower sensitivity for viability (63,64).

The lower sensitivity may be because of the inability to deliver the substrate necessary to increase contractile function when there is advanced cytoskeletal disarray, so the dobutamine stress results in an ineffectual or absent contractile response (24). Echocardiography is also better at predicting functional recovery of hypokinetic rather than akinetic segments (65), although this is true of thallium imaging as well (24). As noted by Bonow (24), the ability of LDSE to predict postrevascularization improvements in wall motion more accurately than PET or SPECT may not be surprising because viability is typically defined by improvements in echocardiographically assessed wall motion.

The specificity of dobutamine stress echocardiography (DSE) for the detection of viability is improved by a phenomenon known as the *biphasic response*. The biphasic response is an improvement in wall motion at low doses of dobutamine, but a diminution in function with higher doses (66). It was postulated that this represented a mismatch between limited perfusion because of coronary disease and the increasing metabolic demand from dobutamine, resulting in myocardial ischemia and dysfunction. Hence, at low doses there is improved contractile function (as in LDSE), but at higher doses of dobutamine, the myocardium becomes ischemic and dysfunctional as the demands of contractile function surpass the supply of metabolic substrate. The presence of a biphasic response increases the specificity of DSE for predicting functional recovery to 73% (67) and improves the concurrence with radionuclide imaging (68).

In summary, dobutamine stress echocardiography is widely available and is generally lower in cost compared to both PET and SPECT. It also can be performed quickly and even portably. Concomitant echocardiography also provides other details about ventricular and valvular structure and function. Disadvantages include poor acoustic windows from lung disease, obesity, or immobility. Interpretation can

be difficult if the endocardium is not well delineated or if there is tethering from adjacent abnormal segments *(69)*. Some of these technical
issues can be ameliorated with the use of echocontrast agents. Finally,
as compared to scintigraphic techniques, it has greater specificity,
although less sensitivity.

Cardiac MRI

Cardiac MRI is playing an increasingly important role in the assessment of viability. Improvements in contrast-enhanced MRI have led to
the ability to detect myocardial perfusion and scar with high spatial
resolution. Ischemic wall motion is detected via a dobutamine protocol
similar to DSE. Quantification of a gadolinium-based contrast material
in the myocardium is used to measure myocardial blood flow. Scar is
manifest by hyperenhancement in the ventricular myocardium. Hyperenhancement is seen after myocardial infarction, but not in patients with
nonischemic cardiomyopathies or in normal volunteers *(70)*. In the first
large study of contrast-enhanced MRI by Kim et al., 78% of nonhyper-
enhancing dysfunctional segments improved after revascularization *(71)*.
Furthermore, MRI was more predictive of improvement in ventricular
segments with akinesia and dyskinesia than in areas of hypokinesia,
which is just the converse of PET and SPECT. There was also an
inverse relationship between the burden of hyperenhancement and the
likelihood of improvement in wall motion after revascularization.

Contrast-enhanced dobutamine MRI will likely become an important tool in the detection of myocardial viability. The advantage of
contrast-enhanced dobutamine stress MRI is the ability to combine
measures of baseline and stress wall motion and myocardial perfusion
with myocardial scar visualization. Disadvantages include lack of
wide availability and the inability to accommodate patients with
metallic hardware common to this population, such as pacemakers and
implantable defibrillators.

In summary, PET still is considered the test to which other modalities are compared for predicting viability. The other radionuclide agents
are similar to PET and provide excellent sensitivity, but dobutamine
echocardiography and MRI have superior specificity (Fig. 2).

Problems in Assessing the Accuracy of Methods
to Detect Myocardial Viability

If recovery of ventricular systolic function defines viability, then the
gold standard for judging the accuracy of a diagnostic technique rests
solely on the assessment of postrevascularization ventricular function
(72). However, it is not clear when to assess the impact of surgical

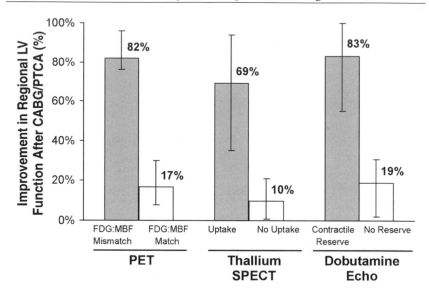

Fig. 2. Analysis of sensitivity and specificity of various modalities for predicting improvement in LV function after revascularization from multiple studies. The positive predictive value of each test is represented by the gray bars, and the inverse of the negative predictive value is represented by the open bars. CABG, coronary artery bypass graft surgery; Echo, echocardiography; FDG, ^{18}F-deoxyglucose; LV, left ventricular; MBF, myocardial blood flow; PET, positron emission tomography; PTCA, percutaneous transluminal coronary angioplasty; SPECT, single-photon emission tomography. (Reproduced with permission from ref. *24*.)

revascularization on ventricular function in the postoperative period, despite the fact that most studies base the accuracy of preoperative viability testing on assessments of ventricular function soon after surgery. Given the potential severity of the cytoskeletal disarray in hibernating myocardium, it is not surprising that full functional recovery may take months. Several studies have demonstrated such delayed recovery after revascularization does take place *(73,74)*. Conversely, viable segments may improve in function without a substantial impact on overall LV function *(75)*. In fact, in one series, the survival of patients undergoing bypass surgery without preoperative viability testing was independent of postoperative improvements in their EF *(76)*.

Completeness of revascularization will also have an impact on the predictive accuracy of tests for postoperative improvements in LV function (Table 2). If there is hypoperfusion of the myocardium from poor runoff, stenosis at the anastomotic site, development of graft atherosclerosis, or progression of native coronary disease distal to the anastamosis, there may not be functional recovery. Similarly, if the graft fails

Table 2
Factors Affecting Improvement in Left Ventricular Function
After Coronary Artery Revascularization

1. Presence and degree of preoperative myocardial hibernation or stunning
2. Coronary anatomy
3. Completeness of revascularization
4. Presence and degree of intraoperative or postoperative myocardial infarction
5. Graft patency
6. Method for determining ventricular function
7. Left ventricular size
8. Time from revascularization to assessment of ventricular function
9. Presence of concomitant myopathy

Adapted from ref. *75.*

and the myocardium becomes infarcted, there will be a lack of functional recovery *(45)*. Trials have shown the predictive accuracy of rest–redistribution Tl 201 is improved with the exclusion of inadequately revascularized segments *(77)*. However, few trials address the completeness of revascularization.

OTHER BENEFITS OF SURGICAL REVASCULARIZATION IN HEART FAILURE

In multivariate models used to predict postrevascularization ventricular function *(43)*, preoperative myocardial viability only accounts for 36% of the variability in the postsurgical EF *(78)*. Therefore, some have questioned whether recovery of ventricular function is the most clinically relevant end point for patients with advanced CAD and heart failure. Statistical improvements in the contraction of segments of myocardium or even in total EF may not easily translate into tangible benefits unless they impact on symptom relief, QoL, or survival. Various studies have examined such end points in addition to postoperative ventricular systolic function.

Symptoms

The identification of viability may identify those most likely to derive symptomatic benefit from surgery. In a study of 36 patients with symptomatic heart failure (a third also had angina) and poor ventricular function (mean EF 28%), the total extent of PET mismatch corresponded linearly with postoperative symptomatic improvement. In fact, those with the largest mismatch had the greatest degree of benefit *(79)*. Improvement in symptoms also paralleled an improvement in survival *(80)*.

Other techniques to identify viability also predict symptomatic improvements. Bax et al. *(81)* used DSE to assess viability in 62 patients, more than half of whom had heart failure as the indication for revascularization. For those patients with four or more viable segments by DSE, the mean NYHA functional class improved from 3.2 to 1.6 ($p < 0.01$) after revascularization and corresponded to an increase in the EF from 27 to 33% ($p < 0.01$). There were no improvements in symptoms or ventricular function in patients with less than four viable segments.

Quality of Life

QoL was investigated in a study of 73 patients (mean EF 28% and mean NYHA class 2.6) who had both PET and DSE prior to bypass surgery. Improvement in exercise capacity correlated with amount of viability by PET but not by echo. The mean NYHA functional class improved from 2.6 to 1.9, but correlated weakly with the viability assessments. Interestingly, QoL scores improved significantly with no correlation to viability *(82)*. The presence of viability contributed to improved symptoms, but QoL may be too complex a measure to be driven solely by symptomatic improvement. In fact, the contribution of the placebo effect of surgery cannot be discounted and was an important confounder in the transmyocardial laser revascularization studies of chronic medically refractory angina.

Survival

Early studies of PET showed 3-year survival was similar to cardiac transplantation with surgical revascularization when viability was present *(83)*. Revascularization of PET-viable territories also decreased nonfatal ischemic events compared to those who were treated medically *(84)*. Other studies have demonstrated decreased incidence of myocardial infarction, cardiac arrest, and death when PET viability was present before revascularization *(85)*. Tl 201 viability has also been shown to improve survival after revascularization *(86–89)* and is independent of age, EF, and number of diseased vessels *(90)*.

Scintigraphic techniques appear comparable when trying to predict survival. For example, ^{13}N-ammonia/^{18}FDG PET and stress/rest ^{99m}Tc-sestamibi SPECT were compared in 103 patients with a mean NYHA class of 2.5 and advanced LV dysfunction (a third had EF <30%). The revascularization team was blinded to the specific test, and the patients received either percutaneous transluminal coronary angioplasty or CABG if there was demonstrable viability; otherwise, they received medical management. The cardiac event-free survival 28 months after revascularization was improved to the same degree regardless of whether SPECT or PET was used to determine viability *(91)*.

Improvements in ventricular geometry may also predict survival and make the use of echocardiographic techniques to assess viability attractive. Using LDSE, an improvement in ventricular geometry predicted a twofold increase in 4-year survival *(92)*. Along with improvements in NYHA class and EF, LDSE viability predicts survival with surgical revascularization when compared to medical management alone *(81,86,93,94)*. Furthermore, LDSE viability was the strongest predictor of survival in a multivariable analysis *(95)*. Lack of echocardiographic viability also predicts an absence of survival benefit with revascularization. In one investigation (Fig. 3), survival from cardiac death after a mean of 40 months was 97% for patients with viability who had revascularization, 69% for those with viability with medical treatment, 50% for those without viability who had revascularization, and 56% for those without viability who were treated medically *(93)*.

A meta-analysis of 24 studies of viability with PET, thallium perfusion, or dobutamine echocardiography was performed to compare the impact of viability testing on prognosis. More than 3000 patients with a mean EF of 32% were followed for more than 2 years. Annual mortality after revascularization with viable myocardium was 3.2% compared to 16% with medical treatment ($p < 0.0001$). If there was demonstrable viability, then the patients with the worst preoperative EF had the greatest degree of benefit. Last, patients with viable myocardium who were treated medically had a death rate of 16% compared with 6.2% (Fig. 4) for patients who had no viability and were treated medically *(96)*.

To conclude, testing for viability to assess suitability for subsequent revascularization of patients with CAD and LV function appears to predict not only improvements in LV function, but also improvements in symptoms and survival. However, the published data to date, as Bonow noted, are generally derived from small, single-center observational trials, with viability treated in a binary fashion and using a mix of surgical and percutaneous revascularization in patients with various degrees of heart failure and angina *(97)*. Furthermore, these studies by and large are retrospective and subject to significant bias because the decision to proceed with surgery was rarely randomized.

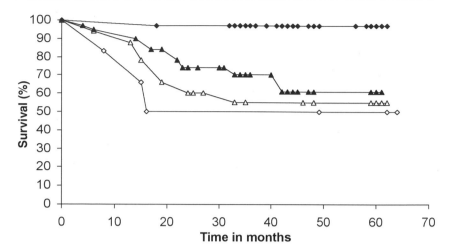

Fig. 3. Effect of myocardial viability by dobutamine echocardiography on survival in 87 consecutive patients with a mean of 2.3 diseased arteries and a mean EF of 25%. Solid diamond, viable myocardium and revascularization; solid triangle, viable myocardium and medical therapy; open triangle, no viable myocardium and medical therapy; open diamond, no viable myocardium and revascularization. (Reproduced with permission from ref. *93*.)

Nonetheless, for the patient with advanced coronary artery disease (and suitable anatomy for revascularization), LV dysfunction, and heart failure, but without angina, revascularization is likely beneficial if viability can be demonstrated. Viability demonstrated by thallium scintigraphy, PET, or dobutamine echocardiography predicts symptomatic improvement, and these modalities are similar in their ability to predict survival after revascularization (Fig. 5). Equally important, patients who lack significant myocardial viability probably do not benefit, and are potentially harmed, from surgery when compared to contemporary medical and device therapies for heart failure.

This body of evidence has contributed to the current recommendations by the American Heart Association/American College of Cardiology (AHA/ACC) for CABG *(98)* in patients with LV dysfunction (*see* Table 3). The choice of method for the preoperative assessment of myocardial viability is ultimately dependent on local expertise and familiarity because the various modalities appear to be comparable (Table 4). Some centers use more than one modality to take advantage of the high sensitivies of certain techniques (i.e., scintigraphic tests) and the high specificities of others (i.e., dobutamine echocardiography or cardiac stress MRI).

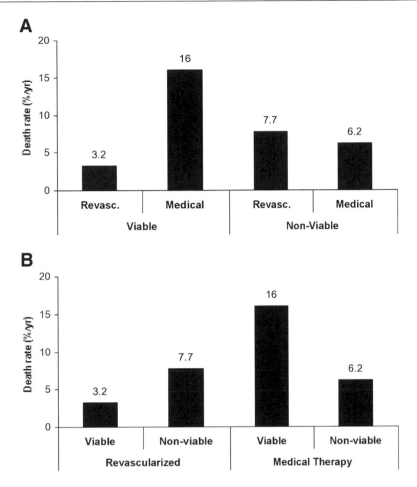

Fig. 4. The results of a meta-analysis of 24 studies using positron emission tomography, thallium 201 perfusion, or dobutamine echocardiography to assess viability in patients with coronary artery disease and left ventricular dysfunction. **(A)** Death rates for patients with and without myocardial viability treated by revascularization (Revasc.) or medical therapy. **(B)** Death rates for patients treated by revascularization or medical therapy with and without demonstrable viability. (Adapted from ref. *96*.)

SURGICAL VENTRICULAR REMODELING

Surgical remodeling of the ventricle, especially when significant ventricular distortion is present, can improve ventricular function and can be performed concomitantly with coronary bypass grafting *(99)*. This procedure, as modified by Dor, involves decreasing the scar size by apposing the surrounding viable myocardium directly or through a pericardial patch *(100)*. By maintaining LV geometry at a lower

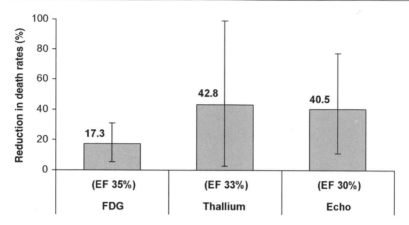

Fig. 5. The results of a meta-analysis of 11 studies of F-18 fluorodeoxyglucose (FDG) positron emission tomography, 6 studies of thallium 201 perfusion imaging, and 7 studies of dobutamine echocardiography on survival in patients with coronary artery disease and LV dysfunction. The mean EF of the patients is listed in parentheses above the modality used to assess viability. The mean decrease in mortality after the revascularization of viable myocardium is represented by the bar graph; the lines represent the 95% confidence intervals. The decrease in mortality is not statistically significantly different between the three modalities for detecting viability. (Adapted with permission from ref. *96.*)

volume, many of the adverse consequences of LV dilation can be pacified *(101,102)*. A study reviewed this approach in 439 patients, 89% of whom had simultaneous bypass surgery, from a variety of surgical centers. Both ventricular function and geometry improved, with the mean EF increasing from 29 to 39% ($p < 0.0001$), and the end systolic volume decreasing from 109 mL/m^2 to 69 mL/m^2 ($p < 0.005$). Most important, in the mortality at 18 months was an acceptable 10.8% *(103)*.

THE FUTURE OF MECHANICAL REVASCULARIZATION IN HEART FAILURE

It still remains that no prospective randomized trial exists to address the problem of revascularization for heart failure and ischemic LV dysfunction. Although current retrospective literature is supportive of surgery in this clinical situation, the evidence is far from definitive. In response to this dilemma, the National Institutes of Health is sponsoring a multicenter prospective randomized trial, the Surgical Treatment for Ischemic Heart Failure (STICH) study. It is recruiting patients with

Table 3
ACC/AHA/ASNC Consensus Recommendations
for Radionuclide Techniques to Assess Myocardial Viability

Indication	Test	Class	Level of evidence
1. Predicting improvement in regional and global LV function after revascularization	Stress–redistribution–reinjection	I	B
	Rest–redistribution imaging	I	B
	Perfusion plus PET FDG imaging	I	B
	Resting sestamibi imaging	I	B
	Gated SPECT sestamibi imaging	IIa	B
	Late Tl 201 redistribution imaging (after stress)	IIb	B
2. Predicting improvement in heart failure symptoms after revascularization	Perfusion plus PET FDG imaging	IIa	B
3. Predicting improvement in natural history after revascularization	Tl 201 imaging (rest–redistribution and stress–redistribution–reinjection)	I	B
	Perfusion plus PET FDG imaging	I	B

ACC, American College of Cardiology; AHA, American Heart Association; ASNC, American Society of Nuclear Cardiology; LV, left ventricular; PET, positron emission tomography; FDG, ^{18}F-deoxyglucose; SPECT, single-photon emission computed tomography; Tl 201, thallium 201. Recommendation class: I, conditions for which there is evidence for and/or general agreement that the procedure or treatment is useful and effective; IIa, the weight of evidence or opinion is in favor of the procedure or treatment. IIb, usefulness/efficacy is less well established by evidence/opinion. Level of evidence B: Data derived from a single randomized clinical trial or nonrandomized studies. (Adapted from ref. 49.)

Table 4
ACC/AHA Guidelines for the Indications for CABG
in Patients With Poor LV Function

Class I
  1. Significant left main coronary artery stenosis
  2. Left main equivalent: significant (≥70%) stenosis of the proximal
      LAD and proximal left circumflex artery
  3. Proximal LAD stenosis with two- or three-vessel disease
Class IIa
  Poor LV function, with significant viable noncontracting
  revascularizable myocardium and without any of the above
  anatomic patterns
Class III
  Poor LV function, without evidence of intermittent ischemia
  and without evidence of significant revascularizable viable
  myocardium

ACC, American College of Cardiology; AHA, American Heart Association; CABG, coronary artery bypass graft surgery; LV, left ventricular; LAD, left anterior descending coronary artery.

Recommendations class: I, conditions for which there is evidence for and/or general agreement that the procedure or treatment is useful and effective; IIa, the weight of evidence or opinion is in favor of the procedure or treatment; III, conditions for which there is evidence and/or general agreement that the procedure or treatment is not useful/effective and in some cases can be harmful. (Adapted from ref. *98*.)

ischemic LV dysfunction with an EF less than 35%, CAD amenable to surgical revascularization, and NYHA class 2–4 heart failure at 50 centers with a goal enrollment of 2800 patients. The overall study design is to randomly assign patients, stratified by presence or absence of angina and by the presence or absence of a large akinetic territory, either to surgery or to continued medical therapy. Those with large akinetic territories will be eligible to undergo surgical ventricular restoration (SVR; i.e., surgical remodeling).

Patients without angina will be divided into two groups: 1600 patients with SVR-ineligible anatomy and 600 patients who are SVR eligible. The SVR ineligible will be randomly assigned to medical therapy vs CABG alone. The SVR eligible will be randomly assigned to one of three arms: medical therapy, CABG alone, or CABG and SVR. Finally, in a subgroup study of 600 patients with angina, those with heart failure and a large area of akinesis will be randomly assigned to conventional CABG alone or CABG and SVR.

The trial will have a minimum follow-up of 3 years. The study has an 89% power to demonstrate a 20% reduction in the combined end point of all-cause death for CABG compared to medical therapy. For SVR-eligible patients, the study has a 90% power to detect a 20% difference in the end point of survival free of hospitalization for cardiac causes when compared to CABG alone or medical therapy. All screened patients who meet inclusion criteria for any of the trial's arms but who refuse study entry will be followed in a registry.

The study will also include an investigation of the noninvasive assessment of viability with cardiac MRI, radionuclide imaging, and echocardiography. There will be postoperative assessments of LV function at 4 months and 2 years. The modalities will be assessed for their ability to predict clinical outcomes both individually and in comparison to one another. Substudies will analyze cost, QoL, neurohormonal mediators, proinflammatory cytokines, natriuretic peptides, and polymorphisms in genotype expression. When completed, this study will surely be a landmark effort in refining the evaluation of patients with ischemic heart failure and defining the roles of medical therapy, revascularization, and surgical ventricular remodeling in their subsequent management.

REFERENCES

1. http://www.americanheart.org/downloadable/heart/1075102824882HDSStats2004 UpdateREV1-23-04.pdf. American Heart Association, Heart Disease and Stroke Statistics—2004 update. Accessed 1/30/04.
2. Pitt B, Zannad F, Remme WJ, et al. for the RALES Study Investigators. The effect of spironolactone on morbidity and mortality in patients with severe heart failure. Randomized Aldactone Evaluation Study Investigators. N Engl J Med 1999;341: 709–717.
3. Packer M, Coats AJ, Fowler MB, et al. of the Carvedilol Prospective Randomized Cumulative Survival Study Group. Effect of carvedilol on survival in severe chronic heart failure. N Engl J Med 2001;344:1651–1658.
4. Hjalmarson A, Goldstein S, Fagerberg B, et al. Effects of controlled-release metoprolol on total mortality, hospitalizations, and well-being in patients with heart failure: the Metoprolol CR/XL Randomized Intervention Trial in congestive heart failure (MERIT-HF). MERIT-HF Study Group. JAMA 2000;283:1295–1302.
5. Publication Committee for the VMAC Investigators (Vasodilatation in the Management of Acute CHF). Intravenous nesiritide vs nitroglycerin for treatment of decompensated congestive heart failure: a randomized controlled trial. JAMA 2002;287:1531–1540.
6. Moss AJ, Zareba W, Hall WJ, et al. of the Multicenter Automatic Defibrillator Implantation Trial II Investigators. Prophylactic implantation of a defibrillator in patients with myocardial infarction and reduced ejection fraction. N Engl J Med 2002;346:877–883.
7. Abraham WT, Fisher WG, Smith AL, et al. of the MIRACLE Study Group. Multicenter InSync Randomized Clinical Evaluation. Cardiac resynchronization in chronic heart failure. N Engl J Med 2002;346:1845–1853.

8. Bradley DJ, Bradley EA, Baughman KL, et al. Cardiac resynchronization and death from progressive heart failure: a meta-analysis of randomized controlled trials. JAMA 2003;289:730–740.

9. The Veterans Administration Coronary Artery Bypass Surgery Cooperative Study Group. Eleven-year survival in the Veterans Administration randomized trial of coronary artery bypass surgery for stable angina. N Engl J Med 1984;311: 1333–1339.

10. Detre KM, Takaro T, Hultgren H, Peduzzi P. Long-term mortality and morbidity results of the Veterans Administration randomized trial of coronary artery bypass surgery. Circulation 1985;72(suppl):V84–V89.

11. The Veterans Administration Coronary Artery Bypass Surgery Cooperative Study Group. Eighteen-year follow-up in the Veterans Affairs cooperative study of coronary artery bypass surgery for stable angina. Circulation 1992;86:121–130.

12. European Coronary Surgery Study Group. Coronary artery bypass surgery in stable angina pectoris: survival at 2 years. Lancet 1979;1:889.

13. Passamani E, Davis KB, Gillespie MJ, Killip T, for the CASS Investigators. A randomized trial of coronary artery bypass surgery: survival of patients with a low ejection fraction. N Engl J Med 1985;312:1665–1671.

14. Myers WO, for the CASS registry. Improved survival of surgically treated patients with triple vessel coronary artery disease and severe angina pectoris. J Thorac Cardiovasc Surg 1989;97:487–495.

15. Caracciolo EA, Davis KB, Sopko G, et al. Comparison of surgical and medical group survival in patients with left main coronary artery disease. Circulation 1995;91:2325–2334.

16. Alderman EL, Bourassa MG, Cohen LS, et al. Ten-year follow-up of survival and myocardial infarction in the randomized Coronary Artery Surgery Study. Circulation 1990;82:1629–1646.

17. Bounos EP, Mark DB, Pollock BG, et al. Surgical survival benefits for coronary disease patients with left ventricular dysfunction. Circulation 1988;78(suppl): I151–I157.

18. Elefteriades JA, Tolis G, Levi E, Mills LK, Zaret BL. Coronary artery bypass grafting in severe left ventricular dysfunction: excellent survival with improved ejection fraction and functional state. J Am Coll Cardiol 1993;22:1411–1417.

19. Baker DW, Jones R, Hodges J, Massie BM, Konstam MA, Rose EA. Management of heart failure: the role of revascularization in the treatment of patients with moderate or severe left ventricular systolic dysfunction. JAMA 1994;272: 1528–1534.

20. Christakis GT, Weisel RD, Fremes SE, et al. Coronary artery bypass grafting in patients with poor ventricular function. J Thorac Cardiovasc Surg 1992;103: 1083–1092.

21. Rahimtoola SH. The hibernating myocardium. Am Heart J 1998;117:211–221.

22. Rahimtoola SH. A perspective on the three large multicenter randomized clinical trials of coronary bypass surgery for chronic stable angina. Circulation 1985;72:V-123.

23. Braunwald E, Rutherford JD. Reversible ischemic left ventricular dysfunction: evidence for the "hibernating myocardium." J Am Coll Cardiol 1986;8:1467.

24. Bonow RO. Identification of viable myocardium. Circulation 1996;94:2674–2680.

25. Ross J. Myocardial perfusion-contraction matching: implications for coronary heart disease and hibernation. Circulation 1991;83:1076.

26. Iskandrian AS, Schelbert HR. Myocardial viability assessment. J Nucl Med 1994; 35(suppl):1S–3S.

27. Dilsizian V, Bonow RO. Current diagnostic techniques of assessing myocardial viability in patients with hibernating and stunned myocardium. Circulation 1993; 87:1–20.
28. Schelbert HR. Merits and limitations of radionuclide approaches to viability and future developments. J Nucl Cardiol 1;S86–S96.
29. Ausma J, Cleutjens J, Thone F, Flameng W, Ramaekers F, Borgers M. Chronic hibernating myocardium: interstitial changes. Mol Cell Biochem 1995;147:35–42.
30. Elsässer A, Schlepper M, Klövekorn WP, et al. Hibernating myocardium: an incomplete adaptation to ischemia. Circulation 1997;96:2920–2931.
31. Braunwald E, Bristow MR. Congestive heart failure: 50 years of progress. Circulation 2000;102:IV14–IV23.
32. Helfant RH, Pine R, Meister SG, Feldman MS, Trout RG, Banka VS. Nitroglycerine to unmask reversible asynergy. Correlation with post-coronary artery bypass ventriculography. Circulation 1974;50:108.
33. Crawford MH, Amon KW, Vance WS. Exercise two-dimensional echocardiography. Quantification of left ventricular performance in patients with severe angina pectoris. Am J Cardiol 1983;51:1.
34. Stadius M, AcAnulty JH, Culter J, Rösch J, Rahimtoola SH. Specificity, sensitivity, and accuracy of the nitroglycerine ventriculogram as a predictor of surgically reversible wall motion abnormalities [abstract]. Am J Cardiol 1980;45:399.
35. Dyke SH, Cohn PF, Gorlin R, Sonnenblick EH. Detection of residual myocardial function in coronary artery disease using post-extra systolic potentiation. Circulation 1974;50:694–699.
36. Cohn LH, Collins JJ, Cohn PF. Use of the augmented ejection fraction to select patients with left ventricular dysfunction for coronary revascularization. J Thorac Cardiovasc Surg 1976;72:835–840.
37. Nesto RW, Cohn LH, Collins JJ, Wynne J, Holman L, Cohn PF. Inotropic contractile reserve: a useful predictor of increased 5 year survival and improved postoperative left ventricular function in patients with coronary artery disease and reduced ejection fraction. Am J Cardiol 1982;50:39.
38. Rozanski A, Berman D, Gray R, et al. Preoperative prediction of reversible myocardial asynergy by postexercise radionuclide ventriculography. N Engl J Med 1982;307:212–216.
39. Schelbert HR. Metabolic imaging to assess myocardial viability. J Nucl Med 1994; 35(suppl):8S–14S.
40. Bax JJ, Wijns W, Cornel JH, Visser FC, Boersma E, Fioretti PM. Accuracy of currently available techniques for prediction of functional recovery after revascularization in patients with left ventricular dysfunction due to chronic coronary artery disease: comparison of pooled data. J Am Coll Cardiol 1997;30: 1451–1460.
41. Di Carli MF, Hachamovitch R, Berman D. The art and science of predicting postrevascularization improvement in left ventricular (LV) function in patients with severely depressed LV function. Circulation 2002;40:1744–1747.
42. Tillisch J, Brunker R, Marshal R, et al. Reversibility of cardiac wall-motion abnormalities predicted by positron tomography. N Engl J Med 1986;314:884.
43. Beanlands RSB, Ruddy TD, deKemp RA, et al. Positron emission tomography and recovery following revascularization (PARR-1): the importance of scar and the development of a prediction rule for the degree of recovery of left ventricular function. J Am Coll Cardiol 2002;40:1735–1743.
44. Wackers FJ. Myocardial perfusion imaging to assess myocardial viability. J Myocardial Ischemia 1994;6:41–44.

45. McGhie AI, Weyman A. Searching for hibernating myocardium: time to reevaluate investigative strategies? Circulation 1996;94:2685–2688.
46. Manyari DE, Knudtson M, Kloiber R, Roth D. Sequential thallium-201 myocardial perfusion studies after successful percutaneous translumenal coronary angiography: delayed resolution of exercise-induced scintigraphic abnormalities. Circulation 1988;77:86–95.
47. Kiat H, Berman DS, Maddahi J, et al. Late reversibility of tomographic myocardial thallium-201 defects: an accurate marker of myocardial viability. J Am Coll Cardiol 1988;12:1456–1463.
48. Yang LD, Berman DS, Kiat H, et al. The frequency of later reversibility in SPECT thallium-201 stress-redistribution studies. J Am Coll Cardiol 1989;15:334–340.
49. Klocke FJ, Baird MG, Lorell BH, et al. ACC/AHA/ASNC guidelines for the clinical use of cardiac radionuclide imaging—executive summary: a report of the American College of Cardiology/American Heart Association Task Force on Practice Guidelines (ACC/AHA/ASNC Committee to Revise the 1995 Guidelines for the Clinical Use of Cardiac Radionuclide Imaging). J Am Coll Cardiol. 2003; 42:1318–1333.
50. Kayden DS, Sigal S, Soufer R, Mattera J, Zaret BL, Wackers FJ. Thallium-201 for assessment of myocardial viability: quantitative comparison of 24-hour redistribution imaging with imaging after reinjection at rest. J Am Coll Cardiol 1991; 19:1121.
51. Dilsizian V, Rocco TP, Freedman NM, Leon MB, Bonow RO. Enhanced detection of ischemic but viable myocardium by the reinjection of thallium after stress-redistribution imaging. N Engl J Med 1990;323:141–146.
52. Zimmerman R, Mall G, Rauch B, et al. Residual ^{201}Tl activity in irreversible defects as a marker or myocardial viability. Circulation 1995;91:1016–1021.
53. Perrone-Filardi P, Pace L, Prastaro M, et al. Assessment of myocardial viability in patients with chronic coronary artery disease: rest-4-hour-24-hour 201Tl tomography versus dobutamine echocardiography. Circulation 1996;94: 2712–2719.
54. Bonow RO, Dilsizian V, Cuocolo A, Bacharach SL. Identification of viable myocardium in patients with chronic coronary artery disease and left ventricular dysfunction: comparison of thallium scintigraphy with reinjection and PET imaging with ^{18}F-fluorodeoxyglucose. Circulation 1991;83:26–37.
55. Kitsiou AN, Srinivasan G, Quyyumi AA, Summers RM, Bacharach SL, Dilsizian V. Stress-induced reversible and mild-to-moderate irreversible thallium defects: are they equally accurate for predicting recovery of regional left ventricular function after revascularization? Circulation 1998;98:501–508.
56. Dilsizian V, Perrone-Filardi P, Arrighi JA, et al. Concordance and discordance between stress–redistribution–reinjection and rest–redistribution thallium imaging for assessing viable myocardium: comparison with metabolic activity by positron emission tomography. Circulation 1993;88:941–952.
57. Medrano R, Lowry R, Young JB, et al. Assessment of myocardial viability with 99mTc sestamibi in patients undergoing cardiac transplantation: a scintigraphic/ pathological study. Circulation 1996;94:1010–1017.
58. Matsunari I, Fujino S, Taki J, et al. Quantitative rest technetium-99m tetrofosmin imaging in predicting functional recovery after revascularization: comparison with rest-redistribution thallium-201. J Am Coll Cardiol 1997;29:1226–1233.
59. Gunning MG, Anagnostopoulos C, Knight CJ, et al. Comparison of ^{201}Tl, ^{99m}Tc-tetrofosmin, and dobutamine magnetic resonance imaging for identifying hibernating myocardium. Circulation 1998;98:1869–1874.

60. Kauffman GJ, Boyne TS, Watson DD, Smith WH, Beller GA. Comparison of rest thallium-201 imaging and rest technetium-99m sestamibi imaging for assessment of myocardial viability in patients with coronary artery disease and severe left ventricular dysfunction. J Am Coll Cardiol 1996;27:1592–1597.
61. Udelson JE, Coleman PS, Metherall J, et al. Predicting recovery of severe regional ventricular dysfunction. Comparison of resting scintigraphy with ^{201}Tl and ^{99m}Tc-sestamibi. Circulation 1994;89:2552–2561.
62. Cheitlin MD, Armstrong WF, Aurigemma GP, et al. ACC/AHA/ASE 2003 Guideline Update for the Clinical Application of Echocardiography: summary article. A report of the American College of Cardiology/American Heart Association Task Force on Practice Guidelines (ACC/AHA/ASE Committee to Update the 1997 Guidelines for the Clinical Application of Echocardiography). J Am Soc Echocardiogr 2003;10:1091–1110.
63. Panza JA, Dilsizian V, Laurienzo JM, Curiel RV, Katsiyiannis PT. Relation between thallium uptake and contractile response to dobutamine: implications regarding myocardial viability in patients with chronic coronary artery disease and left ventricular dysfunction. Circulation 1995;91:990–998.
64. Perrone-Filardi P, Pace L, Prastaro M, et al. Assessment of myocardial viability in patients with chronic coronary artery disease: rest-4-hour-24-hour ^{201}Tl tomography vs dobutamine echocardiography. Circulation 1996;94:2712–2719.
65. Smart SC. The clinical utility of echocardiography in the assessment of myocardial viability. J Nucl Med 1994;35(suppl):49S–58S.
66. Chen C, Li L, Chen LL, et al. Incremental doses of dobutamine induce a biphasic response in dysfunctional left ventricular regions subtending coronary stenoses. Circulation 1995;92:756–766.
67. Afridi I, Kleiman NS, Raizner AE, Zoghbi WA. Dobutamine echocardiography in myocardial hibernation: optimal dose and accuracy in predicting recovery of ventricular function after coronary angioplasty. Circulation 1995;91:663–670.
68. Senior R, Lahiri A. Enhanced detection of myocardial ischemia by stress dobutamine echocardiography utilizing the "biphasic" response of wall thickening during low and high dose dobutamine infusion. J Am Coll Cardiol 1995;26:26–32.
69. Hansen TH, Segar DS. The use of dobutamine stress echocardiography for the determination of myocardial viability. Clin Cardiol 1996;19:607–612.
70. Wu E, Judd RM, Vargas JD, Klocke FJ, Bonow R, Kim RJ. Visualization of presence, location, and transmural extent of healed Q-wave and non-Q-wave myocardial infarction. Lancet 2001;357:21–28.
71. Kim RJ, Wu E, Rafael A, et al. The use of contrast-enhanced magnetic resonance imaging to identify reversible myocardial dysfunction. N Engl J Med 2000;343:1445–1453.
72. McGhie AI, Weyman A. Searching for hibernating myocardium. Time to reevaluate investigative strategies? Circulation 1996;94:2685–2688.
73. Luu M, Stevenson LW, Brunken RC, Drinkwater DM, Schelbert HR, Tillisch JH. Delayed recovery of revascularized myocardium after referral for cardiac transplantation. Am Heart J 1990;119:668.
74. Marwick TH, MacIntyre WJ, Lafont A, Nemec JJ, Salcedo EE. Metabolic responses of hibernating and infracted myocardium to revascularization: a follow-up study of regional perfusion, function, and metabolism. Circulation 1992;85:1347–1353.
75. Iskandrian AS, Heo J, Stanberry C. When is myocardial viability an important clinical issue? J Nucl Med 1994;35(suppl):4S–7S.
76. Samady H, Elefteriades JA, Abbott BG, Mattera JA, McPherson CA, Wackers FJ. Failure to improve left ventricular function after coronary revascularization for

ischemic cardiomyopathy is not associated with worse outcome. Circulation 1999; 100:1298–1304.

77. Ragosta M, Beller GA, Watson D, Kaul S, Gimple LW. Quantitative planar rest-redistribution Tl-201 imaging in detection of myocardial viability and prediction of improvement in left ventricular function after coronary bypass surgery in patients with severely depressed left ventricular function. Circulation 1993;87: 1630–1641.

78. Di Carli MF, Hachamovitch R, Berman DS. The art and science of predicting postrevascularization improvement in left ventricular (LV) function in patients with severely depressed LV function. J Am Coll Cardiol 2002;40:1744–1747.

79. Di Carli M, Asgarzadie F, Schelbert HR, et al. Quantitative relation between myocardial viability and improvement in heart failure symptoms after revascularization in patients with ischemic cardiomyopathy. Circulation 1995;92:3436–3444.

80. Di Carli MF, Davidson M, Little R, et al. Value of metabolic imaging with positron emission tomography for evaluating prognosis in patients with left ventricular dysfunction. Am J Cardiol 1994;73:527–533.

81. Bax JJ, Poldermans D, Elhendy A, et al. Improvement of left ventricular ejection fraction, heart failure symptoms and prognosis after revascularization in patients with chronic coronary artery disease and viable myocardium detected by dobutamine stress echocardiography. J Am Coll Cardiol 1999;34:163–169.

82. Marwick TH, Zuchowski C, Lauer MS, Secknus M, Williams MJ, Lytle BW. Functional status and quality of life in patients with heart failure undergoing coronary bypass surgery after assessment of myocardial viability. J Am Coll Cardiol 1999;33:750–758.

83. Louie HW, Laks H, Milgalter E, et al. Ischemic cardiomyopathy: criteria for coronary revascularization and cardiac transplantation. Circulation 1991;84(suppl): III-290–III-295.

84. Lee KS, Marwick TH, Sevastian AC, et al. Prognosis of patients with left ventricular dysfunction, with and without viable myocardium after myocardial infarction: relative efficacy of medical therapy and revascularization. Circulation 1994;90:2687–2694.

85. Eitman D, Al-Aouar Z, Kanter HL, et al. Clinical outcome of patients with advanced coronary artery disease after viability studies with positron emission tomography. J Am Coll Cardiol 1992;20:559–565.

86. Pasquet A, Robert A, D'Hondt AM, Dio R, Melin JA, Vanoverschelde JLJ. Prognostic value of myocardial ischemia and viability in patients with chronic left ventricular ischemic dysfunction. Circulation 1999;100:141–148.

87. Gioia G, Powers J, Heo J, Iskandrian AS, Russell J, Cassell D. Prognostic value of res-redistribution tomographic thallium-201 imaging in ischemic cardiomyopathy. Am J Cardiol 1995;75:759–762.

88. Chan RKM, Raman J, Lee KJ, et al. Prediction of outcome after revascularization in patients with poor left ventricular function. Ann Thorac Surg 1996;61: 1428–1434.

89. Cuocolo A, Petretta M, Nicolai E, et al. Successful coronary revascularization improves prognosis in patients with previous myocardial infarction and evidence of viable myocardium at thallium-201 imaging. Eur J Nucl Med 1998;25:60–68.

90. Pagley PR, Beller GA, Watson DD, Gimple LW, Ragosta M. Improved outcome after coronary bypass surgery in patients with ischemic cardiomyopathy and residual myocardial viability. Circulation 1997;96:793–800.

91. Siebelink HJ, Blanksma PK, Crijns HJG, et al. No difference in cardiac event-free survival between positron emission tomography-guided and single-photon

emission computed tomography-guided patient management. Am Coll Cardiol 2001;37:81–88.

92. Senior R, Lahiri A, Kaul S. Effect of revascularization on left ventricular remodeling in patients with heart failure from severe chronic ischemic left ventricular dysfunction. Am J Cardiol 2001;88:624–629.

93. Senior R, Kaul S, Lahiri A. Myocardial viability on echocardiography predicts long-term survival after revascularization in patients with ischemic congestive heart failure. J Am Coll Cardiol 1999;33:1848–1854.

94. Afridi I, Grayburn PA, Panza JA, Oh JK, Zoghbi WA, Marwick TH. Myocardial viability during dobutamine echocardiography predicts survival in patients with coronary artery disease and severe left ventricular systolic function. J Am Coll Cardiol 1998;32:921–926.

95. Chaudry FA, Tauke JT, Alessandrini RS, Vardi G, Parker MA, Bonow RO. Prognostic implications of myocardial contractile reserve in patients with coronary artery disease and left ventricular dysfunction. J Am Coll Cardiol 1999;34: 730–738.

96. Allman KC, Shaw LJ, Hachamovitch R, Udelson JE. Myocardial viability testing and impact of revascularization on prognosis in patients with coronary artery disease and left ventricular dysfunction: a meta-analysis. J Am Coll Cardiol 2002; 39:1151–1158.

97. Bonow R. Myocardial viability and prognosis in patients with ischemic left ventricular dysfunction. J Am Coll Cardiol 2002;39:1159–1162.

98. Eagle KA, Guyton RA, Davidoff R, et al. ACC/AHA Guidelines for Coronary Artery Bypass Graft Surgery: a report of the American College of Cardiology/ American Heart Association Task Force on Practice Guidelines (Committee to Revise the 1991 Guidelines for Coronary Artery Bypass Graft Surgery). American College of Cardiology/American Heart Association. J Am Coll Cardiol 1999;34:1262–1347.

99. Cooley DA, Frazier OH, Duncan JM, Reul GJ, Krajacer Z. Intracavitary repair of ventricular aneurysm and regional dyskinesia. Ann Surg 1992;215:417–423.

100. Dor V, Saab M, Coste P, Kornaszewska M, Montiglio F. Left ventricular aneurysm: a new surgical approach. Thorac Cardiovasc Surg 1989;37:11–19.

101. Kono T, Sabbah, HN, Stein PD, Brymer JF, Khaja F. Left ventricular shape as a determinant of functional mitral regurgitation in patients with severe heart failure secondary to either coronary artery disease or idiopathic dilated cardiomyopathy. Am J Cardiol 1991;68:355–359.

102. White HD, Norris RM, Brown MA, Brandt PW, Whitlock RM, Wild CJ. Left ventricular end-systolic volume as the major determinant of survival after recovery from myocardial infarction. Circulation 1987;76:44–51.

103. Athanasuleas CL, Stanley AW Jr, Buckberg GD, Dor V, DiDonato M, Blackstone EH, and the RESTORE group. Surgical anterior ventricular endocardial restoration (SAVER) in the dilated remodeled ventricle after anterior myocardial infarction. J Am Coll Cardiol 2001;37:1199–1209.

3

Aortic Valve Surgery With Severe Left Ventricular Dysfunction

Blasé A. Carabello, MD, FACC

INTRODUCTION

In most patients with severe aortic stenosis, management is relatively straightforward. Prognosis is excellent even in patients with severe valve obstruction as long as they are asymptomatic. However, once the classic symptoms of angina, syncope, dyspnea, or other symptoms of congestive heart failure (CHF) develop, prognosis dramatically worsens *(1,2)*. Because 75% of symptomatic patients will die within 3 years of the onset of the symptoms unless the aortic valve is replaced, the onset of symptoms is a compelling reason to perform aortic valve

From: *Contemporary Cardiology: Surgical Management of Congestive Heart Failure*
Edited by: J. C. Fang and G. S. Couper © Humana Press Inc., Totowa, NJ

replacement. In many asymptomatic patients, left ventricular (LV) hypertrophy normalizes wall stress, and LV systolic function is normal. However, the increase in wall thickness necessary to compensate the increased pressure term of the Laplace equation (stress equals the pressure times the radius divided by twice the thickness) results in reduced LV compliance and diastolic dysfunction *(3)*. Typically, diastolic dysfunction precedes systolic dysfunction; thus, when congestive symptoms do arise, systolic function is usually normal.

Because the general awareness of the importance of the symptoms has increased since the 1970s and because of the ease of echocardiographic surveillance, most patients with aortic stenosis develop symptoms and receive medical attention while systolic function is still normal. However, some patients still present for the first time with advanced CHF and reduced ejection fraction (EF). Because reduced ejection performance indicates poor prognosis for almost all other heart diseases, the patient with aortic stenosis presenting with CHF and systolic dysfunction often raises concerns about the risks of aortic valve replacement or even whether the patient is a surgical candidate.

CAUSES OF SYSTOLIC DYSFUNCTION

The major determinants of EF are preload, afterload, and contractility. In aortic stenosis, it is conceivable that the left ventricle might become so stiff that sarcomere stretch (preload) is reduced despite increased filling pressure. However, there is currently no evidence that reduced preload is a contributor to reduced systolic function in patients with aortic stenosis. Rather, afterload access alone or in combination with reduced contractility is the usual cause of reduced EF *(4,5)*. Huber and colleagues *(4)* suggested that, in approx 75% of patients with aortic stenosis and reduced EF, afterload mismatch plays some role, and in most patients it plays a dominant role in depressing ejection performance. It seems clear that, when afterload mismatch is the major cause for LV dysfunction, prognosis following surgery is excellent *(5,6)*. When the aortic valve is replaced, aortic orifice area increases, afterload falls, and ejection performance increases. Following surgery, symptoms abate, and lifestyle and life span improve dramatically.

Much more problematic is that group of patients with aortic stenosis and reduced ejection performance for whom contractile dysfunction, often in league with afterload mismatch, is the major cause of reduced EF. Because contractility is often irreversibly depressed in this group of patients, prognosis is much less favorable than in the group of patients for whom afterload mismatch is the prime contributor to LV dysfunction *(5)*.

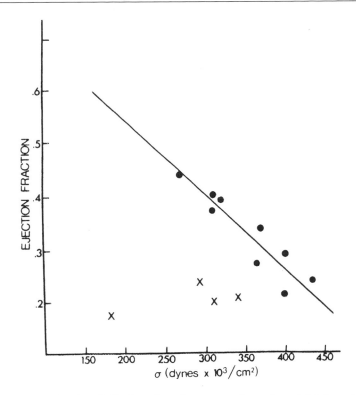

Fig. 1. Ejection fraction (EF) plotted against mean circumferential left ventricular wall stress σ for group 1 (good outcome) (●) and group 2 (bad outcome) (X). Group 2 patients fell below and to the left of group 1 patients, indicating lower EF despite less σ. This is consistent with the concept that left ventricular performance (EF) was depressed in group 1 patients because of afterload mismatch and in group 2 patients because of myocardial failure.

As shown in Fig. 1, in patients with reduced EF for whom reduced performance was primarily the result of increased afterload (increased wall stress), prognosis was excellent; in patients for whom contractile dysfunction played the predominant role, prognosis was poor *(5)*. In general, the computation of wall stress is cumbersome, which has limited its use in clinical practice and even in clinical investigations. However, as shown in Fig. 2, the transaortic pressure gradient performs as a reasonable substitute for afterload. Thus, when gradient is reduced in tandem with reduced EF, prognosis is also reduced because contractility is most severely depressed in those patients with a low gradient *(5)*.

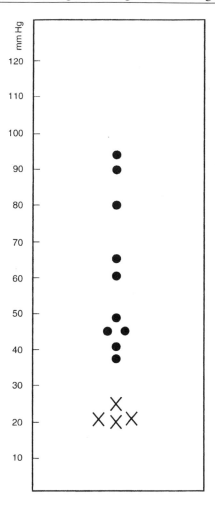

Fig. 2. Mean systolic aortic pressure gradients for patients in group 1 (●) and group 2 (X). Group 2 patients had lower systolic gradients in every case.

Virtually every study that has examined outcome in patients with aortic stenosis has demonstrated that low gradient combined with low EF has a poor prognosis *(5–8)*. A study by the Mayo Clinic demonstrated a 21% operative risk in such patients, and only 50% survived for 4 years *(8)*. Nonetheless, that study and others also demonstrated that many patients in this category do benefit from surgery. A study by the Cleveland Clinic retrospectively matched patients with low EF and low gradient who underwent aortic valve replacement to a similar group who underwent medical therapy *(9)*. Almost all patients on medical therapy died; most patients undergoing aortic valve replacement survived for at least 3 years. This was the first study to demonstrate a survival benefit of aortic valve replacement in this group of patients with an unfavorable prognosis.

WHICH PATIENTS WITH LOW GRADIENT, LOW EJECTION FRACTION WILL BENEFIT FROM AORTIC VALVE REPLACEMENT?

Currently, it is unknown whether all patients with low EF and low gradient benefit from aortic valve replacement. However, it has become common practice to try to separate patients with severe valve stenosis with low gradient and low EF from those patients with less-severe stenosis by manipulating their hemodynamics. Logically, if severe stenosis has caused ventricular dysfunction, aortic valve replacement should be beneficial. On the other hand, if a ventricle weakened from some other cause, such as coronary disease, is unable to open a mildly stenotic valve (aortic pseudostenosis), its replacement with a prosthesis that is also inherently at least mildly stenotic should be of little advantage. Unfortunately, it has become clear that aortic valve area at rest alone cannot make this distinction. In the group with severe stenosis that has presumably led to muscle damage and LV dysfunction and in the group with aortic valve pseudostenosis, calculated aortic valve area may be reduced equally. In the Cleveland Clinic study *(9)*, no systematic attempt was made to separate these two kinds of patients. Thus, it is possible (although improbable) that patients with mild stenosis do benefit from aortic valve replacement. However, unless there is proof that patients with mild stenosis do benefit from valve replacement, it seems wise to separate those patients with true aortic stenosis and offer an aortic valve replacement to them.

As noted, it is clear that calculation of aortic valve area at rest is insufficient to divorce true aortic stenosis from aortic pseudostenosis. Thus, it has become common practice to increase forward flow, reexamine hemodynamics, and recalculate aortic valve area. Both dobutamine and nitroprusside have been used to manipulate hemodynamics pharmacologically to try to make the distinction between severe aortic stenosis and aortic pseudostenosis. When dobutamine is used, the positive inotropic response increases the force of contraction and forward output. In true stenosis, the increase in gradient is proportionate to the increase in cardiac output, and the valve area remains constant or increases only slightly *(10)*. In aortic valve pseudostenosis, increased forward flow presumably increases the aortic valve orifice such that flow increases out of proportion to gradient, and the newly calculated valve area increases substantially (>0.3 cm or to a valve area >1.0 cm^2).

Alternatively, nitroprusside can be infused to make the distinction. As shown in Fig. 3, the concept in the use of a vasodilator is that the aortic valve and the total peripheral resistance form two resistances to flow in series *(11–13)*. If the stenotic valve is the primary and most severe resistance to outflow, infusion of a vasodilator will decrease total peripheral resistance, but flow cannot increase through the stenotic valve. As such, there will be a fall in downstream pressure and an increase in gradient with little change in output. In this case, aortic valve area does not increase or may even decrease. On the other hand, if it is the total peripheral resistance that is the major resistor (the valve is not severely stenotic, therefore it is aortic pseudostenosis), then vasodilatation decreases total peripheral resistance, resulting in increased flow through the mildly stenotic valve; the gradient changes little, and the newly calculated valve area increases substantially.

An inherent risk in the use of sodium nitroprusside to make this determination is the potential for fall in downstream pressure in patients with true stenosis. Thus, the drug must be used with caution, increasing the dose in tiny increments while monitoring hemodynamics carefully. It also should be pointed out that if dobutamine is used, there is the risk of precipitating angina in patients with concomitant coronary disease. Thus, it is helpful to know the coronary anatomy before hemodynamic manipulation.

AORTIC VALVE RESISTANCE

In cases of either true or pseudoaortic stenosis, the aortic valve area is flow dependent, increasing as flow increases, albeit the increase is small in true stenosis. Increased aortic valve area with increased flow may indicate a true increase in aperture as greater flow forces greater leaflet separation, or it may be the calculation rather than the valve area itself that is flow dependent *(14)*. One potential reason for this is that the discharge coefficients for the Gorlin formula for calculating aortic valve area were never determined for that valve *(15)*.

These problems have led investigators to use aortic valve resistance as another marker for stenosis severity *(11,12)*. Resistance is simply gradient divided by flow and utilizes no discharge coefficients. Its usefulness has been studied many times, with different investigators coming to disparate conclusions about the usefulness of valve resistance as a gage of aortic stenosis severity. In some studies, resistance was substantially less flow dependent than was valve area when transvalvular

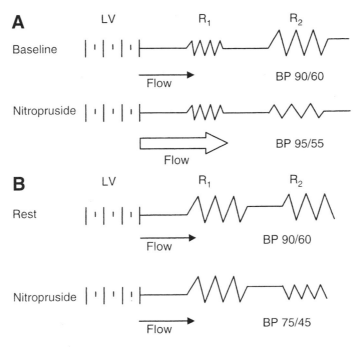

Fig. 3. (A) In this figure depicting aortic pseudostenosis, R_2 (total peripheral resistance) exceeds the resistance offered by a mildly stenotic aortic valve (R_1). When nitroprusside is infused, both resistances become low, and cardiac output increases substantially. **(B)** In the lower panel depicting true aortic stenosis, at rest both R_1 and R_2 are large. However, following nitroprusside infusion, R_2 decreases, but R_1 dose not, resulting in no increase in outflow from the left ventricle, but a fall in blood pressure (which is the product of cardiac output and total peripheral resistance).

flow was altered *(16)*. In other studies, flow dependence was quite variable *(17)*. It could be that this variability itself may be a useful tool. In separating valve types, in rigid valves with little flexibility (truly severely stenotic valves) resistance should change more with flow than valve area (gradient increases more than flow), because area is based on the square root of gradient. On the other hand, in flexible pseudostenotic valves, resistance varies less than aortic valve area *(11)*. Thus, resistance, valve area, and their respective changes to increased flow may all help separate truly stenotic from less-stenotic valves.

OVERALL DIAGNOSTIC STRATEGY

It is clear the transvalvular gradient can be measured or calculated accurately echocardiographically. If the echocardiographic approach is pursued, patients with low EF and low gradient should be studied at rest and then following infusion of dobutamine. Valve area should be recalculated following infusion. If area increases by more than 0.3 cm², pseudostenosis is likely present. If infusion of dobutamine causes a substantial increase in gradient, valve area is likely to remain constant or increases only slightly, indicating the presence of truly severe aortic stenosis. If the patient's left ventricle fails to respond to dobutamine with little change in gradient or output, severe muscle dysfunction without inotropic reserve is present, and such patients have a poor prognosis irrespective of stenosis severity *(18)*.

Although the usefulness of echocardiography is unchallenged, I personally prefer cardiac catheterization in the diagnosis of this group of patients. Because dobutamine may cause myocardial ischemia and therefore decrease rather than increase cardiac function, it is (in my opinion) wise to know the coronary status prior to infusion. This is most easily judged following coronary arteriography. In addition, a right heart catheterization gives important data regarding hemodynamics and their improvement or lack of improvement following pharmacological intervention. Although not the norm, nitroprusside infusion is useful as discussed in the section on which patients benefit from aortic valve replacement. If patients respond to nitroprusside with an increase in cardiac output, a small or no increase in gradient, and an improvement in hemodynamics, severe aortic valve disease is virtually excluded. Furthermore, these results give reassurance that the patient can be treated successfully as an outpatient with vasodilator drugs, drugs usually contraindicated in patients with severe aortic stenosis.

The combined use of aortic valve resistance and aortic valve area during pharmacological manipulation should be explored further. In the patient for whom valve resistance increases dramatically with an increase in flow and the valve area remains relatively constant, it is highly likely that severe obstruction exists, and these patients should be the best candidates for aortic valve replacements. On the other hand, when resistance remains relatively unchanged but valve area increases dramatically, pseudoaortic stenosis is probably present. It should be emphasized that avoiding operation on such patients is based on logic, not fact. It is possible but unlikely that even patients with mild stenosis might improve following aortic valve replacement by relief of mild obstruction to outflow. However, it seems unlikely that the large randomized trial necessary to demonstrate the utility or futility of aortic valve replacement in pseudostenosis will occur.

SURGICAL CONSIDERATIONS

When the decision is made to perform aortic valve replacement, it seems reasonable that all other comorbidities be corrected first. Otherwise, the risk may be prohibitive. Furthermore, of major concern is the type of substitute valve that is placed. Debated in many studies is whether valve size ultimately makes a difference in outcome for patients with aortic stenosis *(8,19,20)*. Some studies have indicated higher mortality and poorer regression of LV hypertrophy when smaller valve sizes with larger gradients are inserted. The hemodynamic logic behind use of valves with the best hemodynamics is obvious, yet some studies have demonstrated that valve size has not affected the outcome.

Irrespective of this debate, it seems most unwise to leave even partial hemodynamic obstruction in patients with such weakened ventricles. If the patient begins with only a 25 mmHg transvalvular gradient, a residual gradient of 10 mmHg represents 40% of the original gradient. Alternatively, one could argue that the additional ischemic time required to implant stentless valves or homografts with better hemodynamics outweighs the hemodynamic advantages of these valves. Clearly, the decision rests with the preferences of the operating surgeon, but logic dictates that the valve with the best hemodynamic profile be implanted in this group of patients.

SUMMARY

For most patients with aortic stenosis, the onset of the symptoms of angina, syncope, or CHF indicates the need for aortic valve replacement. Following surgery in patients who have recently become symptomatic, the outcome is excellent. Although reduced systolic function is usually an indicator of worse prognosis in most types of heart disease, it is not so for patients with aortic stenosis. For those patients whose ejection performance is reduced because of the high afterload presented by the obstructing valve and for whom the left ventricle can still generate a high systolic gradient, prognosis is excellent. Following aortic valve replacement, afterload decreases, ejection performance improves, and symptoms abate.

The most problematic group of patients with aortic stenosis is that group with a low EF, low gradient, and severe LV contractile dysfunction. Although risk is clearly increased, many such patients do benefit, both symptomatically and with improved mortality, from aortic valve replacement. It seems wise (until further data are available) to separate patients with severe valvular obstruction from those with only mild obstruction prior to consideration for surgery.

Using the logic that it is those patients with the severest obstruction who should gain the most benefit from valve replacement, hemodynamic manipulation should be provided either in the echocardiographic or catheterization laboratories. Patients who have a large increase in valve area when cardiac output is increased probably have only mild stenosis and probably will not benefit from aortic valve replacement. Those patients who increase output and increase gradient have severe obstruction and should be the group most likely to benefit. Those patients who fail to augment their inotropic state apparently have the poorest LV function and reserve and poor prognosis.

REFERENCES

1. Ross J Jr, Braunwald E. Aortic stenosis. Circulation 1968;38(suppl V):V-61–V-67.
2. Kelly TA, Rothbart RM, Cooper CM, Kaiser DL, Smucker ML, Gibson RS. Comparison of outcome of asymptomatic to symptomatic patients older than 20 years of age with valvular aortic stenosis. Am J Cardiol 1988;61:123–130.
3. Hess OM, Ritter M, Schneider J, Grimm J, Turina M, Krayenbuehl HP. Diastolic stiffness and myocardial structure in aortic valve disease before and after valve replacement. Circulation 1984;69:855–865.
4. Huber D, Grimm J, Koch R, Krayenbuehl HP. Determinants of ejection performance in aortic stenosis. Circulation 1981;64:126–134.
5. Carabello BA, Green LH, Grossman W, Cohn LH, Koster JK, Collins JJ Jr. Hemodynamic determinants of prognosis of aortic valve replacement in critical aortic stenosis and advanced congestive heart failure. Circulation 1980;62:42–48.
6. Lund O. Preoperative risk evaluation and stratification of long-term survival after valve replacement for aortic stenosis. Reasons for earlier operative intervention. Circulation 1990;82:124–139.
7. Brogan WC, Grayburn PA, Lange RA, Hillis LD. Prognosis after valve replacement in patients with severe aortic stenosis and a low transvalvular pressure gradient. J Am Coll Cardiol 1993;21:1657–1660.
8. Connolly HM, Oh JK, Schaff HV, et al. Severe aortic stenosis with low transvalvular gradient and severe left ventricular dysfunction: Result of aortic valve replacement in 52 patients. Circulation 2000;101:1940–1946.
9. Pereira JJ, Lauer MS, Bashir M, et al. Survival after aortic valve replacement for severe aortic stenosis with low transvalvular gradients and severe left ventricular dysfunction. J Am Coll Cardiol in press.
10. deFilippi CR, Willett DL, Brickner ME, et al. Usefulness of dobutamine echocardiography in distinguishing severe from nonsevere valvular aortic stenosis in patients with depressed left ventricular function and low transvalvular gradients. Am J Cardiol 1995;75:191–194.
11. Cannon JD, Zile MR, Crawford FA, Carabello BA. Aortic valve resistance as an adjunct to the Gorlin formula in assessing the severity of aortic stenosis in symptomatic patients. J Am Coll Cardiol 1992;20:1517–1523.
12. Carabello BA. Selection of patients for operation: the asymptomatic patient and the patient with poor LV function. Adv Cardiol.
13. Ford LE, Feldman T, Chiu YC, Carroll JD. Hemodynamic resistance as a measure of functional impairment in aortic valvular stenosis. Circ Res 1990;66:1–7.

14. Tardif J, Rodrigues, AG, Hardy J, et al. Simultaneous determination of aortic valve area by the Gorlin formula and by transesophageal echocardiography under different transvalvular flow conditions. Evidence that anatomic aortic valve area does not change with variations in flow in aortic stenosis. J Am Coll Cardiol 1997;29:1296–1302.

15. Gorlin R, Gorlin SG. Hydraulic formula for calculation of the area of the stenotic mitral valve, other cardiac valves, and central circulatory shunts: I. Am Heart J 1951;41:1–29.

16. Bermejo J, Garcia-Fernandez MA, Torrecilla EG, et al. Effects of dobutamine on Doppler echocardiographic indexes of aortic stenosis. J Am Coll Cardiol 1996;28: 1206–1213.

17. Shively BK, Charlton GA, Crawford MH, Chaney RK. Flow dependence of valve area in aortic stenosis: relation to valve morphology. J Am Coll Cardiol 1998; 311998:654–660.

18. Monin JL, Monchi M, Gest V, Duval-Moulin AM, Dubois-Rande JL, Gueret P. Aortic stenosis with severe left ventricular dysfunction and low transvalvular pressure gradients. J Am Coll Cardiol 2001;37:2101–2107.

19. Milano AD, De CM, Mecozzi G, et al. Clinical outcome in patients with 19-mm and 21-mm St. Jude aortic prostheses: comparison at long-term follow-up. Ann Thorac Surg 2002;73:37–43.

20. Arom KV, Goldenberg IF, Emery RW. Long-term clinical outcome with small size standard St. Jude medical valves implanted in the aortic position. J Heart Valve Dis 1994;3:531–536.

4   Mitral Valve Surgery With Severe Left Ventricular Dysfunction

Vinay Badhwar, MD
and Steven F. Bolling, MD

CONTENTS

INTRODUCTION

The management of patients with congestive heart failure (CHF) has become an international health care problem. In the ever-aging population, advances in basic cardiac care that have extended the average life expectancy have also left more people living with chronic cardiac disease than ever before. In the United States alone, nearly 4.9 million suffer from heart failure, yet of the 500,000 new patients diagnosed annually, fewer than 3000 are offered transplantation because of limitations of age, comorbid conditions, and donor availability.

From: *Contemporary Cardiology: Surgical Management of Congestive Heart Failure*
Edited by: J. C. Fang and G. S. Couper © Humana Press Inc., Totowa, NJ

Therapeutic limitations have left a significant number of these patients and their physicians searching for alternate options. Despite improvements in the medical management of CHF, more than 50% of patients continue to die within 3 years of presentation *(1,2)*. Furthermore, when patients with heart failure develop mitral regurgitation (MR), their 1-year survival has been reported as low as 30%.

This has prompted a renewed interest in the surgical management of MR in cardiomyopathy. Interventions that restore mitral competency in these patients can now be performed with low mortality and provide significant improvements in symptomatology and long-term survival. The following briefly reviews the pathological alterations of the mitral valve in the failing ventricle, outlines essentials of preoperative preparation, and discusses the principles of effective mitral replacement and repair surgery with severe left ventricular (LV) dysfunction.

MITRAL VALVE ALTERATIONS IN HEART FAILURE

Fundamental to the management of MR in heart failure is a firm understanding of the functional anatomy of the mitral valve. The mitral valve apparatus is the physiological union of the annulus, leaflets, chordae tendinae, papillary muscles, and the entire left ventricle. Accordingly, the integrity of this union plays a vital role in the maintenance of normal mitral and ventricular geometry.

MR can be classified into anatomic MR or geometric MR (Table 1). Etiologies of anatomic MR are limited to primary valvular abnormalities. These include infectious, rheumatic, and degenerative changes that alter the structural integrity of the leaflets or apparatus and manifest as perforation, prolapse, stenosis, or a combination. These valvular-based alterations result in valvular-based MR.

Geometric MR, however, results from a structural distortion of the left ventricle, leading to leaflet distraction and a disruption of the zone of coaptation. Whether ischemic or nonischemic, the geometric distortion of the annular–ventricular complex alters the physiological coordination of the mitral apparatus. These ventricular-based alterations result in ventricular-based MR.

Geometric MR is a significant and common complication of cardiomyopathy. It may affect all patients with heart failure as a preterminal or terminal event. Its presence is associated with escalations in CHF symptoms, progressive ventricular dilatation, and significant reductions in long-term survival *(3)*. As the ventricle fails, the geometric dilatation of the left ventricle gives rise to progressive dilatation of the mitral

Table 1
Classification of Mitral Regurgitation

Anatomic MR	
Cause	Primary defect of leaflet or annulus
Etiology	Rheumatic
	Degenerative
	Infectious
Geometric MR	
Cause	Distortion of the annular–ventricular apparatus
Etiology	Ischemia (acute, chronic)
	Dilated cardiomyopathy

annulus, and regurgitation ensues as a consequence of incomplete leaflet coaptation. In ischemic cardiomyopathy, the functional MR from annular dilatation is compounded by ischemic changes to the subvalvular structures of the left ventricle. The phrase *papillary muscle dysfunction* does not simply refer to an isolated disorder of the papillary muscle, but to a disturbance in the coordination between the lateral ventricular walls and the mitral valve apparatus. Thus, the combination of annular dilatation and subvalvular ischemic changes furthers the distortion of ventricular geometry and the perturbation of mitral valve function (Fig. 1).

Regardless of etiology, the progression to heart failure is accompanied by a loss of the normal ellipsoid architecture of the ventricle. Over time, the geometric alterations of the failing left ventricle are guided by the law of Laplace, and thus all patients, ischemic and nonischemic alike, remodel in a similar manner. The left ventricle attains a more spherical configuration, the interpapillary distance widens, and the anterior and posterior papillary muscles become distracted in opposing directions (Fig. 2). The resulting chordal tension leads to apical displacement of the zone of coaptation, increases in leaflet tethering forces, and incomplete mitral closure during systole *(4,5)*. These structural ventricular changes may also lead to limited diastolic leaflet excursion because of reduced anterior motion relative to the posteriorly displaced papillary muscles. This occurs independent to inflow volume and without varying mitral orifice area *(6)*.

The preoperative adaptations to severe MR in cardiomyopathy include increases in ventricular preload, wall tension, and stroke volume. With nearly half of the stroke volume ejected into the left atrium during presystole, the contractile efficiency of the ventricle is

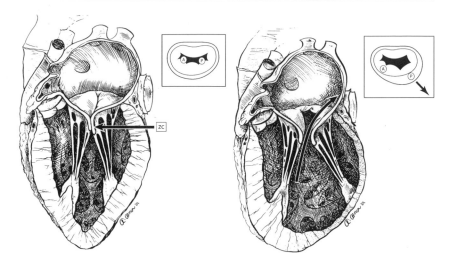

Fig. 1. Note the structural changes that occur from the normal to the ischemic left ventricle. With ischemic damage and thinning of the ventricular wall, there is lateral tethering and displacement of the papillary muscle, resulting in an eccentric jet of mitral regurgitation. This illustrates the concept that ischemic mitral regurgitation results from "lateral wall dysfunction," which if left untreated, may progress to global left ventricular dysfunction and heart failure.

limited even further. The reduction in effective cardiac output combined with increases in left ventricle wall stress serves to restrict coronary flow reserve further. Thus, regardless of the preoperative ejection fraction (EF), surgical elimination of the regurgitant flow results in augmented effective cardiac output, reduced ventricular volume and wall stress, and improved coronary flow reserve.

The firm understanding of the precise mechanism of MR allows effective preoperative and operative management.

PREOPERATIVE PREPARATION

Prior to surgical intervention, myopathic patients with MR require careful evaluation and preoperative management. The process of preoperative investigation should coincide with optimizing the patient's medical management. This should entail an aggressive regimen of diuretic and vasodilator therapy to minimize ventricular afterload and normalize circulating volume. For patients with severe heart failure, a brief period of inotropic therapy for ventricular resuscitation may be

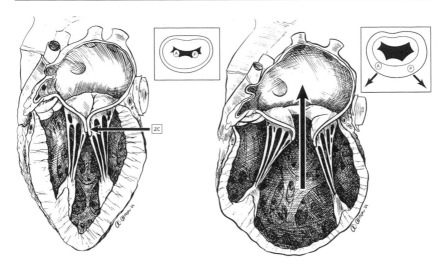

Fig. 2. Note the geometric changes that occur from the normal to the failing left ventricle. With the ventricular and annular dilation of heart failure, the mitral leaflets cannot adequately cover the enlarged mitral orifice. Geometric mitral regurgitation results from a combination of annular dilatation, papillary muscle displacement, increased leaflet tethering forces, and weakened leaflet-closing forces.

necessary for preoperative optimization. Inability to be weaned from this support is often indicative of severe myocardial injury and poor overall prognosis with any surgical therapy other than mechanical ventricular assistance or transplantation. Moreover, markedly elevated pulmonary artery pressures, right ventricular failure, or debilitating ascites should be considered relative contraindications for mitral surgery to avoid unremitting postcardiotomy right ventricle failure.

Physical examination of MR in cardiomyopathy typically reveals a hyperdynamic cardiac impulse and a characteristic blowing holosystolic murmur that may radiate from the apex to the axilla, back, or neck. However, with severely depressed ventricular function, these clinical findings may be inconspicuous. Radiographically, patients usually have an enlarged cardiac silhouette indicative of LV or atrial enlargement. Typical electrocardiogram findings include left atrial enlargement and ventricular hypertrophy.

If ischemia is suspected, coronary angiography should be performed prior to mitral surgery to identify the extent of native coronary disease or to assess the patency of grafts in those patients who have had prior revascularization. Should occlusions be detected, a study to assess myocardial viability in the distribution of the occluded vessel is advocated to determine if a preoperative percutaneous or a concomitant surgical revascularization procedure is warranted. In this situation, perhaps the most important correlate of successful surgical recovery is the quantification of myocardial viability. Prior to subjecting hearts with limited ventricular function to the temporary stunning of cardiopulmonary bypass, a determination of myocardial contractile reserve is essential. Not only is this useful to ensure the patient can be safely separated from bypass, but also this information is predictive of recovery of ventricular function and long-term survival following operation (7).

Although thallium 201 perfusion scans may distinguish myocytes with membrane integrity from scar, dynamic contrast magnetic resonance imaging (MRI), positron emission tomographic (PET) scanning, and dobutamine stress echocardiography (DSE) have emerged as reliable methods to identify preoperative myocardial viability and predict postoperative function. With the use of systemically administered ^{18}F-deoxyglucose (FDG) to identify aerobic cellular activity, PET scanning detects mismatches between myocardial blood flow and myocyte function to identify hypoperfused FDG-positive areas of the myocardium as viable or hibernating. Despite the high specificity of PET scanning, its cost and relative lack of availability have limited its widespread use. DSE involves the administration of incremental doses of dobutamine and observing for changes in segmental wall thickness and recruitment of segmental ventricular function. A biphasic response to the introduction and withdrawal of inotropy can be highly predictive of contractile reserve and an indicator of the patient's functional recovery following cardiopulmonary bypass. Although this is less expensive and more widely available than a PET scan or dynamic MRI, it requires the expertise of a trained cardiologist and may be observer dependent. Therefore, the optimal test for myocardial viability remains dependent on the facilities available at a particular institution (7–9).

A transthoracic echocardiogram is often the most helpful preliminary investigation to assess ventricular function and estimate the severity of MR. Left ventricular performance is best inferred from the diameter of the left ventricle at end systole. Measurements of end-systolic dimension are less dependent on preload than EF and thus provide a more accurate assessment of contractile function.

Once MR is documented, it is essential to define clearly the mitral pathoanatomy by transesophageal echocardiography. A detailed understanding of leaflet and chordal excursion, including the character of the regurgitant jet, is helpful to plan the correct operative approach effectively. In the majority of these patients, geometric left ventricle distortion results in a symmetric central jet from mitral annular dilation. Restoring geometry with reduction annuloplasty can readily repair this defect. In cases of anatomic distortion of the valve anatomy, the regurgitant jet may be eccentrically located. These patients often require a partial resection and reconstruction to correct leaflet prolapse or chordal rupture.

Although routine echo color Doppler may provide a semiquantitative analysis of MR, this method is often sensitive to load conditions, driving pressure, jet eccentricity, and left atrial size and thus may lead to incorrect estimations of the true degree of MR. Proximal flow convergence analysis, which calculates the regurgitant volume by measuring the flow proximal to the mitral valve orifice, may be a preferable method to quantify the extent of regurgitation accurately in patients with heart failure *(10–13)*.

The optimal choice of operative technique is dependent on the type of MR, the quality of available leaflet tissue, and the anatomy of the subvalvular structures. With effective management and workup, the operative strategy should be formulated preoperatively, with final confirmation made only after intraoperative inspection of the mitral apparatus.

Regardless of the etiology of MR, the resultant volume overload of the already failing left ventricle begets more MR and further ventricular dilatation, commencing a downward spiral of ventricular function. This may explain why surgical geometric restoration that preserves the annular–subvalvular continuity serves not only to reestablish valvular competency, but also to improve ventricular function.

MITRAL VALVE REPLACEMENT IN HEART FAILURE

Historically, the surgical approach to MR was prosthetic mitral valve replacement (MVR), yet little was understood of the interdependence of ventricular function and annulus–papillary muscle continuity. As a result, patients with low EFs who underwent a classical MVR with removal of the subvalvular apparatus had prohibitively high mortality rates *(14–16)*.

In an attempt to explain these outcomes, the concept of a beneficial "pop off" effect of MR was conceived. This idea erroneously proposed that mitral incompetence provided a low-pressure relief during systolic ejection from the failing ventricle, and that removal of this effect through MVR was responsible for the deterioration in ventricular function. Consequently, MVR in patients with LV dysfunction went into disfavor.

Once it began to be understood that the mitral apparatus was anatomically and functionally contiguous with the ventricle, techniques of mitral surgery were developed to preserve subvalvular integrity. Mounting laboratory and clinical evidence supporting these concepts led surgeons to embrace valve-sparing techniques (17–19). The significant improvements in short- and long-term survival that accompanied these adaptations ushered in the modern era of mitral surgery.

There has been much interest in comparisons between MVR with and without chordal preservation (CP) to elucidate the role subvalvular structures play in mitral and ventricular function. It has been learned that excision or exclusion of the subvalvular structures at the time of MVR results in a series of mechanical and geometric perturbations. This involves changes in myocardial wall thickness at the transsection sites that are accompanied by inhomogeneous local shortening, loss of normal systolic torsional deformation, and increased regional wall stress (20,21). Following chordal transsection, the depression of ventricular function at the defunct papillary muscle base also results in slowed relaxation that may contribute to diastolic dysfunction (22).

Conversely, CP at the time of MVR renders significant hemodynamic benefits, especially in the setting of depressed LV function. The improved ventricular geometry with CP results in a reduction of ventricular wall stress, enhancements in regional wall motion, and diminutions of end-systolic and end-diastolic volumes compared to MVR without CP (23–25). Patients with intact subvalvular continuity have increased EFs and superior LV performance, and perhaps most important, patients with CP have improved long-term survival over those without CP (19,26). These findings have paved the way for effective mitral surgery in patients with severe LV dysfunction.

The techniques used to maintain subvalvular continuity remain dependent, however, on the etiology of MR and the valvular anatomy. Destruction or scarring of the subvalvular apparatus by endocarditis or severe rheumatic disease may make repair impossible and the preservation of native structures difficult. Although these are less common in heart failure than with other etiologies, the preservation of subvalvular continuity is equally important to maintain ventricular geometry and function (27). Thus, techniques have evolved to adapt to the pathology encountered intraoperatively.

The majority of techniques involve keeping the posterior leaflet and chordae intact and resuspending the anterior chordae to the debrided annulus. These preserved chordae can be transfixed to the anterior annulus (28) or to both trigones (29) or transposed to the posterior annulus (30). When extensive calcification requires debridement and removal of the posterior leaflet, the anterior leaflet may be transposed to reinforce the posterior annulus prior to prosthesis implantation *(31)*. Alternatively, reconstruction of the subvalvular apparatus at the time of MVR can be readily performed with Gore-Tex or polytetrafluoroethylene (PTFE). These sutures permit resuspension of the papillary muscles in anatomic continuity with the debrided annulus. This material becomes readily incorporated with endothelial coverage and has excellent long-term durability *(32–34)*. Replacement sutures equal to or slightly longer than the excised chordae effectively lower wall stress and preserve global LV function and geometry *(35)*.

Concerns have been raised with total CP MVR regarding obstruction of the left ventricular outflow tract (LVOT) as well as prosthesis impingement because of retained subvalvular structures. These significant complications have directed some to advocate partial CP, usually of only the posterior leaflet *(36,37)*. However, subsequent laboratory and clinical evidence has revealed that much of the geometric and functional benefit of subvalvular integrity is lost with only partial CP. Total preservation results in improved ejection performance, less systolic wall stress, less left ventricle strain, and lower mortality when compared to MVR with partial CP *(38–40)*.

It has also been noted that all prostheses implanted with intact subvalvular structures have an element of flow restriction. When CP is utilized, stented bioprostheses have lower restrictive properties than mechanical prostheses. Frustration with impingement and obstruction have led some surgeons to implant mechanical bileaflet valves in the antianatomic position with PTFE chordal reconstruction, and some even to abandon regressively CP altogether *(41)*.

Much of these mechanical concerns pertain to MVR in patients with normal ventricular volumes. Those with severe LV dysfunction who require prosthetic valve replacement may avoid the issues of LV outflow obstruction because of the widening of the aorto–mitral angle associated with ventricular dilatation. Furthermore, if the mitral valve must be replaced in the setting of severe LV dysfunction, attempts at native or PTFE CP should be utilized because of its clear geometric advantage and long-term benefit in this group. The limited life span of patients with severe LV dysfunction, combined with the improved durability of most third-generation porcine and pericardial valves, make the bioprosthesis the valve of choice when necessary for managing MR in end-stage heart failure.

Despite the noted benefits of MVR with CP, the possibility of prosthesis-related complications, the increased morbidity of anticoagulation therapy, and the 7–15% mortality associated with MVR have made mitral repair the treatment of choice for MR in cardiomyopathy whenever possible.

GEOMETRIC MITRAL RECONSTRUCTION IN HEART FAILURE

The resurgence of interest in mitral repair surgery over the past decade has provided long-term outcome data supporting its superiority to MVR for the treatment of MR (42–45).

Repaired valves have clear benefits over prostheses in terms of endocarditis risk, need for anticoagulation, stroke incidence, and operative mortality. With the valve-related advantages aside, mitral repair has demonstrated improvements over MVR in terms of cardiac function as well as long-term survival (26). Decreased left ventricle volumes, improved left ventricle performance, and stable or enhanced EFs have all been reported following repair. Patients with repairs also have better systolic and diastolic function compared to those with MVR with subvalvular preservation (44). The superior conservation of ventricular geometry may explain why immediate intraoperative left ventricle function is preserved after repair, but is depressed after MVR (42). Beyond these recognized benefits over MVR, the resulting lower length of stay following repair has also made it a cost-effective treatment for MR (46,47).

One explanation for the inferiority of MVR is the rigid fixation of the mitral annulus. The normal annulus is a dynamic structure that undergoes dorsiflexion and contraction. Thus, the insertion of a rigid prosthesis impairs its normal three-dimensional function. Furthermore, as the left ventricle base consists of the mitral annulus and the LVOT orifice, when the ventricle contracts against an immobile prosthesis, the valve occupies more of the LV in systole, and a relative narrowing of the LVOT results. This antiphysiological fixation of the mitral annulus following MVR may explain why left ventricle function is better served with mitral reconstruction (48–50).

In patients with cardiomyopathy, the etiology of MR is most often caused by mitral annular dilatation and geometric distortion of the mitral apparatus. Accordingly, the most significant determinant of leaflet coaptation and MR is the diameter of the annulus (51,52). The LV dimension is less important because the lengths of the chordae and papillary muscles are similar in myopathic hearts regardless whether MR is present. This may explain why mitral reconstruction can be applied to patients with reduced EFs. Therefore, the primary goal of effective repair in these patients must be to reestablish the zone of coaptation by flexible mitral annular remodeling.

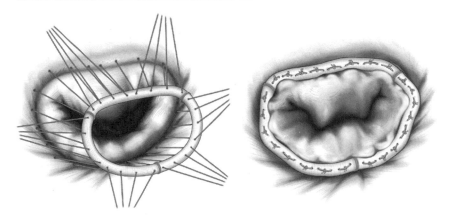

Fig. 3. Successful augmentation of the zone of coaptation and prevention of recurrent MR can be achieved by implanting an undersize circumferential annuloplasty ring.

At the University of Michigan, 145 patients with end-stage cardiomyopathy and refractory severe MR have undergone geometric mitral reconstruction with an undersize flexible annuloplasty ring (Fig. 3). All patients were in New York Heart Association (NYHA) class III or IV heart failure despite receiving maximal medical therapy. Patients had severe LV systolic dysfunction as defined by an EF of less than 25%, with a mean of 14%. On immediate postoperative echocardiograms, the mean transmitral gradient has been only 3 ± 1 mmHg (range 2–6 mmHg). The overall operative mortality has been 3.5%. There were five 30-day mortalities: one intraoperative death because of right ventricular failure, one from a cerebrovascular accident, one from CHF, and two from multisystem organ failure. Only five patients have required intra-aortic balloon counterpulsation (3.5%), and no patient has required mechanical LV assistance. The duration of follow-up of these patients has been between 1 and 75 months, with a mean of 38 months. There have been 27 late deaths: 12 from sudden ventricular arrhythmias, 9 from progression of CHF but without MR, 3 related to complications from other operative procedures, 2 that progressed to transplantation, and 1 suicide. The 1-, 2-, and 5-year actuarial survival is 82, 71, and 57%, respectively.

At 24-month assessment, all patients were in NYHA class I or II. Their mean EF had increased from 14% preoperatively to 26%. NYHA symptoms were reduced from a preoperative mean of 3.2 ± 0.2 to 1.8 ± 0.4 postoperatively. These improvements paralleled subjective

Table 2
Matched Preoperative and Postoperative Echocardiographic Data
at 24 Months Following Mitral Reconstruction for Heart Failure

ECHO parameter	Preoperative	Postoperative (24 mo)	p
End diastolic volume (mL)	281 ± 86	206 ± 88	<0.001
Ejection fraction (%)	16 ± 5	26 ± 8	0.008
Regurgitant fraction (%)	70 ± 12	13 ± 10	<0.001
Cardiac output (L/min)	3.1 ± 1.0	5.2 ± 0.8	0.001
Sphericity index (D/L)	0.82 ± 0.10	0.74 ± 0.07	0.005

functional improvements reported by all patients. Echocardiographically, there were marked improvements in regurgitant fraction, end-diastolic volume, cardiac output, and sphericity index (Table 2). Although significant undersizing of the mitral annulus was employed to overcorrect for the zone of coaptation, no systolic anterior motion of the anterior leaflet or mitral stenosis was noted in these patients.

The technique of undersizing in mitral reconstruction avoids systolic anterior motion in these myopathic patients likely because of widening of the aorto–mitral angle in these hearts with increased left ventricle size. Furthermore, acute remodeling of the base of the heart with this reparative technique may also reestablish the somewhat normal geometry and ellipsoid shape the left ventricle. As evidenced by the decreased sphericity index and left ventricle volumes seen in these patients, the geometric restoration of mitral reconstruction not only effectively corrects MR, but also achieves surgical unloading of the ventricle (53–55).

In our study, patients with MR and severe refractory heart failure were selected to undergo geometric mitral reconstruction regardless of etiology. No patients required coronary revascularization. There were no differences in operative mortality, immediate postoperative recovery, or 1-year survival between patients with ischemic or nonischemic cardiomyopathy. However, it has been observed that those with ischemic etiologies do have a comparative decrease in long-term survival despite negative preoperative viability studies. This may represent the relative inability of the myocardium to reverse remodel in these patients. There were also slightly more late sudden deaths observed in this subpopulation, which may suggest a potential role for automatic implantable cardioverter defibrillator therapy in patients with ischemic cardiomyopathy who are not suitable for revascularization.

Mitral reconstruction can now be performed with reproducible long-term results and minimal operative mortality (56–60). The physiological

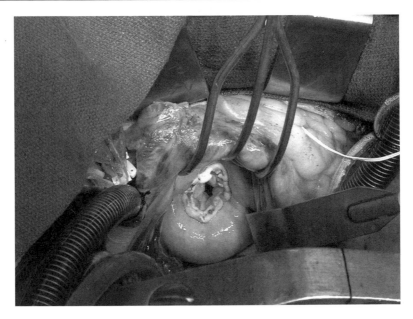

Fig. 4. Technique of geometric mitral reconstruction: bicaval cannulation, approaching the mitral valve through the interatrial groove, and the use of a self-retaining retractor greatly enhances exposure. Multiple circumferential annular sutures are placed, followed by the implantation of an undersize flexible ring. Note the reduced size of the annulus after successful reconstruction.

improvement in contractile efficiency and cardiac output affords patients significant improvements in functional status and quality of life. The straightforward technique of this geometric remodeling operation (Fig. 4) has resulted in some surgeons accepting a policy of "no EF is too low" for mitral reconstruction. Intermediate-term outcomes have attained the level of those obtained from transplantation, but without the need for immunosuppression.

Other groups have corroborated these encouraging results. The following studies illustrate that mitral surgery can be readily performed in the presence of dilated or ischemic cardiomyopathy. Each of these studies indicated that mitral surgery can be performed safely in the setting of severe LV dysfunction.

Chen et al. reported a series of 81 patients in Boston with MR and dilated cardiomyopathy managed with mitral repair *(56)*. In this series, 77% underwent concomitant coronary revascularization, and at follow-up, LVEF improved from 24 to 32%, with an improvement in the mean NYHA class from 3.3 to 1.6. Survival in their study was 73, 58, and 38 at 1, 3, and 5 years, respectively.

Bishay et al. examined 35 patients in Cleveland who underwent mitral repair and 9 who underwent MVR in the setting of severe LV dysfunction *(57)*. They reported LVEF improvements from 28 to 36% and mean NYHA class reductions from 2.9 to 1.2 at follow-up. Survival was 89, 86, and 67% at 1, 2, and 5 years, respectively.

In Chieti, Italy, Calafiore et al. reported a series of 49 patients with dilated cardiomyopathy; 29 underwent mitral repair, and 20 had MVR, with a mortality of 4.2% and comparable long-term survival *(58)*. Bitran et al. from Jerusalem, Israel, reported on 21 patients with ischemic cardiomyopathy and EF below 25% who underwent mitral repair with concomitant coronary revascularization with no early mortality *(59)*. At 3-year follow-up, 67% of the patients were in NYHA class I–II, with a late mortality of 14%.

SUMMARY

Mitral reconstruction in conjunction with medical management may now be offered to all patients with MR and cardiomyopathy as a first-line therapy for heart failure, and it should now be included in the armamentarium of every heart failure surgeon.

Advances in diagnostic and surgical techniques for the management of MR have resulted in improved long-term outcomes and survival rates. Although renewed approaches to mitral surgery in severe LV dysfunction have been successful, more effort is needed to encourage the early referral of patients with MR before ventricular deterioration occurs. With knowledge of the natural history of regurgitation and its negative impact on ventricular remodeling and long-term survival, it behooves us to withhold surgical therapy until heart failure appears *(61–64)*. With this renewed multidisciplinary approach to MR, repairs may be made earlier and impact the survival of heart failure with a modicum of prevention.

REFERENCES

1. Tavazzi L. Epidemiology of dilated cardiomyopathy: a still undetermined entity. Eur Heart J 1997;18:4–6.
2. Hunt SA. Current status of cardiac transplantation. JAMA 1998;280:1692–1698.
3. Blondheim DS, Jacobs LE, Kotler MN, Costacurta GA, Parry WR. Dilated cardiomyopathy with mitral regurgitation: decreased survival despite a low frequency of left ventricular thrombus. Am Heart J 1991;122(3 part 1):763–771.
4. Hashim SR, Fontaine A, He S, et al. A three-component force vector cell for in vitro quantification of the force exerted by the papillary muscle on the left ventricular wall. J Biomech 1997;30:1071–1075.
5. Dagum P, Timek TA, Green GR, et al. Coordinate-free analysis of mitral valve dynamics in normal and ischemic hearts. Circulation 2000;102(19 suppl 3): III62–III69.

6. Otsuji Y, Gilon D, Jiang L, et al. Restricted diastolic opening of the mitral leaflets in patients with left ventricular dysfunction: evidence for increased valve tethering. J Am Coll Cardiol 1998;32:398–404.

7. Marwick TH, Zuchowski C, Lauer MS, et al. Functional status and quality of life in patients with heart failure undergoing coronary bypass surgery after assessment of myocardial viability. J Am Coll Cardiol 1999;33:750–758.

8. DiCarli MF, Maddahi J, Roshsar S, et al. Long-term survival of patients with coronary artery disease and left ventricular dysfunction: implications for the role of myocardial viability assessment in management decisions. J Thorac Cardiovasc Surg 1998;116:997–1004.

9. Senior R, Kaul S, Lahiri A. Myocardial viability on echocardiography predicts long-term survival after revascularization in patients with ischemic congestive heart failure. J Am Coll Cardiol 1999;33:1848–1854.

10. Spain MG, Smith MD, Grayburn PA, et al. Quantitative assessment of mitral regurgitation by Doppler color flow imaging: angiographic and hemodynamic correlations. J Am Coll Cardiol 1989;13:585–590.

11. Cape EG, Yoganathan AP, Weyman AE, et al. Adjacent solid boundaries alter the size of regurgitant jets on Doppler color flow maps. J Am Coll Cardiol 1991;17:1094–1102.

12. Boltwood CM, Tei C, Wong M, et al. Quantitative echocardiography of the mitral complex in dilated cardiomyopathy: the mechanism of functional mitral regurgitation. Circulation 1983;68:498–508.

13. Hansen A, Haass M, Zugck C, et al. Prognostic value of Doppler echocardiographic mitral inflow patterns: implications for risk stratification in patients with chronic congestive heart failure. J Am Coll Cardiol 2001;37:1049–1055.

14. Pitarys CJ II, Forman MB, Panayiotou H, et al. Long-term effects of excision of the mitral apparatus on global and regional ventricular function in humans. J Am Coll Cardiol 1990;15:557–563.

15. Phillips HR, Levine FH, Carter JE, et al. Mitral valve replacement for isolated mitral regurgitation: analysis of clinical course and late postoperative left ventricular ejection fraction. Am J Cardiol 1981;48:647–654.

16. David TE, Uden DE, Strauss HD. The importance of the mitral apparatus in left ventriuclar function after correction of mitral regurgitation. Circulation 1983;68 (3 part 2):II76–II82.

17. Sarris GE, Cahill PD, Hansen DE, et al. Restoration of left ventricular systolic performance after reattachment of the mitral chordae tendineae. The importance of valvular–ventricular interaction. J Thorac Cardiovasc Surg 1988;95:969–979.

18. Miki S, Ueda Y, Tahata T, et al. 1988: Mitral valve replacement with preservation of chordae tendinae and papillary muscles. Updated in 1995. Ann Thorac Surg 1995;60:225–226.

19. Okita Y, Miki S, Ueda Y, et al. Left ventricular function after mitral valve replacement with or without chordal preservation. J Heart Valve Dis 1995;4(suppl 2): S181–S192.

20. DeAnda A Jr, Komeda M, Nikolic SD, et al. Left ventricular function, twist, and recoil after mitral valve replacement. Circulation 1995;92(9 suppl):II458–II466.

21. Moon MR, DeAnda A Jr, Daughters GT II, et al. Effects of chordal disruption on regional left ventricular torsional deformation. Circulation 1996;94(9 suppl): II143–II51.

22. Takayama Y, Holmes JW, LeGrice I, et al. Enhanced regional deformation at the anterior papillary muscle insertion site after chordal transsection. Circulation 1996;93:585–593.

23. Straub U, Feindt P, Huwer H, et al. Postoperative assessment of chordal preservation and changes in cardiac geometry following mitral valve replacement. Eur J Cardiothorac Surg 1996;10:734–740.

24. Straub U, Huwer H, Kalweit G, et al. Improved regional left ventricular performance in mitral valve replacement with orthotopic refixation of the anterior mitral leaflet. J Heart Valve Dis 1997;6:395–403.

25. Natsuaki M, Itoh T, Tomita S, et al. Importance of preserving the mitral subvalvular apparatus in mitral valve replacement. Ann Thorac Surg 1996;61:585–590.

26. David TE, Armstrong S, Sun Z. Left ventricular function after mitral surgery. J Heart Valve Dis 1995;4(suppl 2):S175–S180.

27. Essop MR, Kontozis L, Sareli P. Preoperative left ventricular systolic dysfunction correlates with the adverse postoperative consequences of annular–papillary disconnection in the course of mitral valve replacement for stenosis. J Heart Valve Dis 1998;7:431–437.

28. Rose EA, Oz MC. Preservation of anterior leaflet chordae tendinae during mitral valve replacement. Ann Thorac Surg 1994;57:768–769.

29. Miki S, Kusuhara K, Ueda Y, et al. Mitral valve replacement with preservation of the chordae tendinae and papillary muscles. Ann Thorac Surg 1988;45:28–34.

30. Feikes HL, Daugharthy JB, Perry JE, et al. Preservation of all chordae tendinae and papillary muscle during mitral valve replacement with a tilting disc valve. J Card Surg 1990;5(2):81-5.

31. Casselman FP, Gillinov AM, McDonald ML, et al. Use of the anterior mitral leaflet to reinforce the posterior mitral annulus after debridement of calcium. Ann Thorac Surg 1999;68:261–262.

32. Minatoya H, Okabayashi H, Shimada I, et al. Pathologic aspects of polytetrafluoroethylene sutures in human heart. Ann Thorac Surg 1996;61:883–887.

33. Kobayashi J, Sasako J, Bando K, et al. Ten-year experience of chordal replacement with expanded polytetrafluoroethylene in mitral valve repair. Circulation 2000;102(19 suppl 3):III30–III34.

34. Sintek CF, Khonsari S. Use of extended polytetrafluoroethylene (ePTFE) chordae to re-establish annular–papillary connection after mitral valve excision. J Heart Valve Dis 1996;5:362–364.

35. Reimink MS, Kunzelman KS, Cochran RP. The effect of chordal replacement suture length on function and stresses in repaired mitral valves: a finite element study. J Heart Valve Dis 1996;5:365–375.

36. Esper E, Ferdinand FD, Aronson S, et al. Prosthetic mitral valve replacement: late complications after native valve preservation. Ann Thorac Surg 1997;63:541–543.

37. Greenwood JP, Nolan J, Mackintosh AF. Late, intermittent obstruction of a mitral prosthesis by chordal remnants. Eur J Cardiothorac Surg 1997;12:804–806.

38. Moon MR, DeAnda A Jr, Daughters GT II, et al. Effects of mitral valve replacement on regional left ventricular systolic strain. Ann Thorac Surg 1999;68:894–902.

39. Yun KL, Sintek CF, Miller DC, et al. Randomized trial of partial vs complete chordal preservation methods of mitral valve replacement. A preliminary report. Circulation 1999;100(19 suppl):II90–II94.

40. Yu Y, Gao C, Li G, et al. Mitral valve replacement with complete mitral leaflet retention: operative techniques. J Heart Valve Dis 1999;8:44–46.

41. Fontaine AA, He S, Stadter R, et al. In vitro assessment of prosthetic valve function in mitral valve replacement with chordal preservation techniques. J Heart Valve Dis 1996;5:186–198.

42. Ren JF, Aksut S, Lightly GW Jr, et al. Mitral valve repair is superior to valve replacement for the early preservation of cardiac function: relation of ventricular geometry to function. Am Heart J 1996;131:974–981.

43. Lawrie GM. Mitral valve repair vs replacement. Current recommendations and long-term results. Cardiol Clin 1998;16:437–448.

44. Corin WJ, Sutsch G, Mukakami T, et al. Left ventricular function in chronic mitral regurgitation: preoperative and postoperative comparison. J Am Coll Cardiol 1995;25:113–121.

45. Lee EM, Shapiro LM, Wells FC. Importance of subvalvular preservation and early operation in mitral valve surgery. Circulation 1996;94:II117–II123.

46. Pagani FD, Benedict MB, Marshall BL, et al. The economics of uncomplicated mitral valve surgery. J Heart Valve Dis 1997;6:466–469.

47. Barlow CW, Imber CJ, Sharples LD, et al. Cost implications of mitral valve replacement vs repair in mitral regurgitation. Circulation 1997;96(9 suppl): II90–II93.

48. Komoda T, Hertzer R, Oellinger J, et al. Mitral annular flexibility. J Card Surg 1997;12:102–109.

49. Komeda M, Glasson JR, Bolger AF, et al. Three-dimensional dynamic geometry of the normal canine mitral annulus and papillary muscles. Circulation 1996;94 (9 suppl):II159–II163.

50. Komoda T, Hertzer R, Sinlawaski H, et al. Effects of prosthetic valve replacement on mitral annular dynamics and the left ventricular base. ASAIO J 2001;47: 60–65.

51. Rosario LB, Stevenson LW, Solomon SD, et al. The mechanism of decrease in dynamic mitral regurgitation during heart failure treatment: importance of reduction in the regurgitant orifice size. J Am Coll Cardiol 1998;32:1819–1824.

52. Kono T, Sabbah HN, Rosman H, et al. Left ventricular shape is the primary determinant of functional mitral regurgitation in heart failure. J Am Coll Cardiol 1992;20:1594–1598.

53. Bolling SF, Deeb GM, Brunsting LA, et al. Early outcome of mitral valve reconstruction in patients with end-stage cardiomyopathy. J Thorac Cardiovasc Surg 1995;109:676–683.

54. Bach DS, Bolling SF. Improvement following correction of secondary mitral regurgitation in end-stage cardiomyopathy with mitral annuloplasty. Am J Cardiol 1996;78:966–969.

55. Bolling SF, Pagani FD, Deeb GM, et al. Intermediate-term outcome of mitral reconstruction in cardiomyopathy. J Thorac Cardiovasc Surg 1998;115:381–388.

56. Chen FY, Adams DH, Aranki SF, et al. Mitral valve repair in cardiomyopathy. Circulation 1998;98:II-124–II-127.

57. Bishay ES, McCarthy PM, Cosgrove DM, et al. Mitral valve surgery in patients with severe left ventricular dysfunction. Eur J Cardiothorac Surg 2000;17: 213–221.

58. Calafiore AM, Gallina S, DiMauro M, et al. Mitral valve procedure in dilated cardiomyopathy: repair or replacement? Ann Thorac Surg 2001;71:1146–1152.

59. Bitran D, Merrin O, Klutstein MW, et al. Mitral valve repair in severe ischemic cardiomyopathy. J Card Surg 2001;16:79–82.

60. deVarennes B, Haichin R. Impact of preoperative left ventricular ejection fraction on postoperative left ventricular remodeling after mitral valve repair for degenerative disease. J Heart Valve Dis 2000;9:313–318.

61. Ling LH, Enriquez-Sarano M, Seward JB, et al. Clinical outcome of mitral regurgitation due to flail leaflet. N Engl J Med 1996;335:1417–1423.

62. Ofili E, Oduwole A, Lapa-Bula R. Surgical timing for mitral valve regurgitation. Echocardiography 2000;17:285–292.
63. Carabello BA. The pathophysiology of mitral regurgitation. J Heart Valve Dis 2000;9:600–608.
64. Smolens IA, Pagani FD, Deeb GM, et al. Prophylactic mitral reconstruction for asymptomatic mitral regurgitation. Ann Thorac Surg 2001;72:1210–1215.

5

Tricuspid Valve Surgery in Right Heart Failure

James P. Greelish, MD,
Bradley J. Phillips, MD,
James C. Fang, MD,
and John G. Byrne, MD

CONTENTS

INTRODUCTION

Tricuspid valve disease is often found in combination with other valvular pathology. Tricuspid regurgitation (TR), the most common tricuspid valvular condition, is commonly asymptomatic, although progressive, in nature. With time, it may lead to right ventricular (RV) enlargement, annular dilatation, and systolic dysfunction. Clinical symptoms and the degree of RV impairment usually determine whether

From: *Contemporary Cardiology: Surgical Management of Congestive Heart Failure*
Edited by: J. C. Fang and G. S. Couper © Humana Press Inc., Totowa, NJ

medical or surgical therapy is most appropriate. However, operative intervention should be carefully considered; there is an unusually high mortality rate associated with tricuspid valve surgery, ranging from 19 to 25% (1–3). In this chapter, we review the pathophysiology and surgical therapy of the tricuspid valve for the management of RV failure.

ANATOMY OF THE RIGHT HEART AND TRICUSPID VALVE

The right heart serves as a collection chamber. The right atrium can be divided into three sections: the atrial appendage, the vestibule, and the tricuspid valve. The appendage is a triangular-shape structure that is frequently used for venous cannulation during cardiac surgery and marks the location of the sinus node. The atrioventricular node lies within the triangle of Koch, defined by the septal annulus posteriorly, the ostium of the coronary sinus on the right, and the tendon of Todaro on the left (Fig. 1). The bundle of His travels through the central fibrous body and into the membranous part of the interventricular septum. Misplaced sutures in this region can result in various degrees of heart block. Temporary atrial and ventricular pacing wires are routinely placed at the conclusion of most tricuspid operations for this reason.

The vestibule of the right atrium has two embryologically distinct areas: (1) a smooth-walled posterior part, called the sinus venarium, that receives blood from the venae cavae/coronary sinus and (2) a rough-walled anterior region that has internal muscular ridges (musculi pectinati). These two parts of the atrial vestibule are separated externally by the sulcus terminalis (i.e., terminal groove) and internally by the crista terminalis. A prominent feature of this area is the fossa ovalis. This fetal remnant of the foramen ovale is a thumbprint-size translucent depression facing the inferior vena cava.

The three leaflets of the tricuspid valve reflect their anatomical location: septal, anterior, and posterior. All three leaflets are folds of endocardium strengthened by fibrous tissue. The leaflets are continuous with the tricuspid ring and join at their zones of apposition or commissures; they are tethered by fan-shaped chords arising from prominent papillary muscles (Fig. 2) (4). The individual leaflets are ill defined from a surgical standpoint, and their exact papillary relationships can vary. However, a trifoliate relationship almost always exists despite the various fibrous interconnections.

Classically, the largest anterior leaflet extends from the subpulmonary conus; the septal leaflet attaches to the membranous and muscular septum. The posterior leaflet bridges the space between the

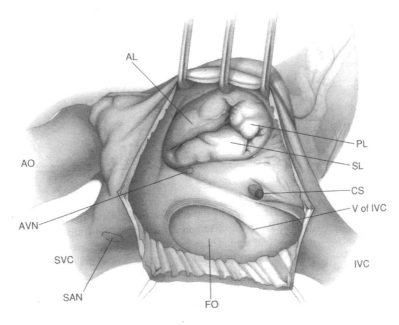

Fig. 1. The right heart. AL, anterior leaflet; PL, posterior leaflet, AO, aorta, SL, septal leaflet, AVN, atrioventricular node; SVC, superior vena cava; FO, fossa ovalis; CS, coronary sinus; V of IVC, valve of inferior vena cava; SAN, sinoatrial node; IVC, inferior vena cava. (Reproduced with permission from ref. *4*.)

intraventricular septum and the anterolateral wall. These leaflets are anchored at their periphery to a fibrous "annulus" and centrally by chordae tendinae. Although chordae of the anterior leaflet generally attach to a dominant papillary muscle, the chordae of the septal and posterior leaflets attach directly to the ventricular myocardium. These direct ventricular attachments are unique in valvular anatomy and help to define the true identity of this valve in congenital anomalies.

It is also important to realize that a well-formed tricuspid annulus does not exist. Instead of having a distinct, collagenous band surrounding the valve orifice (as seen in other valves), the tricuspid valve lies within an atrioventricular groove, a fibrofatty tissue plane separating the right atrium from its ventricle, that folds in on itself to form the base of the tricuspid valve leaflets. The orifice of this annulus is larger than that of the mitral valve (approx 3.1–4.0 cm in diameter). In general, annular dilatation is the most common mechanism of TR.

The right ventricle is a thin-wall structure with its free wall normally measuring less than 5 mm thick. The outlet portion of the right

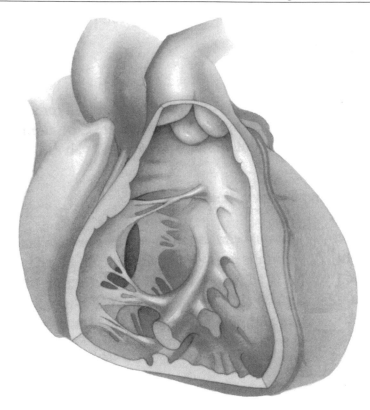

Fig. 2. The right ventricle. (Reproduced with permission from ref. *4*.)

ventricle is composed of the muscular infundibulum, which supports the leaflets of the pulmonary valve. The geometry of the RV chamber is difficult to characterize, but some have likened it to a triangular bellows with the apex at the pulmonic valve and the base formed by the diaphragmatic surface of the heart. The right ventricle has a smaller mass than the left, but is much more compliant and therefore able to accommodate large diastolic volumes.

The coronary anatomy of this region also has significance in right-sided heart failure. RV dysfunction from coronary artery disease is usually a result of extension of an inferoposterior transmural infarction. Given that the blood supply to the right ventricle is most commonly derived from the right coronary artery and acute marginal branches (i.e., "right-sided dominance"), an inferior myocardial infarction (MI) from proximal right coronary occlusion usually leads to RV dilatation *(5,6)*. TR can also occur with an inferoseptal infarction because, as described above, some tricuspid chordae are septophilic (i.e., directly attached to the ventricular septum). This "ischemic TR" is usually responsive to coronary revascularization. Only in isolated cases has tricuspid valve surgery been attempted for intractable regurgitation after an inferior MI *(7)*. Although RV infarction commonly accompanies inferior MI, the right ventricle is generally resistant to permanent dysfunction and usually recovers.

PATHOPHYSIOLOGY OF RIGHT-SIDED FAILURE

The right ventricle normally propels blood toward a low-resistance pulmonary bed. When an elevated pulmonary vascular resistance (PVR) challenges the ventricle, systolic failure may ensue. This inability to overcome additional afterload stress differentiates the right ventricle from its left-sided counterpart and is an important consideration when planning a surgical procedure that results in the right ventricle pumping against near-systemic pressures (i.e., the Fontan operation for hypoplastic left ventricular [LV] syndromes).

The most common cause of RV dysfunction, and subsequent TR, is LV failure. Elevation of the LV end-diastolic pressure (LVEDP) passively creates secondary pulmonary hypertension. If severe enough, the right ventricle will fail, manifested by ventricular enlargement and tricuspid annular dilatation. Secondary TR in this situation will further exacerbate RV failure by decreasing the forward cardiac output.

The geometric relationship of the cardiac chambers to one another, the shared ventricular septum, and pericardial constraint produce ventricular interdependence. RV shape is unlike that of the left: Both the RV free wall and the interventricular septum are concave. On the right side of the heart, the free wall moves toward the septum in a near-parallel fashion, which is commonly referred to as a *bellows effect*. Classically, the septum normally moves to the left during systole and to the right during diastole. However, in the presence of RV volume overload (i.e., TR), an abnormal "paradoxical" motion occurs. The septum moves to the left during both systole and diastole, which reduces systolic shortening in the dimension of the septum to the LV free wall and decreases the LV stroke volume and ejection fraction (EF). Louie et al. *(8)* demonstrated this concept in a study of volume- and pressure-loaded right ventricles. They studied 10 patients with severe TR following tricuspid valve resection to elucidate the impact of pure volume overload on LV function. They found that the LVEF was significantly less compared to age-matched controls ($51 \pm 4\%$ vs $60 \pm 4\%$, $p < 0.001$); LV end-diastolic volumes were similar between groups (84 ± 26 vs 77 ± 20 mL, p not significant). In contrast, pressure-loaded right ventricles (in patients with pulmonary hypertension) had normal resting LVEFs because of augmented systolic shortening despite relative ventricular underfilling. These investigators have also demonstrated that severe TR results in marked right atrial distension, reversal of the normal interatrial curvature, and compression of the left atrium (left atrium cross-sectional area: 5.9 ± 2.2 vs 8.6 ± 1.2 cm^2/m^2, $p < 0.005$). In this manner, the volume-overloaded right ventricle also decreases left atrial preload and consequently LV stroke volume (9).

Because the left and right ventricles share a common, space-limiting envelope (i.e., the pericardium), there are other consequences of RV dilatation. When the pericardium is intact, expansion of one ventricle will have an impact on the diastolic function of the other. In this way, RV dilatation can mimic tamponade, leading to an increased RV end-diastolic pressure and decreased LV diastolic volume. In this manner, right-sided failure can mimic pericardial heart disease. In fact, classic findings of pericardial constraint such as diastolic pressure equalization, a "dip-and-plateau" or "square-root" sign, pulsus paradoxus, and Kussmaul's sign have all been documented in patients with RV failure. In fact, sporadic cases of misdiagnosis have led to pericardial surgery (10).

When the right atrial and RV end-diastolic pressure exceed the pulmonary capillary wedge and LVEDP, advanced RV failure is present. The presence of a noncompliant right atrial waveform (i.e., an M or W wave) with a Y descent deeper than the X descent is also highly specific (11). In the absence of pericardial or valvular disease, these findings are rather specific for RV failure.

The neurohormonal profile of right-sided heart failure has also been characterized (12,13). In a group of patients with advanced right heart failure from carcinoid heart disease (right atrial pressure 16 mmHg, cardiac index 1.9 L/min/m^2), preoperative atrial natriuretic peptide levels were markedly elevated and paralleled the clinical signs of right heart failure. All patients demonstrated significant and dramatic reductions of atrial natriuretic peptide levels following tricuspid valve replacement (Fig. 3).

SURGICAL APPROACHES TO THE TRICUSPID VALVE

When severe TR is early in its course, medical therapy (diuresis, digoxin, and salt restriction) can usually control symptoms and maintain compensated hemodynamics. However, in the advanced stages of TR, the right ventricle begins to fail from chronic volume overload (and pressure overload when pulmonary hypertension is present). At

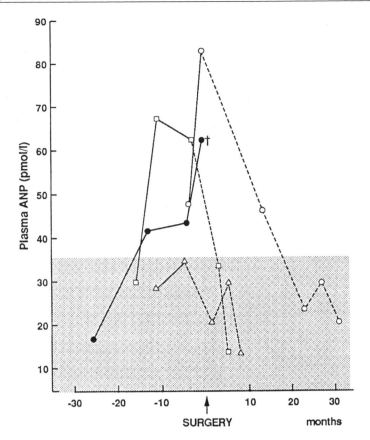

Fig. 3. Plasma atrial natriuretic peptide (ANP) levels in TR. Solid line, preoperative; dashed line, postoperative; open circles, case 1; closed circles, case 2; open triangle, case 3; open square, case 4, †, death postoperatively. (Reproduced with permission from ref. *12.*)

this point, the right heart becomes a passive conduit, and the circulation becomes univentricular. Fluid administration and elevated central venous pressures (to increase RV end-diastolic volume) may be necessary to support the cardiac output *(14)*. In the presence of severe pulmonary hypertension, an atrial septostomy may be required simply to maintain left ventricular preload. Maintaining A-V synchrony and avoiding agents that reduce preload, such as nitroglycerin and morphine, are also useful *(15)*. Inotropic support (e.g., milrinone, dobutamine, isoproterenol) may be required.

When right heart dysfunction is secondary to left-sided failure, treatment of the left-sided disease should take precedent. In this setting, surgical therapy of secondary TR may serve as an adjuvant to surgical therapy of the left ventricle (i.e., coronary bypass or mitral valve repair). Rarely is it indicated to operate solely on the tricuspid valve when the regurgitation is secondary to left heart disease. In contrast, when TR is primary (i.e., endocarditis), valve repair or replacement is warranted when medical therapy cannot control symptoms.

The tricuspid valve is usually approached through a median sternotomy. A right anterolateral thoracotomy may alternatively be performed in reoperative cases. Minimally invasive approaches have also been described, but may require femoral cannulation. Most patients requiring surgery for tricuspid disease have enlarged right atriums, making visualization of the tricuspid valve easier. Bicaval venous cannulation is performed in the standard manner, and arterial cannulation is obtained via the aorta. After initiation of bypass, the patient is cooled, and the aorta is cross-clamped. All other procedures are performed prior to addressing the tricuspid valve (e.g., coronary artery bypass graft, aortic valve, mitral valve, etc.).

The mitral valve can be reached through a transseptal incision, thereby avoiding a second atriotomy. Generally, we perform tricuspid procedures during rewarming after the aortic cross-clamp has been removed. Prior to this, snares are secured around the superior vena cava and inferior vena cava venous cannulae to avoid inadvertent blood flow. This technique creates a relatively dry field, with the exception of blood draining from the coronary sinus. Although previously considered the standard method of diagnosis, we have not found it helpful to assess the degree of regurgitation by finger palpation through the right atrium; we rely primarily on preoperative and intraoperative echocardiography.

Once the anatomy of this region has been identified, the valve itself is inspected. Asymmetric dilatation in the posterior region is commonly present and is a consequence of the septal leaflet's annular structure fixation to the fibrous skeleton of the heart. Therefore, Cohn *(16)* and others *(17–20)* have suggested techniques to reduce the clinical role of this region. In Cohn's technique, a partial annuloplasty is performed in the region of the posterior annulus using a sizing obturator to avoid unnecessary constriction (Fig. 4). This method is a variation of the classic annuloplasty technique initially proposed by De Vega *(21)*. De Vega's method utilizes a double continuous suture placed from the anteroseptal commissure to the posteroseptal commissure in a clockwise fashion. This suture is nearly circumferential and ends in the region of the conduction bundle, placing the atrioventricular node in jeopardy (Fig. 5). The Kay-Wooler repair also tries to reduce the tricuspid annulus in the posterior region. This technique approximates and opposes the annulus at the posterior leaflet, thus "bicuspidizing" the tricuspid valve (Fig. 6) *(19)*.

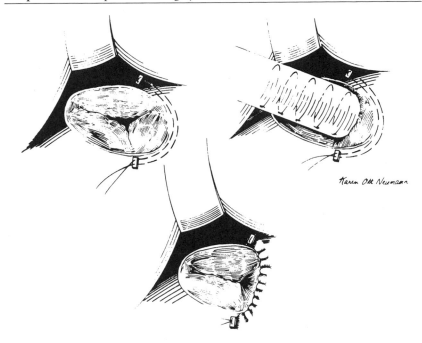

Fig. 4. Modified De Vega annuloplasty. (Reproduced with permission from ref. *16*.)

When 3 to 4+ TR exists, some surgeons elect to repair the valve with a ring annuloplasty. This repair utilizes a structured band to reduce annular dimension. The ring is sized to the septal leaflet and secured carefully to avoid the bundle of His. Ring types most commonly used are those described by Carpentier-Edwards and colleagues *(22)*, Duran and Ubago *(23)*, and McCarthy and Cosgrove *(24)* (Fig. 7).

Ring annuloplasty and commisurotomy may be indicated for rheumatic-induced tricuspid stenosis (TS). The fused commissures, which can be identified by their fan chordae, are incised with a scalpel, taking care not to enter the annulus proper. To avoid iatrogenically induced regurgitation, commissurotomy should be limited to one or two commissures; we usually do not incise the anteroseptal commissure because this area is most likely to develop insufficiency. When performed, commisurotomy should be combined with a ring to ensure durability.

If the tricuspid valve has to be replaced, we excise or imbricate the anterior and posterior leaflets. Imbrication has the distinct advantage of allowing the surgeon to retain the subvalvular apparatus, an important principle of mitral valve surgery. Sutures are placed in the septal leaflet proper to avoid the specialized conductive tissue (Fig. 8). Valve competency is tested by infusing saline into the right ventricle and

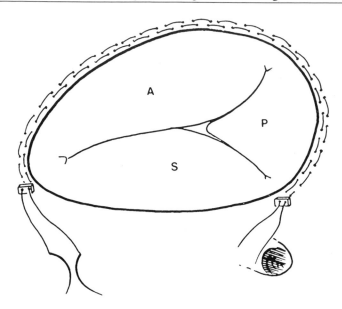

Fig. 5. De Vega annuolplasty. A, anterior leaflet; P, posterior leaflet; S, septal leaflet. (Reproduced with permission from ref. *81.*)

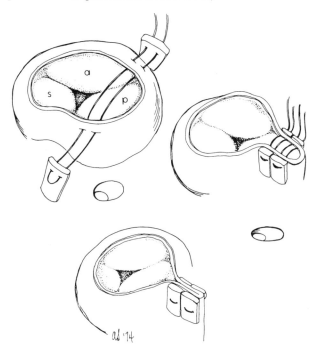

Fig. 6. Kay or Wooler annuloplasty. a, anterior leaflet; p, posterior leaflet; s, septal leaflet. (Reproduced with permission from ref. *82.*)

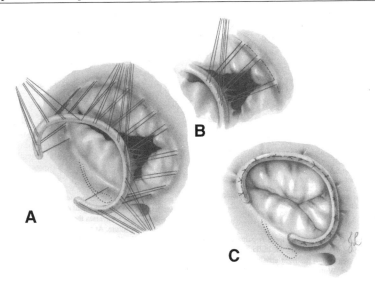

Fig. 7. Carpentier ring annuloplasty. A, anchoring mattress sutured; B, reducing the size of the annulus; C, restoring the valve to its normal configuration. (Reproduced with permission from ref. *4*.)

assessing leaflet coaptation. If this proves satisfactory, the atrium is closed, and the patient is weaned from bypass with transesophageal echocardiographic confirmation prior to decannulation. In 88 patients treated by reparative techniques at the Brigham and Women's Hospital, 72 patients had suture annuloplasty (69 De Vega, 3 Kay-Wooler); 16 had ring annuloplasty (all 16 had 4+ TR; 15 Carpentier-Edwards, 1 Duran). There were 79 patients in New York Heart Association class III or IV, and 82 patients underwent concomitant mitral valve replacement. The operative mortality was 11.5%. A 2-year follow-up was available for 53 patients: TR was absent in 7, "trace TR" was present in 28, and "mild TR" was identified in 18 *(16)*.

In general, many of the left ventricular hemodynamic benefits derived from mitral valve repair can also be seen in the right ventricle with tricuspid repair *(25)*. Although the tricuspid valve is more forgiving of surgical technique, valve repair has been associated with a higher incidence of residual insufficiency compared to replacement. The decision of repair vs replacement is typically based on the degree of regurgitation. In general, we follow the American College of Cardiology/American Heart Association guidelines: Mild TR is treated conservatively; moderate TR is treated with annuloplasty; and severe TR is treated with replacement *(26)*. When a valve is required, a bioprosthesis theoretically can avoid the

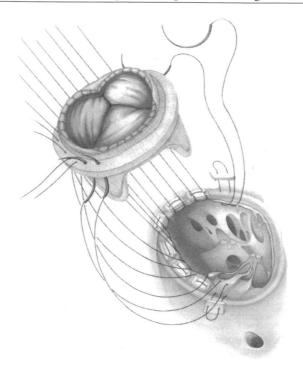

Fig. 8. Tricuspid valve replacement. (Reproduced with permission from ref. *4*.)

risk of mechanical thrombosis *(27)*. Valve durability is also much greater in the tricuspid position than it is in the aortic or mitral positions *(28–30)*. Also, mechanical valve replacement requires placement of permanent epicardial pacing wires because percutaneous leads cannot be placed through the mechanical valve. We favor the use of long-term anticoagulation for mechanical and biologic tricuspid valves. In our opinion, the relatively low flow rate through the valve orifice increases the likelihood of valvular thrombi. Others, however, limit anticoagulation to only those patients with mechanical valves *(31)*.

RIGHT HEART FAILURE CAUSED BY SPECIFIC CLINICAL CONDITIONS

The surgical approach to right heart failure generally involves the treatment of tricuspid valve disease (Table 1). Pulmonic valve disease is rarely severe enough to produce right heart failure, and a discussion of its surgical treatment is not reviewed here. TR is the most common form of tricuspid valve disease associated with right heart failure. TS is much more rare, as are mixed stenosis and regurgitation (Tables 2 and 3).

Table 1
Relative Indications for Tricuspid Surgery

1. Medically refractory right-sided heart failure secondary to severe TR
   Postcardiac transplant
   Endocarditis
   Trauma
   Carcinoid heart disease
   Rheumatic
2. Moderate-to-severe TR at time of left heart surgery (i.e., mitral valve or coronary)
3. TS with a valve gradient ≥5 mmHg

Table 2
Primary Causes of Tricuspid Valve Disease

Tricuspid regurgitation
    Endocarditis
    Ebstein's anomaly
    Atrioventricular canal deformity
    Myxomatous degeneration
    Carcinoid heart disease
    Trauma
    Biopsy induced
Tricuspid stenosis
    Congenital tricuspid atresia

Tricuspid Regurgitation

TR is relatively common and can arise from a variety of causes. Primary TR is usually seen with congenital anomalies of the tricuspid valve or acquired leaflet deformities. Secondary TR typically develops in the setting of pressure overload (i.e., primary or secondary pulmonary hypertension) or RV cardiomyopathies (i.e., RV infarction, arrythmogenic RV dysplasia). Functional TR generally becomes evident when the RV systolic pressure becomes greater than 55 mmHg *(26)*. As the degree of regurgitation worsens, the progressive volume overload distends the ventricle and the tricuspid annulus, producing more TR. The right atrial hemodynamic tracing becomes ventricularized with increasing degrees of insufficiency, producing larger and larger V waves (Fig. 9). Eventually, clinical signs of right-sided failure appear: jugular venous distension, hepatic congestion, ascites, and peripheral edema.

Table 3
Secondary Causes of Tricuspid Valve Disease

Tricuspid regurgitation
    Aortic valve disease (stenosis or insuffiency)
    Mitral valve disease (stenosis or regurgitation)
    Congestive heart failure
    Primary pulmonary hypertension
    Pulmonary stenosis
    Right-sided ventricular infarction
    Dilated cardiomyopathy
    Pulmonary embolism
    Marfan syndrome
    Rheumatic heart disease
    Diet drugs: fenfluramine/phentermine
    Arrhythmogenic right ventricular dysplasia
Tricuspid stenosis
    Rheumatic heart disease
    Constrictive pericarditis
    Carcinoid syndrome
    Fibroelastosis
    Endomyocardial fibrosis
    Lupus erythematosus
    Right atrial myxoma

Tricuspid Stensosis

TS produces mechanical obstruction to RV filling (32,33). TS is almost exclusively caused by rheumatic inflammation and accompanies rheumatic mitral stenosis in up to 30% of patients. Rheumatic TS is usually associated with some degree of TR as well. TS may also be secondary to the carcinoid syndrome, endocarditis, and intracardiac tumors. Clinically, TS is not well tolerated. Impairment to RV filling (with mean diastolic gradients as low as 5 mmHg) may produce impressive symptoms of right-sided failure, and the importance of coexisting mitral disease therefore may be overestimated (32,33).

Although medical management of TS (sodium restriction and diuresis) suffices early in its course, the disease is progressive, and surgical therapy is usually required. Operative strategies include open and closed commissurotomy (33). Balloon valvuloplasty has been performed, but with variable success (34). Unfortunately, these techniques are associated with poor long-term outcomes, primarily because of sur-

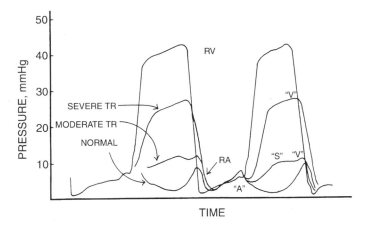

Fig. 9. Pressure tracing of tricuspid regurgitation. RA, right atrium; RV, right ventricle. (Reproduced with permission from ref. *83*.)

gically induced regurgitation. To achieve long-term success, valve replacement is commonly required.

Tricuspid Valve Endocarditis

Tricuspid valve endocarditis results from seeding of the valve leaflets during sustained bacteremia. Surgical indications in tricuspid valve endocarditis include continued sepsis despite appropriate antibiotic coverage, heart failure caused by tricuspid insufficiency, and recurrent multiple pulmonary emboli. Arbulu et al. *(35)* were the first to advocate complete excision of the tricuspid valve (without subsequent replacement). From an infectious disease standpoint, this approach has the distinct advantage of complete extirpation of infected tissue and avoids placement of prosthetic material. Although initially tolerated, this procedure unfortunately produces late-onset right-sided failure in the majority of patients *(35–37)*. In a 20-year follow-up of the originally reported series of 55 patients with intractable right-sided endocarditis who underwent tricuspid valvulectomy without replacement, 2 patients (4%) died in the postoperative period because of right-sided failure. Six patients (11%) required prosthetic valve insertion 2 days to 13 years later for medically refractory right-sided heart failure. Of the 6 who underwent reoperation, 4 (66%) died. Therefore, severe hepatic congestion and the need for reoperative valve replacement have made this approach untenable to some authors *(38)*. An alternative treatment option is to delay valve replacement for 3–9 months. Reparative strategies at time of the original operation have also been successful in treating this challenging group of patients *(4,39)*.

TR After Heart Transplantation

The reported incidence of TR in the heart transplant population varies widely, occurring in 20–83% of patients *(40,41)*. Regardless of the actual incidence, TR after transplantation is generally not severe (either asymptomatic or easily controlled with diuretics). Occasionally, the degree of regurgitation may be severe enough to warrant tricuspid valve surgery *(42,43)*. The etiology of TR in this select population has been attributed to a number of mechanisms: anastomotic technique, ischemic reperfusion injury, iatrogenic damage from endomyocardial biopsies, size mismatch between donor and recipient hearts, and chronic rejection.

The technique of orthotopic heart transplantation commonly performed until the 1990s was that of Lower and Shumway *(44,45)* using a biatrial anastomosis. Although this technique preserved a portion of the recipient's right atrium, the final geometry of the atria were often dilated and distorted and complicated by asynchronous atrial contraction. Before long, reports of TR and mitral regurgitation surfaced (in the context of a normal valve apparatus) *(46,47)*.

The now-contemporary bicaval anastomosis, popularized by Sievers et al. *(48)*, appears to alleviate some of these issues. In their original report, when tested in a prospective randomized trial, the bicaval anastomosis was associated with less TR and smaller right atria during exercise. Sarsam et al. *(49)* found a lower incidence of postoperative right heart failure and right atrial pressure (4.9 mmHg vs 9.6 mmHg, $p < 0.01$) in those transplanted with bicaval anastomoses despite a lack of difference in pulmonary artery pressures.

Percutaneous transvenous endomyocardial biopsy of the transplanted heart is the conventional method to detect allograft rejection *(50)*. It is a generally safe procedure, and major complications, such as cardiac perforation and tamponade, are unusual (<0.4% of cases) *(51)*. However, TR may result from the inadvertent injury of tricuspid valve by the bioptome and may be as frequent as 6% *(52)*. Fortunately, it is generally well tolerated and of modest severity. The need for surgical correction for medically refractory iatrogenic TR is rare *(53)*.

In addition to the aforementioned etiologies, some authors have also attributed the higher incidence of TR in the transplant population to preoperative pulmonary hypertension. Lewen et al. *(54)* found that preoperative pulmonary hypertension (>55 mmHg) was a predictor of late postoperative moderate-to-severe TR (mean 17 months) and was associated with postoperative elevation in the PVR. Other investigators have confirmed these observations *(41)*. When TR does occur in the transplant patient, medical management is usually effective. When medical therapy fails to control symptoms, valve replacement is usually favored over repair to avoid the potential need for repeated operative intervention in an immunocompromised patient.

Rheumatic TR

The most common cause of organic tricuspid disease worldwide is rheumatic fever, typically in association with mitral and/or aortic involvement. Commonly, rheumatic tricuspid disease is both stenotic and with regurgitant. Functional TR reported in these patients is a misnomer; the rheumatic tricuspid annulus is actually structurally weakened by the rheumatic inflammation rather than dilated from RV enlargement. This type of annular pathology may be suspected when normal valve leaflets accompany the regurgitation in a patient with a history of rheumatic fever, a markedly dilated annulus, and severe TR. The regurgitant jet in these cases is frequently large in volume and low in velocity. Rheumatic TR may be exacerbated by rheumatic mitral disease and concomitant pulmonary hypertension.

Distinguishing whether the dilated tricuspid annulus is caused by secondary causes or primary rheumatic weakening may be difficult, but this distinction can influence the surgical approach. A number of authors have recognized the significance of rheumatic weakening of the tricuspid annulus in the absence of rheumatic leaflet damage and have noted that it may manifest well after rheumatic mitral valve surgery *(2,55)* (*see* section on Tricuspid Valve Disease Following Mitral Valve Surgery). Thus, some have advocated tricuspid annuloplasty at the time of rheumatic mitral surgery even if there is no overt tricuspid pathology.

Rheumatic valvular surgery may also be complicated by the restriction–dilation syndrome, described originally by Barlow *(56,57)* (Fig. 10). The pressure and volume overload of the right heart from left-sided heart disease sets into motion a vicious cycle of ventricular dilatation, but pericardial constraint. As the right heart dilates, there is an exaggerated diastolic septal shift to the left, further increases in LVEDP/left atrium pressures, greater pulmonary hypertension, worsening TR, more right heart volume overload, and again more RV dilation. Although LV systolic function may be intrinsically normal under these conditions, the LVEDP will be elevated. Postoperative adhesions will further exacerbate this cycle by precluding compensatory ventricular expansion and exaggerating the septal shift. This

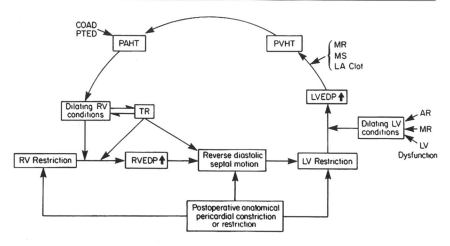

Fig. 10. The restriction–dilation syndrome. LV, left ventricle; RV, right ventricle; TR, tricuspid regurgitation; RVEDP, right ventricular end-diastolic pressure; PAHT, pulmonary artery hypertension; LVEDP, left ventricular end-diastolic pressure; AR, aortic regurgitation; MR, mitral regurgitation; PVHT, pulmonary vein hypertension; MS, mitral stenosis; LA, left atrial; PTED, pulmonary thromboembolic disease; COAD, coronary occlusive arterial disease. (Reproduced with permission from ref. *56*.)

syndrome is possible after any left-sided surgery, but is most commonly seen in rheumatic heart disease (*55–58*). Correction of TR at the time of operative therapy for hemodynamically important left-sided valvular disease will interrupt this cycle.

Tricuspid Valve Disease Following Mitral Valve Surgery

Although early-onset TR following mitral valve surgery may reflect a variety of underlying causes (persistent pulmonary hypertension, mitral prosthetic dysfunction, progressive aortic valve disease, or LV failure), late-onset TR usually reflects intrinsic RV dysfunction and/or tricuspid annular abnormalities (*59–61*). Functional tricuspid insufficiency has been reported in up to 67% of those undergoing left heart surgery and is thought to be from the effects of transmitted afterload from left heart disease (*62–64*). Therefore, conservative management of TR was initially advocated (*65*) because of expected improvements in functional regurgitation after left-sided surgery. However, it is now generally accepted that symptoms of right heart failure and exercise intolerance will persist in a significant number of patients with this approach (*3*). Furthermore, tricuspid valve annuloplasty (or valve replacement) for functional TR at the time of the initial aortic/mitral valve surgery does appear to improve outcomes *(66–68)*.

It is difficult to discern whether TR after mitral valve repair is a primary disorder of the tricuspid apparatus or is secondary to the mitral surgery. Groves et al. *(59)* compared the clinical and echocardiographic characteristics of 26 patients with and without late-onset TR after mitral valve surgery. Both groups had similar pulmonary artery pressures and no evidence of prosthetic valve dysfunction, significant aortic valve disease, or intrinsic tricuspid pathology. Only tricuspid annular diameter and RV size were greater in those patients that developed severe late-onset TR. Similarly, Porter et al. *(64)* reviewed late-onset TR in patients who had previously undergone mitral valve replacement without tricuspid valve surgery for rheumatic heart disease. Again, it was difficult to predict who would go on to develop late-onset TR: The pre- and postoperative pulmonary artery pressures, the predominance of mitral lesions, the prosthetic valve gradients, and the degree of regurgitation were similar in patients with and without late-onset TR.

The decision to operate on patients with late-onset TR following remote left-sided valve surgery is a difficult one. Staab et al. *(69)* reviewed 34 patients who underwent isolated tricuspid valve operations for severe TR following prior left-sided valve surgery. Although 85% of survivors improved symptomatically, the early mortality rate was 8.8%, and the 5-year event-free actuarial survival was only 41.6%. Predictors of poor outcome were increased age and previous cardiac surgery. Outcome did not vary depending on the degree of pulmonary hypertension, LV function, RV size/function, annular diameter, or the use of valve replacement vs repair.

King et al. *(2)* reviewed their series of 16 tricuspid annuloplasties and 16 tricuspid valve replacements 4 months to 14 years after mitral valve surgery. Of patients, 53% required concomitant mitral or aortic valve surgery at the time of reoperation. The in-hospital mortality was 25%, and the 5-year actuarial survival was 44%. Moreover, nearly 54% of those surviving longer than 30 days had little or no improvement in tricuspid valve function following the procedure. They concluded that late-onset TR occurring after left-sided surgery was a signal of RV failure, and restoring valve competence was merely palliative: Patient outcome was primarily determined by RV function.

Given the high incidence of late mortality and poor long-term results, the timing of reoperative tricuspid surgery is crucial and probably should not be considered in advanced degrees of RV dysfunction. This approach reemphasizes the need for early diagnosis and treatment of TR when present at the initial operation *(3,55,60,64)*. Our general policy is to treat moderate or severe TR during the initial aortic or mitral valve operation. We share the opinion that reoperation for late-onset TR following left-sided valvular surgery should be approached with caution.

Traumatic TR

The pathophysiology of traumatic TR is thought to involve a severe and sudden elevation in RV intracavitary pressure, leading to disruption of the valve apparatus. This acute-onset regurgitation, if not diagnosed promptly, leads to volume loading of the right ventricle, ventricular enlargement, and subsequent annular dilatation. In a review of 13 patients with nonpenetrating traumatic tricuspid insufficiency, Miller et al. *(70)* found that the primary mechanism of regurgitation was a flail anterior leaflet. In more than 90% of patients, this was caused by ruptured chords, an avulsed anterior papillary muscle, or a tear in the leaflet proper. Severity of the valvular disease and associated injuries will then dictate the appropriateness of surgical repair. A thorough echocardiographic evaluation should also be undertaken at the time of surgery *(70–72)*.

When feasible, tricuspid valve damage should be repaired electively unless tamponade or heart failure mandates immediate intervention *(72)*. It should be noted that delayed presentation is common; in Miller et al.'s series, the average time to presentation was 9 years. Although valve replacement has traditionally been performed, traumatic lesions are frequently amenable to repair, thereby avoiding a mechanical prosthesis and systemic anticoagulation *(70)*.

Carcinoid Tricuspid Valve Disease

The carcinoid syndrome results from midgut carcinoid tumors metastatic to the liver and/or lung. Once these organs are involved, serotonin and other vasoactive amines are released directly into the systemic venous system, thus bypassing the detoxification that would have normally occurred when delivered via the portal vein. These substances produce vasomotor changes, bronchospasm, diarrhea, and telangiectasias. The mural and valvular endothelium of the right heart are directly exposed to these vasoactive products, resulting in endomyocardial fibrosis, diastolic dysfunction, and tricuspid/pulmonic stenosis/insufficiency. Characteristically, the tricuspid and pulmonic valve leaflets are thickened and restricted in motion or even fixed. TR is almost universal. Right heart failure in the absence of left-sided heart disease is common *(73)*.

The natural history of carcinoid heart disease is ominous *(73,74)*. However, the recent development of somatostatin analogs (serotonin antagonists), catheter-based hepatic embolization, and chemotherapy have dramatically improved symptoms and survival, approaching 50% at 5 years *(74–76)*. Unfortunately, right heart failure from tricuspid or pulmonic valve involvement is a common cause of the high mortality in this disease. Approximately one-third of patients with metastatic disease will suffer from right-sided failure *(12)*.

The primary disease should be controlled prior to operative intervention. Patients with rapid deterioration or multisystem organ failure should be excluded from surgery. At the other end of the spectrum, asymptomatic patients should not undergo surgery purely on the basis of echocardiographic evidence of carcinoid heart disease. Generally, one-third of patients with carcinoid heart disease will eventually present to cardiac surgery *(12)*. Preoperatively, somatostatin should be administered prophylactically to prevent the potential intraoperative complications of hypotension, bronchospasm, and tachycardia that can result from tumor release of vasoactive substances *(77,78)*.

The ability to repair valves affected by carcinoid disease is rare, and patients almost always require valve replacement. Involvement of the pulmonary valve may require combined valve replacement or pulmonary valvotomy/valvectomy to avoid right ventricle outflow obstruction. These last procedures should not be used in the setting of advanced right-sided failure. The type of tricuspid replacement, mechanical or bioprosthetic, remains controversial, but this decision does not appear to affect survival significantly. Reports of carcinoid involvement of bioprosthetic tissue leaflets have been reported *(75,79)* and led some to advocate the use of mechanical valves. In such settings, the risk of anticoagulation must be weighed against the potential risk of serotonin-induced damage to bioprosthetic leaflets *(77)*.

The largest surgical series of patients with carcinoid heart disease was reported by Connolly et al. *(78)*. Of 26 patients with tricuspid surgery (who were compared to historical controls), one-third died within 30 days, and half of these deaths were attributed to cardiovascular causes. Of those who survived, another one-third died late from primarily hepatic failure (up to 1.5 years). One-third survived 2 or more years, compared to an 8% survival in historical controls. Those who survived had an improvement of one to two New York Heart Association functional classes. Predictors of late survival included a lower preoperative somatostatin requirement and a lower preoperative 5-hydroxyindoleacetic acid level. However, those with cardiac involvement generally have more symptoms, higher serotonin levels, and increased urine 5-hydroxyindoleacetic acid levels compared to those without cardiac involvement *(80)*. Therefore, patients with carcinoid heart disease have to be selected carefully for operative intervention.

CONCLUSION

The surgical management of right heart failure is primarily directed at the operative strategies for tricuspid valve regurgitation. Timing of operative intervention for TR should take into account the symptomatic status of the patient, a functional assessment of RV function, and consideration of left heart disease. Because tricuspid disease is generally found in combination with valvular or myocardial disease of the left heart, operative management of tricuspid valve disease should be considered at the time of left heart surgery. Early and aggressive surgical attention to the tricuspid valve combined with appropriate patient selection can lead to an improvement in right heart failure.

REFERENCES

1. Jamieson WR, Edwards FH, Schwartz M, Bero JW, Clark RE, Grover FL. Risk stratification for cardiac valve replacement. National Cardiac Surgery Database. Database Committee of the Society of Thoracic Surgeons. Ann Thorac Surg 1999;67:943–951.
2. King RM, Schaff HV, Danielson GK, et al. Surgery for tricuspid regurgitation late after mitral valve replacement. Circulation 1984;70(3 part 2):I193–I197.
3. Kaul TK, Ramsdale DR, Mercer JL. Functional tricuspid regurgitation following replacement of the mitral valve. Int J Cardiol 1991;33:305–313.
4. Khonsari S. Surgery of the Tricuspid Valve. Cardiac Surgery: Safeguards and Pitfalls in Operative Technique. Lippincott-Raven, Philadelphia, PA: 1997, pp. 105–112.
5. Isner JM, Roberts WC. Right ventricular infarction complicating left ventricular infarction secondary to coronary heart disease. Frequency, location, associated findings and significance from analysis of 236 necropsy patients with acute or healed myocardial infarction. Am J Cardiol 1978;42:885–894.
6. D'Arcy B, Nanda NC. Two-dimensional echocardiographic features of right ventricular infarction. Circulation 1982;65:167–173.
7. Korr KS, Levinson H, Bough EW, et al. Tricuspid valve replacement for cardiogenic shock after acute right ventricular infarction. JAMA 1980;244:1958–1960.
8. Louie EK, Lin SS, Reynertson SI, Brundage BH, Levitsky S, Rich S. Pressure and volume loading of the right ventricle have opposite effects on left ventricular ejection fraction. Circulation 1995;92:819–824.
9. Louie EK, Bieniarz T, Moore AM, Levitsky S. Reduced atrial contribution to left ventricular filling in patients with severe tricuspid regurgitation after tricuspid valvulectomy: a Doppler echocardiographic study. J Am Coll Cardiol 1990;16: 1617–1624.
10. Lorell B, Leinbach RC, Pohost GM, et al. Right ventricular infarction. Clinical diagnosis and differentiation from cardiac tamponade and pericardial constriction. Am J Cardiol 1979;43:465–471.

11. Lopez-Sendon J, Coma-Canella I, Gamallo C. Sensitivity and specificity of hemodynamic criteria in the diagnosis of acute right ventricular infarction. Circulation 1981;64:515–525.

12. Lundin L, Hansson HE, Landelius J, Oberg K. Surgical treatment of carcinoid heart disease. J ThoracCardiovasc Surg 1990;100:552–561.

13. Lundin L, Landelius J. Echocardiography for carcinoid heart disease. Ann NY Acad Sci 1994;733:437–445.

14. Goldstein JA, Vlahakes GJ, Verrier ED, et al. Volume loading improves low cardiac output in experimental right ventricular infarction. J Am Coll Cardiol 1983;2:270–278.

15. Topol EJ, Goldschlager N, Ports TA, et al. Hemodynamic benefit of atrial pacing in right ventricular myocardial infarction. Ann Intern Med 1982;96: 594–597.

16. Cohn LH. Tricuspid regurgitation secondary to mitral valve disease: when and how to repair. J Card Surg 1994;9(2 suppl):237–241.

17. Reed GE, Boyd AD, Spencer FC, Engelman RM, Isom OW, Cunningham JN. Operative management of tricuspid regurgitation. Circulation 1976;54(6 suppl): III96–III98.

18. Bex JP, Lecompte Y. Tricuspid valve repair using a flexible linear reducer. J Card Surg 1986;1:151–159.

19. Kay JH. Surgical treatment of tricuspid regurgitation. Ann Thorac Surg 1992;53: 1132–1133.

20. Minale C, Lambertz H, Messmer BJ. New developments for reconstruction of the tricuspid valve. J Thorac Cardiovasc Surg 1987;94:626–631.

21. De Vega NG. [Selective, adjustable and permanent annuloplasty. An original technic for the treatment of tricuspid insufficiency]. Rev Esp Cardiol 1972;25: 555–556.

22. Carpentier A, Deloche A, Hanania G, et al. Surgical management of acquired tricuspid valve disease. J ThoracCardiovasc Surg 1974;67:53–65.

23. Duran CG, Ubago JL. Clinical and hemodynamic performance of a totally flexible prosthetic ring for atrioventricular valve reconstruction. Ann Thorac Surg 1976; 22:458–463.

24. McCarthy JF, Cosgrove DM. Tricuspid valve repair with the Cosgrove-Edwards annuloplasty system. Ann Thorac Surg 1997;64:267–268.

25. Rabago G, Fraile J, Martinell J, Artiz V. Technique and results of tricuspid annuloplasty. J Card Surg 1986;1:247–253.

26. Bonow RO, Carabello B, de Leon AC Jr, et al. Guidelines for the management of patients with valvular heart disease: executive summary. A report of the American College of Cardiology/American Heart Association Task Force on Practice Guidelines (Committee on Management of Patients With Valvular Heart Disease). Circulation 1998;98:1949–1984.

27. Boskovic D, Elezovic I, Simin N, Rolovic Z, Josipovic V. Late thrombosis of the Björk-Shiley tilting disc valve in the tricuspid position. Thrombolytic treatment with streptokinase. J Thorac Cardiovasc Surg 1986;91:1–8.

28. Jegaden O, Perinetti M, Barthelet M, et al. Long-term results of porcine bioprostheses in the tricuspid position. Eur J Cardiothorac Surg 1992;6:256–260.

29. McGrath LB, Chen C, Bailey BM, Fernandez J, Laub GW, Adkins MS. Early and late phase events following bioprosthetic tricuspid valve replacement. J Card Surg 1992;7:245–253.

30. Treasure T. Which prosthetic valve should we choose? Curr Opin Cardiol 1995; 10:144–149.

31. Braunwald E. Valvular heart disease: tricuspid, pulmonic, and multivalvular disease: tricuspid stenosis. In: Braunwald E., Zipes DP, Libby P. eds. Heart Disease. A Textbook of Cardiovascular Medicine, 6th ed. WB Saunders, Philadelphia, PA, 2001, pp. 1643–1722.

32. Gibson R, Wood P. The diagnosis of tricuspid stenosis. Br Heart J 1955; 17:552–562.

33. Kitchen A, Turner R. Diagnosis and treatment of tricuspid stenosis. Br Heart J 1964;26:354–379.

34. Ribeiro PA, Al Zaibag M, Al Kasab S, et al. Percutaneous double balloon valvotomy for rheumatic tricuspid stenosis. Am J Cardiol 1988;61:660–662.

35. Arbulu A, Thoms NW, Wilson RF. Valvulectomy without prosthetic replacement. A lifesaving operation for tricuspid pseudomonas endocarditis. J Thorac Cardiovasc Surg 1972;64:103–107.

36. Arbulu A, Asfaw I. Tricuspid valvulectomy without prosthetic replacement. Ten years of clinical experience. J Thorac Cardiovasc Surg 1981;82:684–691.

37. Arbulu A, Holmes RJ, Asfaw I. Surgical treatment of intractable right-sided infective endocarditis in drug addicts: 25 years experience. J Heart Valve Dis 1993;2: 129–37; discussion 138–139.

38. Karp RB. Acquired disease of the Tricupid Valve. In: Sabiston DC and Spencer FC, eds. Surgery of the Chest, 5th ed. W. B. Saunders, Philadelphia, PA, pp. 1667–1672.

39. Yee ES, Ullyot DJ. Reparative approach for right-sided endocarditis. Operative considerations and results of valvuloplasty. J Thorac Cardiovasc Surg 1988;96: 133–140.

40. Yankah AC, Musci M, Weng Y, et al. Tricuspid valve dysfunction and surgery after orthotopic cardiac transplantation. Eur J Cardiothorac Surg 2000;17: 343–348.

41. Rees AP, Milani RV, Lavie CJ, Smart FW, Ventura HO. Valvular regurgitation and right-sided cardiac pressures in heart transplant recipients by complete Doppler and color flow evaluation. Chest 1993;104:82–87.

42. Votapka TV, Appleton RS, Pennington DG. Tricuspid valve replacement after orthotopic heart transplantation. Ann Thorac Surg 1994;57:752–754.

43. Stahl RD, Karwande SV, Olsen SL, Taylor DO, Hawkins JA, Renlund DG. Tricuspid valve dysfunction in the transplanted heart. Ann Thorac Surg 1995;59: 477–480.

44. Lower RR, Shumway NE. Studies of the orthotopic homotransplantation of the canine heart. Ann Thorac Surg 1960;11:18–23.

45. Shumway NE, Lower RR, Stofer RC. Transplantation of the heart. Adv Surg 1966;2:265–284.

46. Stevenson LW, Dadourian BJ, Kobashigawa J, Child JS, Clark SH, Laks H. Mitral regurgitation after cardiac transplantation. Am J Cardiol 1987;60:119–122.

47. Angermann CE, Spes CH, Tammen A, et al. Anatomic characteristics and valvular function of the transplanted heart: transthoracic vs transesophageal echocardiographic findings. J Heart Transplant 1990;9:331–338.

48. Sievers HH, Weyand M, Kraatz EG, Bernhard A. An alternative technique for orthotopic cardiac transplantation, with preservation of the normal anatomy of the right atrium. Thorac Cardiovasc Surg 1991;39:70–72.

49. Sarsam MA, Campbell CS, Yonan NA, Deiraniya AK, Rahman AN. An alternative surgical technique in orthotopic cardiac transplantation. J Card Surg 1993;8: 344–349.

50. Caves PK, Stinson EB, Billingham ME, Rider AK, Shumway NE. Diagnosis of human cardiac allograft rejection by serial cardiac biopsy. J Thorac Cardiovasc Surg 1973;66:461–466.

51. Fowles RE, Mason JW. Endomyocardial biopsy. Ann Intern Med 1982;97: 885–894.

52. Braverman AC, Coplen SE, Mudge GH, Lee RT. Ruptured chordae tendineae of the tricuspid valve as a complication of endomyocardial biopsy in heart transplant patients. Am J Cardiol 1990;66:111–113.

53. Huddleston CB, Rosenbloom M, Goldstein JA, Pasque MK. Biopsy-induced tricuspid regurgitation after cardiac transplantation. Ann Thorac Surg 1994;57: 832–836; discussion 836–837.

54. Lewen MK, Bryg RJ, Miller LW, Williams GA, Labovitz AJ. Tricuspid regurgitation by Doppler echocardiography after orthotopic cardiac transplantation. Am J Cardiol 1987;59:1371–1374.

55. Barlow JB. Mitral valve disease: a cardiologic-surgical interaction. Isr J Med Sci 1996;32:831–842, 843–844.

56. Popcock, WA, Antunes MJ, Sareli P, Meyer TE. Late postoperative course and complicatons: emphasis on the "restriction-dilation" syndrome. In: Barlow JB, ed. Perspectives on the Mitral Valve. FA Davis, Philadelphia, PA, 1987, pp. 270–288.

57. Barlow JB. Aspects of tricuspid valve disease, heart failure and the "restriction-dilatation syndrome." Rev Port Cardiol 1995;14:991–1004.

58. Barlow JB. Aspects of mitral and tricuspid regurgitation. J Cardiol Suppl 1991; 25:3–33.

59. Groves PH, Lewis NP, Ikram S, Maire R, Hall RJ. Reduced exercise capacity in patients with tricuspid regurgitation after successful mitral valve replacement for rheumatic mitral valve disease. Br Heart J 1991;66:295–301.

60. Groves PH, Hall RJ. Late tricuspid regurgitation following mitral valve surgery. J Heart Valve Dis 1992;1:80–86.

61. Groves PH, Ikram S, Ingold U, Hall RJ. Tricuspid regurgitation following mitral valve replacement: an echocardiographic study. J Heart Valve Dis 1993;2:273–278.

62. Cohen SR, Sell JE, McIntosh CL, Clark RE. Tricuspid regurgitation in patients with acquired, chronic, pure mitral regurgitation. II. Nonoperative management, tricuspid valve annuloplasty, and tricuspid valve replacement. J Thorac Cardiovasc Surg 1987;94:488–497.

63. Goldman ME, Guarino T, Fuster V, Mindich B. The necessity for tricuspid valve repair can be determined intraoperatively by two-dimensional echocardiography. J Thorac Cardiovasc Surg 1987;94:542–550.

64. Porter A, Shapira Y, Wurzel M, et al. Tricuspid regurgitation late after mitral valve replacement: clinical and echocardiographic evaluation. J Heart Valve Dis 1999;8: 57–62.

65. Braunwald NS, Ross J, Morrow AG. Conservative management of tricuspid regurgitation in patients undergoing mitral valve replacement. Circulation 1967;35 (4 suppl):I63–I69.

66. Brilla C, Hammen M, Jaksch R, Unterberg R, Seboldt H, Karsch KR. [Effect of tricuspid annuloplasty in mitral/aortic valve replacement on the clinical aspects and global function of the right heart chamber]. Thorac Cardiovasc Surg 1988;36: 122–126.

67. Breyer RH, McClenathan JH, Michaelis LL, McIntosh CL, Morrow AG. Tricuspid regurgitation. A comparison of nonoperative management, tricuspid annuloplasty, and tricuspid valve replacement. J Thorac Cardiovasc Surg 1976;72:867–874.

68. Duran CM, Pomar JL, Colman T, Figueroa A, Revuelta JM, Ubago JL. Is tricuspid valve repair necessary? J Thorac Cardiovasc Surg 1980;80:849–860.
69. Staab ME, Nishimura RA, Dearani JA. Isolated tricuspid valve surgery for severe tricuspid regurgitation following prior left heart valve surgery: analysis of outcome in 34 patients. J Heart Valve Dis 1999;8:567–574.
70. Miller FA, Seward JB, Gersh BJ, Tajik AJ, Mucha P. Two-dimensional echocardiographic findings in cardiac trauma. Am J Cardiol 1982;50:1022–1027.
71. Chirillo F, Totis O, Cavarzerani A, et al. Usefulness of transthoracic and transoesophageal echocardiography in recognition and management of cardiovascular injuries after blunt chest trauma. Heart 1996;75:301–306.
72. Doty JR, Cameron DE, Elmaci T, Salomon NW. Penetrating trauma to the tricuspid valve and ventricular septum: delayed repair. Ann Thorac Surg 1999;67: 252–253.
73. Soga J, Yakuwa Y, Osaka M. Carcinoid syndrome: a statistical evaluation of 748 reported cases. J Exp Clin Cancer Res 1999;18:133–141.
74. Moertel CG. Karnofsky memorial lecture. An odyssey in the land of small tumors. J Clin Oncol 1987;5:1502–1522.
75. Knott-Craig CJ, Schaff HV, Mullany CJ, et al. Carcinoid disease of the heart. Surgical management of 10 patients. J Thorac Cardiovasc Surg 1992;104: 475–481.
76. Oberg K, Persson U, Alm G, Eriksson B. Long-term treatment with alpha interferons of patients with malignant carcinoid tumors: the 6 year experience. In: Stewart WE, Schellekens H, eds. The Biology of the Interferon System. Elsevier, Amsterdam, The Netherlands: 1989, pp. 361–384.
77. DiSesa VJ, Mills RM, Collins JJ. Surgical management of carcinoid heart disease. Chest 1985;88:789–791.
78. Connolly HM, Nishimura RA, Smith HC, Pellikka PA, Mullany CJ, Kvols LK. Outcome of cardiac surgery for carcinoid heart disease. J Am Coll Cardiol 1995; 25:410–416.
79. Schoen FJ, Hausner RJ, Howell JF, Beazley HL, Titus JL. Porcine heterograft valve replacement in carcinoid heart disease. J Thorac Cardiovasc Surg 1981;81: 100–105.
80. Robiolio PA, Rigolin VH, Wilson JS, et al. Carcinoid heart disease. Correlation of high serotonin levels with valvular abnormalities detected by cardiac catheterization and echocardiography. Circulation 1995;92:790–795.
81. deRibrolles C. Techniques de correction de L'insuffisance trcuspidienne. In: Bex JP, ed. Pathologie de la valve tricuspide. Masson, Paris: 1981 pp. 24–34.
82. Boyd A, Engleman R, Isom OW, et al. Tricuspid annuloplasty, five and one-half years' experience with 78 patients. J Thorac Cardiovasc Surg 1974;68:344.
83. Grossman W, ed. Cardiac Catheterization and Angiography, 5th ed. Lea and Febiger, Philadelphia, PA: 1996.

6 Pacing in Heart Failure

Uday N. Kumar, MD, Teresa De Marco, MD, and Leslie A. Saxon, MD

CONTENTS

INTRODUCTION

Background

Heart failure is a disease of immense burden and cost to individuals and society. It is estimated that more than 4.5 million people in the United States currently suffer from heart failure, and more than 400,000 cases are newly diagnosed each year *(1)*. The prevalence of the disease increases with age such that nearly 10% of the population will be affected in the ninth decade of life *(2)*. Furthermore, heart failure is the leading cause of hospitalizations of individuals older than 65 years, and it was estimated that there would be more than 1 million hospitalizations for heart failure in 2004, with an economic cost exceeding

From: *Contemporary Cardiology: Surgical Management of Congestive Heart Failure*
Edited by: J. C. Fang and G. S. Couper © Humana Press Inc., Totowa, NJ

$40 billion *(3)*. Given the tremendous scope of heart failure, a great deal of research has gone into finding therapies that can reduce its morbidity and mortality.

Numerous trials have resulted in guidelines that currently recommend the use of β-blockers, angiotensin-converting enzyme (ACE) inhibitors, diuretics, aldosterone antagonists, and digoxin for the treatment of patients with heart failure at various stages of the disease *(4)*. Despite these advances in the pharmacological management of patients with heart failure, it is clear that there still remain a significant number of patients with persistent symptoms who are on maximal medical therapy. More important, heart failure continues to be one of the most progressive and lethal diseases and still directly and indirectly contributes to 250,000 deaths annually *(4)*. It is expected that the personal, societal, and economic burden of heart failure will only grow as the number of individuals over the age of 65 increases in the next few decades. Given this background, device therapies represent a promising new modality in the treatment of patients with heart failure, especially as advances in these device technologies allow them to be studied in a very safe and controlled manner.

Ventricular Dyssynchrony

An important characteristic of heart failure is the presence of dysrhythmias and conduction system abnormalities. Some have estimated that up to 53% of patients with heart failure have an intraventricular conduction delay (IVCD) that can lead to abnormal electrical depolarization and subsequent dyssynchrony between the right and left ventricles *(5)*. Although many efforts have focused on other aspects of heart failure, such as optimization of preload, afterload, and contractility, technological breakthroughs have now made addressing the correction of ventricular dyssynchrony a possibility. This is significant because the consequences of ventricular dyssynchrony, including abnormal interventricular septal wall motion, reduction in stroke volume, reduction in the rate of rise of left ventricular (LV) pressure, diminished diastolic filling times, and prolongation of mitral regurgitation, all contribute to worsening heart failure and can cause symptomatic deterioration *(6–8)*.

To identify patients for whom ventricular dyssynchrony may be a problem, the presence of a bundle branch block (BBB) or IVCD on a standard electrocardiogram (ECG) has been used because these findings are the manifestation of ventricular dyssynchrony. In fact, the presence of a wide QRS complex has been shown to be an independent or contributing risk factor in patients with heart failure, with the degree of conduction delay possibly serving as a marker of disease severity *(5,9–12)*.

Thus, it was hypothesized that, because ventricular dyssynchrony is primarily an aberrance of normal conduction, perhaps pacemakers, which are primarily designed to treat atrioventricular (AV) and sinus node conduction defects, could be modified to help correct ventricular dyssynchrony and its deleterious consequences.

Role of Pacemakers

Numerous pacing strategies using traditional right-sided pacemakers, which have right atrial (RA) and right ventricular (RV) leads, have been attempted to resynchronize electrical depolarization. Attempts to manipulate parameters, such as the AV delay, have yielded inconsistent results and in certain cases have worsened ventricular dyssynchrony *(6–8,13–20)*.

These results subsequently led to investigations of various stimulation sites within the right ventricle, including the apex, septum, and outflow tract, as well as studies looking at LV and biventricular (BV) stimulation using epicardial leads placed through a thoracotomy. Except for a small subset of patients with dilated cardiomyopathy (DCM) for whom traditional right-sided pacing may have a role, results have convincingly demonstrated that LV and BV strategies are far superior in achieving a hemodynamic improvement, in part thought to be because of improvement of ventricular dyssynchrony *(21–26)*.

Figure 1 demonstrates the ECG from a patient enrolled in a resynchronization trial at baseline and after BV stimulation; note the narrowing of the QRS complex with BV stimulation. In terms of specific parameters, improved LV contractility, increased pulse pressure, decreased myocardial oxygen utilization, decreased LV end-diastolic and end-systolic volumes, and improved myocardial performance index have all been seen *(23,25–31)*. Furthermore, improvement in 6-minute walk distances, oxygen uptake at peak exercise, quality-of-life (QoL) scores, and New York Heart Association (NYHA) class has been seen *(31–33)*. Finally, preliminary results from currently ongoing randomized trials have shown that BV resynchronization in patients with heart failure significantly improves myocardial performance and numerous clinical parameters. Perhaps most important, recently reported data comparing resynchronization therapy to medical therapy demonstrated significant improvements in the composite end points of all-cause hospitalization and mortality *(34–37)*.

A   NSR Left BBB

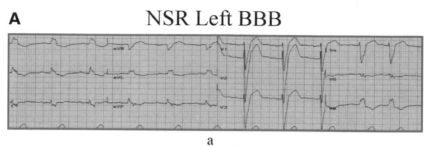

a

B   Atrial Sensed (VDD) BV Stimulation

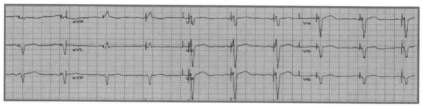

Fig. 1. (A) Baseline electrocardiogram from a patient enrolled in a resynchronization trial demonstrating normal sinus rhythm (NSR) and a left bundle branch block (BBB). (B) Electrocardiogram in the same patient during atrial-sensed (VDD mode) biventricular stimulation showing narrowing of the QRS complex.

An important aspect of recent trials has been the replacement of LV epicardial leads placed via a thoracotomy by coronary venous leads placed percutaneously; initial experience with these leads has been very good in terms of their functioning and in terms of reduced implantation morbidity *(38,39)*. Based on this technological advancement, current investigational systems now incorporate entirely percutaneously placed leads and support various programmable resynchronization therapies.

This chapter reviews the established and emerging indications for pacing devices in the setting of heart failure. The discussion briefly considers the use of standard dual-chamber pacing in DCM and the role of pacing in patients with atrial fibrillation (AF), but mainly focuses on the use of resynchronization therapies in patients with heart failure. Current trials of resynchronization therapies also are reviewed.

STANDARD DUAL-CHAMBER PACING
IN DILATED CARDIOMYOPATHY

Rationale

The effect of standard dual-chamber pacing in DCM is not clearly understood. A potential benefit was suggested in an uncontrolled study of 17 patients with DCM who had medically refractory heart failure and severe symptoms *(15,16)*. Pacing was in the dual mode, dual pacing, dual sensing mode with an AV interval of 100 ms, and patients were followed for up to 5 years. All patients had significant improvements in functional capacity, which was maintained throughout the follow-up period, and in left ventricular ejection fraction (LVEF; 16 vs 26%), which tended to decrease with time. No patient required hospitalization for an exacerbation of heart failure. During the first few months after implantation, cessation of pacing for 2 to 4 hours led to a marked reduction in LVEF; in comparison, pacing withdrawal in later months had a progressively less-deleterious effect *(16)*. The median survival was 22 months, with no patient dying from progressive heart failure. Although much enthusiasm resulted from these data, a well-controlled trial of chronic short AV delay pacing did not find a consistent benefit *(17)*.

Potential Mechanisms

Despite the possible benefit of dual-chamber pacing in DCM, the mechanisms responsible for the improvements seen in some trials are still poorly understood. Possible mechanisms include increased filling time, optimization of left heart mechanical AV delay, and normalization of intraventricular activation, which result in a more coordinated ventricular contraction pattern and an improvement in LVEF *(40)*. When ventricular contraction occurs shortly after atrial contraction, valve closure is optimized, and the time for diastolic mitral regurgitation is minimized. In addition, atrial pacing is less effective than atrial sensing and ventricular pacing (ventricular sensing dual mode, dual pacing [VDD] mode), possibly because of an increase in interatrial conduction delay.

Current and Future Indications

Although the data on dual-chamber pacing in the patient with DCM are limited, it seems likely that a subset of patients will benefit. However, there is no clear method to predict which patients will respond, and thus there are currently no established criteria to identify the patient who will benefit from dual-chamber pacing or to determine when it should be used.

The future in this area may lie with multisite ventricular pacing, including transvenous BV stimulation with standard RA pacing, or through the development of techniques and technologies, which will allow for pacing leads to be placed in the optimal atrial and ventricular sites to minimize conduction delays *(41)*. Data about these types of pacing strategies also remain limited, and there is as yet no consensus on how to optimize the parameters of these systems. However, it is hoped numerous ongoing trials of various pacing strategies in heart failure, described below, will lead to the establishment of guidelines defining when and how a particular pacing strategy should be used in DCM.

PACING IN ATRIAL FIBRILLATION

Background

Paroxysmal or persistent AF occurs in up to 30% of patients with heart failure (42). Low-dose amiodarone is the safest and most efficacious therapy for maintenance of normal sinus rhythm (NSR) and ventricular rate control (43). However, up to 30 to 40% of patients with heart failure will have recurrent AF on low-dose amiodarone or have a side effect or contraindication to amiodarone therapy (42,43).

Drugs with AV nodal blocking properties traditionally used to control the rate response to AF, such as calcium channel blockers or β-blockers, may be contraindicated in some patients with heart failure or not be well tolerated at the doses needed to achieve rate control during activity. In addition, a small percentage of patients with a rapid ventricular response to AF may actually have a tachycardia-mediated cardiomyopathy and will experience improvement in LVEF with control of the ventricular response (44).

Role for Pacemakers

Both rate control (45,46) and rate regularity (46–48) appear to be important to optimize symptom status in patients with AF, particularly in the presence of depressed ventricular function. Both of these objectives can be achieved with radiofrequency ablation of the AV node and pacemaker therapy with traditional RV-based pacemakers. As an example, a controlled trial evaluated the efficacy of this approach in 66 patients with clinical heart failure, AF, and a resting ventricular rate greater than 90 beats per minute; the patients were randomly assigned to pharmacological AV nodal blockade or AV nodal ablation and implantation of a ventricular rate-responsive pacemaker (48). After a 12-month follow-up, patients undergoing AV nodal ablation and a pacemaker had significant reductions in palpitations (78%) and dyspnea with exertion (22%) compared to those receiving pharmacological therapy. There was, however, no difference in overall QoL, NYHA functional class, or objective measures of cardiac function; cardiac performance remained stable over time in both groups. In addition, another long-term observational study found that AV nodal ablation and pacing had no adverse effects on survival (49).

To avoid the need for a pacemaker, AV nodal modification rather than ablation has been proposed. One study addressed this issue by randomly assigning 44 patients with heart failure and uncontrolled AF to AV nodal ablation or modification *(50)*. Nodal modification was associated with a small improvement in exercise tolerance, but no change in LVEF or QoL scores. It also resulted in a substantial risk of late complete heart block. In contrast, nodal ablation was associated with a significant improvement in all of these parameters.

Pacing using an LV lead to achieve cardiac resynchronization could potentially extend the benefit of radio-frequency AV nodal ablation followed by standard pacing in AF and thus merits further clinical study *(51)*.

His Bundle Pacing in Atrial Fibrillation

A still-investigational approach for patients with DCM who have chronic AF and normal ventricular activation (QRS ≤ 120 ms) is direct His bundle pacing. Compared to apical pacing, His bundle pacing produces synchronous ventricular depolarization and improved cardiac function. This was illustrated in a series of 18 patients in whom the ventricular rate during AF was controlled pharmacologically or with ablation; chronic His bundle pacing was accomplished using a single-chamber rate-responsive pacemaker and a screw-in lead *(52)*. After a 23-month follow-up, there was a reduction in LV end-diastolic and end-systolic dimensions, an increase in LVEF from 20 to 31%, and a decrease in the cardiothoracic ratio. However, given the high incidence of an IVCD in these patients, this approach may be limited to only a subset of patients with intact intraventricular conduction who are not pacemaker dependent.

RESYNCHRONIZATION THERAPY

Definition

Pacing modalities that utilize BV or LV stimulation to optimize cardiac pump function through synchronization of ventricular contraction are referred to as *resynchronization* or *ventricular resynchronization* therapy *(53)*. Resynchronization therapies can be present in a single device or in a device equipped with bradycardia pacing support or incorporated into an implantable cardioverter defibrillator (ICD).

Rationale

As briefly outlined in the introduction, the rationale for resynchronization therapy is based on several observational studies that showed that the presence of an IVCD, as manifested by a prolonged QRS, in patients with heart failure caused by systolic dysfunction was associated with a worsening of symptom class status and poorer overall outcome when compared to matched patients with normal intraventricular conduction *(6,9)*. Data from the PATH-CHF trial suggested that a QRS duration of 155 ms had the best positive and negative predictive accuracy for predicting hemodynamic improvement with BV pacing *(54)*. Other studies have shown that the longer the QRS delay at baseline, the greater the response to resynchronization therapy; however, it is unclear if the extent of QRS narrowing because of resynchronization can predict the extent of the response to therapy *(24)*.

Resynchronization therapy is currently approved in Europe for symptomatic heart failure that occurs in the setting of IVCD or BBB. This approval was granted on the basis of several studies of acute resynchronization therapy and data compiled for approx 150 patients receiving BV or LV stimulation for 3 months as part of two nonrandomized studies, InSync and PATH-CHF *(31,32,36)*. Because it is estimated that 20 to 30% of patients with symptomatic heart failure have an IVCD and resultant discordant ventricular contraction, there are many patients who may qualify for resynchronization therapy *(34)*. In fact, it has been estimated that approx 10%% of an unselected group of patients with heart failure would be appropriate candidates for resynchronization therapy *(55)*.

There is also another setting in which resynchronization might be important. It is estimated that approx 8 to 15% of patients with advanced heart failure have pacemakers implanted for symptomatic bradycardia; an additional group of patients with heart failure have an ICD and use the bradycardia feature of the device to pace the right ventricle. Such patients have an increased risk of mortality or urgent transplantation because of progressive pump dysfunction; in one series, the risk at 1 year was 49 vs 15% in patients without a pacemaker *(56)*. This difference may be in part be caused by the dyssynchronous contraction caused by right ventricle-based pacing. Whether such patients would benefit from "upgrading" these devices to resynchronization therapies by the addition of an LV lead is not known.

Results of the DAVID Trial suggested that there may be deleterious effects of chronic right ventricle pacing in patients with impaired LV function *(57)*. The observation that the risk of heart failure hospitalization is higher in patients receiving ventricular pacing challenges us to reconsider whether a more physiological way of pacing can be achieved in bradycardia-indicated patients with depressed LV function. Furthermore, uncontrolled data, reported in patients with AF who were receiving chronic right ventricle pacing, suggested that improvement in symptoms and a reduction in heart failure hospitalizations can be achieved *(58)*.

Data from animal models of heart failure with and without dyssynchrony indicated that dyssynchrony can result in alterations in myocardial protein expression *(59)*. These are the first data to demonstrate evidence of molecular remodeling associated with chronic dyssynchrony.

Potential Mechanisms

EFFECT ON CONTRACTILE FUNCTION

Hemodynamic data acquired in patients with heart failure and BBB during acute BV or LV stimulation have consistently shown improvements in measures of contractile response, such as force of contraction, cardiac output, LVEF, and pulmonary artery pressure, when compared to NSR or right ventricle pacing *(21,23–26,60–62)*. Interestingly, in contrast to other therapies that increase myocardial contractility, BV and LV stimulation appear to reduce myocardial energy demands and myocardial oxygen consumption modestly *(28)*.

In one study of 18 patients with DCM and an IVCD, aortic and LV pressures, dp/dt, and pressure–volume measurements were obtained during acute stimulation at single RV endocardial or single LV epicardial sites or during BV pacing *(25)*. The following observations were made:

- There was an improvement in systolic pressures with LV free wall or BV stimulation, primarily because of an improvement in systolic function; there was no benefit on diastolic filling pressure or relaxation.
- RV apical or septal stimulation did not produce any hemodynamic changes.
- Patients who had the greatest hemodynamic improvement had the longest QRS duration (i.e., the greatest IVCD); however, the QRS duration did not consistently shorten with stimulation. In addition, the conduction delay pattern generally predicted the pacing sites of greatest benefit.

Another study evaluated the effects of acute resynchronization therapy on the coordination of global contraction in 13 patients with DCM and an IVCD, using the novel method of phase analysis applied to equilibrium-gated blood pool scintigraphy *(61)*. During sinus rhythm, ventricular contraction was markedly abnormal, and the degree of interventricular dyssynchrony correlated with the LVEF; the more marked the conduction system delay, the more inhomogeneous was the ventricular contraction. Resynchronization therapy using BV pacing improved measures of ventricular coordination that correlated with acute improvements in LVEF; the degree of interventricular dyssynchrony present in sinus rhythm correlated with the magnitude of improvement in synchrony during BV pacing *(61)*.

Interestingly, although markers of sympathetic activation, such as serum norepinephrine and heart rate variability, often vary directly with the severity of heart failure, these markers have not predictably changed in patients for whom resynchronization therapy appears to improve contractile function *(63–65)*.

REVERSE REMODELING

Based on echocardiographic data, preliminary results from the Multicenter InSync Randomized Clinical Investigation (MIRACLE) trial suggested that BV pacing is associated with reverse remodeling in patients with heart failure *(66,67)*. BV pacing produced very significant reduction in mitral regurgitation jet area and a significant reduction in LV mass, both signs of reverse remodeling. Reverse remodeling, particularly by LV dimension measures, was also seen in the CONTAK CD, VIGOR-CHF, and PATH-CHF trials, in which there were significant reductions in both LV end-systolic and end-diastolic dimensions among patients receiving BV pacing *(66–68)*.

Figure 2 demonstrates improvements in LV systolic volume, diastolic volume, and internal dimension indices observed in the VIGOR-CHF trial after 12 weeks of continuous BV pacing in 34 patients. Figure 3 illustrates changes in LV dimension indices observed in more than 400 patients followed for 6 months in the CONTAK CD trial who were randomly assigned to resynchronization therapy or to no resynchronization therapy. Echocardiograms were analyzed at a single core laboratory in both studies and had excellent intra- and interobserver variability *(67,68)*.

Similar improvements in LV size and thickness have been reported from the MIRACLE trial *(69)*.

Surgical Issues Regarding Implantation of Resynchronization Devices

HISTORY OF IMPLANTATION OF BV SYSTEMS

In the first clinical trials, PATH-CHF and VIGOR-CHF, LV stimulation was achieved using a limited thoracotomy, and an active fixation epicardial lead was placed on the LV. The LV lead body was then tunneled to the pectoral space. The right-sided atrial and ventricular leads were implanted using a transvenous approach. This procedure was associated with additional operative risk because of the underlying

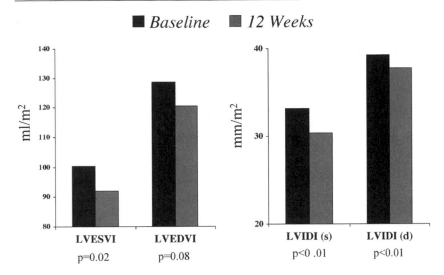

Fig. 2. Improvements in left ventricular systolic and diastolic volume indices and internal dimensions at baseline and after 12 weeks of biventricular (BV) stimulation in the VIGOR-CHF trial. LVESVI, left ventricular end-systolic volume index; LVEDVI, LV end-diastolic volume index; LVIDI, LV internal dimension index during systole (s) or diastole (d).

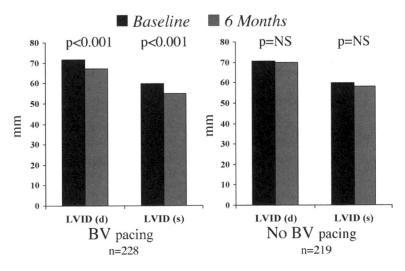

Fig. 3. Changes observed in left ventricular (LV) internal dimension at baseline and after 6 months in the CONTAK CD trial. Improvements in LV internal dimensions were only seen with biventricular (BV) pacing. LVID, LV internal dimension during diastole (d) or systole (s); NS, not significant.

severity of heart failure in the patients undergoing implantation coupled with the need for general anesthesia *(70)*. The expected complications, such as pneumonia and pleural effusions, occurred because of the need for a thoracotomy. In addition, exacerbations of underlying heart failure were observed. The epicardial LV leads were less reliable than endocardial RV or subsequent epicardial coronary sinus leads and had a greater than 10% risk of chronic elevation of capture thresholds *(34–36)*. There were additional concerns about LV epicardial lead placement using a thoracotomy because this approach provides limited epicardial exposure and risks compromise to a bypass conduit in patients with a prior history of coronary artery bypass grafting. Despite these concerns, patients enrolled in these early trials had improvement in the clinical measures of therapy efficacy *(31,36,43,53)*. Yet, the need for a thoracotomy and suboptimal performance of the epicardial lead limited applicability of the therapy to the more advanced heart failure group.

EVOLUTION OF PACING TECHNOLOGY

The coronary sinus provides for the venous drainage from the heart and can be accessed from its os in the inferior septal RA at the tricuspid annulus. The vein then continues as the great cardiac vein along the AV groove, eventually becoming the anterior interventricular vein. There are several other major branch vein tributaries, in some cases extending toward the apex of the LV. These include the posterior, middle cardiac, or lateral veins and the anterior interventricular vein.

Figure 4 demonstrates the normal anatomy of the coronary sinus and branch veins in the right anterior oblique (RAO) and left anterior oblique (LAO) radiographic views, obtained by occlusive venography. There is also marked patient variability in the location of the coronary os, the course of the great cardiac vein, and the extent and course of the major tributaries. This is particularly true in subjects with heart failure with both ischemic and nonischemic etiologies of heart failure. Figure 5A illustrates the coronary sinus anatomy, obtained by occlusive venography, in a patient with ischemic cardiomyopathy. The major branch veins are atretic, tortuous, and narrowed. Figure 5B shows an over-the-wire coronary sinus lead successfully placed in the anterolateral branch of the lateral vein. The types of variabilities seen in these vessels require novel lead designs beyond those used for standard transvenous pacing of the endocardial RA and RV surfaces.

Electrogram recordings from temporary pacing and recording catheters placed in the great cardiac vein, along the AV groove, are frequently used in electrophysiology studies. Recordings of electrical activity along the inferior tricuspid and mitral annulus help target sites

RAO   LAO

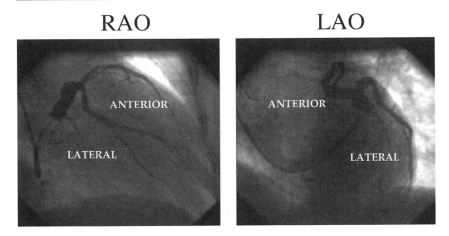

Fig. 4. Fluoroscopic views obtained in the right anterior oblique (RAO) and left anterior oblique (LAO) projections illustrating the coronary sinus branch vein anatomy. In this example, the anterior and lateral cardiac branch veins are seen; the posterior vein is not visualized.

RAO   RAO

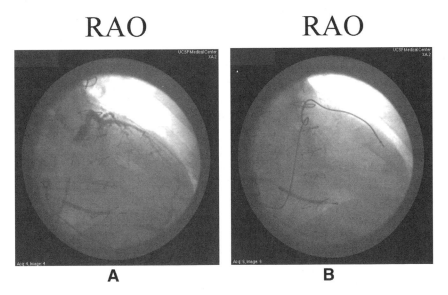

A   **B**

Fig. 5. **(A)** Fluoroscopic right anterior oblique (RAO) occlusive venogram of the coronary sinus showing atretic coronary sinus branch veins. Note the collateral flow to the posterior vein from the anterior interventricular vein. This patient had a prior left anterior descending artery infarction. **(B)** Successful placement of an over-the-wire chronic left ventricular lead in the mid- to apical portion of the anterolateral vein despite the small caliber of the veins. A defibrillation lead is seen in the right ventricular apex.

for ablation of AV nodal reentrant tachycardia accessory pathways
(71). Cannulation of one of the branch vein tributaries allows for
pacing and recording of the LV. Historically, chronic pacing leads
placed in the great cardiac vein or a branch vein have been used to
achieve left atrial (LA) pacing in patients with congenital heart disease
or other anatomic limitations to placement of RA leads. The coronary
sinus leads were more difficult to place and subject to dislodgment
(72). Chronic leads placed in the great cardiac vein were also used in
the early transvenous defibrillators as a component of the shocking
lead defibrillation circuit *(72)*.

In 1997 and 1998, chronic transvenous coronary sinus pacing leads
were incorporated into clinical trials for pacing the LV to achieve LV
stimulation for use in BV or LV resynchronization devices. The earliest transvenous lead, employed in the initial phases of the European
InSync trial, was designed and approved for atrial pacing from the
coronary sinus (Medtronic Inc., Attain™ model 2188). This lead was
placed in a coronary sinus tributary to achieve LV pacing, mostly at the
base of the heart. The lead is a traditional pacing lead maneuvered
using shaped stylets placed through the lumen of the lead. LV pacing
could be achieved in more than 70% of patients using this lead *(31,32)*.
Subsequent modifications to this stylet-driven coronary sinus lead
(Attain™ model 2187) have improved the ability to place leads in several venous tributaries and to advance the lead further toward the apex
of the LV. This has improved lead placement success rates to 90% as
well as resulting in excellent long-term patient thresholds *(66,73)*.

A major breakthrough in lead technology was the development of an
over-the-wire lead designed specifically for coronary sinus branch vein
LV pacing (Guidant Corp., EASYTRAK™), which was incorporated
into clinical trials in 1998. This lead, unlike stylet-driven leads, has an
open lumen that permits atraumatic steerability. The lead is tracked over
a standard 0.014 guide wire to allow access to multiple sites within the
branch veins. In addition, it is small caliber (4 French size), allowing it
to be placed in a more tapered, distal vein location. The distal section of
the lead is flexible with an atraumatic silicone rubber tip. Unlike the
newer stylet-driven leads, this lead has a tined tip, which allows for passive fixation, stabilizing the lead in a terminal vein *(39)*. Acute and
chronic pacing thresholds are excellent, and the implant success rates
exceed 95% in centers with implant experience *(73)*. Figure 6 shows
RAO and LAO radiographic images of an over-the-wire lead placed in
a basal LV location in a patient with ischemic cardiomyopathy; Figure 7
shows an over-the-wire lead in an apical-lateral LV location in a patient
with nonischemic cardiomyopathy.

RAO   LAO

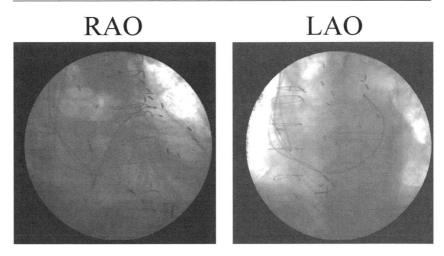

Fig. 6. Fluoroscopic right anterior oblique (RAO) and left anterior oblique (LAO) views of a coronary sinus lead placed in the anterolateral vein of the coronary sinus in a patient with ischemic cardiomyopathy. Despite the fact that the lead could only be advanced to the midbasal left ventricle because of prior bypass surgery, excellent left ventricular sensing and capture thresholds were obtained, and the patient symptomatically improved.

RAO   LAO

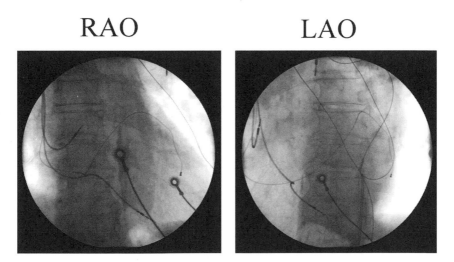

Fig. 7. Fluoroscopic right anterior oblique (RAO) and left anterior oblique (LAO) views of a coronary sinus lead placed in an apical-lateral left ventricular location in a patient with nonischemic cardiomyopathy. The large branch vein caliber allowed advancement of the lead deep into the branch vein. Endocardial right atrial appendage and right ventricular apical leads are also seen.

IMPLANTATION OF THE CORONARY SINUS BRANCH VEIN LV LEAD

Significant care and thoughtful planning need to be taken to implant resynchronization devices successfully with minimal operative morbidity and mortality. The patient population with advanced systolic dysfunction and left BBB are particularly vulnerable to operative complications resulting from excessive procedure times. General anesthesia with endotracheal intubation, excessive contrast use, and fluid administration are all poorly tolerated (investigating officers of COMPANION Steering Committee Implant Guidelines, personal communication, March 12, 2001).

There are several important considerations in the successful placement of a coronary sinus LV lead that extend beyond the need to obtain a stable branch vein lead position with an acceptable pacing threshold. A delivery system must also be used to access the coronary sinus os and provide stability and support in the RA and in the great cardiac vein to permit lead placement in a branch vein. In addition, the coronary sinus branch vein anatomy needs to be at least partially visualized.

After cannulation of a right- or left-sided subclavian or cephalic vein (the left-sided approach is favored in the United States; the right-sided approach is favored in Europe), a flexible guide catheter is placed over an electrophysiology electrode catheter or guide wire into the great cardiac vein. The electrophysiology electrode catheter is advantageous because it allows for both anatomical and electrical documentation of the guide catheter in its proper location in the great cardiac vein. Preformed tip shapes are currently available to accommodate anatomic variations. These guiding sheaths have flexible tips to minimize the risk of vascular trauma and should not be placed without a guiding wire or catheter.

Coronary sinus venography can then be performed with a gentle injection of contrast, either directly through the end of the guiding catheter or with the addition of an occluding balloon to visualize the branch veins and provide a "road map" to facilitate lead placement. Because of retrograde flow from the coronary sinus, a balloon inflation during injection of contrast usually allows more complete visualization of the branch veins, but may be associated with a higher incidence of coronary sinus trauma (39). It is imperative to have a fluoroscopy system capable of both RAO and LAO projections to identify lead position correctly. The lead is then deployed to the branch vein through the guide and placed in a stable position.

Of note, the majority of coronary sinus leads have been placed in the midportion of the ventricle midway between the apex and base, most often in a lateral or anterior-lateral branch vein. It is critically important not only to document acceptable LV lead pacing and sensing thresholds, but also to test for phrenic nerve stimulation, which can occur when pacing from an epicardial LV site. If phrenic nerve stimulation is present, the lead must be maneuvered to an alternative location.

Once an acceptable lead position within a branch vein is achieved, the guide catheter must be removed without dislodgment of the lead. This procedure must be performed under continuous fluoroscopic guidance and with care. A stylet or other stiff wire can be placed partially through the lead to aid in lead stability during guide catheter removal, or the lumenal wire can be left in place. The guide is removed primarily or may be cut and peeled away, depending on guide design. After lead removal, the lead is fixed at the venotomy site and to the fascia using standard practices incorporating lead sleeves.

Most physicians who are experienced in LV lead implants prefer to implant the RA and RV pacing leads prior to coronary sinus lead placement. The rationale for this practice is that it helps to identify the right-sided anatomy as well as provides the capability of RV pacing support in the event that transient heart block is observed during LV lead placement.

The technical difficulties encountered during implants are most commonly related to two issues: (1) difficulty in engaging the coronary sinus os and branch vein to permit advancement of a guiding sheath and (2) difficulty in obtaining a stable branch vein position to allow for acceptable sensing and pacing thresholds without phrenic nerve stimulation (investigating officers of COMPANION Steering Committee Implant Guidelines, personal communication, March 12, 2001). In addition, the variations in coronary sinus anatomy may render identification and cannulation of the os and great cardiac vein difficult. The presence of semilunar valves at the os and in the course of the great cardiac vein may further impede lead placement (74).

The incidence of trauma to the coronary sinus is 2–5%, occurring during some part of the LV lead delivery procedure (investigating officers of COMPANION Steering Committee Implant Guidelines, personal communication, March 12, 2001). The majority of these events involve staining of the coronary sinus intima and do not result in clinical sequelae such as cardiac tamponade. The incidence of coronary sinus perforation resulting in tamponade is less than 1% (66).

LONG-TERM ISSUES

Technology continues to evolve, and improvements in both the LV leads and the delivery tools occur constantly. Thus far, 1-year follow-up data in more than 3000 patients enrolled in US clinical trials indicated

•Symptomatic heart   •LVEF < 0.3-.35
  failure on stable
  medical therapy   •QRS duration > 120 msec
  (90% ACE inhibitors,
  30-60% beta-blockers,   •No indications for
  90% diuretics,   bradycardia pacing
  25-30% amiodarone)
                          •In some trials, indications
•NYHA Class II-IV   for ICD

Fig. 8. Usual inclusion criteria for enrollment in current trials of resynchronization therapy. The percentages given for the various medications represent the percentage of patients enrolled in resynchronization trials who were on these medications.

that the LV leads and resynchronization devices have an excellent track record in terms of system safety and chronic thresholds *(66,73)*.

The issues of the ease and risk of lead extraction have not yet become significant. Leads that acutely dislodge can be replaced successfully, and infected leads generally are removed without difficulty *(66,73)*. There have not yet been a significant number of events to consider this a real, as opposed to theoretical, hazard.

Clinical Trials

General Overview

There are a number of trials evaluating the role of resynchronization therapy in patients with heart failure caused by systolic dysfunction. As demonstrated in Fig. 8, the usual inclusion criteria include symptomatic heart failure that is stable on medical therapy, NYHA class II to IV, LVEF below 35%, QRS duration longer than 120 to 140 ms, and in some trials, an indication for an ICD. Most exclude patients with AF and patients with standard indications for bradycardia rate support. Thus far, the majority of patients enrolled in clinical trials of resynchronization therapies have been on optimal medical therapies for heart failure *(67,73,75)*. The treated patients usually receive LV or BV stimulation in the VDD mode. Figure 9 illustrates the chronological progression of clinical trials of resynchronization therapy using LV or simultaneous BV stimulation.

The identification of appropriate end points for cardiac resynchronization therapy devices and the duration of follow-up required to detect an improvement in heart failure status have been difficult to

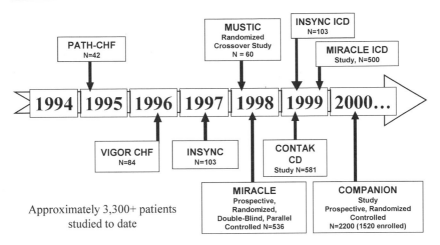

Fig. 9. Chronological progression of clinical trails of resynchronization therapy. See text for the details of specific trails.

determine. The Food and Drug Administration (FDA) initially approved studies having a duration of therapy of 12 weeks to assess the efficacy and safety of cardiac resynchronization therapy. However, as the trials progressed, the FDA considered 6 months a more appropriate duration of therapy and determined that the most appropriate end points should be total mortality and hospitalization. Figure 10 lists the end points of the US trials of chronic resynchronization therapy.

The initial clinical trials of resynchronization therapy utilized an epicardial lead for LV pacing or a transvenous lead that was not specifically designed and tested for long-term LV pacing *(31,34)*. As described in the discussion of pacing technology, the development of a completely transvenous coronary sinus lead designed for long-term LV pacing has simplified the implant procedure and markedly reduced operative risk; it is now used in clinical trials.

Some initial trials have reported results, and many trials are still ongoing. Preliminary data suggested that the improvement in LV function and hemodynamics results in an improvement in functional status in many patients.

CURRENT TRIALS WITH RELEASED DATA

VIGOR-CHF. VIGOR-CHF, a trial now closed to enrollment, included patients with heart failure primarily caused by nonischemic cardiomyopathy and with a left BBB but no indication for conventional

1995 - 2000
- Implant efficacy/safety
- Functional status
  NYHA Class
  Six minute walk
  Quality of life score
  Peak oxygen
    consumption

- Cardiac performance
  Echocardiogram
- Neurohormonal
- Holter

2000 -
- Combined all-cause
  mortality and
  hospitalization

Fig. 10. Clinical end points for US trials of chronic resynchronization therapy.

bradycardia pacemaker therapy *(34)*. The patients were randomly assigned to receive either BV pacing or no pacing for 6x weeks, after which both groups received BV pacing therapy. This was the first US trial of resynchronization therapy, initiated in 1995 when transvenous leads were not yet available. After the introduction of the transvenous lead, this trial failed to complete enrollment and was closed after enrolling only 58 patients. However, all patients had serial echocardiograms at all study points, performed at a single core laboratory. As mentioned in the section on reverse remodeling, there was evidence of reverse remodeling, as shown by significant decreases in LV systolic and diastolic parameters (Fig. 2) *(34)*.

MUSTIC Study. The Multisite Stimulation in Cardiomyopathies (MUSTIC) study is a single-blind, randomized, controlled crossover study involving 131 patients, who were divided into two groups based on their underlying rhythm *(76)*.

Group 1 included 67 patients with NYHA class III heart failure, a QRS duration longer than 150 ms, stable sinus rhythm, and no conventional indications for pacemaker therapy; they were randomly assigned to BV pacing or no BV pacing for 3 months, after which the pacing modes were switched. Forty-eight patients completed both phases of the study. Exercise tolerance, as measured by the 6-minute walk distance, increased by 23% after BV pacing (399 vs 326 m, $p < 0.001$). Other significant improvements included a 32% increase in QoL score, an 8% increase in peak oxygen consumption, and a 66% reduction in hospitalizations. Furthermore, active BV pacing was preferred by 85% of patients.

Group 2 included 64 patients with chronic AF who required a permanent pacemaker because of a slow ventricular rate; the patients were randomly assigned to either single-site RV pacing or BV pacing in the same fashion as in group 1 *(77)*. BV pacing was associated with improvements in exercise tolerance and peak oxygen consumption, but the changes were not as marked as those seen in patients with NSR; there also were no improvements in QoL scores or hospitalization rates. Not all patients were completely pacemaker dependent, however, and thus may not have had the benefit of continuous BV pacing.

MIRACLE Trial. The MIRACLE trial randomly assigned 510 patients with heart failure to BV or no pacing for 6 months *(66,67)*. Data presented on the first 266 patients showed a significantly greater proportion of patients undergoing BV pacing had an improvement in NYHA functional status by at least one class (69 vs 34% for no pacing, $p < 0.001$) and an increase in 6-minute walk distance by 50 meters or more (50 vs 30%).

InSync Trial. The InSync trial was a nonrandomized study that evaluated atrial-synchronous BV pacing in 103 patients with DCM who met the entry criteria for BV pacing *(31,32)*. After a 1-month follow-up, 70% of patients responded with an improvement in NYHA class (≥ 1), an improvement in QoL score, and an increase in 6-minute walk distance (≥ 100 meters); there was further improvement in these parameters at 1 year. Responders to resynchronization had a consistent shortening of QRS duration, an increase in LVEF, and a reduction in LV end-diastolic diameter.

VENTAK CHF/CONTAK CD. VENTAK CHF/CONTAK CD included patients with heart failure who also had an indication for an ICD; it utilized an ICD system designed to provide BV pacing *(34)*. In contrast to VIGOR-CHF, most patients primarily had ischemic cardiomyopathy, reflecting the large percentage of postinfarction ventricular tachycardia (VT) observed in ICD recipients *(78,79)*. Of the more than 500 patients followed, the majority were male, had NYHA class II–IV heart failure, a QRS duration longer than 120 ms, and an indication for an ICD. The patients all had an ICD and were programmed to receive BV pacing or no pacing for 6 months.

Preliminary results from this trial showed that 25% of patients had at least one episode of a life-threatening arrhythmia requiring device discharge. At 1 year, the composite end point (death, heart failure hospitalizations, worsening heart failure requiring other interventions, and VT or ventricular fibrillation [VF] events) was reduced by 21% with BV pacing; the incidence of death was reduced by 23%, worsening heart failure requiring other interventions by 26%, heart failure hospitalizations by 13%, and VT/VF events by 9% *(73)*. BV pacing also improved 6-minute walk distance by an average of 35 meters, peak oxygen consumption by 0.9 mL/kg per minute, and QoL score by 16% compared to baseline. For all three of these measures, patients with the most advanced heart failure showed the most improvement. As mentioned in the section on remodeling, favorable effects on remodeling were observed at 6 months (66).

Figure 11A–D summarizes the results of the major studies of chronic resynchronization therapy, demonstrating the improvements in the clinical end points of QoL score, NYHA functional class, 6-minute walk distance, and peak oxygen consumption (36,53,67,73,76).

COMPANION. The Comparison of Medical Therapy, Pacing, and Defibrillation in Chronic Heart Failure (COMPANION) trial is a recently completed, open-label prospective, multicenter, randomized study that evaluated cardiac resynchronization therapy with and without an ICD compared to standard drug therapies for heart failure (75). The COMPANION trial results were presented at the American College of Cardiology Annual Scientific Sessions in March 2003. The goal of the study was to determine whether optimal drug therapy combined with ventricular resynchronization alone or with an ICD would decrease a combined end point of mortality and all-cause hospitalization when compared to optimal drug therapy alone.

After optimal heart failure therapy was initiated, patients were randomly assigned in a 1:2:2 scheme to drug therapy (control arm) vs drug therapy and cardiac resynchronization therapy vs drug therapy plus cardiac resynchronization therapy coupled with an ICD (Fig. 12). COMPANION was the first study to evaluate cardiac resynchronization therapy with and without an ICD in patients with no history of a significant ventricular arrhythmia. It was also the first completed trial using the heart end points of all-cause hospitalization and mortality as primary end points.

COMPANION enrolled 1520 patients and was halted November 20, 2003, when the prespecified boundaries had been crossed for efficacy. A 19% reduction in time to death or any hospitalization was achieved with resynchronization therapy compared to medical therapy. In addition, more than a 35% reduction was observed in the incidence of heart failure hospitalization. The secondary end point of mortality alone was reduced only in the group receiving a resynchronization defibrillator. As prespecified, the use of heart failure medications was excellent in the COMPANION trial. In addition to ACE inhibitor therapy, more than 65% of COMPANION patients were receiving β-receptor blocker therapy, and more than 50% were taking spironolactone.

The results of COMPANION suggested that the majority of patients eligible for resynchronization therapy should be considered for a resynchronization ICD. It also needs to be emphasized that COMPANION patients were required to have a hospitalization for heart failure worsening in the year prior to enrollment. Patients enrolled in COMPANION therefore had severe symptom class heart failure, and the results of this trial should not be extrapolated to a less-symptomatic group of patients.

ONGOING TRIALS

A number of ongoing trials should provide additional information about the efficacy of resynchronization therapy. The following is a summary of the basic designs of some of these trials.

CARE-HF. The Cardiac Resynchronization for Heart Failure (CARE-HF) trial is a double-blind, controlled study of 800 patients comparing medical therapy to BV pacing (Medtronics Inc., 2003). The end points to be considered include total mortality, peak oxygen consumption, and 6-minute walk distance. The results of CARE-HF will be of great interest when compared to the COMPANION trial results. This will be especially important in assessing the relative risk–cost–benefit analysis of the resynchronization device alone compared to inclusion of ICD capability.

RE-LE-VENT. The Remodeling of Cardiac Cavities by Long-Term Left Ventricular-Based Pacing in Patients With Severe Heart Failure (RE-LE-VeNT) trial will randomly assign 240 patients to medical therapy, LV pacing alone, or BV pacing (St. Jude Medical, 2003). The end points of the RE-LE-VeNT trial are total mortality, quality of life, and various echocardiographic indices.

PACMAN. The Pacing for Cardiomyopathies, a European Study (PACMAN) is a European trial that will compare resynchronization delivered with BV or LV stimulation and outcomes when resynchronization is coupled to an ICD.

EFFICACY IN AF

The effects of resynchronization therapy may be more apparent in patients with heart failure who have established AF. This was illustrated in a report of 37 patients with DCM; the improvements in exercise capacity and LVEF with BV pacing were greater in patients with AF compared to those in sinus rhythm *(51)*. This may have resulted from the combined effects of resynchronization and better heart rate control because of AV nodal ablation.

The Effects of Ventricular Pacing Site Variation on Cardiac Function and Chronic Status in Patients With Chronic Atrial Fibrillation and Ventricular-Based Pacing (PAVE) trial is the first controlled study in

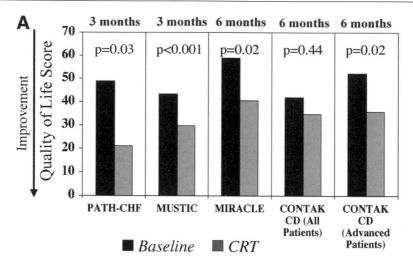

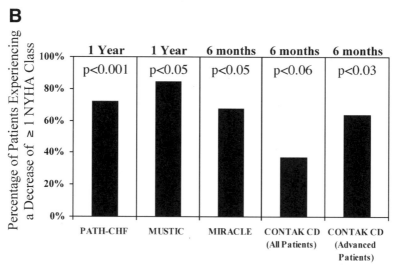

Fig. 11. (A) Improvement in the average quality-of-life score seen in different trials of chronic resynchronization therapy (CRT). Quality-of-life scores were determined using the Minnesota Living With Heart Failure Questionnaire. The advanced patients in the CONTAK CD trial were classified as having NYHA class III heart failure at baseline. **(B)** Improvements in NYHA class seen in different trials of CRT. The advanced patients in the CONTAK CD trial were classified as having NYHA class III heart failure at baseline.

the United States that will evaluate the role of resynchronization therapy in patients with heart failure who have established AF (St. Jude Medical, 2003). The objective is to evaluate exercise capacity and

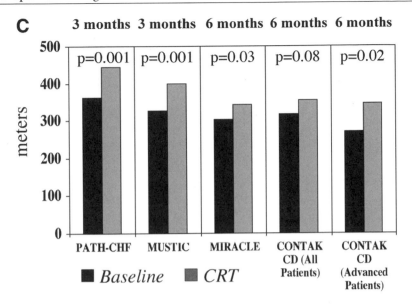

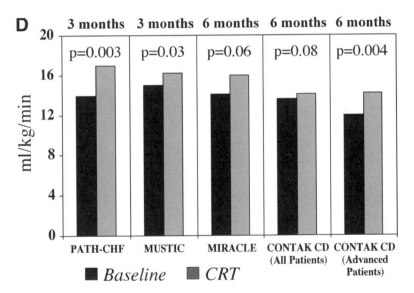

Fig. 11. *(continued)* **(C)** Improvements in the average 6-minute walk distance seen in different trials of CRT. The advanced patients in the CONTAK CD trial were classified as having NYHA class III heart failure at baseline. **(D)** Improvements in the average peak oxygen consumption seen in different trials of CRT. The advanced patients in the CONTAK CD trial were classified as having NYHA class III heart failure at baseline.

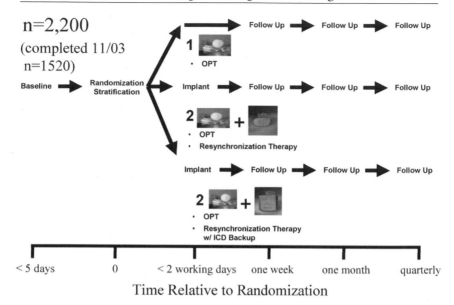

Time Relative to Randomization

Fig. 12. Overview of the study design, enrollment parameters, and randomization scheme for the COMPANION trial. OPT, optimal medical therapy.

global cardiac performance associated with RV vs LV vs BV pacing sites. The trial was closed in October 2003 after enrolling 361 patients and is currently in the follow-up phase. A premarket approval has been submitted to the FDA.

LEFT VENTRICULAR PACING

Although BV pacing is extensively studied, there has also been interest in trying to achieve the same benefit using only LV stimulation. Numerous uncontrolled studies demonstrated a benefit equivalent to BV pacing when acute hemodynamic parameters were considered *(23,25,26,28)*. Based on these preliminary data, to assess the clinical follow-up of LV pacing, a prospective observational study was undertaken in which 33 patients with NYHA class III or IV and a left BBB were assigned to LV or BV pacing for 6 months in a nonrandomized way *(80)*. There was no difference between the two groups in numerous parameters, including improvement in NYHA functional class. However, LV end-diastolic dimension was more significantly decreased in the BV group. Of note, other trials mentioned here, including the RE-LE-VeNT, PACMAN, and PAVE trials, have LV pacing as independent arms in their study designs (St. Jude Medical and Guidant Corp., 2003).

Although LV pacing alone appears to result in similar acute hemodynamic benefit to BV stimulation, a study showed that electrical dispersion is increased with LV pacing alone *(81)*. These data point out that achieving mechanical resynchronization can actually worsen electrical synchrony.

SUMMARY AND FUTURE INDICATIONS

BV pacing to achieve cardiac resynchronization is a promising approach to the therapy of patients with heart failure and an IVCD. Studies completed to date demonstrated that BV stimulation can improve exercise tolerance and NYHA functional class and, most important, the combined end point of time to hospitalization and mortality. Given the very debilitating symptoms that patients with heart failure experience, often despite maximal medical therapy, and the cost of repeat hospitalizations for treatment of exacerbations, the need for an adjunctive therapy such as resynchronization therapy is clear *(82)*. The COMPANION data suggested additional mortality benefit can be obtained with the inclusion of an ICD.

One of the more important and overlooked aspects of resynchronization therapy is its potential to allow maximal optimization of the pharmacological treatment of heart failure. This can be achieved by the ability of the resynchronization device to help support blood pressure and heart rate while also treating arrhythmias. However, the use of resynchronization devices, at present, is limited by the technical skill required to implant resynchronization devices and the need for longer term follow-up. Based on the early data presented and the rapid pace of innovation and development in this field, these limitations are sure to be overcome in the next few years.

REFERENCES

1. American Heart Association. 1999 Heart and Stroke Statistical Update. American Heart Association, Dallas, TX: 1998.
2. Ho KK, Pinsky JL, Kannel WB, Levy D. The epidemiology of heart failure: the Framingham Heart Study. J Am Coll Cardiol 1993;22(4 suppl A):6A–13A.
3. O'Connell JB, Bristow MR. Economic impact of heart failure in the United States: time for a different approach. J Heart Lung Transplant 1994;13:S107–S112.
4. Heart Failure Society of America (HFSA) practice guidelines: HFSA guidelines for management of patients with heart failure caused by left ventricular systolic dysfunction—pharmacological approaches. J Card Fail 1999;5(4):357–382.
5. Aaronson KD, Schwartz JS, Chen TM, et al. Development and prospective validation of a clinical index to predict survival in ambulatory patients referred for cardiac transplant evaluation. Circulation 1997;95:2660–2667.

6. Grines CL, Bashore TM, Boudoulas H, et al. Functional abnormalities in isolated left bundle branch block. The effect of interventricular asynchrony. Circulation 1989;79:845–853.

7. Xiao HB, Lee CH, Gibson DG. Effect of left bundle branch block on diastolic function in dilated cardiomyopathy. Br Heart J 1991;66:443–447.

8. Xiao HB, Brecker SJ, Gibson DG. Effects of abnormal activation on the time course of the left ventricular pressure pulse in dilated cardiomyopathy. Br Heart J 1992;68:403–407.

9. Shamim W, Francis DP, Yousufuddin M, et al. Intraventricular conduction delay: a prognostic marker in chronic heart failure. Int J Cardiol 1999;70:171–178.

10. Xiao HB, Roy C, Fujimoto S, Gibson DG. Natural history of abnormal conduction and its relation to prognosis in patients with dilated cardiomyopathy. Int J Cardiol 1996;53:163–170.

11. Schoeller R, Andresen D, Buttner P, et al. First- or second-degree atrioventricular block as a risk factor in idiopathic dilated cardiomyopathy. Am J Cardiol 1993; 71:720–726.

12. Wilensky RL, Yudelman P, Cohen AI, et al. Serial electrocardiographic changes in idiopathic dilated cardiomyopathy confirmed at necropsy. Am J Cardiol 1988; 62:276–283.

13. Nishimura RA, Hayes DL, Holmes DR Jr, Tajik AJ. Mechanism of hemodynamic improvement by dual-chamber pacing for severe left ventricular dysfunction: an acute Doppler and catheterization hemodynamic study. J Am Coll Cardiol 1995; 25:281–288.

14. Shinbane JS, Chu E, DeMarco T, Sobol Y, et al. Evaluation of acute dual-chamber pacing with a wide range of atrioventricular delays on cardiac performance in refractory heart failure. J Am Coll Cardiol 1997;30:1295–1300.

15. Hochleitner M, Hortnagl H, Ng CK, et al. Usefulness of physiologic dual-chamber pacing in drug-resistant idiopathic dilated cardiomyopathy. Am J Cardiol 1990;66: 198–202.

16. Hochleitner M, Hortnagl H, Hortnagl H, et al. Long-term efficacy of physiologic dual-chamber pacing in the treatment of end-stage idiopathic dilated cardiomyopathy. Am J Cardiol 1992;70:1320–1325.

17. Gold MR, Feliciano Z, Gottlieb SS, Fisher ML. Dual-chamber pacing with a short atrioventricular delay in congestive heart failure: a randomized study. J Am Coll Cardiol 1995;26:967–973.

18. Rosenqvist M, Isaaz K, Botvinick EH, et al. Relative importance of activation sequence compared to atrioventricular synchrony in left ventricular function. Am J Cardiol 1991;67:148–156.

19. Betocchi S, Piscione F, Villari B, et al. Effects of induced asynchrony on left ventricular diastolic function in patients with coronary artery disease. J Am Coll Cardiol 1993;21:1124–1131.

20. Leclercq C, Gras D, Le Helloco A, et al. Hemodynamic importance of preserving the normal sequence of ventricular activation in permanent cardiac pacing. Am Heart J 1995;129:1133–1141.

21. Cazeau S, Ritter P, Bakdach S, et al. Four chamber pacing in dilated cardiomyopathy. Pacing Clin Electrophysiol 1994;17(11 part 2):1974–1979.

22. Foster AH, Gold MR, McLaughlin JS. Acute hemodynamic effects of atriobiventricular pacing in humans. Ann Thorac Surg 1995;59:294–300.

23. Blanc JJ, Etienne Y, Gilard M, et al. Evaluation of different ventricular pacing sites in patients with severe heart failure: results of an acute hemodynamic study. Circulation 1997;96:3273–3277.

24. Saxon LA, Kerwin WF, Cahalan MK, et al. Acute effects of intraoperative multi-site ventricular pacing on left ventricular function and activation/contraction sequence in patients with depressed ventricular function. J Cardiovasc Electrophysiol 1998;9:13–21.
25. Kass DA, Chen CH, Curry C, et al. Improved left ventricular mechanics from acute VDD pacing in patients with dilated cardiomyopathy and ventricular conduction delay. Circulation 1999;99:1567–1573.
26. Auricchio A, Stellbrink C, Block M, et al. Effect of pacing chamber and atrioventricular delay on acute systolic function of paced patients with congestive heart failure. The Pacing Therapies for Congestive Heart Failure Study Group. The Guidant Congestive Heart Failure Research Group. Circulation 1999;99: 2993–3001.
27. Touissaint JF, Ritter P, Lavergne T, et al. Biventricular resynchronization in end-stage heart failure: an eight-month follow-up by phase map radionuclide angiography. Pacing Clin Electrophysiol 1999;22(4 part 2):840.
28. Nelson GS, Berger RD, Fetics BJ, et al. Left ventricular pre-excitation improves mechanoenergetics of patients with dilated cardiomyopathy and ventricular conduction delay. J Am Coll Cardiol 2000;35(2 suppl A):230A.
29. Breithardt O, Stelbrink C, Diem B, et al. Effect of chronic multisite pacing on left ventricular volumes in patients with congestive heart failure. Pacing Clin Electrophysiol 1999;22(4 part 2):732.
30. Stellbrink C, Breithardt OA, Diem B, et al. Acute effects of multisite pacing with different AV delays on diastolic and systolic function in congestive heart failure. Pacing Clin Electrophysiol 1999;22(4 part 2):829.
31. Gras D, Mabo P, Tang T, et al. Multisite pacing as a supplemental treatment of congestive heart failure: preliminary results of the Medtronic Inc. InSync study. Pacing Clin Electrophysiol 1998;21(4 part 2):2249.
32. Gras D, Mabo P, Bucknall C, et al. Responders and nonresponders to cardiac resynchronization therapy: results from the InSync trial. J Am Coll Cardiol 2000;35(2 suppl A):230A.
33. Krahnfeld O, Vogt J, Tenderich G, et al. Changes in QRS-duration in patients with biventricular pacing system for congestive heart failure treatment and clinical outcome. Pacing Clin Electrophysiol 1999;22(4 part 2):733.
34. Saxon LA, Boehmer JP, Hummel J, et al. Biventricular pacing in patients with congestive heart failure: two prospective randomized trials. The VIGOR CHF and VENTAK CHF Investigators. Am J Cardiol 1999;83(5B):120D–130D.
35. Stellbrink C, Auricchio A, Diem B, et al. Potential benefit of biventricular pacing in patients with congestive heart failure and ventricular tachyarrhythmia. Am J Cardiol 1999;83(5B):143D–150D.
36. Auricchio A, Stellbrink C, Sack S, et al. Chronic benefit as a result of pacing in congestive heart failure: results of the PATH-CHF trial. J Card Fail 1999; 5(3 suppl 1):78.
37. Bristow MR, Saxon LA, Boehmer J, et al. for the COMPANION Investigators. Cardiac resynchronization therapy (CRT) reduces hospitalizations, and CRT plus an implantable defibrillator (CRT-D) reduces mortality in chronic heart failure: results of the COMPANION trial. N Engl J Med 2004;350;2140–2150.
38. Auricchio A, Sack S, Stellbrink C, et al. Transvenous left ventricular pacing using a new over the wire coronary venous lead. Pacing Clin Electrophysiol 1999;22(4 part 2):717.
39. Auricchio A, Klein H, Tockman B, et al. Transvenous biventricular pacing for heart failure: can the obstacles be overcome? Am J Cardiol 1999;83(5B):136D–142D.

40. Auricchio A, Salo RW. Acute hemodynamic improvement by pacing in patients with severe congestive heart failure. Pacing Clin Electrophysiol 1997;20 (2 part 1):313–324.
41. Walker S, Levy TM, Coats AJ, et al. Bi-ventricular pacing in congestive cardiac failure. Current experience and future directions. The Imperial College Cardiac Electrophysiology Group. Eur Heart J 2000;21:884–889.
42. Saxon LA. Atrial fibrillation and dilated cardiomyopathy: therapeutic strategies when sinus rhythm cannot be maintained. Pacing Clin Electrophysiol 1997;20 (3 part 1):720–725.
43. Wood MA, Brown-Mahoney C, Kay GN, Ellenbogen KA. Clinical outcomes after ablation and pacing therapy for atrial fibrillation: a meta-analysis. Circulation 2000;101:1138–1144.
44. Roy D, Talajic M, Dorian P, et al. Amiodarone to prevent recurrence of atrial fibrillation. Canadian Trial of Atrial Fibrillation Investigators. N Engl J Med 2000; 342:913–920.
45. Shinbane JS, Wood MA, Jensen DN, et al. Tachycardia-induced cardiomyopathy: a review of animal models and clinical studies. J Am Coll Cardiol 1997;29: 709–715.
46. Daoud EG, Weiss R, Bahu M, et al. Effect of an irregular rhythm on cardiac output. Am J Cardiol 1996;78:1433–1436.
47. Natale A, Zimerman L, Tomassoni G, et al. Impact on ventricular function and quality of life of transcatheter ablation of the atrioventricular junction in chronic atrial fibrillation with a normal ventricular response. Am J Cardiol 1996;78:1431–1433.
48. Brignole M, Menozzi C, Gianfranchi L, et al. Assessment of atrioventricular junction ablation and VVIR pacemaker vs pharmacological treatment in patients with heart failure and chronic atrial fibrillation: a randomized, controlled study. Circulation 1998;98:953–960.
49. Ozcan C, Jahangir A, Friedman PA, et al. Long-term survival after ablation of the atrioventricular node and implantation of a permanent pacemaker in patients with atrial fibrillation. N Engl J Med 2001;344:1043–1051.
50. Twidale N, McDonald T, Nave K, Seal A. Comparison of the effects of AV nodal ablation vs AV nodal modification in patients with congestive heart failure and uncontrolled atrial fibrillation. Pacing Clin Electrophysiol 1998;21(4 part 1): 641–651.
51. Leclercq C, Victor F, Alonso C, et al. Comparative effects of permanent biventricular pacing for refractory heart failure in patients with stable sinus rhythm or chronic atrial fibrillation. Am J Cardiol 2000;85:1154–1156.
52. Deshmukh P, Casavant DA, Romanyshyn M, Anderson K. Permanent, direct His-bundle pacing: a novel approach to cardiac pacing in patients with normal His-Purkinje activation. Circulation 2000;101:869–877.
53. Saxon LA, Kumar UN, De Marco T. Heart failure and cardiac resynchronization therapies: US experience in the year 2000. Ann Noninvasive Electrocardiol 2000; 5:188–194.
54. Kadhiresan V, Vogt J, Auricchio A, et al. Sensitivity and specificity of QRS duration to predict acute benefit in heart failure patients with cardiac resynchronization. Pacing Clin Electrophysiol 2000;23(4 part 2):555.
55. Farwell D, Patel NR, Hall A, et al. How many people with heart failure are appropriate for biventricular resynchronization? Eur Heart J 2000;21:1246–1250.
56. Saxon LA, Stevenson WG, Middlekauff HR, Stevenson LW. Increased risk of progressive hemodynamic deterioration in advanced heart failure patients requiring permanent pacemakers. Am Heart J 1993;125(5 part 1):1306–1310.

57. The DAVID Trial Investigators. Dual chamber pacing or ventricular backup pacing in patients with an implantable defibrillator. JAMA 2002;288:3115–3123.
58. Leon AR, Greenberg JM, Kanuru N, et al. Cardiac resynchronization in patients with congestive heart failure and chronic atrial fibrillation: effect of upgrading to biventricular pacing after chronic right ventricular pacing. J Am Coll Cardiol 2002;39:1258–1263.
59. Spragg DD, Leclercq C, Loghmani M, et al. Regional alterations in protein expression in the dyssynchronous failing heart. Circulation 2003;108:929–932.
60. Leclercq C, Cazeau S, Le Breton H, et al. Acute hemodynamic effects of biventricular DDD pacing in patients with end-stage heart failure. J Am Coll Cardiol 1998;32:1825–1831.
61. Kerwin WF, Botvinick EH, O'Connell JW, et al. Ventricular contraction abnormalities in dilated cardiomyopathy: effect of biventricular pacing to correct interventricular dyssynchrony. J Am Coll Cardiol 2000;35:1221–1227.
62. Kerwin WF, Foster E, Paccanaro M, et al. Effect of chronic biventricular pacing on Doppler measures of myocardial performance correlate with Doppler measures of systolic function. Pacing Clin Electrophysiol 1999;22(4 part 2):732.
63. Saxon LA, DeMarco T, Chatterjee K, et al. The magnitude of sympathoneural activation in advanced heart failure is altered with chronic biventricular pacing. Pacing Clin Electrophysiol 1998;21(4 part 2):499.
64. Dibs SR, Kerwin WF, Godin G, et al. Chronic biventricular pacing does not worsen autonomic imbalance in heart failure. Pacing Clin Electrophysiol 2000; 23(4 part 2):660.
65. Auricchio A, on behalf of the PATH-CHF Investigators. Optimal cardiac resynchronization decreases heart rate and increases heart rate variability in heart failure patients with conduction delay. Pacing Clin Electrophysiol 2000;23(4 part 2): 602.
66. July 10th Circulatory Systems Device Panel (MIRACLE trial). IDE G980219. Available at: www.FDALive, accessed 2001.
67. Saxon LA, De Marco T, Dibs S, et al. Chronic biventricular pacing improves indices of systolic function and reduces left ventricular volume. Pacing Clin Electrophysiol 2000;23(4 part 2);635.
68. De Marco T, Schafer J, Foster E, Saxon LA. Chronic resynchronization therapy results in reverse remodeling in mild to moderate heart failure. J Card Fail 2001; 7(3 suppl 2):58.
69. St John Sutton MG, Plappert TJ, Abraham WT, et al. Cardiac resynchronization therapy results in improvement in echocardiographic parameters in heart failure patients: Evidence from MIRACLE and MIRACLE ICD trials [abstract]. J Cardiac Fail 2002;8:abstract 034.
70. Saxon LA, De Marco T, Chatterjee K, et al. Operative risk associated with chronic biventricular pacemaker implantation in advanced heart failure. Pacing Clin Electrophysiol 1998; 21(4 part 2):498.
71. Leon A, Langberg J. Energy sources for catheter ablation. In: Zipes D, Jalife J, eds. Cardiac Electrophysiology: From Cell to Bedside, 2nd ed. WB Saunders, Philadelphia, PA: 1995.
72. Reynolds D, Belott P. Permanent pacemaker and implantable cardioverter-defibrillator implantation. In: Ellenbogen K, Kay G, Wilkoff B, eds. Clinical Cardiac Pacing and Defibrillation, 2nd ed. WB Saunders, Philadelphia, PA: 2000.
73. July 10th Circulatory Systems Device Panel (CONTAK CD trial). IDE G970259. Available at: www.FDALive, accessed 2002.

74. Hewitt M, Chen J, Ravon CE, Gallagher JJ. Coronary sinus atrial pacing: radiographic considerations. Am J Roentgenol 1981;136:323–328.

75. Bristow MR, Feldman AM, Saxon LA. Heart failure management using implantable devices for ventricular resynchronization: Comparison of Medical Therapy, Pacing, and Defibrillation in Chronic Heart Failure (COMPANION) trial. COMPANION Steering Committee and COMPANION Clinical Investigators. J Card Fail 2000;6:276–285.

76. Cazeau S, Leclercq C, Lavergne T, et al. Effects of multisite biventricular pacing in patients with heart failure and intraventricular conduction delay. N Engl J Med 2001;344:873–880.

77. Data presented at the European Society of Cardiology Scientific Sessions, Amsterdam, The Netherlands, 2000.

78. Buxton AE, Lee KL, Fisher JD, et al. A randomized study of the prevention of sudden death in patients with coronary artery disease. Multicenter Unsustained Tachycardia Trial Investigators. N Engl J Med 1999;341:1882–1890.

79. Moss AJ, Hall WJ, Cannom DS, et al. Improved survival with an implanted defibrillator in patients with coronary disease at high risk for ventricular arrhythmia. Multicenter Automatic Defibrillator Implantation Trial Investigators. N Engl J Med 1996;335:1933–1940.

80. Touiza A, Etienne Y, Gilard M, et al. Long-term left ventricular pacing: assessment and comparison with biventricular pacing in patients with severe congestive heart failure. J Am Coll Cardiol 2001;38:1966–1970.

81. Leclercq C, Faris O, Tunin R, et al. Systolic improvement and mechanical resynchronization does not require electrical synchrony in the dilated failing heart with left bundle-branch block. Circulation 2002;106:1760–1763.

82. Saxon LA, De Marco T. Cardiac resynchronization: a cornerstone in the foundation of device therapy in heart failure. J Am Coll Cardiol 2001;38:1971–1973.

7 Left Ventricular Assist Devices

Paul L. DiGiorgi, MD,
Yoshifumi Naka, MD, PhD,
and Mehmet C. Oz, MD

CONTENTS

INTRODUCTION
INDICATIONS
PATIENT SELECTION
TYPES OF PUMPS
DEVICE SELECTION
POSTOPERATIVE MANAGEMENT
CONCLUSION
REFERENCES

INTRODUCTION

Left ventricular assist devices (LVADs) have become the standard of care for potential heart transplant patients with life-threatening heart failure refractory to medical therapy. Significant advances in both the technology and the clinical experience have taken place. In addition, indications for placement of ventricular assist devices (VADs) have broadened to include patients previously thought unsuitable for device insertion. There is a wide array of devices available and in development. These range from univentricular percutaneous driveline-powered devices to fully implantable total artificial hearts (TAHs). Both patient

From: *Contemporary Cardiology: Surgical Management of Congestive Heart Failure*
Edited by: J. C. Fang and G. S. Couper © Humana Press Inc., Totowa, NJ

and device selection have a great impact on outcome. In addition, the improving long-term success with device support has led to the possibility of permanent support. This review describes indications for VAD placement, reviews current devices, and discusses postoperative management.

INDICATIONS

The traditional indication for VAD support was refractory cardiac failure in patients approved for transplantation. Our patient population has expanded from these patients with chronic heart failure to include a large proportion of patients with acute heart failure. Although some reports have shown better outcomes in stable patients awaiting heart transplant (1,2), acceptable results have been obtained in the emergent patient population (3–8). In addition, our experience suggests similar survival rates between urgent and nonurgent LVAD placements.

There are now several clinical scenarios in which VADs are implanted. These include postcardiotomy cardiogenic shock (PCCS), acute myocardial infarction (AMI), acute decompensation of chronic heart failure, myocarditis, chronic heart failure in transplantation candidates, ventricular arrhythmias, and high-risk cardiac operations.

PCCS patients have shown significant survival benefits if identified early and appropriately treated (8). Because most centers have the capability for short-term but not long-term VAD support/ transplant, we created a network that rapidly identifies and transfers appropriate patients in our region. Initial evaluation optimizes short-term VAD support and transfers patients within 72 hours of decompensation. Long-term LVAD implantation, if necessary, is then performed within 5 days.

AMI patients suffer from cardiogenic shock about 6% of the time and have a mortality of almost 80% (9,10). Even with early revascularization, 1-year survival remains less than 50% (11). Many of these patients suffer either unrecoverable myocardial damage or lack suitable coronary anatomy for revascularization. Advanced mechanical support may be the only therapy available for these patients and can successfully bridge these patients to either recovery or transplant if necessary (12,13).

Patients with long-standing heart failure may decompensate acutely or over longer periods of time. These patients may not have been listed for transplant at the time of failure, although often they are followed at transplant centers. Acute decompensation can be triggered by several etiologies, including new ischemic injuries, arrhythmias, and infections. Patients already listed for heart transplant are the traditional group that has made up VAD populations. These patients tend to do well with VAD placement as rehabilitation can be optimized before transplant *(14)*.

LVAD implantation in acute myocarditis, particularly in young patients, most often is a bridge to recovery rather than transplantation. Unfortunately, it is difficult to determine which patients will benefit from short-term support or require long-term devices with subsequent transplantation *(15)*. Because recovery is more likely in this population, short-term VADs are more often placed, with subsequent transition to long-term VADs if necessary *(3)*. The patient then proceeds along the same treatment algorithm as other VAD patients.

Patients with ventricular arrhythmias are unique in that, aside from the arrhythmia, their native cardiac function may not be significantly compromised. If pharmacological therapy and defibrillators have failed, VAD support may be warranted. Indeed, VAD support has successfully been implemented in this scenario *(16–18)*.

Patients undergoing high-risk cardiac surgery may need mechanical ventricular support if the surgical procedure is not successful. We routinely arrange for LVAD backup for such cases. The patient is screened for transplant candidacy preoperatively in case of the need for LVAD support and heart transplant.

PATIENT SELECTION

The selection process for VAD implantation must reach a balance between highest risk patients who have unacceptably high mortality rates and too conservative an approach passing over patients who would otherwise benefit from VAD support. Judicious use is also important as VAD implantation incurs significant social and financial investment.

According to the US Food and Drug Administration (FDA), approval for transplant is required for VAD implantation, although this may be difficult in the setting of acute cardiac failure. The generally accepted hemodynamic criteria include systolic blood pressure less than 80 mmHg (or mean arterial blood pressure <65 mmHg), pulmonary capillary wedge pressure more than 20 mmHg, systemic vascular resistance more than 2100 dynes*s/cm^5, urine output less than 20 cc per hour (adults) despite diuretics, and a cardiac index of less than 2 L/min/m^2 despite maximal inotropic or intra-aortic balloon pump (IABP) support *(19)*. In addition, some centers are more specific about the use of inotropic agents, requiring at least two at specified doses *(20)*. Several other factors must be taken into account. We use a system of cardiac and extracardiac factors when evaluating a patient for VAD placement (Table 1).

Table 1
Ventricular Assist Device Considerations

1. Transplant candidate
2. Hemodynamic variables
   a. Cardiac index <2 L/min/m²
   b. Systolic blood pressure <80 mmHg
   c. Pulmonary capillary wedge pressure >20 mmHg
   d. On maximized medical therapy
3. Cardiac factors
   a. Right ventricular function
   b. Valvular disease/prosthetic valves
   c. Ischemia/bypass grafts
   d. Arrhythmias
4. Noncardiac factors
   a. Neurological function
   b. Infectious diseases
   c. Prolonged prothrombin time
   d. Oliguria
   e. Blood urea nitrogen
   f. Bilirubin
   g. Pulmonary disease
   h. Body surface area <1.5 m²

Adapted from ref. *20a*.

Cardiac Factors

There are several cardiac factors that must be taken into account when considering VAD placement. Right heart failure (RHF) is one of the most important causes of perioperative mortality *(21,22)*. RHF complicating LVAD placement has been associated with low preoperative mean pulmonary arterial pressure and right ventricle stroke work index *(23)*. Hemodynamic indicators include left atrial pressures less than 10 mmHg, a cardiac index less than 1.8 L/min/m², and a decreasing cardiac index developing in the setting of high pulmonary arterial and central venous pressures *(22)*.

Pulmonary vascular resistance/index and the transpulmonary gradient have been used to predict RHF in the post-heart transplant population *(24–26)*. However, we were unable to distinguish survivors from nonsurvivors using these criteria *(22)*. It should be remembered that normal preoperative pulmonary pressures do not necessarily indicate adequate right heart function. Although a patient may have a normal pulmonary vascular resistance in low cardiac output states, a fixed pulmonary vasculature can translate into pulmonary hypertension and RHF after instituting VAD support.

Although valve disease plays a role in patient selection for VAD implantation, most problems can be addressed at the time of surgery. Aortic insufficiency can cause shunting and loss of forward flow. The degree of aortic insufficiency may be underestimated in the preoperative setting. We therefore recommend intraoperative direct assessment with a left ventricular (LV) vent and believe that all regurgitant flow greater than 1.5 L/min should be addressed.

In patients requiring long-term LVAD support as a bridge to transplant, our preferred strategy is to oversew an incompetent aortic valve. In patients who have the potential for myocardial recovery and subsequent LVAD explant, the valve is repaired by resuspending the prolapsing cusp or by suturing it to the adjacent normal cusp, thereby creating a bicuspid valve. A prosthetic valve should be oversewn to reduce the incidence of thromboembolism.

Mitral stenosis can compromise device inflow and may need to be corrected at the time of implant as well. Repair of other valve pathologies, such as aortic stenosis and mitral regurgitation, should be considered regarding device weaning. A tissue valve should be considered, if replacement is necessary, because of lower risk of thromboembolism and the avoidance of anticoagulation. In addition, bubble studies should be performed and a patent foramen ovale repaired as hypoxia can result from right-to-left shunting after left-sided unloading from an LVAD. Tricuspid stenosis, although rare, should be treated as it will reduce right atrial pressure and improve forward flow through the pulmonary circulation. Correction of tricuspid regurgitation, commonly found, has no benefit unless ascites is present. As LV failure improves on device support, so will right ventricular failure and concomitant tricuspid regurgitation.

Preexisting coronary artery disease (CAD) is common in LVAD candidates. Adequate evaluation of CAD is important to maximize the benefits of VAD implantation. Right-sided bypasses may be necessary when implanting an LVAD to support right ventricular (RV) function. This is especially important for early postoperative RV protection.

In addition, ischemic complications such as angina and arrhythmias may still occur after VAD implantation and can be relieved by coronary bypass. Refractory, malignant arrhythmias themselves can be an indication for VAD implantation (17,18). However, we usually do not perform left-sided bypasses for angina as post-LVAD angina is uncommon. Unless ventricular recovery is likely, left-sided bypasses may not be warranted secondary to a relatively low-flow state after

VAD implantation and the potential for early graft closure. However, there is a possibility that VAD support increases diastolic coronary flows by up to 97% (27). If bypasses are performed, placement of the proximal anastomoses should take into account the LVAD outflow anastomosis site. We, therefore, recommend proximal bypass anastomoses on the lesser curvature of the aorta, providing ample room on the anterolateral aspect of the aorta to accommodate the LVAD outflow graft.

Noncardiac Factors

As more patients with PCCS are evaluated for VAD implantation, neurological status has become an increasingly important and difficult assessment to make and remains an important determinant of mortality in transferred patients (8). It is ethically permissible to discontinue support if patients have unrecoverable neurological function. Ideally, patients should have both thorough neurological and psychiatric evaluations to determine their ability to tolerate mechanical support.

Infection is the Achilles' heal of mechanical support. Infection is the most common complication of long-term VADs and accounts for substantial morbidity and even mortality among VAD patients (14,24,28–31). The location of the infection can have a significant impact on outcome (29). Patients should ideally have negative blood cultures for at least a week prior to VAD implantation. This is especially true for fungal organisms because of the functional T-cell deficiency incurred by these patients (32). Unfortunately, we have been unable to identify either fever or elevated white blood cell count as a risk factor for infection (33). However, others have found elevated white blood cell count, but not fever, as a risk factor for mortality (20,34). As designs and treatments improve, VAD patients with infections do increasingly well posttransplant (28).

In our past experience, renal failure has been the strongest predictor of mortality. We avoid placing devices in patients with serum creatinine levels greater than 5 mg/dL. Patients who have acute cardiac failure may not show an elevated creatinine until later, however. Blood urea nitrogen less than 20 mg/dL has been associated with increased survival (35). We have found urine output to be the best indicator of renal function. Urine output less than 30 mL per hour despite diuretic use has been our most important indicator (33). Although renal impairment is common in this population, recovery during the VAD support period is excellent (22,36,37). In fact, our most recent analysis indicated renal function is no longer predictive of mortality.

Hepatic function is an important factor in post-VAD survival. A prothrombin time greater than 16 seconds is particularly ominous because patients require more blood products. Increased transfusion requirements directly correlate with RHF. Coagulopathies should be aggressively treated with serine protease inhibitors (Aprotinin), vitamin K, and fresh frozen plasma. Hepatic function, evidenced by bilirubin, has been proposed as the best predictor of survival (38). Other studies have failed to associate bilirubin with survival, however (35).

Reoperation can make VAD implantation more challenging technically, but its impact on mortality has varied in published reports (20,33,35,38). We found reoperation was a significant risk factor and use it as part of our screening scale to predict survival postimplant.

Other relative contraindications to VAD implantation include pulmonary failure exclusive of pulmonary edema and malignancy that would preclude survival longer than 2 years. Presently, any condition excluding patients from transplant also excludes them as VAD candidates if this is known preoperatively.

Several studies have attempted to develop simple selection criteria for VAD implantation. These have been based on both unique clinical variables (20) and Acute Physiology and Chronic Health Evaluation II (APACHE II) scores (22). In 1995, we published our own scoring scale (Table 2) (33). Scores were based on seven relatively simple variables, including urine output, central venous pressure, mechanical ventilation, prothrombin time, reoperation, white blood cell count, and temperature. We found scores greater than 5 correlated with increased mortality. It is important to remember that no scoring system serves as an absolute predictor for VAD candidacy or success. In addition, as both technology and patient selection evolve, these systems will become obsolete, and new ones will need to be developed.

By appropriately selecting patients for VAD insertion, lives are saved, end-organ impairment is reduced, and transplantation risks are reduced. Ultimately, the utilization of donor hearts will be maximized.

TYPES OF PUMPS

Extracorporeal

CENTRIFUGAL PUMPS

Centrifugal devices have been the most commonly used pumps for postcardiotomy cardiac support (39). Blood enters axially into the pump, is spun by the magnetically driven blades, and exits peripherally through the outlet port. Although in clinical use for more than 20 years,

Table 2
Risk Factors for Poor Survival After Left
Ventricular Assist Device Placement

Risk factor	Relative risk	Score
Urine output <30 mL per hour	3.9	3
Central venous pressure >20 mmHg	3.1	2
Mechanical ventilation	3.0	2
Prothrombin time >16 seconds	2.4	2
Reoperation	1.8	1
White blood cell count >15,000	1.1	0
Temperature >101.5°F	0	0

Adapted from ref. *166*.

initial enthusiasm waned because of excessive hemolysis. Since then, many new designs have been produced with improved hemodynamics *(40–54)*.

The two most commonly used pumps are the Biomedicus Bio-Pump (Medtronic Inc.) (Fig. 1) and the Sarns/3M Centrifugal System (Sarns/3M). Centrifugal pumps are now considered by many to cause less hemolysis and blood element activation compared to roller pumps *(55–57)*. None of the commonly used pumps has shown significant clinical advantages *(54)*.

Indications for centrifugal pump implantation are extracorporeal membrane oxygenation (ECMO), thoracic aortic surgery, postcardiotomy ventricular failure, bridge to a long-term VAD, and bridge to transplant. Besides thoracic aortic surgery, the major indication has been postcardiotomy ventricular failure *(43,54,58–62)*. Published outcomes have paralleled other short-term devices, with 56 to 68% of patients weaned, and 21 to 44% of patients surviving to discharge *(59,61–63)*. Support duration is shorter than the other commonly used short-term device, the Abiomed BVS 5000 (Abiomed Cardiovascular Inc.), running usually less than 4 days. Popularity of centrifugal pumps has been primarily because of the lower price, ease of use, and greater availability they have historically enjoyed. This may change, however, as more advanced systems like the Abiomed BVS 5000 become more ubiquitous and cost differences diminish *(64)*.

Major limitations include seal disruption, usually within 48 hours, requiring close inspection *(65)*, mandatory anticoagulation, continued sedation with mechanical ventilation, and the inability to ambulate or rehabilitate patients while on the device. In addition, a full-time, bedside

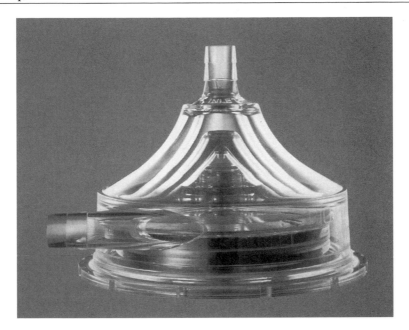

Fig. 1. The centrifugal Biomedicus Biopump. Blood enters the pump apically (top connector) and exits peripherally (lower left connector). (Courtesy of Medtronic Inc., Minneapolis, MN.)

perfusionist is required to run each centrifugal pump system. Finally, the devices are not FDA approved for this purpose. Given these complications and limitations, especially in rehabilitation, centrifugal mechanical assist devices are mainly useful for short-term support in the patient with postcardiotomy ventricular failure and the bridge-to-transplant scenario.

The next generation of centrifugal pumps, however, now in bench and animal testing, is designed for long-term support with partial or total implantability *(66–72)*. Advantages will include their smaller size, potential total implantability, lower energy requirements compared to pusher-plate technologies, and outpatient use. The potential disadvantages of nonpulsatile flow remain to be seen with long-term support.

ABIOMED BVS 5000

The Abiomed BVS 5000 is a short-term uni- or biventricular (BV) support system composed of external pumps driven by a computer-controlled drive console (Fig. 2). The FDA first approved the product in 1992 for postcardiotomy support *(73)*. Since then, the indications for use have grown to include AMI, myocarditis, RV support in conjunction

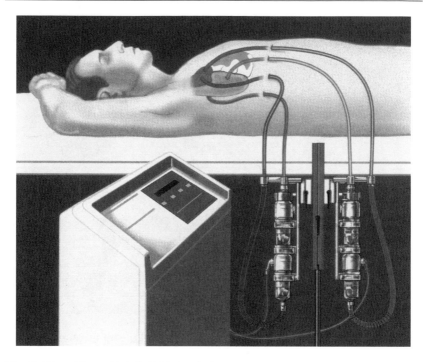

Fig. 2. The Abiomed BVS 5000. Both the pumps and drive console are external. (Courtesy of Abiomed Cardiovascular Inc., Danvers, MA.)

with a long-term LV support device, as a bridge to recovery, and as a bridge to transplant. As a result, the device has become one of the most commonly used means of short-term mechanical cardiac support *(74,75)*. It is the only device approved by the FDA for all patients with potentially reversible heart failure.

Advantages that have made the BVS system popular are the ease of insertion and simplicity in operation, obviating the need for a full-time perfusionist. The system functions reliably for several days, with average support duration between 5 and 9 days. This has been particularly helpful in community hospitals, in which there may be the need to transfer the patient to a transplant center for further treatment *(8,76)*. It has proven its effectiveness in the treatment of both acute myocarditis and PCCS *(3,4,74,77)*. In addition, the cost may be closer to that of centrifugal pumps than previously expected *(64)*. For these reasons, the BVS system has become our standard for bridging patients to longer term devices.

Disadvantages of this device include the requirement for continuous anticoagulation, limited mobility compared to implantable devices, and the requirement to remain in an intensive care unit. Flow rates are also limited compared to other devices. The maximum flow rate of 6 L per minute may not be enough for septic or large patients. Although patients have been supported as long as 90 days, the device is best suited for short-term use (<10 days). For these reasons, we do not use the device if we feel the support period will be longer than 7 days.

THORATEC DEVICE

The Thoratec VAD (Thoratec Laboratories Corp.) consists of an externalized pneumatic pusher-plate pump positioned subcostally and connected to a drive console. The drive is capable of uni- or BV support with flows up to 7 L per minute. The cannulae are tunneled, exiting out the upper abdominal wall and connected to the extracorporeal pump (Fig. 3). The device was first used clinically in 1982 for post-cardiotomy support *(78)* and in 1984 as a bridge to transplantation *(79)*. It has received FDA approval as both a bridge to recovery and a bridge to transplant.

The main advantage of the Thoratec system is the ability to provide long-term BV support. This has become increasingly important with prolonged waiting periods for transplant. The Thoratec system is the only extracorporeal device that is used for long-term support. The paracorporeal position has some particular benefits as well. These include identification of clot and device exchange without invasive surgery. Survival to transplant has been good, up to 74% with support durations longer than 200 days *(80–83)*.

The major limitations of the Thoratec system are the limited mobility and rehabilitation potential because of a large drive console and the need for chronic anticoagulation. New, portable drive units will allow portability, which should overcome the limitations of the original system *(84)*. In addition, the device is not recommended for pediatric patients.

Even with limited portability and the need for chronic anticoagulation, the Thoratec VAD system provides a valuable adjunct to the cardiac assist device armamentarium because of the ability to provide long-term, BV support. At present, we use this device in patients with substantial end-organ injury prior to device insertion and in individuals likely to require BV support

ADULT ECMO

ECMO provides mechanical cardiac support (uni- or biventricular) as well as pulmonary support. Although neonatal use has been very successful, the adult experience has been mixed.

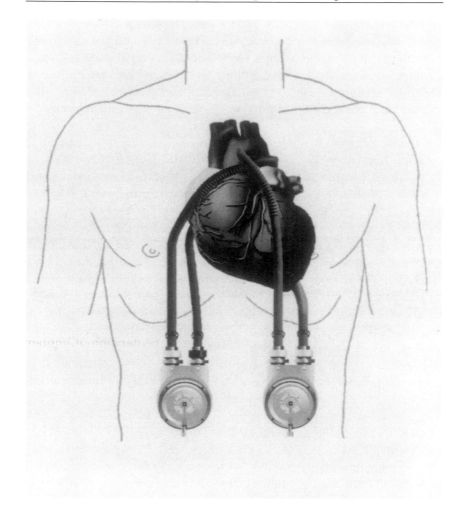

Fig. 3. Thoratec ventricular assist device. Both the pumps and drive console are external. (Courtesy of Thoratec Laboratories Corp., Pleasanton, CA.)

The main indication for ECMO is the need for mechanical assistance when respiratory failure complicates cardiovascular collapse. When initially used for PCCS, survival was low (25%) (85), but with experience and improved circuits, survival increased to 40% (86). ECMO benefits from potential peripheral cannulae insertion and versatility of small consoles. This allows potential implementation in areas outside the operating room for both cardiac and pulmonary support.

Major limitations include requirement for sedation and possible paralysis, heparinization (except in cases of pure respiratory support), and the potential need for an IABP to reduce afterload. A full-time per-fusionist is also necessary to run the equipment. The duration of support is usually only 2 to 3 days, although it can be several days. Complications are common, including leg ischemia, renal failure, bleeding, and oxygenator failure, especially with venoarterial ECMO support.

Overall, the successful use of ECMO in adults has been limited to select centers, and the epidemiological benefits remain minor.

BERLIN HEART

The Berlin heart (Mediport Kardiotechnik) is a pneumatically driven paracorporeal support device capable of providing both uni-ventricular and BV mechanical support. The system has been used in Europe since 1988. The blood pumps come in a variety of sizes, down to stroke volumes of about 10 mL, allowing for pediatric use *(87,88)*. Implantation is usually performed via a sternotomy with or without cardiopulmonary bypass and cardioplegic arrest *(89)*. The cannulae are brought out the epigastrium to connect to the external blood pumps. Various drive consoles have been developed, allowing discharge to home while on ventricular support. The duration of implant averages 2 months and has been more than 500 days.

The Berlin heart can provide BV or univentricular support. It has the advantage of pediatric applications and has proven its reliability and low rate of thromboembolic complications. Newer, portable consoles allow patients to be more mobile with better rehabilitation and home discharge.

Coumadin is mandatory (international normalized ratio [INR] 2.5 to 3.5), along with aspirin and dipyridamole *(89)*. The pumps also require twice-weekly inspection for thrombus formation. These high-maintenance requirements should provide reliable service, however, for extended periods of time. This device is not approved by the FDA, so US use is not yet feasible.

Intracorporeal

INTRA-AORTIC BALLOON PUMP

In use since the 1960s *(90)*, the IABP is the most commonly used cardiac assist device in use today. It is based on diastolic coronary blood flow augmentation and aortic counterpulsation. As a result, myocardial oxygen consumption is decreased by afterload reduction, and coronary blood flow is increased *(91)*. Percutaneous placement was developed by the 1980s, greatly increasing the use of the devices *(92,93)* by enabling placement by nonsurgeons outside the operating room.

It is most commonly used in cardiogenic shock or ongoing myocardial infarction refractory to medical therapy. Preoperatively, IABP support is commonly used to stabilize patients with myocardial ischemia despite medical therapy before proceeding with revascularization. Survival benefit has been shown with preoperative IABP placement, especially in patients with ejection fractions (EFs) less than 25% (94) as well as in those with EFs less than 40% (95). Intraoperatively, it is used for patients who fail weaning from cardiopulmonary bypass despite maximal medical therapy. Insertion of an IABP intraoperatively or postoperatively has been an independent predictor of death. Preoperative insertion has been associated with significantly increased survival (96).

The IABP benefits from relatively rapid and easy insertion without necessarily requiring a surgical approach. The benefits of increased coronary perfusion as well as reduced myocardial oxygen demand are most realized in the ischemic heart, although other forms of cardiomyopathies are also benefited. It does not, however, provide the level of support of other assist devices. Anticoagulation with intravenous heparin is used to prevent thrombotic complications at both the insertion and balloon sites. Postoperative anticoagulation can be started with low-molecular-weight dextran and switched to heparin later.

Vascular complications remain the most common source of morbidity, with rates varying from 9 to 36% (97,98). Most often, this is related to the femoral artery, stressing the importance of common femoral artery insertion (rather than insertion in the superficial femoral artery). Given these complications, however, the IABP has become an important tool in supporting cardiac function without the need for significant surgical intervention.

THORATEC HEARTMATE

The HeartMate LVAD is an implantable, long-term, univentricular cardiac assist device (Fig. 4). It was developed by Thermo Cardiosystems Inc. (TCI) and is now distributed by Thoratec Laboratories. Based on work started in the mid-1960s, the first clinical implantation of the HeartMate took place in 1986. The HeartMate was the first mechanical circulatory support device to be approved by the FDA for bridging to transplant. Both a pneumatically driven (implantable pneumatic) and an electrically powered (vented electric) version exist. Most hospitals now have converted to the portable electric version, allowing discharge to home on support.

Both systems function with a pusher-plate mechanism delivering up to 10 L per minute of flow. The driveline containing the electric

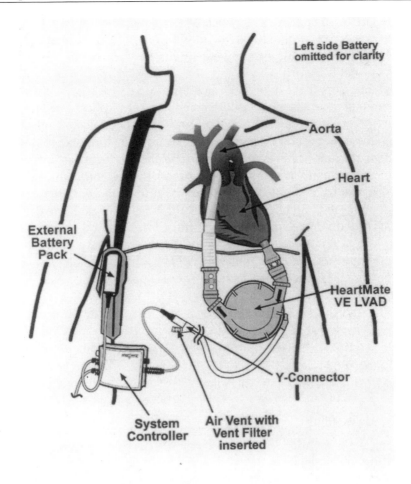

Left side Battery
omitted for clarity

Aorta

Heart

External
Battery
Pack

HeartMate
VE LVAD

Y-Connector

System
Controller

Air Vent with
Vent Filter
inserted

Fig. 4. The HeartMate LVAD. Implantable pump and external drive console. VE, vented electric. (Courtesy of Thoratec Laboratories Corp., Pleasanton, CA.)

cable and an air vent exit the skin to attach to the external drive console. Both inflow and outflow porcine valves are attached to the pump. The inflow cannula is attached to the LV apex, and the outflow is via the ascending aorta. The blood-contacting portion of the pump incorporates titanium microspheres, and the flexible diaphragm is covered with textured polyurethane. This promotes the formation of a pseudointimal layer. This unique surface may be responsible for the low thromboembolic risk associated with the HeartMate despite the lack of anticoagulation *(99–101)*.

The main advantage of the HeartMate is the very low thromboembolic rate (<5%) without anticoagulation *(101–103)*. Patients can be discharged home while awaiting transplant; they can resume almost all their normal activities.

Patients must have a body surface area (BSA) of at least 1.5 m² to accommodate the abdominally placed pump. Proper screening of potential recipients is critical *(33)*. Early complications are related to technique. We prefer a preperitoneal drive implantation to avoid intra-abdominal complications, a long driveline tunnel to avoid infectious complications, and a secure, hemostatic ascending aorta/outflow graft anastomosis to avoid bleeding, dissection, and rupture. Other centers prefer intra-abdominal insertion with the benefit of additional tissue around the driveline, including omentum. The major causes of perioperative mortality are hemorrhage and RHF. These have been reduced with the introduction of aprotinin (Bayer) and nitric oxide *(104–108)*. If right-sided mechanical support is necessary, a different device would need to be placed.

Although the HeartMate represents the first generation of reliable mechanical cardiac assist devices, it has enjoyed significant clinical success. As a result, the Randomized Evaluation of Mechanical Assistance for the Treatment of Congestive Heart Failure (REMATCH) study was undertaken using the device as an alternative rather than bridge to transplantation *(109)* (*see* section on postoperative management).

NOVACOR N1000PC

The Novacor N1000PC (World Heart Corp.) is a wearable LV assist system with implantable pump and externalized vent tube, controller, and batteries (Fig. 5). Its dual pusher-plate design provides symmetrical movement, minimizing mechanical torque *(110,111)*. The pump is lined with a smooth polyurethane sac and has gelatin-sealed inflow and outflow grafts. The first successful bridge-to-transplant implantation took place in 1984, and it received FDA approval for bridge to transplant in 1998. Inflow comes from the LV apex, and outflow is through the ascending aorta, with flows up to 10 L per minute. Patients can ambulate with little impairment after implantation. Many patients have been successfully discharged from the hospital to await transplant. It also has an excellent mechanical reliability rate with few device failures *(112)*.

Successful outcome requires proper patient selection. Device-specific exclusion criteria include blood dyscrasias, presence of a prosthetic aortic valve, and a recipient BSA less than 1.5 m² *(113)*. Preoperative multisystem organ failure is predictive of poor outcome

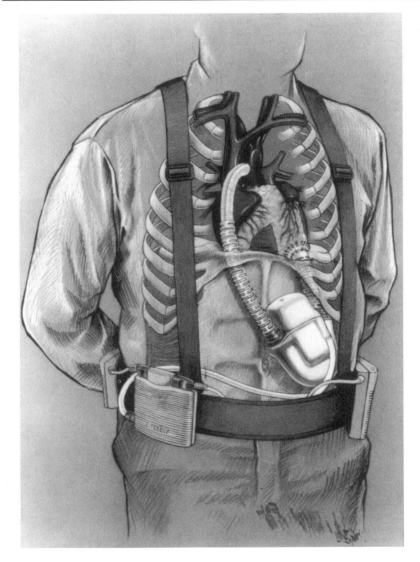

Fig. 5. The Novacor N1000PC. Implantable pump and external drive console. (Courtesy of Baxter Healthcare Corp., Berkeley, CA.)

as well *(33,35,114)*. Like other LVADs, bleeding and RHF are the most significant perioperative complications. Anticoagulation must be maintained with coumadin (INR 2–3) and with aspirin. Despite anticoagulation, the embolic stroke rate associated with the Novacor device has been high (26%). However, recent inflow cannula/conduit modifications have dropped the embolic stroke rate to 12% *(113)*.

TOTAL ARTIFICIAL HEARTS (*SEE ALSO* CHAPTER 13)

The CardioWest TAH (CardioWest Technologies Inc.) is a pneumatic, biventricular, orthotopically implanted TAH with an externalized driveline to its console (Fig. 6). It consists of two spherical polyurethane chambers with polyurethane diaphragms. Inflow and outflow conduits are constructed of Dacron™ and contain Medtronic-Hall™ valves. It began as the Jarvik-7 TAH, used in the early 1980s *(115,116)*. Despite early obstacles, a new investigational device exemption study started in 1993. It is the only TAH approved for use in the United States under the FDA investigational device exemption. The trial showed support durations of 12 to 186 days, with a 93% survival to transplant *(117)*. European experience with the CardioWest TAH has been slightly worse, although encouraging *(118,119)*.

The TAH benefits from having the ability to provide excellent, early support, avoiding irreversible end-organ damage in rapidly decompensating critically ill patients *(117)*. Unlike the other biventricular devices, it obviates the presence of the native heart. This is particularly useful when leaving the native heart in place would be detrimental or impossible (infection or cardiac tumors).

Adequate intrathoracic space is required to accommodate the TAH. Fitting criteria includes BSA greater than 1.7 m^2, cardiothoracic ratio 0.5, LV diastolic dimension above 66 mm, AP distance more than 10 cm, and combined ventricular volume of more than 1500 mL. Careful intraoperative fitting is critical. In addition to size requirements, strict anticoagulation with coumadin, aspirin, Persantine, and Trental is needed *(120)*. Rehabilitation is limited as well because of the large console. A portable console for the CardioWest TAH is in development, however.

New TAHs are in development that will allow full implantability and hospital discharge. The AbioCor TAH (Abiomed Cardiovascular) consists of an internal thoracic pump, internal rechargeable battery, internal electronics, and an external battery pack. External power is delivered via a transcutaneous energy transmission coil located on the chest wall. The pump consists of two ventricles with their corresponding mechanical valves. Its stroke volume is between 60 and 65 cc, with an output of between 4 and 10 L per minute. A centrifugal pump moves hydraulic fluid between each ventricle, providing alternate LV and RV pulsatile flow. There is an atrial balance chamber that adjusts for left and right atrial pressures. As with previous TAHs, fitting is critical. The Abiofit system was developed using three-dimensional computed tomography reconstruction to size patients before implantation. Anticoagulation is

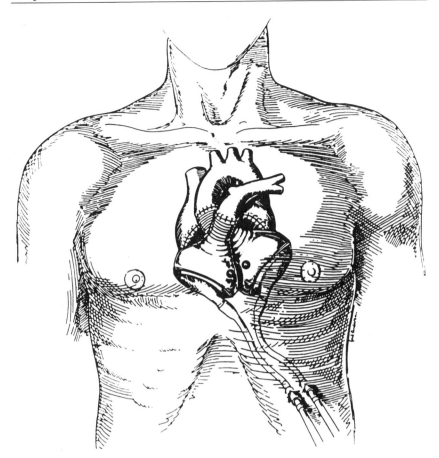

Fig. 6. The CardioWest total artifical heart. Implantable pump and external drive console. (Courtesy of CardioWest Technologies Inc., Tucson, AZ.)

maintained with coumadin and Plavix. The first human implantation took place in July 2001 at Jewish Hospital in Louisville, Kentucky *(121)*. The implantation, part of the initial AbioCor trial, represents the first implantation of a totally implantable TAH. End points include 60-day mortality and quality-of-life measurements, with an anticipated sample size of 15 to 30 patients recruited over 2 years. As of 2004, 5 patients have been implanted, totaling nearly 1 year of support without device malfunction.

AXIAL FLOW PUMPS

Axial flow pumps represent one of the newest generations of assist devices. They can provide full cardiac support in a much smaller pump with fewer moving parts and less blood-contacting surface than pusher-plate devices. In addition to their small size, their design is notable for nonpulsatile flow. Several studies have demonstrated metabolic and neurohumoral changes in organ perfusion compared to pulsatile flow (122–134). However, both clinical and long-term animal studies have failed to show significant differences in morbidity and mortality with axial flow pumps (135–143). The most promising devices are the HeartMate II (Thoratec Laboratories), DeBakey VAD (MicroMed Technology Inc.), and Jarvik 2000 (Jarvik Heart Inc.). These devices weigh between 53 and 176 grams and can generate flows in excess of 10 L per minute.

The Jarvik 2000 axial flow pump, HeartMate II, and the DeBakey axial flow pump all have similar features. Their small size allows implantation into smaller patients than most pulsatile pumps. This also makes placement and explantation easier. With fewer moving parts, there are fewer points of friction, therefore increasing their expected durability. Although there is controversy over long-term nonpulsatile flow, most patients maintain some native cardiac function and therefore continue to have pulsatile blood flow.

Unfortunately, if there is a device failure, there are few options or backup mechanisms in place other than replacement. In addition, because they lack valves, if device malfunction does occur, the patient can develop the equivalent of wide-open aortic insufficiency. The DeBakey pump has already been successfully implanted in a few patients in Europe (144,145). In addition, the HeartMate II and the Jarvik 2000 have been successfully implanted in humans (146).

CARDIAC COMPRESSION DEVICES

Epicardial compression devices support the circulation by compressing the failing heart from its epicardial surface. The Anstadt cup was introduced in 1965 (147) as a cardiac massage device used for cardiac arrest. This early compression device held the heart in place with vacuum, but did not employ any means to synchronize with the cardiac cycle. Feasibility tests resulted in no device-related complications (148).

Newer devices consist of a cup or cuff with an internal inflatable diaphragm, an electrocardiogram sensor/trigger, and a compression driver console. The force generated by the compression device adds to the ventricular pressure generated by the native, contracting myocardium. Diastolic compliance is lessened, however, requiring higher filling pressures to obtain the same preload (149,150).

Both Abiomed and Cardio Technologies Inc. have compression devices under development. The CardioSupport System of Cardio Technologies is undergoing phase I trials in Europe. Early animal studies demonstrated successful support for up to 7 days *(151)*. The compression devices benefit from not having any blood–device interface, reducing the need for anticoagulation. The epicardial application should be relatively easier without the requirement for cardiopulmonary bypass. With variable compression strength, the devices are easily weaned as well. Potential problems include rhythm disturbances and myocardial injury that may result after prolonged use *(152)*.

DEVICE SELECTION

Device selection is invariably influenced by both availability and physician experience. Although much has been published on individual devices, few studies have compared assist devices at a single institution *(64,153)*. There are two major indications for cardiac assist device support: bridge to recovery and bridge to transplant. Destination therapy, although probable, remains investigational.

There are five FDA-approved assist devices in addition to the IABP for these indications. Table 1 summarizes these devices: the Abiomed BVS 5000, the Thoratec device, the Novacor N1000PC, the TCI Heart-Mate Implantable Pneumatic, and the TCI HeartMate Vented Electric LVAD. In addition to the FDA-approved devices, there are several other VADs in development and clinical use. Table 3 summarizes most of the current VADs along with their major characteristics.

Important clinical issues in choosing a device include the expected duration of support, need for biventricular support, cost, device-related risks, patient characteristics, and United Network of Organ Sharing classification rules. Institutional standard of care, ranging from community practice to tertiary heart failure/transplant centers, also influences device selection.

Patients who may require mechanical circulatory support can be divided into three main categories; these different clinical scenarios and patient needs dictate the best type of device to use:

1. Acute profound shock, such as from postcardiotomy cardiac arrest, potentially with end-organ failure and RHF.
2. Decompensated chronic congestive heart failure. These individuals are more chronically ill patients who are transplant candidates.
3. Nontransplant candidates. These patients are not at a transplant center and have potentially recoverable myocardium.

Table 3
Ventricular Assist Devices

Class	Device	Implantable	Long-term	BiVAD capable	Hosp D/C	No AC	Advantage	Disadvantage
TAH	CardioWest	+	+	+			Greatest TAH clinical experience	Fitting required Immobility Infection (10–90%) Emboli (12%)
TAH	Abiomed	+	+	+	+		Totally implantable	Fitting required
TAH	Penn State	+	+	+	+		Totally implantable	Fitting required
Centrifugal	Biomedicus			+			Simple Easy Inexpensive	Bleeding (45%) Embolus (2–63%) Device failure (15%) RF (35%) Bed bound Perfusionist required
External pneumatic	Abiomed			+			Easy Most common	Flow limit 6 L Bleeding (40%) Hospital bound
External pneumatic	Thoratec		+	+			Only FDA-approved long-term BV VAD	Hospital bound BSA limitation Bleeding (42%) Infection (36%) RF (36%) Embolus (8%)

					Advantages	Disadvantages
Pusher plate	Berlin heart	+	+		Low-BSA compatible	Pump cleaning required
Pusher plate	HeartMate VE	+	+	+	Low CVA rate	Infection BSA >1.5
Pusher plate	Novacor	+	+		Reliable (0.8%)	Infection (30–50%) BSA limit CVA (12–26%)
Axial flow	Jarvik	+	+		Small size Small drive line	Nonpulsatile? AI with pump failure rpm only
Axial flow	Heart Mate II	+	+		Small size Small drive line	Nonpulsatile? AI with pump failure
Axial flow	DeBakey	+	+		Small size Small drive line Flow probe 10 L/min	Nonpulsatile? AI with pump failure Fixed pump speed
Epicardial compression	CTI		+	+	Weanable Defibrillation option	Myocardial trauma? Unproven durability
Epicardial compression	Abiomed		+	+	Weanable Defibrillation option	Myocardial trauma? Unproven durability

AC, anticoagulation; AI, aortic insufficiency; BV, biventricular; BSA, body surface area; CVA, cerebrovascular accident; RF, renal failure; rpm, revolutions per minute; TAH, total artifical heart; VAD, ventricular assist device; VE, vented electric.

Patients in profound shock with end-organ dysfunction and RHF need early and reliable support to avoid permanent end-organ damage and increased chances of survival. The preferred devices in such a scenario are the Abiomed BVS 5000, the Thoratec device, and the TAH. These devices provide full BV support, reestablishing near-normal hemodynamics and allowing myocardial recovery *(73)*. Early implementation of BV support is critical in patients with severe BV failure *(3,4,77)*. While on ventricular support, the potential for myocardial recovery and neurological status can be determined. If a prolonged support period is expected, a longer term device should be implanted, such as the Thoratec or TAH. Despite their severe cardiac failure, these patients can be successfully salvaged, with survival rates approaching that of the general cardiac transplantation population *(80,81)*.

Patients who suffer from more chronic congestive heart failure and who are transplant candidates may decompensate before receiving their transplant. In these patients, the potential for long-term support must be considered. Hospital discharge and rehabilitation become important factors in choosing a device for this patient population *(114,154)*. Longer term support with end-organ recovery and better rehabilitation is associated with better long-term survival *(155)*. Therefore, the recommended devices are the implantable HeartMate and the Novacor LVAD. Treatment of RHF, if present, is mandatory. This can be done either medically or with a short-term VAD such as the Abiomed.

Nontransplant candidates may be patients at nontransplant centers or with recoverable cardiac function. Patients at nontransplant centers, who may benefit from a longer term device and transplant workup, can be safely transferred once stabilized on short-term devices *(76)*. Many patients transferred on assist devices are successfully weaned without requiring a long-term implantable LVAD *(8,76)*. The preferred device for use in this setting is the Abiomed BVS 5000. A long-term device can be implanted later as required.

POSTOPERATIVE MANAGEMENT

Early Postoperative Management

There are several factors we have found useful in the postoperative management of LVAD patients. Antibiotic prophylaxis is started preoperatively and continues for at least 3 days postimplant. We treat RHF with milrinone and nitric oxide *(108)*. In addition, we treat vasodilatory hypotension with intravenous arginine vasopressin (Parke-Davis) *(156)*. Aprotinin is continued in the postoperative period until hemorrhage has stopped. Ventricular arrhythmias are managed with appropriate pharmacological agents and cardioversion if necessary.

Late Postoperative Management

Late postoperative care focuses on rehabilitation and monitoring of the immunological changes *(157)* induced by the LVAD while awaiting heart transplantation. Patients with the vented electric TCI LVAD are eligible for discharge to home while awaiting transplant *(154,158,159)*. Patients are followed weekly in the LVAD clinic. Panel-reactive antibody levels are measured in TCI LVAD patients biweekly.

LVAD Explant vs Transplant

Unless in a study, all LVAD patients are listed as heart transplant candidates. Long-term LVAD explantation is considered only if there is significant myocardial recovery evidenced by an exercise testing protocol. The profound ventricular unload provided by LVAD support can lead to reverse remodeling evident at genetic, biochemical, and histological levels *(160,161)*. Our protocol to assess myocardial recovery is to reduce LVAD flow to 2 L per minute while patients exercise on a treadmill. Right heart catheterization and echocardiography is performed to determine the adequacy of ventricular function *(162)*. Although functional recovery allowing LVAD explantation has been reported *(163)*, our experience has shown only a few patients can be successfully weaned from their devices *(164)*.

Destination Therapy

The first generation of mechanical cardiac assist devices, such as the HeartMate and the Novacor devices, have enjoyed good relatively long-term clinical success. Because of increased long-term survival as well as improved quality of life with these devices, the use of the LVAD for permanent support without transplantation (so-called destination therapy) is under exploration.

The REMATCH study was conducted to test this concept in a randomized controlled trial *(109)*. There were 129 nontransplant candidates in New York Heart Association class IV heart failure randomly assigned to receive a HeartMate LVAD or optimal medical therapy. The patients had very advanced heart failure, as evidenced by the low EFs (17%), low systolic blood pressure (101–103 mmHg), elevated creatinines (1.7–1.8 mg/dL), and the need for intravenous inotropes in 65 to 72% of patients. There was a 48% reduction in the risk of death from any cause in the LVAD group compared to the medical therapy group. The 1- and

2-year survival were 52 vs 25% ($p = 0.002$) and 23 vs 8% ($p = 0.09$) for the LVAD and medical therapy groups, respectively *(165)*. Furthermore, of the 54 deaths in the medical therapy group, 50 were attributable to heart failure. In contrast, of the 41 deaths in the LVAD arm, only 1 was thought secondary to ventricular dysfunction. Quality of life (using the Minnesota Living With Heart Failure questionnaire and New York Heart Association class) was also better in the assist device group.

However, there are reasons for caution. The probability for device failure was 35% at 24 months, and sepsis accounted for 17 of the 41 deaths in the device arm. Furthermore, the Kaplan–Meier survival curves began to come together after 24 months, with a mortality of 77% in the device arm. Finally, cost analyses are pending and will be critical before VADs can be considered a routine strategy for permanent therapy in advanced heart failure.

CONCLUSION

LVADs are the standard of care for potential heart transplant patients with life-threatening heart failure refractory to medical therapy. Significant advances in both the technology and clinical experience have taken place. Increasing technological advances, clinical experience, and broadening indications are allowing more patients to benefit from VAD support. Thus, a critical niche can be filled while patients await heart transplant. For some patients, LVADs may even become an alternative to transplant. In turn, this results in more appropriate transplant candidates, increased survival, and better quality of life for patients who would otherwise not survive.

REFERENCES

1. Schmid C, Deng M, Hammel D, Weyand M, Loick HM, Scheld HH. Emergency vs elective/urgent left ventricular assist device implantation. J Heart Lung Transplant 1998;17:1024–1028.
2. Deng MC, Weyand M, Hammel D, et al. Selection and outcome of ventricular assist device patients: the Muenster experience. J Heart Lung Transplant 1998;17:817–825.
3. Chen JM, Spanier TB, Gonzalez JJ, et al. Improved survival in patients with acute myocarditis using external pulsatile mechanical ventricular assistance. J Heart Lung Transplant 1999;18:351–357.
4. Marelli D, Laks H, Amsel B, et al. Temporary mechanical support with the BVS 5000 assist device during treatment of acute myocarditis. J Card Surg 1997;12: 55–59.
5. Minami K, El Banayosy A, Posival H, et al. Improvement of survival rate in patients with cardiogenic shock by using nonpulsatile and pulsatile ventricular assist device. Int J Artif Organs 1992;15:715–721.

6. Copeland JG, Smith RG, Arabia FA, Nolan PE, Banchy ME. The CardioWest total artificial heart as a bridge to transplantation. Semin Thorac Cardiovasc Surg 2000;12:238–242.

7. Hendry PJ, Masters RG, Mussivand TV, et al. Circulatory support for cardiogenic shock due to acute myocardial infarction: a Canadian experience. Can J Cardiol 1999;15:1090–1094.

8. Helman DN, Morales DL, Edwards NM, et al. Left ventricular assist device bridge-to-transplant network improves survival after failed cardiotomy. Ann Thorac Surg 1999;68:1187–1194.

9. Goldberg RJ, Gore JM, Thompson CA, Gurwitz JH. Recent magnitude of and temporal trends (1994–1997) in the incidence and hospital death rates of cardiogenic shock complicating acute myocardial infarction: The second National Registry of Myocardial Infarction. Am Heart J 2001;141:65–72.

10. Goldberg RJ, Gore JM, Alpert JS, et al. Cardiogenic shock after acute myocardial infarction. Incidence and mortality from a community-wide perspective, 1975 to 1988. N Engl J Med 1991;325:1117–1122.

11. Hochman JS, Sleeper LA, White HD, et al. One-year survival following early revascularization for cardiogenic shock. JAMA 2001;285:190–192.

12. Mueller HS. Role of intra-aortic counterpulsation in cardiogenic shock and acute myocardial infarction. Cardiology 1994;84:168–174.

13. Champsaur G, Ninet J, Vigneron M, Cochet P, Neidecker J, Boissonnat P. Use of the Abiomed BVS System 5000 as a bridge to cardiac transplantation. J Thorac Cardiovasc Surg 1990;100:122–128.

14. Sun BC, Catanese KA, Spanier TB, et al. One hundred long-term implantable left ventricular assist devices: the Columbia Presbyterian interim experience. Ann Thorac Surg 1999;68:688–694.

15. Houel R, Vermes E, Tixier DB, Le Besnerais P, Benhaiem-Sigaux N, Loisance DY. Myocardial recovery after mechanical support for acute myocarditis: is sustained recovery predictable? Ann Thorac Surg 1999;68:2177–2180.

16. Farrar DJ, Hill JD, Gray LA, Galbraith TA, Chow E, Hershon JJ. Successful biventricular circulatory support as a bridge to cardiac transplantation during prolonged ventricular fibrillation and asystole. Circulation 1989;80(5 part 2):III147–III151.

17. Holman WL, Roye GD, Bourge RC, McGiffin DC, Iyer SS, Kirklin JK. Circulatory support for myocardial infarction with ventricular arrhythmias. Ann Thorac Surg 1995;59:1230–1231.

18. Swartz MT, Lowdermilk GA, McBride LR. Refractory ventricular tachycardia as an indication for ventricular assist device support. J Thorac Cardiovasc Surg 1999;118:1119–1120.

19. Oz MC, Rose EA, Levin HR. Selection criteria for placement of left ventricular assist devices. Am Heart J 1995;129:173–177.

20. Swartz MT, Votapka TV, McBride LR, Lohmann DP, Moroney DA, Pennington DG. Risk stratification in patients bridged to cardiac transplantation. Ann Thorac Surg 1994;58:1142–1145.

20a. Williams MR, Oz MC. Indications and patient selection for mechanical ventricular assistance. Ann Thorac Surg 2001;71:S86–S91.

21. Nakatani S, Thomas JD, Savage RM, Vargo RL, Smedira NG, McCarthy PM. Prediction of right ventricular dysfunction after left ventricular assist device implantation. Circulation 1996;94(9 suppl):II216–II221.

22. Gracin N, Johnson MR, Spokas D, et al. The use of APACHE II scores to select candidates for left ventricular assist device placement. Acute Physiology and Chronic Health Evaluation. J Heart Lung Transplant 1998;17:1017–1023.

23. Fukamachi K, McCarthy PM, Smedira NG, Vargo RL, Starling RC, Young JB. Preoperative risk factors for right ventricular failure after implantable left ventricular assist device insertion. Ann Thorac Surg 1999;68:2181–2184.

24. Springer WE, Wasler A, Radovancevic B, et al. Retrospective analysis of infection in patients undergoing support with left ventricular assist systems. ASAIO J 1996; 42:M763–M765.

25. Cloy MJ, Myers TJ, Stutts LA, Macris MP, Frazier OH. Hospital charges for conventional therapy vs left ventricular assist system therapy in heart transplant patients. ASAIO J 1995;41:M535–M539.

26. Macris MP, Myers TJ, Jarvik R, et al. In vivo evaluation of an intraventricular electric axial flow pump for left ventricular assistance. ASAIO J 1994;40: M719–M722.

27. Tedoriya T, Kawasuji M, Sakakibara N, Takemura H, Watanabe Y, Hetzer R. Coronary bypass flow during use of intraaortic balloon pumping and left ventricular assist device. Ann Thorac Surg 1998;66:477–481.

28. Sinha P, Chen JM, Flannery M, Scully BE, Oz MC, Edwards NM. Infections during left ventricular assist device support do not affect posttransplant outcomes. Circulation 2000;102(19 suppl 3):III194–III199.

29. Holman WL, Skinner JL, Waites KB, Benza RL, McGiffin DC, Kirklin JK. Infection during circulatory support with ventricular assist devices. Ann Thorac Surg 1999;68:711–716.

30. Argenziano M, Catanese KA, Moazami N, et al. The influence of infection on survival and successful transplantation in patients with left ventricular assist devices. J Heart Lung Transplant 1997;16:822–831.

31. Herrmann M, Weyand M, Greshake B, et al. Left ventricular assist device infection is associated with increased mortality but is not a contraindication to transplantation. Circulation 1997;95:814–817.

32. Ankersmit HJ, Tugulea S, Spanier T, et al. Activation-induced T-cell death and immune dysfunction after implantation of left-ventricular assist device. Lancet 1999;354:550–555.

33. Oz MC, Goldstein DJ, Pepino P, et al. Screening scale predicts patients successfully receiving long-term implantable left ventricular assist devices. Circulation 1995;92(9 suppl):II169–II173.

34. Pennington DG, McBride LR, Peigh PS, Miller LW, Swartz MT. Eight years' experience with bridging to cardiac transplantation. J Thorac Cardiovasc Surg 1994;107:472–480.

35. Farrar DJ. Preoperative predictors of survival in patients with Thoratec ventricular assist devices as a bridge to heart transplantation. Thoratec ventricular assist device principal investigators. J Heart Lung Transplant 1994;13(1 part 1): 93–100.

36. Friedel N, Viazis P, Schiessler A, et al. Recovery of end-organ failure during mechanical circulatory support. Eur J Cardiothorac Surg 1992;6:519–522.

37. Frazier OH, Macris MP, Myers TJ, et al. Improved survival after extended bridge to cardiac transplantation. Ann Thorac Surg 1994;57:1416–1422.

38. Reinhartz O, Farrar DJ, Hershon JH, Avery GJ Jr, Haeusslein EA, Hill JD. Importance of preoperative liver function as a predictor of survival in patients supported with Thoratec ventricular assist devices as a bridge to transplantation. J Thorac Cardiovasc Surg 1998;116:633–640.

39. Pae WE Jr, Miller CA, Matthews Y, Pierce WS. Ventricular assist devices for postcardiotomy cardiogenic shock. A combined registry experience. J Thorac Cardiovasc Surg 1992;104:541–552.

40. Pennington DG, Merjavy JP, Swartz MT, Willman VL. Clinical experience with a centrifugal pump ventricular assist device. Trans Am Soc Artif Intern Organs 1982;28:93–99.
41. Bianchi JJ, Swartz MT, Raithel SC, et al. Initial clinical experience with centrifugal pumps coated with the Carmeda process. ASAIO J 1992;38:M143–M146.
42. Coselli JS, LeMaire SA, Ledesma DF, Ohtsubo S, Tayama E, Nose Y. Initial experience with the Nikkiso centrifugal pump during thoracoabdominal aortic aneurysm repair. J Vasc Surg 1998;27:378–383.
43. Curtis JJ, Walls JT, Wagner-Mann CC, et al. Centrifugal pumps: description of devices and surgical techniques. Ann Thorac Surg 1999;68:666–671.
44. Mann FA, Wagner-Mann CC, Curtis JJ, Demmy TL, Turk JR. A calf model for left ventricular centrifugal mechanical assist. Artif Organs 1996;20:670–677.
45. Wagner-Mann C, Curtis J, Mann FA, Turk J, Demmy T, Turpin T. Subchronic centrifugal mechanical assist in an unheparinized calf model. Artif Organs 1996; 20:666–669.
46. Curtis J, Wagner-Mann C, Mann F, Demmy T, Walls J, Turk J. Subchronic use of the St. Jude centrifugal pump as a mechanical assist device in calves. Artif Organs 1996;20:662–665.
47. Magovern GJ Jr, Christlieb IY, Kao RL, et al. Recovery of the failing canine heart with biventricular support in a previously fatal experimental model. J Thorac Cardiovasc Surg 1987;94:656–663.
48. Naganuma S, Yambe T, Sonobe T, Kobayashi S, Nitta S. Development of a novel centrifugal pump: magnetic rotary pump. Artif Organs 1997;21:746–750.
49. Ohtsubo S, Naito K, Matsuura M, et al. Initial clinical experience with the Baylor-Nikkiso centrifugal pump. Artif Organs 1995;19:769–773.
50. Taguchi S, Yozu R, Mori A, Aizawa T, Kawada S. A miniaturized centrifugal pump for assist circulation. Artif Organs 1994;18:664–668.
51. Takami Y, Ohara Y, Otsuka G, Nakazawa T, Nose Y. Preclinical evaluation of the Kyocera Gyro centrifugal blood pump for cardiopulmonary bypass. Perfusion 1997;12:335–341.
52. Nakazawa T, Ohara Y, Benkowski R, et al. A pivot bearing-supported centrifugal pump for a long-term assist heart. Int J Artif Organs 1997;20:222–228.
53. Curtis JJ, Walls JT, Schmaltz RA, et al. Improving clinical outcome with centrifugal mechanical assist for postcardiotomy ventricular failure. Artif Organs 1995; 19:761–765.
54. Curtis JJ. Centrifugal mechanical assist for postcardiotomy ventricular failure. Semin Thorac Cardiovasc Surg 1994;6:140–146.
55. Nishinaka T, Nishida H, Endo M, Miyagishima M, Ohtsuka G, Koyanagi H. Less blood damage in the impeller centrifugal pump: a comparative study with the roller pump in open heart surgery. Artif Organs 1996;20:707–710.
56. Yoshikai M, Hamada M, Takarabe K, Okazaki Y, Ito T. Clinical use of centrifugal pumps and the roller pump in open heart surgery: a comparative evaluation. Artif Organs 1996;20:704–706.
57. Morgan IS, Codispoti M, Sanger K, Mankad PS. Superiority of centrifugal pump over roller pump in paediatric cardiac surgery: prospective randomised trial. Eur J Cardiothorac Surg 1998;13:526–532.
58. Noon GP, Ball JW Jr, Papaconstantinou HT. Clinical experience with BioMedicus centrifugal ventricular support in 172 patients. Artif Organs 1995;19:756–760.
59. Noon GP, Ball JW Jr, Short HD. Bio-Medicus centrifugal ventricular support for postcardiotomy cardiac failure: a review of 129 cases. Ann Thorac Surg 1996;61: 291–295.

60. Noon GP, Lafuente JA, Irwin S. Acute and temporary ventricular support with BioMedicus centrifugal pump. Ann Thorac Surg 1999;68:650–654.

61. Hoy FB, Mueller DK, Geiss DM, et al. Bridge to recovery for postcardiotomy failure: is there still a role for centrifugal pumps? Ann Thorac Surg 2000;70: 1259–1263.

62. Joyce LD, Kiser JC, Eales F, King RM, Overton JW Jr, Toninato CJ. Experience with generally accepted centrifugal pumps: personal and collective experience. Ann Thorac Surg 1996;61:287–290.

63. Magovern GJ Jr. The biopump and postoperative circulatory support. Ann Thorac Surg 1993;55:245–249.

64. Couper GS, Dekkers RJ, Adams DH. The logistics and cost-effectiveness of circulatory support: advantages of the Abiomed BVS 5000. Ann Thorac Surg 1999;68:646–649.

65. Curtis JJ, Boley TM, Walls JT, Demmy TL, Schmaltz RA. Frequency of seal disruption with the Sarns centrifugal pump in postcardiotomy circulatory assist. Artif Organs 1994;18:235–237.

66. Hart RM, Filipenco VG, Kung RT. A magnetically suspended and hydrostatically stabilized centrifugal blood pump. Artif Organs 1996;20:591–596.

67. Nojiri C, Kijima T, Maekawa J, et al. Recent progress in the development of Terumo implantable left ventricular assist system. ASAIO J 1999;45:199–203.

68. Ohtsuka G, Nakata K, Yoshikawa M, et al. Long-term in vivo left ventricular assist device study for 284 days with Gyro PI pump. Artif Organs 1999;23: 504–507.

69. Schima H, Schmallegger H, Huber L, et al. An implantable seal-less centrifugal pump with integrated double-disk motor. Artif Organs 1995;19:639–643.

70. Wakisaka Y, Taenaka Y, Chikanari K, Okuzono Y, Endo S, Takano H. Development of an implantable centrifugal blood pump for circulatory assist. ASAIO J 1997;43:M608–M614.

71. Waters T, Allaire P, Tao G, et al. Motor feedback physiological control for a continuous flow ventricular assist device. Artif Organs 1999;23:480–486.

72. Yamazaki K, Litwak P, Tagusari O, et al. An implantable centrifugal blood pump with a recirculating purge system (Cool-Seal system). Artif Organs 1998;22: 466–474.

73. Guyton RA, Schonberger JP, Everts PA, et al. Postcardiotomy shock: clinical evaluation of the BVS 5000 biventricular support system. Ann Thorac Surg 1993;56: 346–356.

74. Jett GK. Abiomed BVS 5000: experience and potential advantages. Ann Thorac Surg 1996;61:301–304.

75. Wassenberg PA. The Abiomed BVS 5000 biventricular support system. Perfusion 2000;15:369–371.

76. McBride LR, Lowdermilk GA, Fiore AC, Moroney DA, Brannan JA, Swartz MT. Transfer of patients receiving advanced mechanical circulatory support. J Thorac Cardiovasc Surg 2000;119:1015–1020.

77. Samuels LE, Kaufman MS, Thomas MP, Holmes EC, Brockman SK, Wechsler AS. Pharmacological criteria for ventricular assist device insertion following post-cardiotomy shock: experience with the Abiomed BVS system. J Card Surg 1999; 14:288–293.

78. Pennington DG, Bernhard WF, Golding LR, Berger RL, Khuri SF, Watson JT. Long-term follow-up of postcardiotomy patients with profound cardiogenic shock treated with ventricular assist devices. Circulation 1985;72(3 part 2): II216–II226.

79. Hill JD, Farrar DJ, Hershon JJ, et al. Use of a prosthetic ventricle as a bridge to cardiac transplantation for postinfarction cardiogenic shock. N Engl J Med 1986; 314:626–628.
80. Farrar DJ, Hill JD. Univentricular and biventricular Thoratec VAD support as a bridge to transplantation. Ann Thorac Surg 1993;55:276–282.
81. Farrar DJ, Hill JD, Pennington DG, et al. Preoperative and postoperative comparison of patients with univentricular and biventricular support with the Thoratec ventricular assist device as a bridge to cardiac transplantation. J Thorac Cardiovasc Surg 1997;113:202–209.
82. Korfer R, El Banayosy A, Arusoglu L, et al. Temporary pulsatile ventricular assist devices and biventricular assist devices. Ann Thorac Surg 1999;68:678–683.
83. Farrar DJ. The Thoratec ventricular assist device: a paracorporeal pump for treating acute and chronic heart failure. Semin Thorac Cardiovasc Surg 2000;12: 243–250.
84. Farrar DJ, Buck KE, Coulter JH, Kupa EJ. Portable pneumatic biventricular driver for the Thoratec ventricular assist device. ASAIO J 1997;43:M631–M634.
85. Pennock JL, Pierce WS, Wisman CB, Bull AP, Waldhausen JA. Survival and complications following ventricular assist pumping for cardiogenic shock. Ann Surg 1983;198:469–478.
86. Stolar CJ, Delosh T, Bartlett RH. Extracorporeal Life Support Organization 1993. ASAIO J 1993;39:976–979.
87. Hetzer R, Loebe M, Potapov EV, et al. Circulatory support with pneumatic para-corporeal ventricular assist device in infants and children. Ann Thorac Surg 1998; 66:1498–1506.
88. Ishino K, Alexi-Meskishvili V, Hetzer R. Myocardial recovery through ECMO after repair of total anomalous pulmonary venous connection: the importance of left heart unloading. Eur J Cardiothorac Surg 1997;11:585–587.
89. Loebe M, Hennig E, Muller J, Spiegelsberger S, Weng Y, Hetzer R. Long-term mechanical circulatory support as a bridge to transplantation, for recovery from cardiomyopathy, and for permanent replacement. Eur J Cardiothorac Surg 1997;11 (suppl):S18–S24.
90. Kantrowitz A, Tjonneland S, Freed PS, Phillips SJ, Butner AN, Sherman JL. Initial clinical experience with intraaortic balloon pumping in cardiogenic shock. JAMA 1968;203:113–118.
91. Powell WJ, Daggett WM, Magro AE, et al. Effects of intra-aortic balloon counter-pulsation on cardiac performance, oxygen consumption, and coronary blood flow in dogs. Circ Res 1970;26:753–764.
92. Bregman D, Nichols AB, Weiss MB, Powers ER, Martin EC, Casarella WJ. Percutaneous intraaortic balloon insertion. Am J Cardiol 1980;46:261–264.
93. Subramanian VA, Goldstein JE, Sos TA, McCabe JC, Hoover EA, Gay WA. Preliminary clinical experience with percutaneous intraaortic balloon pumping. Circulation 1980;62(2 part 2):I123–I129.
94. Dietl CA, Berkheimer MD, Woods EL, Gilbert CL, Pharr WF, Benoit CH. Efficacy and cost-effectiveness of preoperative IABP in patients with ejection fraction of 0.25 or less. Ann Thorac Surg 1996;62:401–408.
95. Schmid C, Wilhelm M, Reimann A, et al. Use of an intraaortic balloon pump in patients with impaired left ventricular function. Scand Cardiovasc J 1999;33: 194–198.
96. Torchiana DF, Hirsch G, Buckley MJ, et al. Intraaortic balloon pumping for cardiac support: trends in practice and outcome, 1968 to 1995. J Thorac Cardiovasc Surg 1997;113:758–764.

97. Busch T, Sirbu H, Zenker D, Dalichau H. Vascular complications related to intraaortic balloon counterpulsation: an analysis of 10 years experience. Thorac Cardiovasc Surg 1997;45:55–59.

98. Sirbu H, Busch T, Aleksic I, Friedrich M, Dalichau H. Ischaemic complications with intra-aortic balloon counter-pulsation: incidence and management. Cardiovasc Surg 2000;8:66–71.

99. Rose EA, Levin HR, Oz MC, et al. Artificial circulatory support with textured interior surfaces. A counterintuitive approach to minimizing thromboembolism. Circulation 1994;90(5 part 2):II87–II91.

100. Dasse KA, Frazier OH, Lesniak JM, Myers T, Burnett CM, Poirier VL. Clinical responses to ventricular assistance vs transplantation in a series of bridge to transplant patients. ASAIO J 1992;38:M622–M626.

101. Slater JP, Rose EA, Levin HR, et al. Low thromboembolic risk without anticoagulation using advanced-design left ventricular assist devices. Ann Thorac Surg 1996;62:1321–1327.

102. McCarthy PM, Smedira NO, Vargo RL, et al. One hundred patients with the HeartMate left ventricular assist device: evolving concepts and technology. J Thorac Cardiovasc Surg 1998;115:904–912.

103. Goldstein DJ. Thermo Cardiosystems ventricular assist devices. In: Goldstein DJ, Oz MC, eds. Cardiac Assist Devices. Futura, Armonk, NY: 2000, pp. 307–321.

104. Salamonsen RF, Kaye D, Esmore DS. Inhalation of nitric oxide provides selective pulmonary vasodilatation, aiding mechanical cardiac assist with Thoratec left ventricular assist device. Anaesth Intensive Care 1994;22:209–210.

105. Goldstein DJ, Seldomridge JA, Chen JM, et al. Use of aprotinin in LVAD recipients reduces blood loss, blood use, and perioperative mortality. Ann Thorac Surg 1995;59:1063–1067.

106. Chang JC, Sawa Y, Ohtake S, et al. Hemodynamic effect of inhaled nitric oxide in dilated cardiomyopathy patients on LVAD support. ASAIO J 1997;43:M418–M421.

107. Wagner F, Dandel M, Gunther G, et al. Nitric oxide inhalation in the treatment of right ventricular dysfunction following left ventricular assist device implantation. Circulation 1997;96(9 suppl):II-6.

108. Argenziano M, Choudhri AF, Moazami N, et al. Randomized, double-blind trial of inhaled nitric oxide in LVAD recipients with pulmonary hypertension. Ann Thorac Surg 1998;65:340–345.

109. Rose EA, Moskowitz AJ, Packer M, et al. The REMATCH trial: rationale, design, and end points. Randomized Evaluation of Mechanical Assistance for the Treatment of Congestive Heart Failure. Ann Thorac Surg 1999;67:723–730.

110. Portner PM, Oyer PE, Jassawalla JS, et al. An implantable permanent left ventricular assist system for man. Trans Am Soc Artif Intern Organs 1978;24:99–103.

111. Portner PM, Oyer PE, Pennington DG, et al. Implantable electrical left ventricular assist system: bridge to transplantation and the future. Ann Thorac Surg 1989;47:142–150.

112. Lee J, Miller PJ, Chen H, et al. Reliability model from the in vitro durability tests of a left ventricular assist system. ASAIO J 1999;45:595–601.

113. Ramasamy N, Vargo RL, Kormos RL, Portner PM. The Novacor left ventricular assist system. In: Goldstein DJ, Oz MC, eds. Cardiac Assist Devices. Futura, Armonk, NY: 2000, pp. 323–340.

114. Kormos RL, Murali S, Dew MA, et al. Chronic mechanical circulatory support: rehabilitation, low morbidity, and superior survival. Ann Thorac Surg 1994;57: 51–57.

115. Anderson FL, DeVries WC, Anderson JL, Joyce LD. Evaluation of total artificial heart performance in man. Am J Cardiol 1984;54:394–398.

116. DeVries WC, Anderson JL, Joyce LD, et al. Clinical use of the total artificial heart. N Engl J Med 1984;310:273–278.

117. Copeland JG, Arabia FA, Banchy ME, et al. The CardioWest total artificial heart bridge to transplantation: 1993 to 1996 national trial. Ann Thorac Surg 1998;66: 1662–1669.

118. Arabia FA, Copeland JG, Smith RG, et al. International experience with the CardioWest total artificial heart as a bridge to heart transplantation. Eur J Cardio-thorac Surg 1997;11(suppl):S5–S10.

119. Copeland JG, Pavie A, Duveau D, et al. Bridge to transplantation with the CardioWest total artificial heart: the international experience 1993 to 1995. J Heart Lung Transplant 1996;15(1 part 1):94–99.

120. Copeland JG, Arabia FA, Smith R, Nolan P. The CardioWest total artificial heart. In: Goldstein DJ, Oz MC, eds. Cardiac Assist Devices. Futura, Armonk, NY: 2000, pp. 341–355.

121. SoRelle R. Cardiovascular news. Totally contained AbioCor artificial heart implanted July 3, 2001. Circulation 2001;104:E9005–E9006.

122. Angell James JE, Daly M. Effects of graded pulsatile pressure on the reflex vaso-motor responses elicited by changes of mean pressure in the perfused carotid sinus-aortic arch regions of the dog. J Physiol 1971;214:51–64.

123. Gaer JA, Shaw AD, Wild R, et al. Effect of cardiopulmonary bypass on gastro-intestinal perfusion and function. Ann Thorac Surg 1994;57:371–375.

124. Hickey PR, Buckley MJ, Philbin DM. Pulsatile and nonpulsatile cardio-pumonary bypass: review of a counterproductive controversy. Ann Thorac Surg 1983;36:720–737.

125. Hornick P, Taylor K. Pulsatile and nonpulsatile perfusion: the continuing con-troversy. J Cardiothorac Vasc Anesth 1997;11:310–315.

126. Levine FH, Philbin DM, Kono K, et al. Plasma vasopressin levels and urinary sodium excretion during cardiopulmonary bypass with and without pulsatile flow. Ann Thorac Surg 1981;32:63–67.

127. Moores WY, Gago O, Morris JD, Peck CC. Serum and urinary amylase levels following pulsatile and continuous cardiopulmonary bypass. J Thorac Cardio-vasc Surg 1977;74:73–76.

128. Noris M, Morigi M, Donadelli R, et al. Nitric oxide synthesis by cul-tured endothelial cells is modulated by flow conditions. Circ Res 1995;76: 536–543.

129. Taylor KM, Wright GS, Bain WH, Caves PK, Beastall GS. Comparative studies of pulsatile and nonpulsatile flow during cardiopulmonary bypass. III. Response of anterior pituitary gland to thyrotropin-releasing hormone. J Thorac Cardio-vasc Surg 1978;75:579–584.

130. Taylor KM, Wright GS, Reid JM, et al. Comparative studies of pulsatile and nonpulsatile flow during cardiopulmonary bypass. II. The effects on adrenal secretion of cortisol. J Thorac Cardiovasc Surg 1978;75:574–578.

131. Watkins WD, Peterson MB, Kong DL, et al. Thromboxane and prostacyclin changes during cardiopulmonary bypass with and without pulsatile flow. J Thorac Cardiovasc Surg 1982;84:250–256.

132. Sezai A, Shiono M, Orime Y, et al. Major organ function under mechanical sup-port: comparative studies of pulsatile and nonpulsatile circulation. Artif Organs 1999;23:280–285.

133. Sezai A, Shiono M, Orime Y, et al. Comparison studies of major organ micro-circulations under pulsatile- and nonpulsatile-assisted circulations. Artif Organs 1996;20:139–142.

134. Sezai A, Shiono M, Orime Y, et al. Renal circulation and cellular metabolism during left ventricular assisted circulation: comparison study of pulsatile and nonpulsatile assists. Artif Organs 1997;21:830–835.

135. Wakisaka Y, Taenaka Y, Chikanari K, et al. Long-term evaluation of a nonpulsatile mechanical circulatory support system. Artif Organs 1997;21:639–644.

136. Taenaka Y, Tatsumi E, Sakaki M, et al. Peripheral circulation during nonpulsatile systemic perfusion in chronic awake animals. ASAIO Trans 1991;37:M365–M366.

137. Sakaki M, Taenaka Y, Tatsumi E, Nakatani T, Takano H. Influences of nonpulsatile pulmonary flow on pulmonary function. Evaluation in a chronic animal model. J Thorac Cardiovasc Surg 1994;108:495–502.

138. Reddy RC, Goldstein AH, Pacella JJ, Cattivera GR, Clark RE, Magovern GJ. End organ function with prolonged nonpulsatile circulatory support. ASAIO J 1995;41:M547–M551.

139. Macha M, Litwak P, Yamazaki K, et al. Survival for up to 6 months in calves supported with an implantable axial flow ventricular assist device. ASAIO J 1997;43:311–315.

140. Kawahito K, Damm G, Benkowski R, et al. Ex vivo phase 1 evaluation of the DeBakey/NASA axial flow ventricular assist device. Artif Organs 1996;20:47–52.

141. Hindman BJ, Dexter F, Smith T, Cutkomp J. Pulsatile vs nonpulsatile flow. No difference in cerebral blood flow or metabolism during normothermic cardio-pulmonary bypass in rabbits. Anesthesiology 1995;82:241–250.

142. Hindman BJ, Dexter F, Ryu KH, Smith T, Cutkomp J. Pulsatile vs nonpulsatile cardiopulmonary bypass. No difference in brain blood flow or metabolism at 27°C. Anesthesiology 1994;80:1137–1147.

143. Dapper F, Neppl H, Wozniak G, et al. Effects of pulsatile and nonpulsatile perfusion mode during extracorporeal circulation—a comparative clinical study. Thorac Cardiovasc Surg 1992;40:345–351.

144. Wieselthaler GM, Schima H, Hiesmayr M, et al. First clinical experience with the DeBakey VAD continuous-axial-flow pump for bridge to transplantation. Circulation 2000;101:356–359.

145. Potapov EV, Loebe M, Nasseri BA, et al. Pulsatile flow in patients with a novel nonpulsatile implantable ventricular assist device. Circulation 2000;102(19 suppl 3):III183–III187.

146. Westaby S, Banning AP, Jarvik R, et al. First permanent implant of the Jarvik 2000 heart. Lancet 2000;356:900–903.

147. Anstadt GL, Blakemore WS, Baue AE. A new instrument for prolonged mechanical massage [abstract]. Circulation 1965;31(suppl II):43.

148. Anstadt MP, Bartlett RL, Malone JP, et al. Direct mechanical ventricular actuation for cardiac arrest in humans. A clinical feasibility trial. Chest 1991;100: 86–92.

149. Artrip JH, Yi GH, Levin HR, Burkhoff D, Wang J. Physiological and hemo-dynamic evaluation of nonuniform direct cardiac compression. Circulation 1999;100(19 suppl):II236–II243.

150. Artrip JH, Yi GH, Shimizo J, et al. Maximizing hemodynamic effectiveness of biventricular assistance by direct cardiac compression studied in ex vivo and in vivo canine models of acute heart failure. J Thorac Cardiovasc Surg 2000;120: 379–386.

151. Perez-Tamayo RA, Anstadt MP, Cothran RL, et al. Prolonged total circulatory support using direct mechanical ventricular actuation. ASAIO J 1995;41:M512–M517.
152. Anstadt MP, Perez-Tamayo RA, Banit DM, et al. Myocardial tolerance to mechanical actuation is affected by biomaterial characteristics. ASAIO J 1994;40: M329–M334.
153. El Banayosy A, Arusoglu L, Kizner L, et al. Novacor left ventricular assist system vs HeartMate vented electric left ventricular assist system as a long-term mechanical circulatory support device in bridging patients: a prospective study. J Thorac Cardiovasc Surg 2000;119:581–587.
154. DeRose JJ, Umana JP, Argenziano M, et al. Implantable left ventricular assist devices provide an excellent outpatient bridge to transplantation and recovery. J Am Coll Cardiol 1997;30:1773–1777.
155. Ashton RC, Goldstein DJ, Rose EA, Weinberg AD, Levin HR, Oz MC. Duration of left ventricular assist device support affects transplant survival. J Heart Lung Transplant 1996;15:1151–1157.
156. Argenziano M, Choudhri AF, Oz MC, Rose EA, Smith CR, Landry DW. A prospective randomized trial of arginine vasopressin in the treatment of vasodilatory shock after left ventricular assist device placement. Circulation 1997;96 (9 suppl):II-90.
157. Ankersmit H-J, Itescu S. Immunobiology of left ventricular assist devices. In: Goldstein DJ, Oz MC, eds. Cardiac Assist Devices. Futura, Armonk, NY: 2000, pp. 193–211.
158. Morales DL, Catanese KA, Helman DN, et al. Six-year experience of caring for forty-four patients with a left ventricular assist device at home: safe, economical, necessary. J Thorac Cardiovasc Surg 2000;119:251–259.
159. Catanese KA, Goldstein DJ, Williams DL, et al. Outpatient left ventricular assist device support: a destination rather than a bridge. Ann Thorac Surg 1996;62: 646–652.
160. Levin HR, Oz MC, Chen JM, Packer M, Rose EA, Burkhoff D. Reversal of chronic ventricular dilation in patients with end-stage cardiomyopathy by prolonged mechanical unloading. Circulation 1995;91:2717–2720.
161. Frazier OH, Benedict CR, Radovancevic B, et al. Improved left ventricular function after chronic left ventricular unloading. Ann Thorac Surg 1996;62:675–681.
162. Foray A, Williams D, Reemtsma K, Oz M, Mancini D. Assessment of submaximal exercise capacity in patients with left ventricular assist devices. Circulation 1996;94(9 suppl):II222–II226.
163. Mueller J, Wallukat G, Weng Y, et al. Predictive factors for weaning from a cardiac assist device. An analysis of clinical, gene expression, and protein data. J Heart Lung Transplant 2001;20:202.
164. Mancini DM, Beniaminovitz A, Levin H, et al. Low incidence of myocardial recovery after left ventricular assist device implantation in patients with chronic heart failure. Circulation 1998;98:2383–2389.
165. Rose EA, Gelijns AC, Moskowitz AJ, et al. Long-term use of a left ventricular assist device for end-stage heart failure. N Engl J Med 2001;345:1435–1443.
166. Oz MC, Argenziano M, Catanese KA, et al. Bridge experience with long-term implantable left ventricular assist devices. Are they an alternative to transplantation? Circulation 1997;95:1844–1852.

8 Left Ventricular Volume Reduction Surgery for Idiopathic Dilated Cardiomyopathy

Richard Lee, MD, MBA,
Mohammed A. Quader, MD,
Katherine J. Hoercher, RN,
and Patrick M. McCarthy, MD

CONTENTS

INTRODUCTION
THEORY AND SURGICAL TECHNIQUE
EARLY RESULTS
PRESENT STATUS
FUTURE ROLE
CONCLUSION
REFERENCES

INTRODUCTION

In the United States alone, 4.8 million people suffer from congestive heart failure (CHF). Approximately 550,000 new cases of CHF are diagnosed each year *(1)*. As the population ages, the magnitude of this problem is projected to increase *(2)*. After diagnosis, despite improvements in medical management, 5-year mortality is 60% for men and

From: *Contemporary Cardiology: Surgical Management of Congestive Heart Failure*
Edited by: J. C. Fang and G. S. Couper © Humana Press Inc., Totowa, NJ

45% for women *(1)*. There are 150,000 people in the end stage of this disease, and there is a 5-year mortality that approaches 100% despite the use of angiotensin II-converting enzyme inhibitors *(3)*. Approximately half of these patients have heart failure from idiopathic, infectious, or valvular etiologies unrelated to coronary artery disease *(4)*.

Nearly 2500 heart transplants each year offer hope to a fraction of these patients, but the majority are faced with a short, limited life. In an effort to improve symptoms and survival in these patients, several innovative strategies have been attempted. One of the most widely publicized has been left ventricular (LV) volume reduction, the Batista procedure *(5)*. This chapter discusses the theory and technique of the surgery, the early results, the present status, and the future role of ventricular reconstruction in nonischemic, end-stage CHF.

THEORY AND SURGICAL TECHNIQUE

Ventricular reconstruction for ischemic heart disease was performed as early as 1934 by Claude Beck *(6)* and was performed clinically without cardiopulmonary bypass by Charles Bailey in 1957 *(7)*. One year later, Denton Cooley performed the procedure on cardiopulmonary bypass *(8)*. Vincent Dor expanded the indications to include akinetic as well as dyskinetic myocardial segments in 1985 *(9)*. However, it was not until 1994 that Randas Batista popularized the concept of ventricular volume reduction to nonischemic myocardial segments in patients with idiopathic cardiomyopathy, Chagas disease, or valvular disease *(5)*.

Batista's bold move was based on Laplace's law (Wall tension = Pressure × Radius/2 × Wall thickness), where wall stress is a function of chamber diameter. He also observed that muscle mass is proportional to the cube of the radius in animal hearts. He postulated that an increase in the left ventricle diameter would require a compensatory cubic increase in muscle mass to maintain normal LV function. The partial left ventriculectomy attempted to restore the diameter of the left ventricle by excising a portion of the lateral LV wall, usually between the papillary muscles, or with papillary muscle transection and reimplantation (Fig. 1). This would reduce wall stress and decrease the hypertrophic demand placed on the myocardium. The procedure was most commonly accompanied by a mitral valve repair or replacement. Although the concept of the surgical technique was straightforward, the actual application varied widely. In addition, the geometry of the left ventricle led to a variable mass of tissue excised.

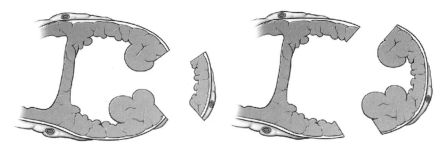

Fig. 1. The partial left ventriculectomy is performed by a wedge-shape excision of myocardium, usually between papillary muscles. However, it often leads to a variable amount of excised myocardium.

EARLY RESULTS

From its inception, the partial left ventriculectomy was plagued by high early mortality. Batista's earliest series in Brazil did not have adequate follow-up to draw any conclusions. However, in 1997, combined results from Brazil and Buffalo General Hospital in New York reported on 120 patients undergoing partial left ventriculectomy *(10)*. The 30-day mortality was 22%, and 2-year survival was 55%. Although all of the patients were in New York Heart Association (NYHA) class IV preoperatively, 57% of the survivors were in NYHA class I, and 33% were in NYHA class II. Unfortunately, only 23 of the 120 patients underwent surgery in Buffalo and had adequate follow-up.

In the same year, McCarthy et al. at the Cleveland Clinic in Ohio reported on 53 patients undergoing partial left ventriculectomy *(11)*. Preoperatively, 60% were in NYHA class IV, and 40% were in NYHA class III. We had only 1 perioperative death (1.9%). However, 15% of our patients required a left ventricular assist device (VAD). With aggressive application of VADs and transplantation, at 11 months actuarial survival was 87%, and freedom from relisting for heart transplantation was 72%. Of the discharged patients, 35% were in NHYA class I, and 32% were in class II.

In 1998, Moreira et al. reported the San Paulo experience in Brazil *(12)*. Left ventriculectomy was performed in 27 patients, 11 in NYHA class III and 16 in NYHA class IV. Hospital mortality was 14.8%, and survival between 6 and 24 months was 59.2%. However, in survivors, NYHA class improved from 3.6 to 1.4. Gradinac had a similar experience in Belgrade with 22 patients *(13)*. The 1-year survival was 68%, but NYHA class improved from 3.8 to 1.4 in those who survived.

Although there were clearly some patients who benefited from the operation, the high early mortality and unpredictable results tempered the initial enthusiasm for the widespread application of this procedure.

In May 2000, the Cleveland Clinic presented its late experience with the partial left ventriculectomy (14). Sixty-two patients underwent partial left ventriculectomy between May 1996 and December 1998. All patients were in NYHA class III (38%) or IV (63%), with 95% transplant candidates. LV end-diastolic diameter (LVEDD) was reduced from 8.4 to 5.9 cm. LV end-diastolic volume (LVED) index was reduced from 133 to 64 mL. Ejection fraction (EF) increased from 16 to 31%. There were only 2 (3.2%) hospital deaths.

Unfortunately, these excellent perioperative results were not durable. Survival was 80% at 1 year and 60% at 3 years. Event-free survival (EFS) was 49% at 1 year and 26% at 3 years. Eleven patients (18%) received left VADs as rescue therapy, and 8 received a heart transplant. Thirty-two patients returned to class IV heart failure. Freedom from class IV was 57% at 1 year and 42% at 3 years. Although there was a small group of patients who appeared to benefit from the operation, we concluded that early and late failures precluded the widespread application of the partial left ventriculectomy. Subsequently, we abandoned the procedure because of the high surgical mortality, concern for diastolic dysfunction, return of heart failure, and occasional postoperative malignant ventricular arrhythmia.

A number of reports helped elucidate some of the reasons that partial left ventriculectomy was unsuccessful. Using mathematical modeling, the group at Columbia found that the geometric rearrangement associated with this operation led to a reduction in wall stress for a given level of pressure generation, thus implying an increase in the efficiency with which wall stress is transduced into intraventricular pressure. However, changes in systolic function were accompanied by offsetting changes in diastolic function; consequently, overall pump function (the Frank-Starling relationship) was depressed (15).

Gorcsan et al. found that partial left ventriculectomy did increase EF and right ventricular ejection by reducing ventricular volumes, but it also resulted in an increase in LV stiffness (16). This may explain why postoperative estimates of LV performance varied with the degree of myocardial fibrosis (16). This may also explain why the effect varied with the preoperative function of the resected segment (17). Artrip et al. found a beneficial effect on this relationship of resecting dyskinetic tissue, an equivocal effect of akinetic scar resection, and a negative effect of removing contracting myocardium (17).

PRESENT STATUS

Despite this information, a few centers persisted with partial left ventriculectomy, especially when transplantation was not a realistic option. An elective international registry reported on 287 patients undergoing partial left ventriculectomy at 48 institutions *(18)*. Several risk factors for EFS, defined by absence of death or ventricular failure that required a VAD or listing for transplantation, were identified. The 1-year EFS was 58% after elective operations, but only 19% after emergent operations. Preoperative NYHA class IV led to a 2-year EFS of 39%. When the preoperative NYHA class was less than IV, EFS was 59% at 2 years. The experience of the center also had a strong impact on outcome. After 20 cases, the 1-year EFS was 69%, as compared to 46% before 20 cases. As few as 5 cases in a single hospital led to a better outcome. Other indicators for a worse outcome included fractional shortening below 5% and duration of preoperative symptoms longer than 9 years. Previous reports have also implicated postoperative mitral regurgitation *(19)* and extent of interstitial fibrosis *(20)* as prognostic indicators.

Suma and members of the RESTORE group reported a series of 82 patients undergoing partial left ventriculectomy for nonischemic cardiomyopathy *(21)*; 40% were in NYHA class III, and 60% were in class IV. During this experience, they changed several aspects of treatment. These included a change to ventriculectomy on-pump on a beating heart, mitral valve replacement via the left ventriculotomy, resection limited to the area between the papillary muscles, and a more targeted resection location based on intraoperative echocardiography. This led to an anterior resection in 12 patients. Overall hospital mortality was 20%, but was only 8% for elective surgeries. When the site was selectively chosen rather than the standard site, hospital mortality decreased from 33 to 15%. The 4-year survival was 53% overall, but 0% for emergencies and 69% for elective procedures. The survivors remain in NYHA class I or II with only 1 patient with a left VAD awaiting transplant.

At the Cleveland Clinic, we recently reviewed our 5-year outcomes from the 62 patients who underwent partial left ventriculectomy between May 1996 and December 1998 *(22)*. Mean follow-up was 3.3 ± 1.9 years. Survival at 1, 2, and 5 years was 82, 78, and 52%, respectively. Survival was similar for patients on preoperative ionotropic support: 84, 80, and 56% at 1, 2, and 5 years, respectively. The risk of death consisted of two phases, an early phase that peaked at

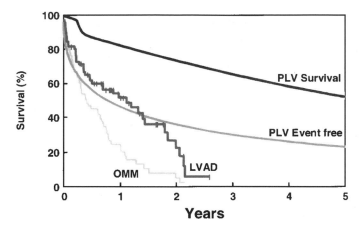

Fig. 2. Comparison of the REMATCH trial results and the Cleveland Clinic results after partial left ventriculectomy (PLV). OMM stands for optimal medical management in the REMATCH trial. LVAD represents the outcome of patients after implantation of a left ventricular device in the REMATCH trial.

4 months and a constant-hazard phase of 11% per year. EFS was 46, 41, and 23% at 1, 2, and 5 years, respectively.

FUTURE ROLE

Although the results of the partial left ventriculectomy have precluded its widespread application, it has shown that certain patients can benefit from ventricular volume reduction, even in nonischemic myocardial disease. To put the results of the partial left ventriculectomy into perspective, we compared them to the results of the Randomized Evaluation of Mechanical Assistance for the Treatment of Congestive Heart Failure (REMATCH) trial (Fig. 2). In patients with similar NYHA classifications, 2-year survival was 23% after left VAD placement in the REMATCH trial. In comparison, at the Cleveland Clinic, 5-year EFS for patients after partial left ventriculectomy was 23%.

Perhaps more important, the partial left ventriculectomy showed that some patients do benefit from LV volume reduction. From lessons learned with dynamic cardiomyoplasty and partial left ventriculectomy, two new devices have been developed either to prevent myocyte overstretch and provide passive LV constraint (Acorn cardiac support device [CSD; ACORN Cardiovascular Inc.]) or reshape the left ventricle altogether without removal of functioning myocardium (Myosplint) *(23)*.

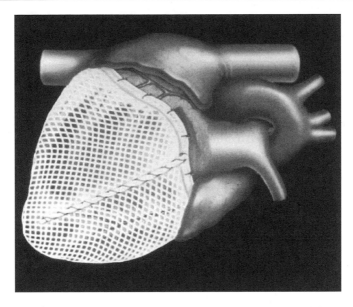

Fig. 3. The Acorn cardiac support device is a custom-made meshlike polyester jacket surgically placed around the ventricles of the heart.

Acorn Cardiac Support Device

The first example of such a device is the Acorn CSD, a custom-made meshlike polyester jacket that is surgically placed around the ventricles of the heart (Fig. 3). Constructed from a compliant woven mesh, it is designed to provide both flexibility and strength. The design of the mesh permits bidirectional compliance of the fabric, which allows it to conform easily to the heart, hence allowing the heart to return to a more normal ellipsoidal shape *(24)*. CSD placement is often performed with concomitant valve repair or coronary artery bypass.

Preclinical studies with CSDs have been reported from two different heart failure models. In an intracoronary microembolization canine heart failure model, Saavedra et al. showed that long-term use of a CSD resulted in decreased end-diastolic and end-systolic volumes and shifted the end-systolic pressure volume relation to the left, compatible with reverse remodeling *(25)*. Chaudrey et al., in a canine heart failure model, showed improved LV diastolic function and chamber sphericity, decreased wall stress, and no evidence of functional mitral regurgitation *(26)*.

In CSD testing on the ovine heart failure model, Power et al. reported similar findings of improved cardiac function, as evidenced by increased EF, fractional shortening, positive dp/dt, and negative dp/dt *(27)*. Sabbah et al. found downregulation of a stretch-mediated p21 ras and sarcoplasmic reticulum adenosine triphosphatase after wrap placement in the canine model. This suggests that the CSD can alter gene expression and promote reverse remodeling *(28)*.

The effect of CSD on akinetic area development following acute myocardial infarction in an ovine model was investigated. Following a baseline magnetic resonance imaging study after creation of an anterior infarct in 10 sheep, a CSD was placed in 5 sheep, with 5 remaining animals serving as controls. The terminal study done at 2 months postinfarction revealed a significantly diminished area of akinesis in the CSD group, with the relative area of akinesis following a similar pattern *(29)*.

Konertz et al. *(30)* examined the safety and efficacy of the CSD in a series of 27 patients suffering from cardiomyopathy and with a mean NYHA of 2.6 ± 0.1. Of these, 16 received concomitant cardiac surgery, principally mitral valve repair or replacement. The remaining 11 patients received a CSD only. In the CSD-only group, 5 of the 11 patients experienced adverse events, including 2 deaths, during an average follow-up of 12.2 ± 1.1 months, but none of the events were device related. Follow-up at 3 and 6 months reflected a significant improvement from pretreatment in EF (21 to 28 and 33%) and NYHA functional class (2.5 to 1.6 and 1.7), as well as a significant decrease in LVEDD (74 to 68 and 65 mm) and left ventricular end-systolic volume (LVESD) (65 to 62 and 57 mm).

Raman et al. *(31)* reported similar findings in a cohort of five patients undergoing CSD with concomitant coronary artery bypass graft. Midterm outcomes at 12-month follow-up demonstrated a significant decrease in LVEDD and LVESD, with an improvement in LVEF and NYHA functional class *(31)*.

From these early studies, it appears the CSD is useful for preventing further cardiac dilation and improves symptoms of heart failure without device-related morbidity or mortality. A randomized, prospective clinical trial of the CSD is currently under way in Europe, the United States, and Australia.

Myosplint

The Myosplint was designed to change the geometry of the left ventricle to decrease wall stress and improve hemodynamics. The implant consists of two epicardial pads and a transventricular tension member. The two pads are located on the surface of the heart, with the load-bearing tension member passing through the ventricle, connecting the pads and drawing the ventricular walls toward one another. Typically,

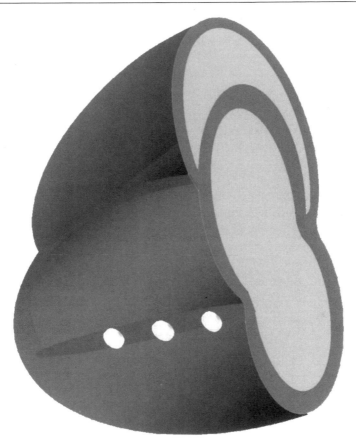

Fig. 4. The Myosplint consists of two epicardial pads and a transventricular tension member. The two pads are located on the surface of the heart with the load-bearing tension member passing through the ventricle connecting the pads and drawing the ventricular walls toward one another. The three Myosplints are tightened to create a bilobular ventricular shape.

three Myosplints are placed on the beating heart, from the lateral left ventricle through the posterior intraventricular septum. The splints are then tightened to create a bilobular shape (Fig. 4).

The Myosplint was initially studied in the canine heart failure model to assess outcomes at 1 month following application. In this trial, heart failure was induced in 15 dogs over a period of 27 days *(32)*. Of these, 7 animals underwent sham surgery, and 8 animals received the Myosplint device. By three-dimensional echocardiographic calculations, LVEF significantly increased from 19% at baseline to 36% acutely and remained at 39% at 1 month after Myosplint implant. Also, LVEDV and LVESV significantly decreased and were sustained at 1 month. End-systolic wall stress (EDWS) significantly decreased by 39% acutely and by 31% at 1 month. Also, EDWS was significantly reduced by 30% acutely and by 41% at 1 month.

Chronic human studies were first performed in seven patients with dilated cardiomyopathy who were NYHA class III–IV. LVEDD in this group ranged from 72 to 102 mm. Mitral valve regurgitation was mild in three patients and moderate in four cases. Four patients underwent concomitant mitral valve repair at the time of Myosplint implant. At 3-month follow-up, one patient experienced worsening heart failure attributed to unrepaired and significant mitral regurgitation. The remaining six patients showed improvement in symptoms of heart failure, with two of the patients removed from the transplant waiting list. This early experience demonstrated that Myosplint implantation can be safely performed without significant adverse affects; however, these investigators noted that mitral valve repair should be done in any patient undergoing the Myosplint implant *(33)*.

The long-term effect of Myosplint therapy on cardiac function awaits results from a larger, randomized study. The Myosplint is undergoing US Food and Drug Administration feasibility testing, with a total of 40 patients enrolled to date.

CONCLUSION

The Batista procedure was unpredictable, suffered from many early failures, worsened diastolic function, and gave only temporary relief to highly selected patients. However, the Batista "concept" of LV reconstruction for idiopathic dilated cardiomyopathy may prove to be a useful adjunct for selected patients with congestive heart failure if patient selection, surgical techniques, or therapeutic devices can be refined.

REFERENCES

1. Levy D, Kenchaiah S, Larson MG, et al. Long-term trends in the incidence and survival with heart failure. N Engl J Med 2002;347:1397–1402.
2. Loop FD. Coronary artery surgery: the end of the beginning. Eur J Cardiothorac Surg 1998;14:554–571.
3. Swedberg K, Kjekshus J, Snapinn S. Long-term survival in severe heart failure in patients treated with enalapril. Ten year follow-up of CONSENSUS I. Eur Heart J 1999;20:136–139.
4. McMurray JJ, Stewart S. Epidemiology, aetiology and prognosis of heart failure. Heart 2000;83:596–602.
5. Batista RJV, Santos JLV, Takeshita N, et al. Partial left ventriculectomy to improve left ventricular function in end-stage heart disease. J Card Surg 1996;11:96–97.
6. Beck CS. Operation for aneurysm of the heart. Ann Surg 1944;120:34–50.

7. Likoff W, Bailey CP. Ventriculoplasty: excision of myocardial aneurysm. JAMA 1958;915–928.

8. Cooley DA, Collins HA, Morris GC, et al. Ventricular aneurysm after myocardial infarction: surgical excision with the use of cardiopulmonary bypass. JAMA 1958; 167:557.

9. Dor V, Kreitmann P, Jourdan J, et al. Interest of physiological closure (circumferential plasty on contractile areas) of left ventricle after resection and endocardectomy for aneurysm of akinetic zone comparison with classical technique about a series of 209 left ventricular resections. J Cardiovasc Surg 1985;26:73.

10. Batista RJV, Verde J, Nery P, et al. Partial left ventriculectomy to treat end-stage heart disease. Ann Thorac Surg 1997;64:634–638.

11. McCarthy PM, Starling RC, Wong J, et al. Early results with partial left ventriculectomy. J Thorac Cardiovasc Surg 1997;114:755–765.

12. Moreira LF, Stolff NAG, Bocchi EA, et al. Partial left ventriculectomy with mitral valve preservation in the treatment of dilated cardiomyopathy. J Thorac Cardiovasc Surg 1998;115:800–807.

13. Gradinac S, Miric M, Popovic Z, et al. Partial left ventriculectomy for idiopathic dilated cardiomyopathy: early results and 6-month follow-up. Ann Thorac Surg 1998;66:1963–1968.

14. Franco-Cereceda A, McCarthy PM, Blackstone EH, et al. Partial left ventriculectomy for dilated cardiomyopathy: is this an alternative to transplantation? J Thorac Cardiovasc Surg 2001;121:879–893.

15. Dickstein ML, Spotnitz HM, Rose EA, Burkhoff D. Heart reduction surgery: an analysis of the impact on cardiac function. J Thorac Cardiovasc Surg 1997;113:1032–1040.

16. Gorcsan J 3rd, Feldman AM, Kormos RL, Mandarino WA, Demetris AJ, Batista RJ. Heterogeneous immediate effects of partial left ventriculectomy on cardiac performance. Circulation 1998;97:839–842.

17. Artrip JH, Oz MC, Burhoff D. Left ventricular volume reduction surgery for heart failure: a physiologic perspective. J Thorac Cardiovasc Surg 2001;122:775–782.

18. Kawaguchi AT, Suma H, Konertz W, et al. Partial left ventriculectomy: the Second International Registry Report 2000. J Card Surg 2001;16:10–23.

19. Bhat G, Dowling RD. Evaluation of predictors of clinical outcome after partial left ventriculectomy. Ann Thorac Surg 2001;72:91–95.

20. Kawaguchi AT, Bergsland J, Ishibashi-Ueda H, et al. Partial left ventriculectomy in patients with dilated failing ventricle. J Card Surg 1998;13:335–342

21. Suma H, the RESTORE group. Left ventriculoplasty for nonischemic dilated cardiomyopathy. Semin Thorac Cardiovasc Surg 2001;13:514–521.

22. Hoercher KJ, Starling RC, McCarthy PM, Blackstone EH, Young JB. Partial left ventriculectomy: lessons learned and future implications for surgical trials. Circulation 2002;106:II-418.

23. Kaplon R, Lombardi P. Passive constraint and new shape-change devices for heart failure. Semin Thorac Cardiovasc Surg 2002;14:150–156.

24. Oz MC. Passive ventricular constraint for the treatment of congestive heart failure. Ann Thorac Surg 2001;71:S185–S187.

25. Saavedra FW, Tunn R, Mishima T, et al. Reverse remodeling and enhanced adrenergic reserve from a passive external ventricular support in experimental dilated heart failure. Circulation 2000;102(suppl II):II-501.

26. Chaudry PA, Mishima T, Sharov VG, et al. Passive epicardial containment prevents ventricular remodeling in heart failure. Ann Thorac Surg 2000;70:1275–1280.

27. Power J, Raman J, Byrne M. Passive ventricular constraint is a trigger for a significant degree of reverse remodeling in an experimental model of degenerative heart failure and dilated cardiomyopathy. Circulation 2000;102(suppl II):II-502.
28. Sabbah HN, Gupta RC, Sharov VG, et al. Prevention of progressive left ventricular dilation with the Acorn cardiac support device (CSD) down regulates stretch-mediated P21ras, attenuates myocardial hypertrophy, and improves sarcoplasmic reticulum calcium cycling in dogs with heart failure. Circulation 2000;102 (suppl II):II-683.
29. Pilla JJ, Blom AS, Brockman DJ, et al. Ventricular constraint using the Acorn cardiac support device reduces myocardial akinetic area in an ovine model of acute infarction. Circulation 2002;106(12 suppl 1):I207–I211.
30. Konertz WF, Shapland JE, Hotz H, et al. Passive containment and reverse remodeling by a novel textile cardiac support device. Circulation 2001;104:I-270–I-275.
31. Raman JS, Hata M, Storere JM, et al. The mid-term results of ventricular containment (Acorn Wrap) for end stage ischemic cardiomyopathy. Ann Thorac Cardiovasc Surg 2001;5:278–281.
32. McCarthy PM, Takagaki M, Ochiai Y, et al. Device-based change in left ventricular shape: a new concept for the treatment of dilated cardiomyopathy. J Thorac Cardiovasc Surg 2001;122:482–490.
33. Schenk S, Reichenspurner H, Boehm DH, et al. Myosplint implant and shape-change procedure: intra- and peri-operative safety and feasibility. J Heart Lung Transplant 2002;21:680–686.

9
Surgical Management of Hypertrophic Cardiomyopathy

William G. Williams, MD,
E. Douglas Wigle, MD,
Harry Rakowski, MD,
Anthony C. Ralph-Edwards, MD,
and Leonard Schwartz, MD

Contents

DEFINITIONS

Hypertrophic cardiomyopathy (HCM) is a genetic disorder characterized by ventricular hypertrophy in the absence of an identifiable cause for the hypertrophy (1–4). The hypertrophy is usually asymmetric and involves the interventricular septum in 90% of patients. Most commonly, the outflow septum (i.e., subaortic area) is the major focus

From: *Contemporary Cardiology: Surgical Management of Congestive Heart Failure*
Edited by: J. C. Fang and G. S. Couper © Humana Press Inc., Totowa, NJ

of hypertrophy, but the midventricular or apical septum may occur in isolation or concomitantly. Rarely (5%) the right ventricle is involved. The extent of the hypertrophy varies tremendously and accounts for different manifestations of the disease (1–5). The hypertrophy is associated with myocardial fiber disarray on microscopy.

The disorder is an inherited autosomal dominant mutation or arises by spontaneous mutation. HCM is a heterogeneous disorder of the sarcomere, and to date 10 genes and more than 200 mutations have been described affecting β-myosin heavy chain, cardiac myosin-binding protein C, cardiac troponin T, troponin I, α-tropomyosin, regulatory myosin light chains, actin, and titin (4,6,7). Although not practical as yet, genetic screening may provide better detection and outcome prediction. The troponin T and some β-myosin heavy-chain mutations have been associated with a poor outcome.

PREVALENCE

Within the general population, HCM may affect as many as 1 per 500 individuals and represents about one-quarter the prevalence of all forms of congenital heart disease (3,4,7). However, many individuals with HCM are asymptomatic and may remain so indefinitely.

CLASSIFICATION OF HCM

The clinical manifestations of HCM are varied and dependent on the extent and location of the hypertrophy and the secondary effects of the hypertrophy (8). Based on hemodynamic criteria, patients may have either an obstructive or nonobstructive form of the disease (Table 1). The obstruction may occur at rest, with provocation (latent), or intermittently (labile). The degree of obstruction varies directly with the inotropic state of the heart and inversely with the systemic vascular resistance and preload.

CLINICAL PRESENTATION

The clinical manifestations of HCM are extremely varied. Many patients are asymptomatic (3–5,9). Symptoms in children are very uncommon, although they are not immune to sudden death (10,11). Symptoms may first develop during adolescence, possibly because of an accelerated growth of myocardial hypertrophy. Most patients become symptomatic in their fourth or fifth decade. Because of the dynamic nature of the obstructive form of HCM, symptoms will vary in intensity from day to day, depending on normal variation in periph-

Table 1
Hemodynamic Characteristics of Hypertrophic Cardiomyopathy

Nonobstructive HCM
   Abnormal diastolic function
      Impaired relaxation and impaired compliance
   Normal or supernormal systolic function
   Impaired systolic (end-stage) systolic function
      secondary to myocardial fibrosis
Obstructive HCM
   Subaortic obstruction
   Midventricular obstruction
   Apical obstruction

eral vascular resistance. The most common presenting symptoms are dyspnea and fatigue; angina; palpitations; and presyncope, syncope, and sudden death.

Dyspnea and Fatigue

Dyspnea and fatigue are the most common symptoms and may be caused by poor diastolic filling of the left ventricle, from reduced compliance secondary to the hypertrophy or to impaired diastolic relaxation. With increased myocardial fibrosis late in the course of the disease, the ventricle may dilate, and compliance may further deteriorate.

In patients with obstruction, the associated mitral valve insufficiency (see Physiology of Obstructive HCM section) increases left atrial (LA) pressure, which results in exercise intolerance, dyspnea, fatigue, and atrial arrhythmias.

Angina

Extensive hypertrophy may result in inadequate blood supply to the endocardium. Concomitant arteriosclerosis of the coronary arteries will lead to regional ischemia, with the hypertrophied area at increased risk. In about 5% of patients with HCM, one or more of the coronary arteries may have an intramyocardial course. The intramyocardial segment is compressed by the surrounding muscle contraction during each systole. The systolic obstruction affects the diastolic flow pattern and has been linked to angina as well as an increased risk of sudden death (10,11).

Palpitations

Poor diastolic function of the left ventricle and the presence of mitral regurgitation will lead to atrial dilation and the onset of supraventricular arrhythmias. Patients with a LA diameter greater than

50 mm are at increased risk of atrial fibrillation (AF). The onset of supraventricular arrhythmias usually precipitates a marked increase in symptoms. The onset of AF also increases the risk of stroke.

Ventricular arrhythmias may occur with HCM and are an ominous sign of increased risk of sudden death *(12–17)*. The mechanism of ventricular arrhythmias is not completely understood, but precipitating factors include the marginal blood supply, myocardial fibrosis, and in some patients, an intramyocardial coronary artery.

Presyncope, Syncope, and Sudden Death

The cause of syncope in these patients may be outflow obstruction, vasovagal reflexes, or arrhythmias, including ventricular tachycardia (VT) or fibrillation (VF). A history of sudden death is not uncommon among patients with HCM and among their families. Syncope is a risk factor for sudden death, and the septal thickness has been correlated with the risk of sudden death *(12,18)*. Brief periods of VT may not be associated with an increased risk of sudden death *(16)*.

HCM accounts for about one-third of sudden deaths among young athletes *(4)*. The outcome of 16 patients with HCM who were resuscitated from VT or VF demonstrated that they are at increased risk of further fatal arrhythmia *(19)*.

PHYSIOLOGY OF OBSTRUCTIVE HCM

Patients with asymmetric septal hypertrophy develop left ventricular (LV) outlet obstruction at the apex, the midventricle, or most commonly in the subaortic area *(1,8,20)*. In the most common variant of subaortic stenosis, the thickened septal wall protrudes into the left ventricular outflow tract (LVOT) just caudal to the aortic valve and opposite the mitral valve annulus and anterior mitral leaflet *(21)*. The thickened septum narrows the subaortic outflow. To maintain a normal cardiac output, the left ventricle must contract more vigorously to force blood through the diminishing diameter of the subaortic channel. Consequently, there is flow acceleration in the subaortic outflow tract, and a pressure gradient develops between the body of the left ventricle and the aorta. The left ventricle responds to this increased systolic pressure demand by hypertrophy, and the hypertrophy occurs in the body of the left ventricle as well as in the septum. Therefore, a vicious circle occurs consisting of the hypertrophied septum obstructing the outflow tract, causing increased LV work and subsequent hypertrophy, which aggravates the outflow obstruction further.

The flow acceleration in the subaortic outflow tract affects the mitral valve and left atrium *(22)*. The mitral valve leaflet, usually the anterior one, is "lifted" by the venturi forces of flow acceleration toward the ventricular septum in midsystole, much as the airflow over an airplane wing lifts the airplane into the air *(23)*. The anterior mitral valve leaflet displacement into the outflow tract is referred to as *systolic anterior motion* (SAM). Because the leaflet of the valve is displaced toward the septum during systole, it prevents normal coaptation and results in mitral regurgitation. The regurgitant jet is typically posteriorly directed and occurs late in systole. The degree of regurgitation is affected by the severity of the obstruction: Factors that increase contractility or decrease peripheral resistance will increase the severity of mitral regurgitation. Although the regurgitation is typically posteriorly directed, intrinsic valve anomalies, such as leaflet prolapse, may cause centrally or anteriorly directed jets of regurgitation.

It is very important to recognize that the regurgitation associated with subaortic obstruction occurs after SAM–septal contact and will therefore resolve when the outlet obstruction is relieved. In contrast, mitral regurgitation that occurs prior to SAM–septal contact is unrelated to the obstruction and will persist after relief of the obstruction. Many patients will have regurgitation because of a combination of intrinsic valve anomalies and SAM.

TREATMENT FOR HCM

Medical Treatment

Many patients remain asymptomatic or have mild symptoms and therefore do not require treatment. They should, however, be assessed for the risk of sudden death. Patients who are symptomatic because of nonobstructive HCM are managed medically with drugs that improve compliance, such as β-blockers, which slow the heart rate and improve ventricular filling. Calcium channel blockers improve diastolic relaxation and may improve filling as well. The combination of β-blockers and verapamil should be used cautiously because the combination may produce excessive atrioventricular (AV) nodal block. Some have also advocated the use of the sodium channel blocker disopyramide because of its negative inotropic effects. However, its routine use is often limited by excessive anticholinergic side effects.

Antiarrhythmic drugs may be indicated for patients at risk of AF or of sudden death. Amiodarone is most commonly used, and its efficacy has been supported by McKenna and others *(24,25)*. However, a comparison of antiarrhythmics vs implantable defibrillators for patients with HCM who have been resuscitated following near-fatal ventricular arrhythmias suggested that the defibrillators may be more effective *(26)*.

Anticoagulants should be considered for patients with AF as they are at risk of stroke.

Implantable Defibrillators

Patients with HCM and resuscitation from sudden death, documented VT, or a strong family history of sudden death should be considered for an implantable cardioverter defibrillator (ICD). In a multicenter study of 128 patients with ICDs, Maron et al. reported appropriate defibrillator discharges at a rate of 7% per year *(26)*. However, a similar proportion of patients had inappropriate ICD discharges.

Pacemakers

Patients with HCM may require permanent pacing for control of atrial or ventricular arrhythmias. Furthermore, patients with the obstructive form of HCM may benefit from dual-chamber pacing in other ways, as first reported by McDonald et al. *(27)*. The mechanisms by which pacing may improve symptoms are not clear, but various hypotheses have been proposed and include the induction of paradoxical septal motion through asynchronous depolarization, a negative inotropic effect, a reduction in mitral valve SAM, an increase in end-systolic volume, and altered myocardial perfusion. However, the clinical benefit of pacing in HCM is controversial. A prospective randomized double-blind crossover trial recommended that pacing not be used as primary therapy *(28)*. Pacing was associated with some symptomatic improvement and a modest reduction in outflow tract gradient of 40%, but objective exercise testing demonstrated no benefit, and there was no change in LV wall thickness on echocardiographic follow-up. The authors did concede that the elderly patient (>65 years) may benefit from atrioventricular pacing.

Heart Transplantation

It has been estimated that approx 5 to 10% of patients with HCM may reach a terminal end stage with dilated cardiomyopathy *(1–4)*. Thinning of the ventricular walls precedes this stage and leads to markedly dilated atrial and ventricular chambers. Transplantation is the only effective therapy at this stage.

Surgical Myectomy

Patients who are symptomatic with the obstructive form of HCM will benefit from subaortic myectomy *(29–33)*. The usual indications for surgery are medically refractory symptoms or intolerance of effective medications. Some centers would also consider high-risk groups (young patient with a very thick septum or a strong family history of sudden death) as an indication as well. When genetic mapping becomes practical, it may help triage the high-risk groups toward a surgical myectomy.

PREOPERATIVE ASSESSMENT

A careful clinical history and family history are important in assessing risk with and without surgery. Identification of concomitant disease is important because such problems, or the necessity to manage associated pathology surgically, may affect the patient's risk.

The echocardiogram is essential is assessing both the extent and the severity of the hypertrophy and in clarifying the status of the mitral valve *(22,23,34)*. Although this information should be available and reviewed before surgical consultation, a transesophageal echocardiography (TEE) assessment is essential intraoperatively, both before and after the myectomy *(34)*.

In adults suitable for myectomy, the interventricular septum thickness should be greater than 17 mm and may be considerably thicker. The echo measurement is useful in gaging the depth of resection required. The length of the hypertrophied septum is measured to determine the length of the excision. Associated midventricular obstruction, which can be masked by upper septal outflow obstruction, requires a longer resection to a level below the head of the papillary muscles.

The mitral valve should be assessed for the quantity, direction, and timing of regurgitation. Mitral regurgitation secondary to dynamic obstruction occurs after the SAM–septal contact and is typically posteriorly directed. Alterations in this pattern do exist and usually resolve following successful myectomy, but regurgitation unrelated to obstruction may require mitral valve repair or replacement.

Because of the association of coronary artery myocardial bridges with HCM and the potential association with sudden death, every patient considered for surgery should have a coronary angiogram to document the presence or absence of both coronary artery disease and these myocardial bridges.

OPERATIVE TECHNIQUE OF MYECTOMY

Myectomy is performed during cardiopulmonary bypass with single right atrial cannulation and LA venting of the LV. Mild hypothermia is used during bypass, but we avoid cooling until after the myocardium is arrested with blood cardioplegia at normal temperature. Once the cardioplegia arrests the heart at normothermia, the cardioplegia is cooled

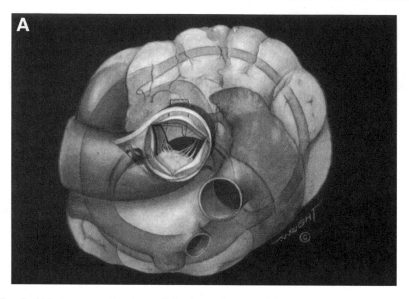

Fig. 1. (A) A surgeon's view of the heart from the patient's right side, looking toward the apex. The ascending aorta is shown open through an oblique aortotomy, exposing the trileaflet aortic valve. The protruding septum narrows the outflow tract opposite the mitral valve. The stippling indicates the thickness of the ventricular septum. The three incisions to complete the myectomy are illustrated and described in the text.

and continued until the myocardium reaches 15°C, generally requiring about 1500 cc. Cooling the beating perfused heart is dangerous because the hypertrophied heart may fibrillate, and cardioplegic perfusion may not be distributed evenly, which leads to poor diastolic relaxation and difficulty in defibrillation following reperfusion. With warm induction cardioplegia, the heart usually recovers spontaneously with reperfusion, with or without terminal warm cardioplegia.

The septal resection is done through an oblique aortotomy extending to, but not across, the sino-tubular junction. Before the myectomy, the outflow tract and mitral and aortic valves should be carefully examined and the septal thickness and length of hypertrophy palpated to confirm the echo findings. Transmural palpation of the free LV wall apex to the septum is a good guide regarding what the septal thickness should be following resection.

The excision requires three incisions into the septum (Fig. 1A). The initial septal subaortic incision is made with a no. 11 scalpel blade and starts 2 mm below the right cusp of the aortic valve and 2 to 3 mm to the right of its nadir. If this incision is started too far to the right, it may

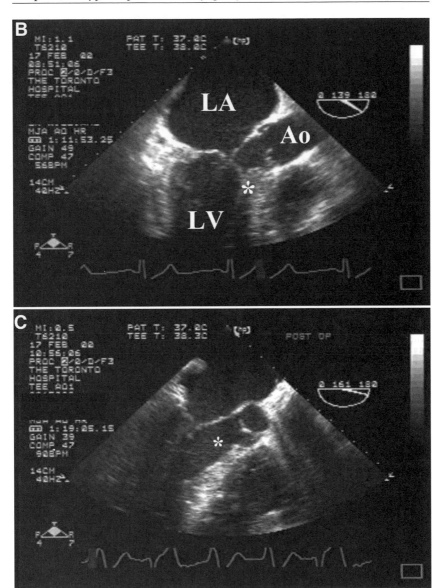

Fig. 1. (B) The systolic anterior motion (SAM) of the mitral valve results in contact of the leaflets with the ventricular septum. The SAM-septal contact obstructs the left ventricular outlet (*) and prevents complete coaptation of the mitral leaflets that results in posteriorly directed mitral regurgitation. **(C)** After successful myectomy, the mitral leaflets close in a normal plane, regurgitation is eliminated, and the left ventricular outlet (*) is no longer obstructed. LA, left atrium; Ao, aorta; LV, left ventricle; * left ventricular outlet.

damage the His bundle. If the hypertrophy is unusually prominent on the right side of the outflow tract, the initial incision may be made further to the right but lower (10 mm from the aortic valve) in the septum and slanted to the left as it extends upward toward the aortic annulus. The depth of this initial incision depends on the estimate, by echo and palpation, of the septal thickness. The depth should leave a residual septal thickness of 8 mm, similar to the LV free wall below the septum. The direction of the initial incision is toward the apex. For right-handed surgeons, the tendency is to direct the incision too far to the left of the apex. To avoid this, the incision can be made with the left hand. The length of the initial incision depends on the extent of the hypertrophy, but generally is 35 to 50 mm long in the adult. For patients with mid-ventricular obstruction, the incision should extend at least to the level of the anteroseptal papillary muscle head. Transmural palpation of the incision is used to judge the adequacy of both its depth and its length.

The second incision is made parallel to the first and 2 mm anterior to the mitral valve insertion. The septum is narrower here than on the right, so the second incision is not as long. Its depth is again determined by palpation, leaving a residual septal thickness of 8 mm.

The third incision is made 2 mm below the aortic annulus and parallel to it. It extends from the proximal extent of the first incision to the proximal extent of the second. The depth of this incision is only 2 mm because a deeper incision would become too shallow. Once the septum is exposed with this incision, it allows a second cut, also 2 mm deep, in a more anterior direction. A third 2-mm incision may be required to establish the depth of the resection, guided by transmural palpation and the depth of the first and second incisions. The purpose of the superficial incisions 2 mm deep is somewhat analogous to a series of short straight lines, each at an angle to one another, creating a circle.

Once the appropriate depth of the third incision is established, the block of muscle to be excised is dissected distally toward the apex, confirming by repeated palpation that the direction and residual septal depth are leaving a residual septal thickness of 5 to 8 mm. Under the right-left aortic commissure, the top of the resection is an acute angle because of the convergence of the annulus. As the dissection continues caudally, the resection more distally under the commissure must be rounded to avoid perforating the septum below the pulmonary valve. On palpation of the residual septum, there should be no difference in thickness compared to the free LV wall below the septum.

The area of the specimen resected should be approximately the area of the aortic valve. On average, the resection measures 25 mm wide, 45 mm long, and 15 mm deep.

Before closing the aortic incision, the mitral and aortic valves are inspected for inadvertent damage. The LV cavity is irrigated to remove any loose pieces of muscle, and the bed of the resection is checked for muscle fragments.

INTRAOPERATIVE POSTMYECTOMY TEE

Once off bypass, the adequacy of the myectomy is checked by TEE *(22,23,34)*. The outflow tract should be a normal diameter, and the mitral valve SAM should be absent, allowing the mitral valve to close in a normal plane of apposition (Fig. 1B,C). On Doppler interrogation, the mitral regurgitation should be considerably less or absent, and the LV outflow gradient should be less than 10 mmHg, with minimal or no increase in gradient after an induced extrasystole. It is not uncommon for some chordal SAM to persist. Color flow Doppler should rule out a ventricular septal perforation and usually identifies divided septal perforators in the base of the resection.

Because the plane of the echo lies at a 30° angle to the plane of the myectomy, the medial wall of the resection appears on TEE as a prominent right-angled divot. Within 1 week of myectomy, this edge of the myectomy atrophies, thereby increasing the outlet diameter.

UNROOFING CORONARY ARTERY MYOCARDIAL BRIDGES

An intramyocardial course of a coronary artery, usually the left anterior descending, may be associated with sudden death, even in patients with HCM without obstruction *(10,11)*. Systolic compression of the coronary may be impressive. Among our surgical patients with obstructive HCM, 26 of 333 (7.8%) had a myocardial bridge. Whether unroofing these bridges decreases the risk of death is unknown, but we attempt to unroof the bridge if a myectomy is performed.

The coronary artery distal to the tunnel is identified, and its superficial (anterior) surface is exposed by sharp dissection. The sharp dissection is then extended proximally by staying along the plane of the artery until it reemerges onto the epicardial surface. The divided myocardium over the artery is usually 3 to 5 mm thick. Unfortunately, the course of the artery may be so deep that trabeculations of the right ventricular cavity are entered. In this situation, after the myocardial bridge has been divided, the opening into the ventricle is repaired by pledgeted sutures placed deep to the coronary.

POSTOPERATIVE MANAGEMENT

Postmyectomy patients are managed very similar to most cardiac patients and benefit from an early extubation protocol *(35)*. They

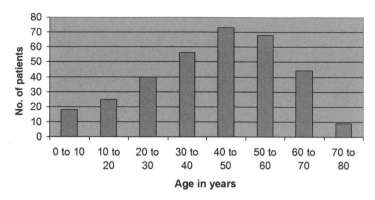

Fig. 2. The histogram illustrates the age range at myectomy by decade. Median age is 44.2 years.

seldom need either inotropic or afterload-reducing drugs. Patients with HCM have increased myocardial contractility and require an adequate preload. They seldom need inotropic support or afterload reduction, and both are generally contraindicated in patients with obstruction.

Postoperative AV block is uncommon (1%). However, all patients should have temporary atrial and ventricular pacing wires placed at the time of surgery with backup ventricular demand pacing capacity. It is not uncommon for postmyectomy patients to require temporary AV pacing for a few hours. Most patients develop left bundle branch block (BBB); therefore, those with preoperative right BBB are at high risk of developing postoperative complete AV block. Overall, about 4 to 5% postmyectomy patients need permanent pacing.

Atrial arrhythmias, typically AF, are not uncommon a few days after myectomy. We routinely use sotalol to prevent or control AF.

SURGICAL RESULTS OF MYECTOMY

Since 1972, we have operated on 333 patients with HCM. The median age at surgery was 44.2 years, with the range 0.2 to 76.4 years (Fig. 2). Men comprised 60.4% of this series. Thirty-eight patients were children (<18 years). Most patients were symptomatic prior to myectomy; the majority (58%) were New York Heart Association (NYHA) class III (Fig. 3). Some younger children with high gradients and very thick septa were operated on in the absence of symptoms. Lesions in addition to HCM were present in 129 (39%) of patients (Table 2). A previous myectomy had been performed in 23 patients. Three of the previous operations were done by an author of this chapter and 20 by other surgeons.

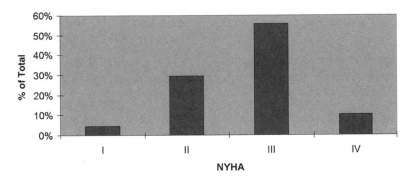

Fig. 3. Preoperative New York Heart Association class.

Table 2
Concomitant Pathology at Time of Surgery

Associated pathology	n	%
None	204	61
Coronary artery	30	9
Mitral disease	29	8
Coronary muscle bridge	26	8
Other	20	6
Midventricular stenosis	15	4
Aortic disease	11	3
RVOTO	8	2
	343*	

*Some patients had more than one associated problem.

There were 6 early deaths (1.8%), and during a follow-up period of 6.7 years (median 5.4, range 0 to 24.4 years), there have been 37 late deaths (Fig. 4). Survival 10 years postmyectomy is estimated as 82% (–3%). Survival is better among the 243 patients who did not require concomitant procedures at the time of myectomy: 86 vs 68% at 10 years after myectomy (Fig. 5).

Older age at myectomy, poorer preoperative NYHA class (Fig. 6), and coronary artery disease appear to be associated with an increased risk of early or late mortality (Table 3). Unroofing of a myocardial coronary artery bridge was not associated with early or late mortality, and there were no deaths among the 6 patients in whom a known myocardial bridge was not unroofed. Permanent pacing, either pre-myectomy (*n* = 14) or postmyectomy (*n* = 24), did not affect overall mortality. Early postoperative complications occurred in 16% of patients,

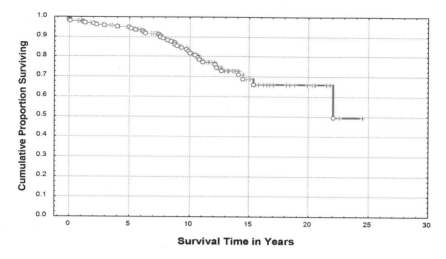

Fig. 4. The Kaplan-Meier plot shows the survival after myectomy for 333 patients with obstructive hypertrophic cardiomyopathy. Survival at 10 years is 82%.

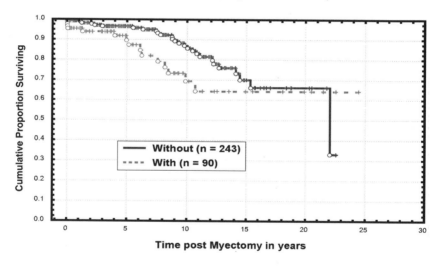

Fig. 5. Survival among patients with concomitant procedures at myectomy was less favorable than those having a myectomy alone.

the most important of which were strokes in 7 patients, 1 of whom had permanent, severe long-term damage.

Symptomatic improvement after myectomy is impressive, with 95% of patients becoming NYHA class I at the most recent follow-up (Fig. 7). Symptomatic improvement persists in most patients.

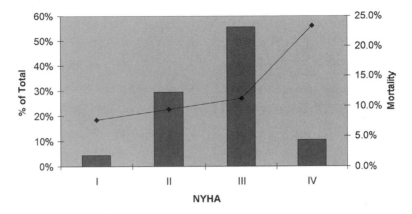

Fig. 6. The total mortality, early and late, is higher among the patients with class IV symptoms prior to myectomy.

Table 3
Risk Factors for Death

	N	Early death	Late death	Total mortality (%)	Mortality without (%)
Coronary artery bypass	30	3	7	33.3	10.9
Age >70 years	9	1	3	44.4	12.0
Mitral valve surgery	13	2	2	30.8	12.2
NYHA class IV	30	3	4	23.3	11.9
Previous myectomy	23	0	6	26.1	11.9
Myocardial bridge unroofing	20	0	0	0.0	13.7
Permanent pacemaker	46	1	7	17.4	12.2

Note: The rightmost column indicates the mortality for all patients without the risk factor in the first column.

Reoperation has been required in only 10 patients, including 3 for recurrent (more likely persistent) outlet obstruction, and one for mid-ventricular obstruction. The median time to reoperation was 3.2 years (range 0 to 19 years). The indications for reoperation are shown in Table 4. The probability of reoperation ($n = 10$) is illustrated by the Kaplan–Meier plot in Fig. 8. Freedom from reoperation is 96 ± 1.5% at 10 years after myectomy.

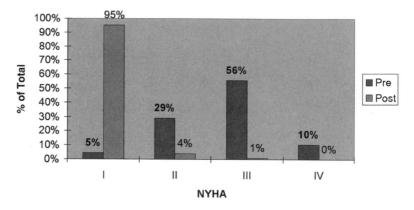

Fig. 7. Symptomatic improvement following myectomy for patients with the obstructive form of hypertrophic cardiomyopathy is impressive, with 95% becoming class I.

Table 4
Indications for Reoperation

	N
Myectomy	3
Heart transplant	2
LV-Ao conduit	1
Mid-ventricular stenosis	1
Mitral valve replacement/maze	1
Aortic valve replacement for SBE	1
Ventricular septal defect and atrial lead recall	1
Total	10

Septal Alcohol Ablation

In 1994, Sigwart introduced a catheter-based treatment for reducing the LVOT obstruction for patients with HCM *(36)*. This was based on the observation that the first septal perforating branch of the left anterior descending artery supplied the area of the intraventricular septum contributing to the production of the LVOT gradient. Sigwart, using standard coronary angioplasty technique, found that temporary occlusion of this branch (up to 30 minutes) resulted in a remarkable decrease in the outflow gradient, with reappearance of the gradient with balloon deflation.

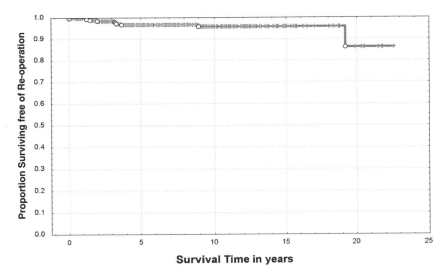

Fig. 8. Only 4% (*n* = 10) of patients required reoperation after myectomy. Among these, only three patients had recurrent outlet obstruction.

To produce a permanent result, he exploited the intraarterial chemical ablation properties of ethyl alcohol *(36)*. The hyperosmolality of ethanol results in acute dehydration of the endothelial cells, with desquamation and occlusion of the injected artery. The rapidity of the toxicity exceeds even that of an acute vascular occlusion, suggesting a direct parenchymal tissue effect as well. The resultant myocardial infarction and scar are extremely well defined histologically in experimental studies and on magnetic resonance imaging in humans. Sigwart slowly injected 3 mL of 95% ethanol through the inflated balloon into the septal branch and deflated the balloon after 5 minutes. The pressure gradient was abolished immediately and did not reappear. In a minority of patients, the proximal septum is supplied by a number of small septal branches rather than by one large branch, and he found that on occasion it was necessary to ablate more than one. The major risk of the procedure is the appearance of conduction abnormalities. In our experience, about 60% develop a right BBB, and in about 10% of cases, complete heart block occurs requiring a permanent pacemaker.

The most important addition to the technique was the introduction of myocardial contrast echocardiography by Faber et al. *(37)*. This involves the forceful bolus injection of 1 mL contrast echo agent through the inflated balloon lumen with on-line continuous echocardiography. This "lights up" the myocardium supplied by the branch, permitting the accurate and specific demarcation of its vascular supply. If this includes the region of SAM–septal contact and no other important other area of supply is identified (such as posterior wall or papillary muscles), then this branch is ablated. The introduction of myocardial contrast echocardiography has reduced the number of branches ablated and resulted in smaller infarct by creatinine kinase measurement, and the need for long-term pacing has become less common. Other complications are rare. Concern regarding the short- and long-term appearance of serious ventricular arrhythmias has not materialized. There have been no documented cases of ventricular septal defects.

The mechanism of relief of the gradient with septal alcohol ablation is complex and temporal (38). It is not unusual for the gradient to disappear completely during the procedure only to reappear in the next few days postprocedure. The immediate effect appears to be because of global changes of LV ejection. There is immediate basal septal dysfunction (hypo- or akinesis) with no change in the mitral valve motion, with the anterior leaflet continuing to move toward the septum. Peak acceleration rate just proximal to the LVOT obstruction is significantly lower, and conduction abnormalities such as the right BBB and the resultant dyssynchrony in LV contraction reduces the acceleration rate even more. The partial reappearance of the gradient early on is almost always temporary, with gradual reduction of the gradient over the succeeding weeks to an average resting value of 9 mmHg at 8 weeks (from 60 mmHg preprocedure) and to an average provocable gradient of 32 mmHg (from 114 mmHg preprocedure).

By 1 year, the average resting gradient is 4 mmHg, and the provocable gradient is 32 mmHg. One group found complete elimination of the LVOT gradient in 67% of patients (39). Regression of LV hypertrophy is present at 1 year and continues for at least 2 years, with LV mass decreasing from a baseline of 301–78 g to 223–5 g at 1 year and 190–58 g at 2 years (40). This long-term benefit is because of LVOT widening as a consequence of the infarction necrosis and replacement fibrosis, which is apparent at 6 weeks, with further widening developing at later follow-up in some cases. We have seen some patients whose improvement has continued beyond 1 year.

In a minority of patients (approx 10%), the LVOT gradient reappears at about 6 weeks even after the usual initial acute reduction. In these patients, peak acceleration rates at follow-up approach baseline values, and the LVOT diameter shows minimal increase from baseline. These patients at the time of the ablation had a smaller septal area opacified by intracoronary contrast injection (3.3–1.9 cm^2) compared to those with a good long-term result (6.5–1.5 cm^2).

Septal alcohol ablation can be considered when there are reasonably large proximal septal perforators (>1.5 mm in diameter) and there are no coexistent abnormalities that require surgical treatment (such as significant myocardial bridging, nonangioplastable coronary disease requiring revascularization, and structural mitral or aortic valvular disease).

SUMMARY

HCM is a myocardial disease that results from a genetic mutation. Protein synthesis is altered in the subaortic region compared to elsewhere in the left ventricular wall *(41,42)*. HCM is not uncommon among the general population, occurring in perhaps 1 in 500 people. Manifestations of the disease are very diverse. The majority of patients are asymptomatic and have a normal life expectancy. However, symptoms from altered diastolic function or from outlet obstruction and associated mitral valve regurgitation may be severe and associated with early death.

Surgical treatment is a useful therapeutic option for some patients with HCM. For those with HCM at high risk of sudden death, an implantable defibrillator should be considered. For the small number of patients with end-stage myocardial dysfunction, heart transplantation may be the only option.

Surgical myectomy for symptomatic patients with the obstructive form of HCM is a low risk (1.8% mortality) procedure, improves symptoms in 95% of patients, and may extend longevity. The results of surgical myectomy are a standard against which the recent advent of catheter alcohol ablation of the blood supply to the septum should be compared *(43,44)*.

REFERENCES

1. Wigle ED, Rakowski H, Kimball BP, Williams WG. Hypertrophic cardiomyopathy. Clinical spectrum and treatment. Circulation 1995;92:1680–1692.
2. Spirito P, Sideman CE, McKenna WJ, Maron BJ. The management of hypertrophic cardiomyopathy. N Engl J Med 1997;336:775–785.
3. Maron BJ. Hypertrophic cardiomyopathy. Lancet 1997;350:127–133.
4. Maron BJ, Salberg L. Hypertrophic Cardiomyopathy: For Patients, Their Families, and Interested Physicians. Futura, New York: 2001.
5. Maron BJ, Casey SA, Poliac LC, et al. Clinical course of hypertrophic cardiomyopathy in a regional United States cohort. JAMA 1999;281:650–655.
6. Maron BJ, Moller JH, Seidman CE, et al. Impact of laboratory molecular diagnostic criteria for genetically transmitted cardiovascular diseases: hypertrophic cardiomyopathy. Long QT syndrome, and Marfan syndrome. Circulation 1998;98:1460–1471.
7. Maron BJ, Gardin JM, Flack JM, Gidding SS, Kurosaki TT, Bild DE. Prevalence of hypertrophic cardiomyopathy in a general population of young adults: echocardiographic analysis of 4111 subjects in the CARDIA study. Circulation 1995;92: 785–789.

8. Wigle ED, Sasson Z, Henderson MA, et al. Hypertrophic cardiomyopathy. The importance of the site and extent of the hypertrophy. A review. Prog Cardiovasc Dis 1985;28:1–83.

9. Hecht GM, Panza JA, Maron BJ. Clinical course of middle-aged asymptomatic patients with hypertrophic cardiomyopathy. Am J Cardiol 1992;69:935–940.

10. Yetman A, Hamilton R, Benson L, McCrindle BW. Factors associated with outcome in children with hypertrophic cardiomyopathy. Can J Cardiol 1997;13:88C.

11. Yetman AT, McCrindle BW, MacDonald C, Freedom RM, Gow R. Myocardial bridging in children with hypertrophic cardiomyopathy—a risk factor for sudden death. N Engl J Med 1998;339:1201–1209.

12. Spirito P, Bellone P, Harris KM, Bernabo P, Bruzzi P, Maron BJ. Magnitude of left ventricular hypertrophy and risk of sudden death in hypertrophic cardiomyopathy. N Engl J Med 2000;342:1778–1785.

13. Maron BJ, Olivotto I, Spirito P, et al. Epidemiology of hypertrophic cardiomyopathy-related death. Circulation 2000;102:858–864.

14. Doevendans PA. Hypertrophic cardiomyopathy: do we have the algorithm for life and death? Circulation 2000;101:1224–1226.

15. Drory Y, Turetz Y, Hiss Y, et al. Sudden unexpected death in persons < 40 years of age. Am J Cardiol 1991;68:1388–1392.

16. Spirito P, Rapezzi C, Autore C, et al. Prognosis of asymptomatic patients with hypertrophic cardiomyopathy and nonsustained ventricular tachycardia. Circulation 1994;90:2743–2747.

17. Elliott PM, Poloniecki J, Dickie S, et al. Sudden death in hypertrophic cardiomyopathy: identification of high risk patient. J Am Coll Cardiol 2000; 36:2212–2218.

18. McKenna WJ, Camm AJ. Sudden death in hypertrophic cardiomyopathy: assessment of patients at high risk. Circulation 1989;80:1489–1492.

19. Elliott PM, Sharma S, Varnava A, Poloniecki J, McKenna WJ. Survival after cardiac arrest or sustained ventricular tachycardia in patients with hypertrophic cardiomyopathy. J Am Coll Cardiol 1999;33:1596–1601.

20. Wigle ED, Rakowski H. Hypertrophic cardiomyopathy: when do you diagnose midventricular obstruction vs apical cavity obliteration with a small nonobliterated area at the apex of the left ventricle? J Am Coll Cardiol 1992;19:525–526.

21. Grigg LE, Wigle ED, Williams WG, Daniel LB, Rakowski H. Transesophageal Doppler echocardiography in obstructive hypertrophic cardiomyopathy: clarification of pathophysiology and importance in intraoperative decision making. J Am Coll Cardiol 1992;20:53–54.

22. Yu E, Chiam C, Siu S, Rakowski H, Wigle ED, O'Kelly B. Left atrial structure and function post myectomy in patients with hypertrophic obstructive cardiomyopathy. Can J Cardiol 1997;13:95C.

23. Yu EHC, Omran AS, Wigle D, Williams WG, Siu SC, Rakowski H. Mitral regurgitation in hypertrophic obstructive cardiomyopathy: relationship to obstruction and relief with myectomy. J Am Coll Cardiol 2000;36:2219–2225.

24. McKenna WJ, Oakley CM, Krikler DM, Goodwin JF. Improved survival with amiodarone in patients with hypertrophic cardiomyopathy and ventricular tachycardia. Br Heart J 1985;53:412–416.

25. Gilligan DM, Missouris CG, Boyd MJ, Oakley CM. Sudden death due to ventricular tachycardia during Amiodarone therapy in familial hypertrophic cardiomyopathy. Am J Cardiol 1991;68:971–973.

26. Maron BJ, Shen W-K, Link MS, et al. Efficacy of implantable cardioverter-defibrillators for the prevention of sudden death in patients with hypertrophic cardiomyopathy. N Engl J Med 2000;342:365–373.

27. McDonald K, McWilliams E, O'Keefe B, Maurer B. Functional assessment of patients treated with permanent dual chamber pacing as a primary treatment for hypertrophic cardiomyopathy. Eur Heart J 1988;9:893–898.

28. Maron BJ, Nishimura RA, McKenna WJ, Rakowski H, Josephson ME, Kieval RS. Assessment of permanent dual-chamber pacing as a treatment for drug-refractory symptomatic patients with obstructive hypertrophic cardiomyopathy. Circulation 1999;99:2927–2933.

29. Williams WG, Wigle ED, Rakowski H, Smallhorn J, Leblanc J, Trusler GA. Results of surgery for hypertrophic obstructive cardiomyopathy. Circulation 1987; 76:V104–V108.

30. Williams WG, Ralph-Edwards AC, Wigle ED. Surgical management of hypertrophic obstructive cardiomyopathy. Cardiol Rev 1997;5:40–49.

31. Theodoro DA, Danielson GK, Feldt RH, Anderson BJ. Hypertrophic obstructive cardiomyopathy in pediatric patients: results of surgical treatment. J Thorac Cardiovasc Surg 1996;112:1589–1599.

32. Heric B, Lytle BW, Miller DP, et al. Surgical management of hypertrophic obstructive cardiomyopathy. Early and late results. J Thorac Cardiovasc Surg 1995;110:195–208.

33. McCully RB, Nishimura RA, Tajik AJ, et al. Extent of clinical improvement after surgical treatment of hypertrophic obstructive cardiomyopathy. Circulation 1999; 99:2927–2933.

34. Grigg LE, Wigle ED, Williams WG, Daniel LB, Rakowski H. Transesophageal echocardiography in obstructive hypertrophic cardiomyopathy: clarification of pathophysiology and importance of intraoperative decision making. J Am Coll Cardiol 1992;53:42–52.

35. Cregg N, Cheng DCH, Karski JM, Williams WG, Webb G, Wigle ED. Morbidity outcome in patients with hypertrophic obstructive cardiomyopathy undergoing cardiac septal myectomy: early-extubation anesthesia vs high-dose opioid anesthesia technique. J Cardiothorac Vasc Anesthesia 1999;13:47–52.

36. Sigwart U. Nonsurgical myocardial reduction for hypertrophic obstructive cardiomyopathy. Lancet 1995;346:211–214.

37. Faber L, Seggewiss H, Fassbender D, et al. Identification of the target vessel (TV) in percutaneous transluminal ablation (PTSMA) in hypertrophic obstructive cardiomyopathy by myocardial contrast echocardiography (MCE) [abstract]. Circulation 1997;96(suppl I):I-639.

38. Flores-Ramirez R, Lakkis NM, Middleton KJ, Killip D, Spencer WH, Nagueh SF. Echocardiographic insight into the mechanisms of relief of left ventricular obstruction after nonsurgical septal reduction therapy in patients with hypertrophic obstructive cardiomyopathy. J Am Coll Cardiol 2001;37:208–214.

39. Woo A, Schwartz L, Wigle ED, Ross J, Rakowski H. Myocardial contrast echocardiography during septal ethanol ablation for obstructive hypertrophic cardiomyopathy. In: Goldberg BB, Raichlen JS, Forsberg F, eds. Ultrasound Contrast Agents. Martin Dunitz: 2000, pp. 197–211.

40. Mazur W, Nagueh SF, Lakkis NM, et al. Regression of left ventricular hypertrophy after nonsurgical septal reduction therapy for hypertrophic obstructive cardiomyopathy. Circulation 2001;103:1492–1496.

41. Li G, Li R-K, Mickle DAG, et al. Elevated insulin-like growth factor-1 and trans-
    forming growth factor-BI and their receptors in patients with idiopathic hyper-
    trophic obstructive cardiomyopathy. Circulation 1998;98:II-144–II-150.
42. Li G, Li R-K, Borger MA, et al. Regional overexpression of IGF-1 and TGF-B1
    in the myocardium of hypertrophic obstructive cardiomyopathy patients. J Thorac
    Cardiovasc Surg 2002;123:89–95.
43. Seggewiss H, Gleichman U, Faber L, et al. Percutaneous transluminal septal
    myocardial ablation in hypertrophic obstructive cardiomyopathy: acute results and
    3 month follow-up in 25 patients. J Am Coll Cardiol 1998;31:252–258.
44. Maron BJ. Role of alcohol septal ablation in treatment of obstructive hypertrophic
    cardiomyopathy. Lancet 2000;355:425–426.

10 Dynamic Cardiomyoplasty and New Prosthetic LV Girdling Devices

Michael A. Acker, MD

CONTENTS

INTRODUCTION

Dynamic cardiomyoplasty (DCMP) is a promising but unproven surgical treatment for patients with end-stage heart failure. Today, the procedure is no longer performed in the Unites States. The procedure, first performed by Alain Carpentier in 1985 *(1)*, involves mobilization of the latissimus dorsi muscle, which is then wrapped circumferentially around the heart. The muscle wrap is then, after a period of training, stimulated to contract in synchrony with cardiac systole. Chronic repetitive stimulation induces biochemical and physiological transformations of the muscle, altering its characteristics toward cardiac muscle. These changes include fatigue resistance, increased aerobic capacity, prolonged contraction duration, diminished size, and reduced maximal power *(2–5)*.

From: *Contemporary Cardiology: Surgical Management of Congestive Heart Failure*
Edited by: J. C. Fang and G. S. Couper © Humana Press Inc., Totowa, NJ

CLINICAL EXPERIENCE WITH DYNAMIC
CARDIOMYOPLASTY

Since 1985, more than 1000 patients have had DCMP performed worldwide. The majority had significant improvement in New York Heart Association (NYHA) functional class and overall quality of life *(6–8)*. Despite this dramatic improvement, consistent objective hemodynamic beneficial effects have not been consistently demonstrated, and a survival advantage has not been proven over medical therapy alone *(9)*. Further clouding the picture have been evolving indications, uncertainty over risk stratification, a past relatively high operative mortality, limitations of a first-generation cardiomyostimulator, concomitant surgery, and a mechanism of action that remains unclear. Lack of a clear survival advantage and ongoing misunderstanding of its mechanism of action hindered its acceptance as a treatment alternative for patients with end-stage heart failure. Recruitment for the definitive phase III US Food and Drug Administration (FDA) study was slow, and the study was terminated early, ending its clinical use in the United States.

In more than several hundred to 1000 patients implanted with Medtronic cardiomyostimulators, consistent clinical improvement has been noted in 80 to 85% of hospital survivors. On the average, the NYHA class improves 1.2 classes. The improvement begins within the first 6 months of surgery and has been sustained for years. Quality-of-life (QoL) measures assessing daily activity, social activity, quality of interaction, and mental health all improve significantly *(10)*. In addition, the number of hospitalizations for heart failure has been seen to decrease *(11)*.

Similar clinical improvement was demonstrated in the phase II FDA trial of DCMP. This was a multicenter prospective trial to evaluate the safety of the device in 68 patients. Outcomes were compared to those of a reference group of medically treated patients with matched demographic, etiologic, clinical, and hemodynamic parameters. In both groups, almost all patients were in NYHA class III heart failure, suffered from either ischemic or idiopathic cardiomyopathy, and were on optimized medical therapy. Operative mortality was 12%. Of the patients, 80% were functionally improved at 6 and 12 months (3 ± 0.1 to 1.7 ± 0.1 NYHA class), which was significantly better than the reference group *(9)*. Patients remained functionally improved to 2 years.

Despite the overwhelming evidence for clinical improvement, consistent evidence of clinically significant hemodynamic benefit is lacking. In the phase II trial, left ventricular ejection fraction (LVEF) increased from $22.7 \pm 1.0\%$ to $25.5 \pm 1.9\%$, and LV stroke work index increased from 26 ± 1 to 30 ± 2 g/m^2 per beat. Both changes were statistically significant. No change, however, was seen in cardiac index, pulmonary capillary wedge pressure, right ventricular (RV)EF, and maximal O_2 consumption. Recent reports continue to demonstrate a small but statistically significant improvement in LVEF *(11–16)*.

The operative mortality associated with cardiomyoplasty has progressively decreased over the last decade. During a FDA phase I feasibility study (1988–1991), 31% of patients did not survive their hospitalization. Many of these patients were NYHA class IV. During the FDA phase II study, in which almost all patients were class III, hospital mortality decreased to 12%. During the recently terminated phase III trial, patients undergoing cardiomyoplasty had a hospital mortality of less than 3% *(10)*. Three-quarters of the hospital deaths were related to progressive heart failure. The remaining deaths were related to sepsis or multisystem organ failure. Deaths that occurred following initial hospital discharge were 80% cardiac in origin, with 38% sudden and 41% nonsudden. Among the approx 20% noncardiac deaths, about half were caused by pneumonia and sepsis; the rest were caused by noncardiac unknown causes *(10)*.

During cardiomyoplasty's initial experience, survival for class IV patients was clearly shown to be much worse than survival for class III. Today, NYHA class IV patients are not considered candidates for DCMP. Actuarial survival appeared to be improving further (1 year 78%, 2 years 70%) for class III patients ($n = 103$) at experienced centers *(10)*.

Furnary et al. *(16)* performed a multivariate analysis of risk factors for poor overall survival in 127 patients who underwent the DCMP from three major centers. They found that predictors of poor results were atrial fibrillation, NYHA class IV status, high pulmonary capillary wedge pressure, and need for intra-aortic balloon pump. When peak oxygen consumption (VO_2) was analyzed, pulmonary capillary wedge pressure and NYHA class were eliminated from the model.

Analysis of 117 patients from the phase II DCMP study group demonstrated VO_2 and LVEF provided independent prognostic information for procedure-related death according to logistic regression analysis *(17)*. Rector et al. *(18)* updated the earlier multicenter analysis ($n = 166$) and found, in addition to VO_2 and LVEF, center experience and significant coronary artery disease (coronary arteries with stenosis lesions <70%) were predictors of cardiac mortality within 2 months after cardiomyoplasty. Moreira et al. *(19)* reported 5-year follow-up on 31 patients post-DCMP. Multivariate analysis of factors influencing outcome showed that preoperative functional class and pulmonary vascular resistance significantly affected long-term survival.

Cardiomyoplasty was originally conceived as a method to assist the heart mechanically during ejection by "squeezing," thereby increasing beat-to-beat EF, stroke volume, and cardiac output. Although a few investigators (20,21) have demonstrated the direct active synchronous assistance of the wrap on the failing heart, convincing hemodynamic evidence of clinically important beat-to-beat systolic assist is at best modest and often not seen at all despite significant improvement in functional status (22). Others have suggested that the primary action is a girdling effect by which the muscle wrap acts to prevent further ventricular remodeling (12,22,23).

There continues to be substantial evidence supporting active systolic assistance in both clinical and animal studies. One year following DCMP in 13 patients, Jatene et al. showed that LVEF increased with stimulator on vs off (20). Cho et al. (24) and Aklog et al. (25) showed augmentation of end-systolic elastance for assisted beats in normal canine hearts. We showed that, in chronic cardiomyopathic canine hearts, active cardiomyoplasty assist will result in a beat-to-beat increase in load-independent indices of contractility (26). In at least some patients Schreuder et al. showed, quite convincingly, that 1 year after DCMP, optimization of stimulation parameters will result in significant beat-to-beat improvement in cardiac function (21).

Although most patients demonstrated no significant change, in about 50% of patients, Hagege et al. saw a decrease in LVEF and dP/dt when the stimulator was turned off for 24 hours, suggesting a heterogeneous response of muscle wrap contraction. This may be related to the individual degree of latissimus dorsi muscle damage (12). Atrophy and fibrosis of the distal part of the latissimus dorsi muscle flap is thought to be caused by ischemia. This contributes to weakening the overall effect of the latissimus dorsi muscle contraction, limiting its ability to improve active systolic assistance.

Carraro et al. (27,28) have developed an intermittent "demand" stimulation protocol that produces and maintains a long-term partial transformation (intermediate fiber type) of the latissimus dorsi muscle. This muscle is relatively fatigue resistant, yet faster and more powerful than a fully transformed muscle. It is a muscle more capable of beat-to-beat assistance of the heart. Arpesella et al. have recently demonstrated in animal study that in situ conditioning and two-stage mobilization improves the distal perfusion and capillary density (29). Kashem et al. also demonstrated in dogs that intermittent stimulation results in a more powerful muscle capable of increased LV assistance (30).

This suggests that cardiomyoplasty should be done in two stages: the first to mobilize the muscle partially and to place electrodes to begin preconditioning in situ and the second stage to complete the muscle flap mobilization, followed by the actual cardiac wrap. Such a strategy, not done in the past, would be expected to result in a more powerful muscle with preserved distal perfusion, avoiding muscle fibrosis seen to date.

EFFECTS OF PASSIVE GIRDLING

Passive girdling effects have been proposed as an additional mechanism of benefit. Carpentier et al. demonstrated a stable cardiothoracic ratio for up to 3 years following DCMP, whereas progressive dilatation would otherwise be anticipated in such patients (6). Capouya et al. reported that placement of an unstimulated wrap around a normal heart followed by rapid ventricular pacing attenuated LV enlargement (23). Our laboratory demonstrated that, in a chronic canine cardiomyopathic model, DCMP limited the remodeling process of ongoing heart failure (26), and this effect can also be demonstrated without chronic systolic assistance (31).

Kass et al. (22) demonstrated in three patients a leftward shift of end-systolic pressure volume relationship and stabilization of the end-diastolic pressure volume relationship at 6 and 12 months after DCMP, suggesting a reversal of the remodeling process. Although no active systolic beat-to-beat assistance could be demonstrated, objective measures of systolic function improved dramatically. Evidence of reverse remodeling has also been demonstrated by Lorusso et al., who reported a significant reduction in left ventricular end-diastolic diameter up to 3 years after DCMP in 22 patients (11).

Hagege et al. (12) reported further evidence that active beat-to-beat assistance is not necessary for overall benefit from DCMP. They reported that in 13 patients, all longer than 1 year after DCMP, there was no change in overall indexes of systolic or diastolic left ventricular function after stopping muscle wrap stimulation for 24 hours. All patients were clinically improved, and overall LVEF was improved. Jondeau et al. reported similar results (14).

Finally, there have been several anecdotal reports of clinical deterioration when the stimulator was dysfunctional for more than 1 to 2 weeks. This speaks more to the importance of synchronous stimulation chronically than its active beat-to-beat assistance.

Kawaguchi and associates showed that mechanical artificial external synchronous systolic compression that mimics DCMP will decrease wall stress and myocardial oxygen consumption (32,33). In acute experiments utilizing unconditioned muscle and normal hearts, Lee et al. (34), Chen et al. (35), and Aklog et al. (25) demonstrated decreased wall stress with active muscle wrap assistance.

Our laboratory demonstrated *(36)*, in a chronic canine cardiomyopathic model, that DCMP results chronically in an improvement in preload recruitable stroke work and myocardial efficiency when compared to control heart failure animals. In addition, muscle wrap stimulation further increased preload recruitable stroke work and myocardial efficiency, and potential energy decreased. This was seen without a change in stroke volume or cardiac output.

Oh et al. postulated that the muscle wrap of DCMP decreases wall stress according to Laplace's law (by increased wall thickness) *(37)*. For this to occur, the muscle wrap must develop and share tension with the myocardium even if there is no change acutely in overall LV function *(37)*. These findings may explain why significant improvement in LVEF and other standard measurements of LV function may not be found in patients who improve clinically.

In some patients with ischemic cardiomyopathy, DCMP may induce increase collateral blood flow to ischemic areas of the ventricle. Mannion et al. demonstrated evidence of this in an ischemic animal model *(38)*, and collaterals have been found in autopsy studies between the myocardium and the muscle wrap *(39)*.

Finally, the possibility that stimulation of the latissimus dorsi nerve may affect the neurohormonal milieu via a central pathway must be investigated. In the future, staged mobilization procedures and new intermittent stimulation protocols may limit muscle damage and produce a stronger, yet still fatigue-resistant, muscle with more potential for powerful cardiac assistance *(27,28,40,41)*.

THE C-SMART TRIAL

The phase III randomized clinical trial, also known as C-SMART (Cardiomyoplasty-Skeletal Muscle Assist Randomized Trial) commenced in June 1995 and was terminated near the end of 1998. Slightly more than 100 patients had been entered into the study. There were to be 400 patients (200 for DCMP and 200 for standard medical therapy) recruited. The study utilized the new Transform cardiomyostimulator (Medtronic Inc.). C-SMART was designed to test the hypothesis that DCMP improves the functional status and quality of life of patients with NYHA class III heart failure compared to a control group with comparable morbidity and mortality evaluated 12 months postenrollment in the trial.

There were 103 patients randomly assigned to C-SMART from 1994 to 1998. At 6 months, 79% of patients with DCMP were NYHA class I or II compared to 25% in the medical group. There was also statistical improvement in QoL scores and 6-minute walk. The 6-month survival was similar between medical and surgical groups *(42)*. Despite these encouraging preliminary results, the trial was halted by Medtronic, the trial's sponsor, because of slowness of recruiting patients. The cardiomyostimulator is no longer produced, and the operation has not been done in the United States since the trial stopped.

Legitimate doubts about the efficacy of DCMP remain. Although patients are improved functionally, no statistically significant hemodynamic or survival benefit has been demonstrated. Many cardiologists and cardiac surgeons agree with Leier, who stated in an editorial, "In short, those who need it, don't survive it and those who survive it, don't need it" *(43)*. Unfortunately, although many patients with class III heart failure can be managed effectively with medication alone, there are clearly many patients on maximal medical therapy whose quality of life and exercise capacity have worsened, yet are not sick enough to consider transplantation. Comparison of Minnesota Living With Heart Failure scores of recent DCMP patients with those of the class II and III patients in the Studies of Left Ventricular Dysfunction (SOLVD) treatment arm demonstrated that the cardiomyoplasty candidates perceived significantly greater limitations of daily living *(11)*, which motivated them to seek a surgical treatment for their heart failure in lieu of medication alone. It is clear that a more potent treatment alternative for these patients must be sought.

Chronic dilatation and remodeling are initial valuable adaptations that allow weakened hearts to achieve near-normal systolic pressure and flows at increased, but still tolerable, diastolic pressures. Although initially adaptive, ongoing remodeling and dilatation is maladaptive and a major risk factor for mortality *(22)*. The remodeled ventricle has a larger chamber with an increased radius of curvature, increased wall stress, increased myocardial oxygen consumption, impaired subendocardial blood flow, impaired myocardial energetics, and increased risk of arrhythmias *(44)*. It is likely that DCMP, through a combination of a chronic elastic constraint and active dynamic assistance, decreases myocardial wall stress and attenuates ventricular dilatation and the remodeling process associated with progressive heart failure (Fig. 1).

It is well accepted that the small, but important, survival benefit attributed to angiotensin-converting enzyme inhibitors in patients with heart failure is secondary to an attenuation of progressive cardiac enlargement. This important but subtle effect was not realized until completion of large prospective randomized studies (SOLVD) *(44)*. What is abundantly clear by now is that DCMP can be shown to limit the remodeling process of heart failure in animal studies and in some patients.

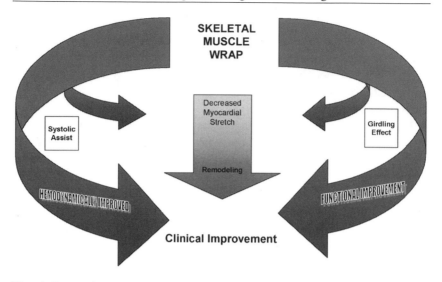

Fig. 1. Dynamic cardiomyoplasty probably acts by at least two mechanisms, ultimately limiting the remodeling process of progressive heart failure.

OTHER STRATEGIES

Stimulated by the potential importance of the passive girdling of the muscle wrap in DCMP, new prosthetic passive girdling devices have been developed. One such device is a polyester jacket (CorCap™, Acorn Cardiovascular Inc.). In animal studies of dilated cardiomyopathy, it promoted reverse remodeling and improved indexes of systolic function. The jacket also has partially reversed the heart failure phenotype on a cellular and molecular level *(45,46)*. It is hypothesized that the CorCap jacket reduces diastolic wall stress (Fig. 2). In an animal model of an acute myocardial infarct, placement of the jacket post-infarct prevents subsequent LV dilatation and remodeling and preserves LV systolic function *(47)*.

During the initial safety trial in Europe, the CorCap was placed in patients with NYHA class III congestive heart failure with dilated cardiomyopathy and was often combined with mitral valve repair. No device-related complications were noted, and very importantly, no cases of constrictive pericarditis developed in over 2 years of follow-up. Although not designed as an efficacy trial, several patients who had the CorCap alone have demonstrated significant improvement in LVEF, with LV volumes stabilizing or reversing. There is currently an ongoing FDA-sponsored phase II multiinstitutional, randomized study of

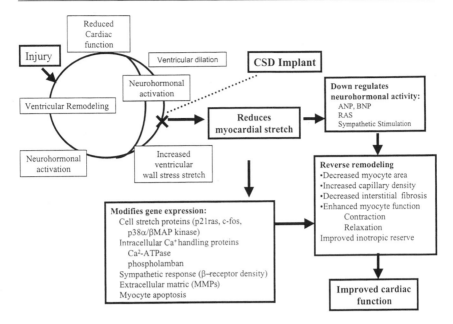

Fig. 2. Decreased myocardial stretch and stress have been demonstrated to modify the heart failure phenotype on global, cellular, and molecular levels. ANP, atrial natriuretic peptide; BNP, brain natriuretic peptide; RAS, renin angiotensin system; MMP, matrix metalloproteinase.

patients with NYHA class III heart failure and dilated ventricles with and without mitral insufficiency (Fig. 3).

Another device still in development is the Myocor Myosplint, which is designed to decrease left ventricular wall stress by changing LV shape, thus improving contractile function. This shape change is accomplished by surgically placing three myosplints perpendicular to the LV long axis, drawing LV walls inward, and creating a symmetric bilobular left ventricle. The bilobular left ventricle has decreased wall stress compared to the original spherical, ellipsoidal shape *(48)*. In contrast to the CorCap, this device decreases wall stress acutely, but is more invasive to place. It has been demonstrated to decrease wall stress in canine models of heart failure and is awaiting human evaluation.

With C-SMART's termination, the potential clinical benefit of cardiomyoplasty will never be totally known. Its ultimate role in the treatment of heart failure depended on the outcome of properly designed randomized controlled studies, such as C-SMART. With termination of the FDA phase III trial, clinical cardiomyopathy has ceased in the United States, although in Europe the procedure is still performed. The

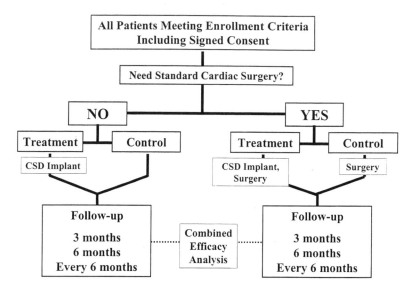

Fig. 3. US multicenter randomized trial of Acorn jacket in patients with NYHA class III heart failure and dilated left ventricles.

lessons learned from cardiomyoplasty (i.e., that an external constraint can be used effectively to limit the remodeling process of heart failure) however, may still prove of larger clinical significance.

REFERENCES

1. Carpentier A, Chacques JC. Myocardial substitution with a stimulated skeletal muscle: first successful clinical case [letter]. Lancet 1985;1:1267.
2. Mannion JD, Bitto T, Hammond RL, et al. Histochemical and fatigue characteristics of conditioned canine latissimus dorsi muscle. Circ Res 1986;58: 298–304.
3. Salmons S, Sreter FA. Significance of impulse activity in the transformation of skeletal muscle type. Nature 1967;263:30–34.
4. Sreter FA, Gergely J, Salmons S, Romanul F. Synthesis by fast muscle of myosin light chains characteristic of slow muscle in response to long-term stimulation. Nature 1973;241:17–19.
5. Clark BJ, Acker MA, McCully K, et al. In vivo ^{31}P-NMR spectroscopy of chronically stimulated canine skeletal muscle. Am J Physiol 1988;254: C-258–C-266.
6. Carpentier A, Chachques JC, Acar C, et al. Dynamic cardiomyoplasty at 7 years. J Thorac Cardiovasc Surg 1993;106:42–52.
7. Moreira LF, Stolf NA, Braile DM, Jatene AD. Dynamic cardiomyoplasty in South America. Ann Thorac Surg 1996;61:408–412.
8. Magovern GJ, Simpson A. Clinical cardiomyoplasty: review of the 10-year United States experience. Ann Thorac Surg 1996;61:413–419.

9. Furnary AP, Jessup M, Moreira LF. Multicenter trial of dynamic cardiomyoplasty for chronic heart failure. The American Cardiomyplasty Group. J Am Coll Cardiol 1996;28:1175–1180.
10. Medtronic dynamic cardiomyoplasty clinical database. 1996.
11. Lorusso R, Milane E, Volterrani M, et al. Cardiomyoplasty as isolated procedure to treat refractory heart failure. Eur J Cardiothorac Surg 1997;363–372.
12. Hagege AA, Desnos M, Fernandez F, et al. Clinical study of the effect of latissimus dorsi muscle flap stimulation after cardiomyoplasty. Circulation 1995;92 (suppl II):II210–II215.
13. Bocchi EA, Bellotti G, Moreira LF. Mid-term results of heart transplantation, cardiomyoplasty and medical treatment of refractory heart failure caused by idiopathic dilated cardiomyopathy. J Heart Lung Transplant 1996;75:736–745.
14. Jondeau G, Dorent R, Dib JC, et al. Dynamic cardiomyoplasty: effect of discontinuing latissimus dorsi stimulation on left ventricular systolic and diastolic performance and exercise capacity. J Am Coll Cardiol 1995;26:129–134.
15. Tasdemir O, Kucukaksu SD, Vural KM, et al. A comparison of early and mid-term results after dynamic cardiomyoplasty in patients with ischemic and idiopathic cardiomyoplasty. J Thorac Cardiovasc Surg 1997;113:173–181.
16. Furnary AP, Chacques JC, Moreira LP, et al. Long-term outcome survival analysis and risk stimulation of dynamic cardiomyoplasty. J Thorac Cardiovasc Surg 1996;112:1640–1650.
17. Phase II Dynamic Cardiomyoplasty Study Group. Factors associated with acute hospital mortality following a latissimus dorsi cardiomyoplasty. Maastricht, The Netherlands, 1994.
18. Rector TS, Benditt D, Chachques J, et al. Retrospective risk analysis for early heart-related death after cardiomyoplasty. The Worldwide Cardiomyoplasty Group. J Heart Lung Transplant 1997;16:1018–1025.
19. Moreira LF, Stolf NA, Bocchi EA, et al. Clinical and left ventricular function outcomes up to 5 years after dynamic cardiomyoplasty. J Thorac Cardiovasc Surg 1995;109:353–362.
20. Jatene AD, Moreira LF, Stolf NA, et al. Left ventricular function changes after cardiomyoplasty in patients with dilated cardiomyopathy. J Thorac Cardiovasc Surg 1991;102:132–139.
21. Schreuder JJ, van der Veen FH, van der Velde ET, et al. Beat-to-beat analysis of left ventricular pressure volume relation and stroke volume by conductance catheter and aortic model flow in cardiomyoplasty patients. Circulation 1995;91:2010–2017.
22. Kass DA, Baughman KL, Pak PH, et al. Reverse remodeling from cardiomyoplasty in human heart failure. Circulation 1995;91:2314–2318.
23. Capouya ER, Gerber RS, Drinkwater DC, et al. Girdling effect of non-stimulated cardiomyoplasty on left ventricular function. Ann Thorac Surg 1993;56:867–871.
24. Cho PW, Levin HR, Curtis WE, et al. Pressure-volume analysis of changes in cardiac function in chronic cardiomyoplasty. Ann Thorac Surg 1993;56:38–45.
25. Aklog L, Murphy MP, Chen FY, et al. Right latissimus dorsi cardiomyoplasty improves left ventricular function by increasing peak systolic elastance. Circulation 1994;90(part II):II-112–II-119.
26. Patel HJ, Lankford EB, Polidori DJ, et al. Dynamic cardiomyoplasty: its chronic and acute effects on the failing heart. J Thorac Cardiovasc Surg 1997;114:169–178.
27. Muneretto C, Carraro U, Barbiero M, et al. Shortened conditioning and lighter

stimulation regimen for dynamic cardiomyoplasty: preliminary results. Basic Appl Myol 1997;7:55–56.

28. Carraro U, Docali G, Barbiero M, et al. Demand dynamic cardiomyoplasty: improved clinical benefits by non-invasive monitoring of LD flap and long-term tuning of its dynamic contractile characteristics by activity-rest regime. Basic Appl Myol 1998;8:11–15.

29. Arpesella G, Carraro V, Mikus PM, et al. Activity–rest stimulation of latissimus dorsi for cardiomyoplasty: 1 year results in sheep. Ann Thorac Surg 1998;66: 1983–1990.

30. Kashem A, Santamore WP, Chiang B, et al. Vascular delay and intermittent stimulation: keys to successful latissimus dorsi muscle stimulation. Ann Thorac Surg 2001;71:1866–1873.

31. Patel HJ, Polidori DJ, Pilla JJ, et al. Stabilization of chronic remodeling by asynchronous cardiomyoplasty in dilated cardiomyopathy: the effects of a conditioned wrap. Circulation 1997;96:3665–3671.

32. Kawaguchi O, Goto Y, Futai S, et al. Mechanical enhancement and myocardial oxygen saving by synchronized dynamic left ventricular compression. J Thorac Cardiovasc Surg 1992;103:573–581.

33. Kawaguchi O, Goto Y, Futaki S, et al. The effects of dynamic cardiac compression on ventricular mechanics and energetics. J Thorac Cardiovasc Surg 1994;107: 850–859.

34. Lee KJ, Dignan RJ, Parmar JM, et al. Effects of dynamic cardiomyoplasty on left ventricular performance and myocardial mechanics in dilated cardiomyopathy. J Thorac Cardiovasc Surg 1991;102:124–131.

35. Chen FY, Aklog L, deGuzman BJ, et al. New technique measures decreased transmural myocardial pressure in cardiomyoplasty. Ann Thorac Surg 1995;60: 1678–1682.

36. Patel HJ, Pilla JJ, Polidori D, et al. Long-term dynamic cardiomyoplasty improves chronic and acute myocardial energetics in a model of left ventricular dysfunction. Circulation 1998;98:II346–II351.

37. Oh JH, Badhwar V, Chiu RC. Mechanism of dynamic cardiomyoplasty. J Card Surg 1996;11:194–199.

38. Mannion JD, Blood V, Bailey W, et al. The effect of basic fibroblast growth factor on blood flow and morphologic features of a latissimus dorsi cardiomyoplasty. J Thorac Cardiovasc Surg 1996;111:19–28.

39. Mott BD, Misawa Y, Lough JO, et al. Clinicopathological correlation of dynamic cardiomyoplasty. Am J Cardiol 1996;11:133E.

40. Carroll SM, Heilman SJ, Steimel RW, et al. Vascular delay improves latissimus dorsi muscle perfusion and muscle function for use in cardiomyoplasty. Plast Reconstr Surg 1997;99:1329–1337.

41. Ianuzzo CD, Ianuzzo SE, Anderson WA. Cardiomyoplasty: transformation of the assisting muscle using intermittent vs continuous stimulation. J Card Surg 1996; 11:293–303.

42. Young JB, Kirklin JK, C-SMART investigators. Cardiomyoplasty-Skeletal Muscle Assist Randomized Trial (C-SMART): 6 month results [abstract]. American Heart Association, 1999.

43. Leier CV. Cardiomyoplasty: is it time to wrap it up? J Am Coll Cardiol 1996;28: 1101–1102.

44. Cohn JN. Structural basis for heart failure: ventricular remodeling and its pharmacologic inhibition. Circulation 1995;91:2504–2507.

45. Chaudhry PA, Mishima T, Sharov UG, et al. Passive epicardial containment prevents ventricular remodeling in heart failure. Ann Thorac Surg 2000;70:1275–1280.
46. Sabbah HN, Chaudhry PA, Paone G, et al. Passive ventricular constraint with Acorn prosthetic jacket prevents progressive left ventricular dilation and improves ejection fraction in dogs with moderate heart failure. Paper presented at: American College of Cardiology Advanced Meeting; March 1999; New Orleans, LA.
47. Pilla JJ, Blom AS, Brockman DJ, et al. Ventricular constraint using the Acorn cardiac support device (CSD) reduces myocardial infarct size in an ovine model of acute infarction. Circulation 2002;106:I207–I211.
48. Takagaki M, McCarthy PM, Ochiai Y, et al. Novel device to change left ventricular shape for heart failure treatment: device design and implantation procedure. ASAIO J 2001;47:244–248.

11 Xenotransplantation

*Joren C. Madsen, MD, DPhil
and Ruediger Hoerbelt, MD*

CONTENTS

INTRODUCTION

Data from the United Network for Organ Sharing (UNOS) indicated that status 1 patients waiting for a heart transplant in the United States have a mortality rate as high as 45% because of the shortage of donor organs *(1)*. The discrepancy between the number of patients waiting for an organ transplant and the number of organs that become available each year is increasing. In 1999, the number of heart transplant candidates on US waiting lists was 4277, but less than 50% received an organ *(1)*. Although it is difficult to determine the overall number of patients who would benefit from cardiac transplantation in the United States if the source of donor organs were unlimited, estimates range from 35,000 to 100,000 patients (reviewed in ref. *2*).

From: *Contemporary Cardiology: Surgical Management of Congestive Heart Failure*
Edited by: J. C. Fang and G. S. Couper © Humana Press Inc., Totowa, NJ

This scarcity of donor organs has led to a strong resurgence of interest in xenotransplantation. However, there are formidable immunological barriers to overcome before the full potential of transspecies organ transplantation can be realized. This chapter primarily examines the immunological barriers to xenotransplantation and the experimental strategies currently employed to overcome them. Because the most excitement in recent years has been in the area of hyperacute rejection and cellular rejection, these two areas are the primary focus of this review. The physiological barriers to cardiac xenotransplantation, although important, are less critical than in liver or kidney xenotransplantation. This subject is reviewed in the Choice of Animal Donor section. Infectious disease issues are summarized at the end of the chapter. The many ethical ramifications of xenotransplantation are beyond the scope of this chapter; excellent reviews are provided in refs. 2–6.

ADVANTAGES OF XENOTRANSPLANTATION

Although the traditional rationale for pursuing xenotransplantation as a treatment for end-stage heart disease has been its promise to provide an unlimited supply of donor organs, there are other advantages that could be realized by bringing xenotransplantation to the clinic. By identifying and preparing the donor and recipient in advance of the transplant, the potentially devastating effects of brain death on the donor organ (7) would be eliminated, and the ischemia/reperfusion injury associated with prolonged preservation times (8) would be greatly reduced. Optimizing the physiological state of the donor organ and the timing of organ procurement would have significant short- and long-term benefits. Indeed, the combined clinical impact of brain death, prolonged preservation times, and associated ischemia/reperfusion injury on whole organ transplantation is highlighted by the fact that kidney allografts from human lymphocyte antigen (HLA)-mismatched living donors survive longer than allografts from HLA-identical cadaveric donors (9).

There is also the exciting potential for modifying the host and the donor organs prior to transplantation, not only to mitigate the vigorous xenogeneic immune response, but also to create "customized" donor organs. From an immunological standpoint, the human host may one day be preconditioned to induce immunological tolerance to the xenograft, for instance, by donor bone marrow transplantation (10) or gene therapy (11). Alternatively, the xenograft could be derived from animals genetically engineered for the lifelong expression of transgenes that mitigate the hyperacute response to natural antibody (12) or that prevent acute vascular rejection (13) (see Prevention of Hyperacute

Rejection section). Most important, scientists have now successfully cloned swine through nuclear transfer from adult somatic cells *(14)* and have been able to "knock out" genes relevant to hyperacute xenograft rejection in the process. This is a major step in bringing xenotransplantation to the clinic (*see* Prevention of Hyperacute Rejection section). Of note, the ability to customize the xenogeneic organ donor genetically may obviate the need for some of the investigative approaches described here.

From a physiological standpoint, gene transfer techniques could be used to overexpress genes of functional value to the organ and donor. For instance, right heart dysfunction/failure might be prevented in a donor heart engineered to overexpress *SERCA2a* (to optimize the utilization of myocardial calcium), β*2-AR* (to improve β-adrenergic signaling), or *Bcl-2* (to block cardiomyocyte apoptosis) *(15)*. Alternatively, an animal heart might be "trained" for implantation into a recipient with fixed pulmonary hypertension by banding or balloon-occluding the main pulmonary artery of the donor prior to procurement *(16,17)*. The resulting pressure load would induce rapid hypertrophy of the right ventricle *(18)*, making it a more suitable organ for a recipient with high pulmonary vascular resistance. Possibilities such as these add to the utility of xenotransplantation.

CHOICE OF ANIMAL DONOR

Early studies of xenotransplantation in several different species demonstrated that hyperacute rejection did not occur in every combination of species, but only in species of great phylogenetic diversity. The greater the phylogenetic distance between species, the more rapid the rejection response was. Realizing this, Calne suggested the terms *concordant*, to describe species combinations in which hyperacute rejection did not occur, and *discordant*, to describe combinations in which it did occur *(19)*. Because hyperacute rejection is the result of preformed, naturally occurring antibodies directed against tissue from other species, these terms have more recently been used to distinguish between (concordant) combinations of species in which there are no preformed natural antibodies (i.e., hamster to rat or monkey to baboon) and (discordant) species combination in which natural antibodies do exist (i.e., guinea pig to rat or pig to baboon).

Understandably, early efforts to apply xenotransplantation in the clinic were directed toward the use of nonhuman primates (chimpanzee) as donors because they were phylogenetically closest to humans and therefore provided concordant xenografts. However, nonhuman primates such as chimpanzees and baboons present other problems that make their use as xenograft donors unlikely. They are small compared to adult humans, their availability is limited, and their potential for transmitting infectious diseases is real. The US Food and Drug Administration has expressed growing concern over the use of nonhuman primate-derived tissues for human transplantation (20).

Most investigators now believe that the pig will be the most suitable source of organs and tissues for humans, even though swine provide discordant xenografts. The advantages of swine include unlimited availability, favorable breeding characteristics, and organs similar in size and function to their human counterparts. Since the late 1970s, a herd of miniature swine has been bred selectively to homozygosity at the porcine major histocompatibility complex (MHC) (21,22). These partially inbred miniature swine provide a number of unique advantages as potential xenograft donors. In contrast to domestic swine, which reach 450 kg, adult miniature swine achieve weights of 120 to 140 kg, making it possible to obtain a miniature swine organ of appropriate size for any potential human recipient.

To identify which miniature swine would donate the best size-matched heart for a particular human recipient, our laboratory performed a morphometric study of the miniature swine heart using transthoracic echocardiography. By comparing the morphometric measurements of aortic annulus diameter in the miniature swine with normative human data, we were able to develop a nomogram, relating swine length to human height, to make the prediction (Fig. 1) (23).

The physiology of the porcine circulatory system is similar to that of humans. To address whether a size-matched miniature swine heart would meet the physiological needs of a human host, we performed a preliminary analysis of the hemodynamic parameters of ejection fraction, stroke volume, and cardiac output in pigs chosen as the appropriate size to donate hearts to a 70-kg human. Swine were placed on cardiopulmonary bypass to vary preload and afterload conditions independent of the right and left ventricles at a fixed heart rate. We found that left ventricular performance was never limiting in the face of high volume and pressure loads. Right ventricular performance was also maintained with increased right ventricular afterload. However, progressive volume loading of the right ventricle under conditions of fixed systemic afterload eventually led to dilatation of the tricuspid annulus and tricuspid regurgitation. These data suggest that the function of a size-matched cardiac xenograft from a miniature swine would be adequate to meet the hemodynamic requirements of a human recipient, but efforts should be made to avoid volume overload in the early postoperative period (23).

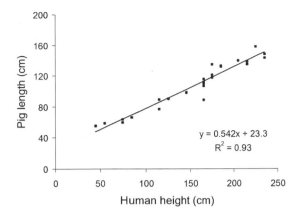

Fig. 1. Swine-to-human cardiac size-matching nomogram. Swine aortic dimensions are highly correlated with a pig's body length. By analogy, human aortic annulus diameter is also highly correlated with a person's height. By comparing echocardiographic swine data to normative human data, we were able to construct a size-matching nomogram. This nomogram predicts the best size-matched pig for a prospective human cardiac xenograft recipient by matching for aortic annulus diameter. (Reproduced with permission from ref. *23*.)

There are additional advantages to using MHC-inbred miniature swine as xenograft donors. Swine express blood groups equivalent to human ABO blood groups. To diminish an immune response against AB antigens, group H (equivalent to human blood group O) miniature swine have been selectively bred for the purpose of transplantation. From the perspective of genetic engineering, incorporating transgenes into a line of pigs from the same inbred herd would permit quicker crossbreeding than possible if different breeding stocks were used. Also, because the major MHC of inbred miniature swine donors has been fully characterized *(24–26)*, a strategy of introducing relevant porcine MHC genes into the bone marrow of human recipients before transplantation could be undertaken possibly to induce tolerance. This process, termed *molecular chimerism*, has proven effective in prolonging the survival of allografts *(11,27)*. Finally, whereas primates may harbor infectious agents such as herpes B virus that can be lethal for human recipients, pigs can be bred to exclude serious human pathogens *(28)*.

HISTORY OF XENOTRANSPLANTATION

Keith Reemtsma introduced xenotransplantation to clinical medicine in 1963 when he performed the first chimpanzee-to-human renal transplant *(29)*. The following year, James Hardy attempted the first human cardiac xenotransplant in the first reported attempt to transplant a heart of any sort into a human recipient *(30)*. The chimpanzee heart that Hardy grafted into his 68-year-old patient dying of end-stage heart failure survived for approx 1 hour after the cessation of cardiopulmonary bypass, but was subsequently "judged incapable of accepting the large venous return" because of an obvious size mismatch *(30)*. In retrospect, the rapidity of spontaneous cardiac dysfunction strongly implicated hyperacute rejection as the mediator of graft loss. Although others have attempted cardiac xenotransplantation, none achieved patient or graft survival *(31)*. These early failures, combined with the dramatic increase in available organ donors because of the widespread acceptance of the concept of brain death in the late 1960s *(32)*, led to a diminished interest in xenotransplantation over the next 15 years.

In 1984, clinical interest in xenotransplantation was rekindled when Bailey transplanted an ABO-incompatible baboon heart into a neonate born with hypoplastic left heart syndrome *(33)*. Using an intensive immunosuppression regimen and a baboon donor selected for eliciting the weakest xenogeneic response in mixed lymphocyte cultures, Bailey and colleagues successfully avoided hyperacute rejection. However, on postoperative day 20, the patient succumbed to an infection, most likely related to the high levels of immunosuppression necessary to abrogate hyperacute rejection. Postmortem microscopic analysis revealed a mononuclear cellular infiltrate with capillary thrombosis suggestive of acute vascular rejection.

Since Bailey et al.'s report *(33)*, there have been at least two attempts at pig-to-human heart transplantation in addition to attempts at pig-to-human liver *(34)* and islet cell *(35)* and baboon-to-human bone marrow transplantation *(36)*, but none of these endeavors resulted in a clear-cut clinical benefit. Perhaps the most encouraging xenotransplantation results to date are in the treatment of neurological disorders *(37,38)*, for which fetal pig neural cells transplanted into the brain of a patient suffering from Parkinson's disease survived over 7 months with appropriate growth of nonhuman dopaminergic neurons using only cyclosporine for immunosuppression *(39)*.

Although advances in the clinical arena have been modest, enormous progress has been made in the scientific investigation of xenotransplantation. Not only have the immunological barriers to successful xenotransplantation been more clearly defined, but also the potential solutions to these problems have increased in number and promise.

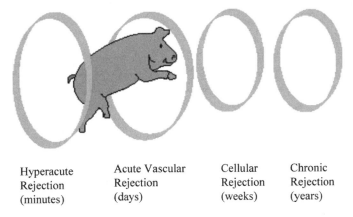

Hyperacute	Acute Vascular	Cellular	Chronic
Rejection	Rejection	Rejection	Rejection
(minutes)	(days)	(weeks)	(years)

Fig. 2. Immunological obstacles in pig-to-primate transplantation. Xenografts will have to pass through four immunological "hoops" (phases) of the host response before long-term graft acceptance can be achieved. (Modified with permission from ref. *185*.)

IMMUNOLOGICAL OBSTACLES

The earliest and perhaps most devastating immunological barrier to xenotransplantation is that of *hyperacute rejection*, which results from the binding of natural antibody to the vascular endothelium of the donor, fixation of complement, activation of the endothelium, and finally the initiation of the coagulation cascade. As illustrated in Fig. 2, other important but less well-understood immunological barriers include (1) acute vascular rejection (also called delayed xenograft rejection or acute humoral xenograft rejection), which probably involves multiple pathways, including antibodies and/or immune cells binding to endothelium and endothelial cell activation; (2) cellular rejection, which involves mechanisms similar in nature, albeit stronger in intensity, to those responsible for clinical allograft rejection; and (3) chronic rejection, which remains enigmatic in both allogeneic and xenogeneic transplantation, but would likely develop following pig organ transplantation in a human unless all immune mechanisms of rejection had been overcome. Because little is known about chronic xenograft rejection, it is not discussed further.

Hyperacute Rejection

When a heart is transplanted from one species into a phylogenetically disparate species (i.e., pig to primate), an extremely fulminant immunological reaction ensues within minutes of organ reperfusion.

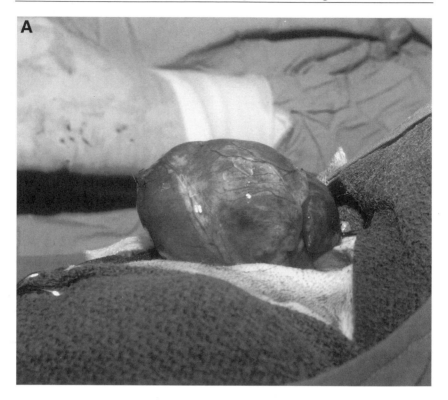

Fig. 3. (A) Photograph taken of a normal pig heart transplanted into the neck of an untreated baboon just after the arterial and venous anastomoses are opened.

The once-normal-appearing myocardium becomes dusky and cyanotic, with diminished, if not absent, contractility (Fig. 3). Widespread intravascular thrombosis and interstitial hemorrhage characteristic of a hypercoagulable state mark the histology of this hyperacute rejection response (Fig. 4). The three major physiological components responsible for this hyperacute rejection response are (1) binding of preformed xenoreactive natural antibodies to carbohydrate moieties on the vascular endothelium of the donor organ, (2) activation of the complement cascade within the recipient, and (3) endothelial cell activation.

PREFORMED NATURAL ANTIBODIES

It was realized as early as the mid-1960s that hyperacute rejection was caused by antibody-mediated complement activation (40,41). However, it was not until the early 1990s that it became clear just

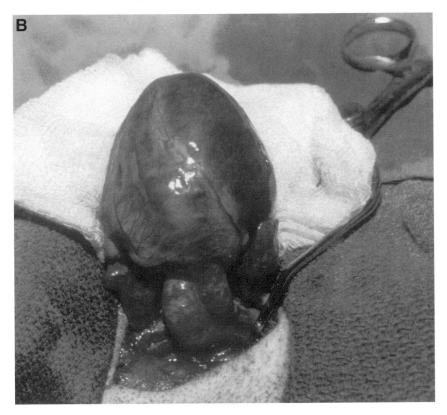

Fig. 3. (B) Photograph of the same pig heart taken 10 minutes after reestablishment of blood flow showing the dusky, cyanotic appearance typical of hyperacute rejection.

what porcine antigen was targeted by human natural antibodies. Although it might be imagined that human natural antibodies would recognize a wide array of antigens on pig organs, it has been documented that more than 80% of human complement-fixing natural antibodies recognize a single structure, Galα1-3Gal, a carbohydrate structurally similar to blood group antigens A and B. It was the seminal work of Good and Cooper *(42,43)* and Galili and colleagues *(44,45)* that clearly established the Galα1-3Gal terminal residue (abbreviated as αGal) on pig endothelium as the determinant responsible for binding the major portion of preformed human natural antibodies.

Expression of the αGal epitope is governed by the presence of an α-galactosyltransferase (αGT) enzyme that catalyzes the reaction *(44)*

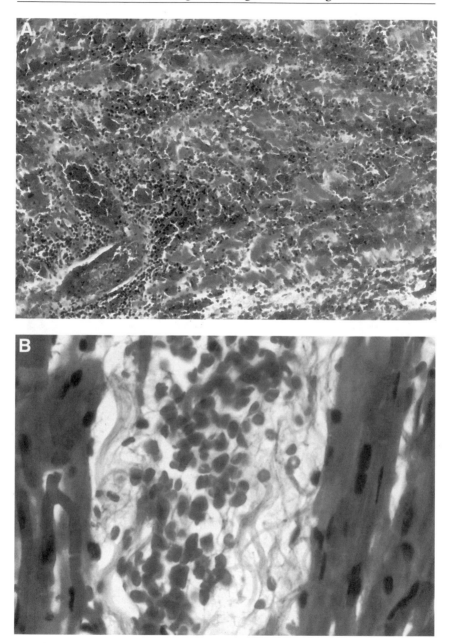

Fig. 4. Photomicrograph of a myocardial biopsy from a hyperacutely rejected pig heart stained with hematoxylin and eosin showing **(A)** interstitial hemorrhage and **(B)** intravascular thrombosis.

$$\text{Gal}\beta1\text{-4GlcNAc-R} + \text{UDP} - \text{Gal}\alpha^{\alpha1,3GT} >$$
$$\text{Gal}\alpha1\text{-3Gal}\beta1\text{-4GlcNAc-R} + \text{UDP}$$

This enzyme is found in New World monkeys and all lower order mammals (including swine). As a result, these species express the αGal epitope on their vascular endothelium and do not have circulating anti-αGal antibody. In contrast, humans and all higher order primates (e.g., chimpanzees, baboons, and Old World monkeys) have lost the gene for αGT. The lack of constitutive αGal expression in these higher order species permits the formation of antibodies directed against the endothelial αGal determinant.

These anti-αGal antibodies are not a constitutive part of the immunoglobulin repertoire of the developing fetus and therefore do not exist at birth. Transplantation of a porcine organ into a newborn baboon that lacks xenoreactive antibodies but has an intact complement system does not result in hyperacute rejection *(46)*. It is believed that, like the natural antibodies that bind blood group antigens, immunoglobulins that bind to the αGal epitope develop as a consequence of exposure to environmental microorganisms that express the same carbohydrate determinants *(47)*. Parenthetically, the loss of the α-galactosyltransferase gene during evolution may have provided a survival advantage by allowing the development of anti-αGal antibodies that could defend against environmental pathogens, including viruses that express this determinant *(48)*.

The majority of natural antibody responsible for binding the αGal epitope on the pig endothelium is of the immunoglobulin (Ig)M isotype; it accounts for as much as 4% of the total circulating IgM in humans *(49)*. It is highly likely that only IgM (but not IgG) natural antibodies can cause hyperacute rejection, probably because the greater number of receptors on the IgM compared to IgG antibodies increase its binding avidity sufficiently to trigger complement activation *(49,50)*. Interestingly, when humans are exposed to pig tissue, either through extracorporeal perfusion of a pig organ, pig islet cell, or bone marrow transplantation, the rise in levels of anti-αGal IgG is significantly greater than the corresponding rise in anti-αGal IgM *(51)*. It is thought that these IgG anti-αGal antibodies may promote antibody-dependent cell-mediated cytotoxicity by binding natural killer cells and macrophages through the Fc portion of the antibody. This mechanism of xenograft destruction is probably more important in acute vascular rejection than in hyperacute rejection (*see* Acute Vascular Rejection section). Although antibodies to foreign alloantigens may exist in prospective recipients because of prior exposure, preformed IgG antibodies directed against foreign MHC molecules do not seem to play a major role in hyperacute rejection *(52)*, but may become important in acute vascular rejection *(53)*.

COMPLEMENT ACTIVATION

The development of hyperacute rejection depends on the activation of complement. In some models of discordant xenotransplantation (i.e., guinea pig to rat), complement is activated through the alternative pathway in the absence of preformed antibody *(54–56)*. However, in what is considered the most clinically relevant model, pig to primate, complement is activated through the classical pathway after binding of natural antibody and formation of antigen–antibody complex *(57,58)*. In either case, the terminal event in the complement cascade is the formation of the membrane attack complex (MAC), which mediates cytolysis by forming pores in cell membranes *(59–61)*. However, the MAC is probably not the only complement component implicated in hyperacute rejection. Inflammatory mediators such as C3b and terminal complement proteins undoubtedly contribute to the process *(62,63)*.

In humans, the vigor of the complement cascade is regulated by a number of endothelial proteins, including decay-activating factor (DAF or CD55), membrane cofactor protein (MCP or CD46), and CD59. These complement regulatory proteins are membrane glycoproteins that act as inhibitors at several key points in the cascade at which the activation of both pathways may be halted. Of major importance in discordant xenotransplantation is the fact that these regulatory proteins are effective only with complement proteins of their own species *(64)*. Indeed, part of the reason why the hyperacute rejection response is so intense and universal in pig-to-human transplantation is that the species-specific pig complement regulatory proteins in the xenograft are unable to control human complement proteins, resulting in uncontrolled activation of the host's complement system. This concept is the basis for the creation of transgenic animals expressing human complement regulatory proteins, with the hope that organs from such animals would resist injury by human complement (*see* Genetic Engineering section).

TYPE I ENDOTHELIAL CELL ACTIVATION

Resting endothelium and the molecules expressed on the surface of quiescent endothelial cells perform several important functions, including prevention of intravascular coagulation and platelet aggregation. The binding of xenoreactive antibodies and activation of complement on the endothelial surface stimulates the resting endothelium to initiate a rapid, protein-synthesis-independent response referred to as *type I endothelial cell activation (65)*. This response is manifested by (1) a change in endothelial cell shape *(66)*, (2) the loss of heparan sulfate from the cell surface *(67)*, and (3) the elaboration of proinflammatory cytokines, chemokines, and adhesion molecules *(68)*.

Reconfiguration of endothelial cell shape causes the cells to separate from one another, forming gaps that allow intravascular fluid to extravasate and platelets to be activated through contact with matrix. The loss of heparan sulfate increases sensitivity to oxidant-mediated injury and gives rise to procoagulant changes on the endothelial surfaces. The elaboration of inflammatory mediators also contributes to vasoconstriction and to direct injury by polymorphonuclear leukocytes. The attachment and activation of platelets leads to the release of a variety of vasoactive substances, such as thromboxane A_2, that constrict vascular smooth muscle and alter regional blood flow. Together, these changes account for the early intravascular thrombosis and extravascular hemorrhage observed in hyperacute rejection.

Prevention of Hyperacute Rejection

The pharmacological immunosuppressive agents currently used to treat allogeneic rejection have no effect in the prevention of hyperacute rejection. Therefore, new and different approaches have been devised to overcome early xenogeneic rejection. Because the two principal factors that precipitate hyperacute rejection are xenogeneic antibodies and complement, these circulating plasma constituents and their receptors have been targeted for elimination or inhibition in attempts to prevent this process.

DEPLETION OR INHIBITION OF ANTI-αGAL ANTIBODY

Four primary methods of depleting or inhibiting anti-αGal antibody and prolonging experimental xenograft survival have been described. They include (1) plasmapheresis *(69–71)*, (2) donor organ perfusion *(57,72)*, (3) extracorporeal immunoadsorption *(73)*, and (4) oligosaccharide infusion *(74)*. Although effective to varying degrees at removing or inactivating natural xenogeneic antibodies, none of these techniques has proven successful in preventing their return. Xenoreactive antibodies usually return within 24 to 48 hours in untreated recipients and between 5 and 7 days in immunosuppressed hosts.

Plasmapheresis represents an effective, albeit nonspecific, method of removing xenogeneic antibody. Plasmapheresis can effectively remove IgM antibodies and, when combined with other therapies such as splenectomy, T-cell depletion, and pharmacological immunosuppression, has resulted in prolongation of pig kidney or heterotopic heart grafts up to 23 days in baboons *(75)*. However, in addition to preformed anti-αGal antibodies, plasmapheresis also eliminates useful proteins that contribute to hemostasis and antimicrobial defense. Furthermore, plasma exchange can cause paradoxical thrombosis secondary to an increase in the synthesis of acute phase-reactant proteins *(76)*. For these reasons, methods have been developed that selectively target xenogeneic antibodies for removal or inactivation.

Donor organ perfusion is more selective than plasmapheresis in removing natural antibodies directed against αGal. This technique involves connecting a vascularized organ from the prospective donor (e.g., a swine liver) to the recipient's (e.g., baboon) circulatory system through catheter connections and then perfusing the organ with three or more of the recipient's circulating blood volumes. During this process, the recipient's xenogeneic antibodies are adsorbed out of the recipient's circulation and onto the vascular endothelium of the donor organ, which is then discarded. A second organ from the donor swine (e.g., a heart) is then transplanted into the antibody-depleted recipient baboon. Cooper et al. *(72)* used porcine kidneys to absorb out natural antibody in baboon recipients that subsequently received pig hearts. Survival of the cardiac xenografts was prolonged from 3 hours in untreated controls to 4–5 days in the group treated with donor organ perfusion.

Although donor organ perfusion is effective in depleting natural antibody, its clinical utility has been reduced by the development of immunoaffinity columns that are more specific, efficient, and safe. Extracorporeal immunoadsorption uses synthetic immunoaffinity columns containing αGal oligosaccharides (Fig. 5). When placed in-line with the recipient's circulation, these highly specific immunoaffinity columns deplete only those antiswine antibodies detrimental to the transplant *(73,77)*. More than 99% of anti-αGal IgM and 97% of anti-αGal IgG can be depleted by this technique *(75)*. Unfortunately, like donor organ perfusion, extracorporeal immunoadsorption is unable to prevent the return of the anti-αGal antibodies. Indeed, even with adjunctive therapy (i.e., pharmacological immunosuppression and splenectomy), the reduction in natural antibody is always transient and is sometimes followed by a rebound within several days to levels of antibody higher than that observed at baseline *(62,63)*.

Another experimental approach involves treating the recipient with continuous intravenous infusion of synthetic or natural αGal oligosaccharides to inhibit natural antibody *(78)*. The infused oligosaccharides are bound by circulating anti-αGal antibodies that are no longer free to attack a subsequently transplanted organ. The infused sugar, however,

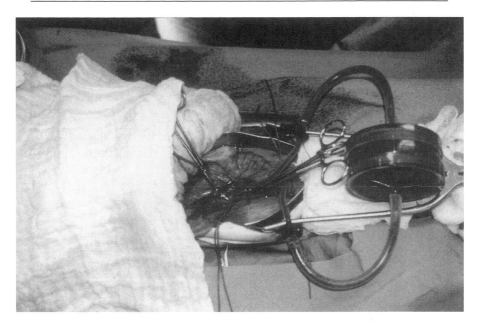

Fig. 5. Perfusion of an αGal oligosaccharide immunoaffinity column with baboon blood. Blood enters the column via a cannula connected to the aorta, and it is returned to the animal by way of a cannula connected to the inferior vena cava. This technique has supplanted liver perfusion for adsorption of natural antibody in nonhuman primates.

is rapidly excreted, making this tactic limited by the difficulty and expense of synthesizing large quantities of oligosaccharides. This problem may be solved by new enzymatic methods to produce the relevant oligosaccharides *(78)*. An alternative to the use of αGal oligosaccharides, either in immunoaffinity columns or as intravenous infusions, is murine-derived antiidiotypic antibodies. Initial studies with these murine antibodies directed against human antipig antibodies have shown them to be effective in temporarily inhibiting circulating anti-αGal antibodies in baboons *(79,80)*. Better results have been obtained using bovine serum albumin conjugated to Gal oligosaccharides *(81)* or multiple Gal molecules conjugated to a poly-L-lysine backbone (GAS914) (D. K. C. Cooper, personal communication, June 2001).

In summary, the ideal technique to remove or inactivate preformed natural xenogeneic antibodies and prevent their return without jeopardizing the baseline immunological properties of circulating nonxenogenic antibodies has not been achieved. More recent efforts to have an impact on natural antibody have concentrated on attempts to eliminate or tolerize the B cells that produce the αGal antibodies by genetic engineering *(82–84)* (*see* Genetic Engineering section).

Suppressing Complement Activation

Attempts to control complement activation in the host have made use of systemic treatment with either purified cobra venom factor or soluble complement receptor type 1 (sCR1). By activating C3b, purified cobra venom factor is very effective in depleting complement and temporarily protecting a discordant xenograft from hyperacute rejection *(85,86)*. However, even with the addition of concomitant pharmacological immunosuppression, treatment with cobra venom factor typically delays rejection by only a matter of days. Within 1 week, xenografts usually develop the histopathological features of acute vascular rejection and fail. The longest survival of a pig organ in a nonhuman primate treated with cobra venom factor has been 27 days *(87)*.

The sCR1is also effective in suppressing complement activation and prolonging the survival of discordant xenografts *(88,89)*. The sCR1 molecule is a soluble form of the human complement receptor 1*(90)*, which is found on most lymphohematopoietic cells. By competitively binding to complement receptor 1, sCR1 inhibits both the classic and alternative pathways of complement activation. Discordant xenografts have survived for more than 3 weeks in recipients treated with sCR1 *(88)*. However, like purified cobra venom factor, the protection afforded the xenograft by sCR1 is temporary.

Genetic Engineering

Perhaps the most significant advance in providing long-term suppression of complement activation has been achieved using genetically engineered swine. Using microinjection techniques, transgenic swine have been created that express human complement regulatory proteins on their vascular endothelium *(91,92)* (Fig. 6). Because these regulatory proteins are species specific, functioning effectively only with the complement proteins of their own species, it was hypothesized that organs from swine that express human regulatory proteins would successfully inhibit the activation of human complement.

The concept of expressing human inhibitors of complement in the pig originated with Dalmasso and colleagues *(64)* and was based on earlier work by Medof et al. *(93)*. When human decay accelerating factor (hDAF or CD55) was incorporated into porcine endothelial cells in vitro, it rendered the pig endothelial cells resistant to cytotoxicity mediated by human complement in a dose-dependent fashion. Of note, the level of functional hDAF expressed on pig endothelial cells that

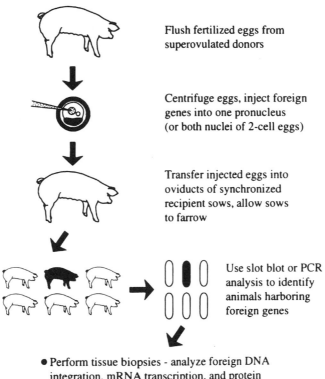

Flush fertilized eggs from
superovulated donors

Centrifuge eggs, inject foreign
genes into one pronucleus
(or both nuclei of 2-cell eggs)

Transfer injected eggs into
oviducts of synchronized
recipient sows, allow sows
to farrow

Use slot blot or PCR
analysis to identify
animals harboring
foreign genes

● Perform tissue biopsies - analyze foreign DNA
integration, mRNA transcription, and protein
production

● Establish transgenic lines to study gene regulation
in progeny

Fig. 6. Creation of transgenic swine. mRNA, messenger ribonucleic acid. (Courtesy of Stem Cell Sciences, Melbourne, Australia.)

was required to abrogate hyperacute rejection was much higher than that normally present on human endothelial cells *(94,95)*. However, exactly how much higher the levels of hDAF must be to prevent hyperacute rejection is unclear.

White and colleagues *(91,96)* have successfully bred transgenic swine that express hDAF on their vascular endothelium. When hearts from these hDAF pigs were heterotopically transplanted into nonimmunosuppressed cynomolgus monkeys, hyperacute rejection was successfully avoided. The hDAF hearts survived for up to 5 days (range 97–126 hours); control hearts from nontransgenic pigs survived for an average of 1.6 days (range 0.4–101 hours) *(97)*. Adding pharmaco-

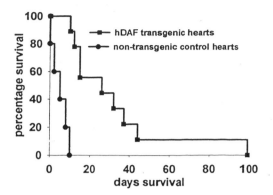

Fig. 7. Survival of hearts from hDAF transgenic swine ($n = 9$; median survival 26 days) and normal controls ($n = 5$; median survival 5 days) transplanted heterotopically into immunosuppressed cynomolgus monkeys. (Reproduced with permission from ref. *98*.)

logical immunosuppression (cyclosporine, cyclophosphamide, and methlyprednisolone) extended hDAF heterotopic cardiac xenograft survival to a median of 40 days *(97)*, with one hDAF heart surviving for 99 days *(98)* (Fig. 7).

Kuwaki and colleagues further intensified the immunosuppressive regimen by adding pretransplant T-cell depletion with low CD2, the costimulation inhibitor anti-CD154, and continuous anticoagulation with heparin. Using this regimen, heterotopic hDAF heart grafts survived in baboons for up to 139 days, which is the longest survival of a non-life-supporting, pig-to-primate organ to date *(99)*. White and colleagues demonstrated that hearts from hDAF transgenic pigs transplanted orthotopically into immunosuppressed baboons were not hyperacutely rejected and were capable of maintaining an adequate cardiac output for up to 39 days *(12,100)*.

Transgenic swine have also been created which express CD59 *(101)*. When hearts from CD59 transgenic pigs were transplanted into baboons, there was diminished complement activation, as demonstrated by the markedly reduced deposition of the MAC *(101)*. Orthotopic transplantation of CD59-expressing pig hearts into baboons treated with plasmapheresis, steroids, and cyclosporine resulted in up to 2-week survival compared to the 24- to 30-hour survival of nonengineered control hearts *(102)*.

Transgenic swine have been produced that express both hDAF and human CD59 proteins on their vascular endothelium. Early results suggested that the survival times of hearts from these double-transgenic swine do not exceed the survival times of hDAF-expressing hearts *(103)*. However, organ-specific expression of the transgenes in the double-transgenic animals was less than that observed in human tissue; therefore, improved results might be observed with better expression of the two transgenes *(104)*.

A second approach to genetic engineering donor swine is competitive glycosylation, which involves inserting a gene that competes with or masks the αGal epitope with an overabundance of another oligosaccharide epitope *(105,106)*. For instance, the α1,2-fucosyltransferase (or H-transferase) gene, which humans use to form the blood group O antigen, has been transferred into mice *(107)* and swine *(108)*. In vitro experiments confirmed that, by competing successfully for substrate with the galactosyltransferase enzyme, transfer of the H-transferase gene reduced the expression of αGal to a remarkable degree (<5% of its original expression) *(107,108)*. However, it is unclear at present what percentage of αGal expression must be eliminated before hyperacute rejection is completely prevented.

Nuclear Transfer (Cloning). Another exciting approach is to eliminate or knock out the gene that codes for the αGT enzyme in the porcine donor. That would eliminate the αGal epitopes and theoretically leave no target for human anti-αGal antibodies *(109)*. Reports have shown that knocking out the α1,3GT gene in the pig is feasible. Using nuclear transfer technique, two groups have produced piglets in which one copy of the α1,3GT gene was disrupted *(110,111)*. They isolated somatic cells from porcine fetuses for production of donor cell lines and replaced the endogenous allele for α1,3GT with a targeting vector. Successful knockout at the α1,3GT locus was confirmed by reverse transcription polymerase chain reaction (RT-PCR) and Southern blot analyses *(110)*. Several lines of cells with the desired knockout were produced, and subsequently the deoxyribonucleic acid (DNA) content of the prepared cells was transferred into in vitro-matured oocytes. The nuclear transfer embryos were finally transferred to the oviducts of the recipient female pig. α1,3GT-null pigs with both α1,3GT-alleles inactivated (homozygotes) have been created through natural breeding of male and female heterozygous knockout animals and by targeted disruption of both alleles of the α1,3GT gene in cloned pigs *(112)*.

Initial studies using the first three homozygous (double α1,3GT knockout) donors available (provided by R. Prather, Missouri, and Infigen, Wisconsin) were performed in the laboratory of David H. Sachs. Baboons received hearts, kidneys, thymokidneys, or kidneys plus vascularized thymic lobes *(113)* from homozygous α1,3GT-knockout pigs. The recipients received either standard immunosuppression or a tolerance induction protocol (see Mixed Chimerism). Standard immunosuppression consisted of anticoagulants, steroids, T-cell depletion, mycophenolate mofetil, and anti-CD154 monoclonal antibody with or without cobra venom factor during the first 2 weeks. The tolerance protocol included thymectomy and transplantation of vascularized xenogeneic thymic tissue, either as a vascularized thymic lobe transplant or as part of a composite thymokidney, in which autologous donor thymic tissue had been implanted 6 to 12 weeks prior to transplantation.

These preliminary studies produced two exciting findings. First, even with no antibody or complement depletion, organs from homozygous α1,3GT-knockout donor suffered no hyperacute rejection and survived for over 81 days (99). Second, when immunosuppression was weaned off recipients undergoing the tolerance protocol, excellent organ function was maintained for more than 81 days (113). The success of these pioneering experiments represents a quantum leap forward in bringing xenotransplantation to the clinic.

B-Cell Tolerance. A genetic engineering approach to eliminating natural antibodies can also be aimed at inducing tolerance to αGal antibody-producing B cells in the recipient. This approach involves introducing a functional αGT gene into host autologous bone marrow-derived cells by retroviral gene transfer, resulting in the expression of αGal epitopes at the cell surface. Because it is presumably the absence of the αGT gene in Old World primates and humans that permits the production of αGal antibodies, introduction of the αGT gene into the bone marrow of these animals should inhibit their production (114).

To test this hypothesis, Iacomini and colleagues (83) used αGT knockout mice, which, like humans, make αGal antibody (115). Bone marrow from αGT knockout mice was transduced with the gene encoding pig αGT. This transduced marrow, which now expressed αGal epitopes, was then used to reconstitute lethally irradiated syngeneic αGT knockout mice. In contrast to unmodified αGT knockout mice, the αGT knockout mice reconstituted with αGT-transduced marrow failed to produce anti-αGal antibodies and showed no return of these antibodies (83). Furthermore, they made no anti-αGal antibody in response to a subsequent challenge with pig cells (116). This represents the first demonstration that production of preexisting natural antibodies can be inhibited by a gene therapy approach (114).

In summary, creation of a pig lacking both α1,3GT alleles has brought xenotransplantation much further toward clinical applicability.

The $\alpha1,3GT$ knockout donor organs appear resistant to hyperacute rejection without the need for removal or inhibition of natural antibodies or complement. This opens the field for further exploration of other ill-defined barriers to xenotransplantation, namely, acute vascular rejection and cellular rejection.

Acute Vascular Rejection

Even when hyperacute rejection is prevented in discordant species combinations using one or more of the methods described above, vigorous rejection still develops days to weeks following transplantation. This delayed rejection response is characterized by the same diffuse intravascular coagulation and lack of cellular infiltrate seen in hyperacute rejection. The timing and histology of this process is suggestive of an induced humoral response that, like hyperacute rejection, targets the vascular endothelium. Indeed, there is an emerging consensus that acute vascular rejection is initiated by returning or residual anti-αGal antibodies in addition to xenoreactive antibodies induced to other swine cell surface molecules, such as donor MHC antigens *(53,117,118)*.

TYPE II ENDOTHELIAL CELL ACTIVATION

Like hyperacute rejection, the primary component in the pathophysiology of acute vascular rejection is endothelial activation. However, unlike hyperacute rejection, endothelial activation occurs more slowly, allowing time for new gene transcription and protein synthesis by the endothelium. Furthermore, it is controversial whether this activation requires complement *(53)*. This delayed endothelial activation is sometimes referred to as type II activation because it represents a different process from the type I endothelial activation associated with hyperacute rejection.

The exact sequence of events that leads to acute vascular rejection remains unclear. Xenogeneic antibodies appear to play a predominant role *(53)*. In addition to antibody, there are cellular elements that can initiate type II endothelial cell activation through the elaboration of cytokines *(119)*. Most notable are monocytes and natural killer cells, which activate endothelial cells through the production of tumor necrosis factor-α and interferon-γ, respectively *(83,120)*.

There are two predominant physiological consequences of type II endothelial activation. One is the generation of a procoagulant state caused by the loss of thrombomodulin and other regulators of thrombosis, such as heparan sulfate *(121–123)*. Thrombomodulin normally binds thrombin and leads to the activation of protein C, which has anticoagulant effects *(124)*. Downregulation of endothelial thrombomodulin results in loss of these anticoagulant mechanisms. Heparan sulfate produces its antithrombotic effect by binding or complexing to antithrombin III, thereby interfering with thrombin activity. Loss of heparan sulfate from the endothelial cell surface results in the loss of anticoagulant activity via antithrombin III inhibition of blood coagulation proteases and the induction of tissue factor activity *(67,124–127)*.

The other physiological consequence of type II endothelial activation is the upregulation of a large number of proinflammatory genes encoding molecules such as interleukin (IL)-1, E-selectin, P-selectin, intercellular adhesion molecule I, and vascular cell adhesion molecule 1. In addition, the activated endothelial cells secrete IL-1, IL-6, and IL-8 as well as platelet-activating factor and plasminogen activator inhibitor. IL-1 is stimulatory to the endothelium and functions to activate monocytes. IL-8 is a chemoattractant for leukocytes, and it mimics some of the functions of C5a. Platelet-activating factor serves to activate neutrophils and platelets. Secretion of plasminogen activator inhibitor inhibits the naturally occurring action of tissue plasminogen activator and results in a decrease in the fibrinolytic activity on the endothelial cell surface. This provides the physiological basis for the pathological findings of platelet aggregation and clot formation in acute vascular rejection. Of note, these events are thought to be in part the consequence of an increase in transcriptional activity mediated by nuclear factor-κB (NF-κB) *(128–131)*.

Prevention of Acute Vascular Rejection

Because of the importance of antibody in acute vascular rejection, current therapies to control this immune response have been primarily directed against B cells. Treatment protocols have included cyclophosphamide, leflunomide, brequinar, 15-deoxyspergualin, and methotrexate *(62)*. However, these regimens are not without substantial toxicity and mortality. Based on current knowledge, inducing robust tolerance to αGal *(83)* or even eliminating the αGal saccharide on donor endothelium (αGT knockout) may still not prevent acute vascular rejection because antibodies other than those directed against αGal are contributory *(132)*.

NF-κB and Protective Genes

Given the large number of proinflammatory genes that are upregulated in type II endothelial activation as a consequence of the transcriptional factor NF-κB *(128–130,133,134)*, Bach *(65)* suggested that targeting NF-κB for inhibition would be an ideal way to prevent acute vascular rejection. NF-κB is present in the cytoplasm of quiescent endothelial cells and is associated with an inhibitory protein, IkBα *(134–136)*. On type II endothelial activation, IkBα is degraded, which releases and activates NF-κB *(137–139)*. NF-κB is then translocated to the nucleus, where it binds to the targeted DNA sequence and activates transcription of various proinflammatory and prothombotic genes.

In studying ways of inhibiting NF-κB, Cooper and colleagues *(140)* investigated the role of antiapoptotic genes in endothelial cells. Their in vitro findings demonstrated that three genes, *A20*, *bcl-2*, and *bcl-xl*, not only prevented apoptosis, but also were effective at blocking the upregulation of NF-κB. The expression of these "protective" genes in endothelial cells blocked the upregulation of the proinflammatory genes in vitro *(65)*. Further evidence that these particular genes exert a protective influence comes from studies in a hamster-to-rat cardiac xenograft model in which recipients were treated with daily cobra venom factor and cyclosporine. All the surviving xenografts expressed the antiapoptotic genes in their endothelium, whereas the endothelium from hearts that were rejected did not *(141)*.

Based on these results, Bach and colleagues argued that acute vascular rejection could be prevented by the expression of protective genes *(141)*, including the stress-response gene *HO-1 (142)*, on the graft vasculature. This is illustrated by the observation that hearts from *HO-1*-deficient (*HO-1*$^{(/()}$) mice transplanted into rats treated with cobra venom factor and cyclosporine underwent acute vascular rejection, whereas hearts from wild-type (*HO-1*$^{+/+}$) mice transplanted under the same regimen survived long term *(142)*. The exact molecular mechanism responsible for the cytoprotective effects of *HO-1* remains unclear. However, recent studies have suggested that carbon monoxide contributes in a critical manner to the overall antiinflammatory actions of *HO-1 (143)*.

Goodman and colleagues suggested that genetic modifications of donor animals by the transgenic expression of protective genes that inhibit NF-κB and prevent apoptosis might be used to prevent acute vascular rejection *(144)*. Another genetic engineering approach to the prevention of acute vascular rejection would be overexpression of antithrombotic molecules on the surface of resting endothelium (i.e., thrombomodulin) of the donor so that these antithrombotic molecules would not be lost during the initial phase of endothelial cell activation *(65,68,123)*.

Cellular Rejection

Accumulating evidence indicates that T cells can reject a xenograft with equal or even greater vigor than they reject an allograft *(145,146)*. This may be caused in part by a more diverse array of T-cell receptors capable of recognizing xenoantigens than alloantigens *(63)*. As in allotransplantation, T cells are able to respond both to direct presentation of xenogeneic antigens *(147)* and to xenogeneic peptides indirectly presented by self-antigen-presenting cells *(148)*. Furthermore, porcine endothelial cells are capable of directly presenting xenogeneic MHC antigens to human T cells and elicit a markedly stronger response than the allogeneic antiendothelial response *(149)*. In addition to T cells, NK cells, macrophages, and neutrophils have all been shown to play an active role in xenograft rejection (reviewed in refs. *53* and *63*).

Prevention of Cellular Rejection

It is clear that controlling T-cell-mediated rejection will be essential in bringing xenotransplantation to the clinic. Some of the nonspecific immunosuppressive agents that have been developed to suppress cellular immunity to allografts are likely to have a suppressive effect on the cellular response to discordant xenografts. However, the intensity of immunosuppression that would be required to prevent the rejection of a xenograft would be so great it would make the associated complications of infection, neoplasm, and drug-related side effects intolerable. Indeed, in pig-to-primate xenograft recipients, the high level of immunosuppression required to achieve even moderate survival has resulted in numerous deaths because of infection and drug-specific complications *(100,150)*.

Many scientists and transplant physicians feel that the success of clinical xenotransplantation will likely depend on developing ways to induce immunological tolerance in the human recipient to pig antigens *(145)*. Thus far, three experimental approaches to inducing T-cell tolerance across a xenograft barrier have been attempted: mixed chimerism, molecular chimerism, and thymic transplantation.

MIXED CHIMERISM

A promising way to induce tolerance across a xenogeneic barrier is by establishing mixed hematopoietic chimerism in the host through infusion of donor bone marrow at the time of organ transplantation. *Mixed chimerism* refers to a state in which both donor and host bone marrow progenitor cells coexist and populate the peripheral circulation with hematopoietic cells of multiple lineages *(10,151)*. By way of comparison, *full chimerism* refers to a state in which all hematopoietic elements are derived from the donor. Full chimerism is achieved by ablating the host's hematopoietic system, usually through lethal irradiation, then reconstituting the host with allogeneic bone marrow. This strategy is useful for the treatment of some hematopoietic malignancies. However, full chimerism is neither necessary nor desirable for solid organ transplantation tolerance, partly because it requires a highly toxic myeloablative conditioning regimen.

Mixed chimerism can be achieved with much less toxicity and will still induce a state of donor-specific tolerance, as demonstrated by the pioneering work of Owen, Medawar, and others (reviewed in refs. *10* and *152*). Also, mixed chimerism is associated with the presence of residual host antigen-presenting cells, which is essential to ensure immunocompetence in the recipient because mature T-cell populations of both host and donor origin are restricted to the recognition of foreign antigens in the context of host MHC antigens *(153)*.

The establishment of mixed chimerism induces central deletional tolerance by actively "tricking" the recipient's immune system into treating donor antigens as self-antigens *(154)*. To achieve this goal, the host, until recently, has received some form of whole body irradiation to make "space" for a subsequent donor bone marrow transfusion. Once hematopoietic stem cells contained in the donor bone marrow engraft, they coexist with recipient stem cells and give rise to cells of all hematopoietic lineages. In addition, hematopoietic progenitor cells seed the thymus, giving rise to both T cells and dendritic cells *(155)*. Because hematopoietic cells from both the recipient and the donor collocate to the thymus, both self-reactive and donor-reactive T cells are eliminated by negative selection (the process that defines the phrase "central deletional tolerance") *(156)*. Consequently, the newly developing T-cell repertoire in mixed chimeras is tolerant toward the donor and remains so as long as chimerism persists *(157)*.

Based on the strategy of mixed chimerism developed in mouse models of xenotransplantation and successfully applied to large animal models of concordant xenotransplantation, Sachs and colleagues have investigated this strategy in the pig-to-nonhuman primate model (reviewed in refs. *10* and *63* and illustrated in Fig. 8). The early preparative regimen of lethal irradiation used to make space for the donor marrow has been supplanted by less-toxic nonmyeloablative methods. One such regimen involves depleting mature host T cells using antithymocyte globulin, anti-CD154 monoclonal antibody, cyclosporine, and

Pre-Op   Post-Op

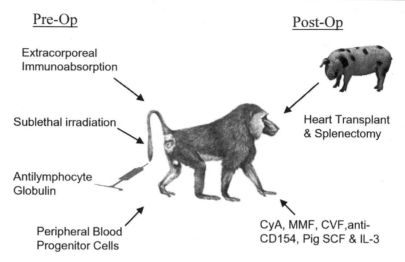

Extracorporeal
Immunoabsorption

Sublethal irradiation   Heart Transplant
                                                           & Splenectomy

Antilymphocyte
Globulin

Peripheral Blood   CyA, MMF, CVF,anti-
Progenitor Cells   CD154, Pig SCF & IL-3

Fig. 8. A protocol for xenogeneic tolerance induction through mixed chimerism. Natural antibody is depleted through the extracorporeal immunoabsorption of the anti-αGal antibody on a solid matrix column that bears the α1,3Gal sugar moiety. Low-toxicity nonmyeloablative whole body radiation. Antithymocyte globulin and/or anti-T-cell monoclonal antibodies are used to remove mature T cells from the recipient. Cyclosporine (CyA) is added to immunosuppress any residual T cells in the posttransplant period. On day 0, the recipient receives high-dose cytokine-mobilized peripheral blood progenitor cells and a heart transplant from the same donor miniature swine. Splenectomy is performed and cobra venom factor (CVF) is added to diminish natural antibody effects. Recombinant cytokines (stem cell factor [SCF] and IL-3) are administered for 2 weeks after the preparative regimen to aid engraftment of the pig progenitor cells. (Modified from ref. *63* with permission.)

mycophenolate mofetil. Large numbers of cytokine-mobilized miniature swine peripheral blood progenitor cells (3×10^{10}/kg) are infused at the time of organ transplantation *(132)*, along with species-specific growth factors (pig recombinant stem cell factor and IL-3) to promote the survival of the pig cells *(83,158,159)*. To prevent antibody-mediated rejection of the porcine hematopoietic cells, extracorporeal immunoadsorption of anti-Gal antibodies *(57,160–162)*, in addition to cobra venom factor and host splenectomy, have been employed *(163,164)*.

Using this regimen, porcine cells have been detectable in conditioned baboons on occasion for more than 20 days by flow cytometry and for at least 1 month by PCR *(165,166)*. Invariably, however, there was return of anti-αGal antibodies, which coincided with loss of the pig cells. This precluded subsequent organ transplantation. Current efforts are therefore focusing on attempts to increase the engraftment of porcine hematopoietic progenitor cells in primate recipients using bone marrow from αGal knockout animals *(167)*.

MOLECULAR CHIMERISM

Successful engraftment of allogeneic or xenogeneic bone marrow cells carries with it the induction of tolerance to any other tissues or organs from the bone marrow donor. However, because of the difficulty encountered in inducing porcine cells to engraft in nonhuman primates, an alternative approach to tolerance has been developed that utilizes gene therapy techniques. Genes from the donor, coding for donor MHC antigens, are inserted into bone marrow cells of the host to induce T-cell unresponsiveness to those immunogenic molecules *(168)*. This strategy, termed *molecular chimerism*, is similar in concept to attempts at achieving B-cell tolerance by transducing autologous bone marrow cells with the αGT gene (discussed in the Hyperacute Rejection section). It is so named because molecular rather than cellular chimerism is established *(114)*.

This approach has induced prolonged acceptance of allogeneic skin grafts transplanted across an isolated MHC class I barrier in mice *(169,170)*. Furthermore, reconstitution of porcine recipients with autologous bone marrow transduced with an allogeneic MHC class II gene permitted successful renal transplantation in a fully mismatched miniature swine treated with a short course of cyclosporine *(11,27)*.

Based on these encouraging results, primates were reconstituted with autologous bone marrow transduced with porcine class II genes *(171)*. The transgene was detected for more than 12 weeks by PCR in most animals. When kidney xenografts were transplanted from pigs expressing the same MHC class II as the transgene, they succumbed to antibody-mediated rejection. However, late T-cell-dependent responses to the porcine xenografts were prevented, suggesting that the gene transfer led to diminution or possibly tolerance to some T-cell responses *(171)*.

THYMIC TRANSPLANTATION

The difficulty in coercing xenogeneic hematopoietic cells to migrate to the recipient thymus and induce deletional tolerance through a strategy of mixed chimerism might be overcome by replacing the recipient thymus with the thymus from the xenogeneic organ donor after host T-cell depletion and thymectomy. Support for this notion comes from studies in which thymectomized, T-cell-depleted mice transplanted with discordant pig thymic grafts not only demonstrated functional recovery of murine CD4 T cells in the pig thymic grafts *(172,173)*, but also became tolerant to donor xenogeneic skin grafts *(174)*.

In summary, the benefits of achieving immunological tolerance to xenografts have far-reaching implications. One of the major advantages of successful application of this strategy would be the avoidance of long-term immunosuppression, which has been implicated in the appearance of posttransplantation lymphoproliferative disease and other malignancies. Loss of transplanted organs from chronic rejection may not be a significant factor because the grafted organ presumably would escape the persistent immunological bombardment implicated in chronic rejection *(175)*. For further reading on this subject, excellent reviews are given in refs. *53, 63, 176,* and *177.*

INFECTIOUS DISEASE OBSTACLES

The possibility that an animal organ donor will pass an infectious agent (xenozoonoses) to a human xenograft recipient and that the infection may be passed to the human population in general has been the center of much debate *(6,178)*. On the one hand, transplanting a pig organ into a human patient bypasses many natural defenses or barriers to infection. Furthermore, the immunosuppression required to prevent xenograft rejection may result in a further reduction in the host's resistance to infections. Most concern has revolved around the transfer of porcine endogenous retroviruses (PERVs) *(179,180)*. These retroviruses are similar to human endogenous retroviruses, which are present in all human cells. Data have shown that PERVs are able to infect human cells in vitro *(181)*.

On the other hand, no known passage of PERVs to humans has ever occurred in vivo, and no human disease associated with PERVs (or for that matter human endogenous retroviruses) has ever been observed *(182)*. Also, using gnotobiotic techniques of delivering piglets, early weaning from the sow, and pathogen-free housing facilities may result in pigs actually representing less of an infectious threat than the current human donor pool for hearts, which frequently carries cytomegalovirus and Epstein-Barr virus, as well as hepatitis and human immunodeficiency virus *(2,176,183)*.

It is generally felt that the potential infection risk associated with successful discordant xenotransplantation remains uncertain, and that knowledge regarding both known and novel xenozoonoses must be expanded before progressing to major clinical trials of pig-to-human heart transplantation. For further reading, excellent reviews are given in refs. *2* and *184.*

SUMMARY

Within a relatively short time, a significant number of barriers to xenotransplantation have been identified and potential solutions generated. However, the survival rates for pig-to-primate heart transplantation remain modest at best, with the longest functioning heterotopic heart transplant surviving only 139 days *(99)*, and the longest functioning orthotopic heart transplant surviving only 39 days *(12,100)*. The most significant recent development has been the generation of α1,3GT double-knockout cloned pigs, which appears to have solved the problem of hyperacute rejection. Although prevention of hyperacute rejection will not, in and of itself, induce long-term acceptance of xenografts, it represents a major achievement and allows for further exploration of acute vascular rejection and cellular rejection. It is anticipated that refined tolerance induction strategies will be able to mitigate the problems of acute vascular rejection and cellular rejection. Taken together, these advances give hope that xenotransplantation will fulfill its promise of alleviating the suffering of the thousands of patients now on transplant waiting lists around the world.

ACKNOWLEDGMENTS

We thank Dr. David K. C. Cooper for his constructive critique of the manuscript. This work was supported in part by grants from the National Heart, Lung, and Blood Institute (R01 HL67110, R01 HL54211, R01 HL71932, P01 HL18646) and the National Institute of Allergy and Infectious Disease (P01 AI50157) of the National Institutes of Health.

REFERENCES

1. United Network for Organ Sharing. Waiting List Data. 2001. United Network for Organ Sharing, Washington DC, 2001.
2. Cooper DKC, Keogh AM, Brink J, et al. Report of the Xenotransplantation Advisory Committee of the International Society for Heart and Lung Transplantation: the present status of xenotransplantation and its potential role in the treatment of end-stage cardiac and pulmonary diseases. J Heart Lung Transplant 2000;19: 1125–1165.
3. Vanderpool HY. Critical ethical issues in clinical trials with xenotransplants. Lancet 1998;351:1347–1350.
4. Pierson RN III, White DJ, Wallwork J. Ethical considerations in clinical cardiac xenografting. J Heart Lung Transplant 1993;12:876–878.
5. Cooper DKC, Lanza RP. Xeno—The Promise of Transplanting Animal Organs Into Humans, 1st ed. Oxford University Press, New York: 2000.

6. Sachs DH, Colvin RB, Cosimi AB, et al. Xenotransplantation—caution, but no moratorium. Nat Med 1998;4:372–373.
7. Pratschke J, Wilhelm MJ, Kusaka M, et al. Brain death and its influence on donor organ quality and outcome after transplantation. Transplantation 1999;67:343–348.
8. Laskowski I, Pratschke J, Wilhelm MJ, Gasser M, Tilney NL. Molecular and cellular events associated with ischemia/reperfusion injury. Ann Transplant 2000;5:29–35.
9. Terasaki PI. The HLA-matching effect in different cohorts of kidney transplant recipients. Clin Transpl 2000;497–514.
10. Sykes M, Sachs DH. Mixed chimerism. Philos Trans R Soc Lond B Biol Sci 2001;356:707–726.
11. Sonntag KC, Emery DW, Yasumoto A, et al. Tolerance to solid organ transplants through transfer of MHC class II genes. J Clin Invest 2001;107:65–71.
12. Vial CM, Ostlie DJ, Bhatti FN, et al. Life supporting function for over 1 month of a transgenic porcine heart in a baboon. J Heart Lung Transplant 2000;19: 224–229.
13. Salama AD, Delikouras A, Pusey CD, et al. Transplant accommodation in highly sensitized patients: a potential role of Bcl-xL and alloantibody. Am J Transplant 2001;1:260–269.
14. Polejaeva IA, Chen SH, Vaught TD, et al. Cloned pigs produced by nuclear transfer from adult somatic cells. Nature 2000;407:86–90.
15. Hajjar RJ, del Monte F, Matsui T, Rosenzweig A. Prospects for gene therapy for heart failure. Circ Res 2000;86:616–621.
16. Jonas RA, Giglia TM, Sanders SP, et al. Rapid, two-stage arterial switch for transposition of the great arteries and intact ventricular septum beyond the neonatal period. Circulation 1989;80:I203–I208.
17. Bonhoeffer P, Carminati M, Parenzan L, Tynan M. Non-surgical left ventricular preparation for arterial switch in transposition of the great arteries. Lancet 1992; 340:549–550.
18. Anversa P, Ricci R, Olivetti G. Quantitative structural analysis of the myocardium during physiologic growth and induced cardiac hypertrophy: a review. J Am Coll Cardiol 1986;7:1140–1149.
19. Calne RY. Organ transplantation between widely disparate species. Transplant Proc 1970;2:550.
20. US Department of Health and Human Services Public Health Service. Guidance for industry: public health issues posed by the use of nonhuman primate xenografts in humans. Federal Regulations 64, 16743–16744 (1999).
21. Sachs DH. MHC homozygous miniature swine. In: Swindle MM, Moody DC, Phillips LD, eds. Swine as Models in Biomedical Research. Iowa State University Press, Ames: 1992, pp. 3–15.
22. Sachs DH. The pig as a potential xenograft donor. Pathol Biol 1994;42:217–228.
23. Allan JS, Rose GA, Choo JK, et al. Morphometric analysis of miniature swine hearts as potential human xenografts. Xenotransplantation 2001;8:90–93.
24. Sullivan JA, Oettinger HF, Sachs DH, Edge AS. Analysis of polymorphism in porcine MHC class I genes: alterations in signals recognized by human cytotoxic lymphocytes. J Immunol 1997;159:2318–2326.
25. Gustafsson K, Leguern C, Hirsch F, Germana S, Pratt K, Sachs DH. Class II genes of miniature swine. IV. Characterization and expression of two allelic class II DQB cDNA clones. J Immunol 1990;145:1946–1951.
26. Gustafsson K, Germana S, Hirsch F, Pratt K, Leguern C, Sachs DH. Structure of miniature swine class II DRB genes: conservation of hypervariable amino acid

residues between distantly related mammalian species. Proc Natl Acad Sci USA 1990;87:9798–9802.

27. Emery DW, Sablinski T, Shimada H, et al. Expression of an allogeneic MHC DRB transgene, through retroviral transduction of bone marrow, induces specific reduction of alloreactivity. Transplantation 1997;64:1414–1423.

28. Fishman JA. Infection and xenotransplantation. Developing strategies to minimize risk. Ann NY Acad Sci 1998;862:52–66.

29. Reemtsma K, McCracken BH, Schlegel JV, Pearl M. Heterotransplantation of the kidney: two clinical experiences. Science 1964;143:700–702.

30. Hardy JD, Chavez CM, Kurrus FD, et al. Heart transplantation in man. Developmental studies and report of a case. JAMA 1964;188:1132–1140.

31. Taniguchi S, Cooper DK. Clinical xenotransplantation: past, present and future. Ann R Coll Surg Engl 1997;79:13–19.

32. Beecher HK, Adams RD, Barger AC, et al.. A definition of reversible coma. JAMA 1968;205:85–88.

33. Bailey LL, Nehlsen-Cannarella WSL, Concepcion W, Jolley WB. Baboon-to-human cardiac xenotransplantation in a neonate. JAMA 1985;254:3321–3329.

34. Makowka L, Cramer DV, Hoffman A, et al. The use of a pig liver xenograft for temporary support of a patient with fulminant hepatic failure. Transplantation 1995;59:1654–1659.

35. Groth CG, Korsgren O, Wennberg L, et al. Xenoislet rejection following pig-to-rat, pig-to-primate, and pig-to-man transplantation. Transplant Proc 1996;28:538–539.

36. Ildstad ST. Xenotransplantation for AIDS. Lancet 1996;347:761–766.

37. Brevig T, Holgersson J, Widner H. Xenotransplantation for CNS repair: immunological barriers and strategies to overcome them. Trends Neurosci 2000;23:337–344.

38. Subramanian T. Cell transplantation for the treatment of Parkinson's disease. Semin Neurol 2001;21:103–115.

39. Deacon T, Schumacher J, Dinsmore J, et al. Histological evidence of fetal pig neural cell survival after transplantation into a patient with Parkinson's disease. Nat Med 1997;3:350–353.

40. Perper RJ, Najarian JS. Experimental renal heterotransplantation. III. Passive transfer of transplantation immunity. Transplantation 1967;5:514–533.

41. Hoffmann MW, Heath WR, Ruschmeyer D, Miller JFAP. Deletion of high-avidity T cells by thymic epithelium. Proc Natl Acad Sci U S A 1995;92:9851–9855.

42. Bravery CA, Batten P, Yacoub MH, Rose ML. Direct recognition of SLA- and HLA-like class II antigens on porcine endothelium by human T cells results in T cell activation and release of interleukin-2. Transplantation 1995;60:1024–1033.

43. Cooper DKC, Good AH, Koren E, et al. Identification of alpha-galactosyl and other carbohydrate epitopes that are bound by human anti-pig antibodies: relevance to discordant xenografting in man. Transplant Immunol 1993;1:198–205.

44. Galili U, Macher BA, Buehler J, Shohet SB. Human natural anti-α-galactosyl IgG. II. The specific recognition of $\alpha(1-_3)$ linked galactose residues. J Exp Med 1985;162:573–582.

45. Galili U, Rachmilewitz EA, Peleg A, Flechner I. A unique natural human IgG antibody with anti-alpha-galactosyl specificity. J Exp Med 1984;160:1519–1531.

46. Minanov OP, Itescu S, Neethling FA, et al. Anti-Gal IgG antibodies in sera of newborn humans and baboons and its significance in pig xenotransplantation. Transplantation 1997;63:182–186.

47. Galili U, Mandrell RE, Hamadeh RM, Shohet SB, Griffiss JM. The interaction between the human natural anti-α?galactosyl IgG (anti-Gal) and bacteria of the human flora. Infect Immunol 1988;57:1730–1737.
48. Rother RP, Fodor WL, Springhorn JP, et al. A novel mechanism of retrovirus inactivation in human serum mediated by anti-alpha-galactosyl natural antibody. J Exp Med 1995;182:1345–1355.
49. Parker W, Bruno D, Holzknecht ZE, Platt JL. Characterization and affinity isolation of xenoreactive human natural antibodies. J Immunol 1994;153:3791–3803.
50. Sandrin MS, Vaughan HA, Dabkowski PL, McKenzie IF. Anti-pig IgM antibodies in human serum react predominantly with Gal(alpha 1-3)Gal epitopes. Proc Natl Acad Sci U S A 1993;90:11,391–11,395.
51. Galili U, Tibell A, Samuelsson B, Rydberg L, Groth CG. Increased anti-Gal activity in diabetic patients transplanted with porcine islet cells. Transplant Proc 1996; 28:564–566.
52. Bartholomew A, Latinne D, Sachs DH, et al. Utility of xenografts: lack of correlation between PRA and natural antibodies to swine. Xenotransplantation 1997;4: 34–39.
53. Cascalho M, Platt JL. The immunological barrier to xenotransplantation. Immunity 2001;14:437–446.
54. Miyagawa S, Hirose H, Shirakura R, et al. The mechanism of discordant xenograft rejection. Transplantation 1988;46:825–829.
55. Gambiez L, Weill BJ, Chereau C, Calmus Y, Houssin D. The hyperacute rejection of guinea pig to rat heart xenografts is mediated by preformed IgM. Transplant Proc 1990;22:1058.
56. Johnston PS, Wang MW, Lim SML, Wright LJ, White DJG. Discordant xenograft rejection in an antibody-free model. Transplantation 1992;54:573–577.
57. Sablinski T, Latinne D, Bailin M, et al. Xenotransplantation of pig kidneys to nonhuman primates: I. Development of the model. Xenotransplantation 1995;2: 264–270.
58. Dalmasso AP, Vercelolotti GM, Fischel RJ, Bolman RM, Bach FH, Platt JL. Mechanism of complement activation in the hyperacute rejection of porcine organs transplanted into primate recipients. Am J Pathol 1992;140:1157–1166.
59. Müller-Eberhard HJ. Complement: chemistry and pathways. In: Gallin JI, Goldstein IM, Snyderman R, eds. Inflammation. Basic Principles and Clinical Correlates. Raven Press, New York: 1992, pp. 33–61.
60. Frank MM. Complement system. In: Frank MM, Austen KF, Claman HN, Unanue ER, eds. Samter's Immunological Diseases. Little, Brown and Company, Boston: 1995, pp. 331–352.
61. Abbas AK, Lichtman AH, Pober JS. The complement system. In: Abbas AK, Lichtman AH, Pober JS, eds. Cellular and Molecular Immunology, 2nd ed. WB Saunders, Philadelphia, PA: 1994, pp. 225–315.
62. Auchincloss H, Sachs DH. Xenogeneic transplantation. Annu Rev Immunol 1998; 16:433–470.
63. Sachs DH, Sykes M, Robson SC, Cooper DKC. Xenotransplantation. In: Dixon FJ, ed. Advances in Immunology. Academic Press, San Diego, CA: 2001, pp. 129–233.
64. Dalmasso AP, Vercelolotti GM, Platt JL, Bach FH. Inhibition of complement-mediated endothelial cell cytotoxicity by decay-accelerating factor: potential for prevention of xenograft hyperacute rejection. Transplantation 1991;52: 530–533.

65. Bach FH. Xenotransplantation: problems and prospects. Annu Rev Med 1998;49: 301–310.
66. Saadi S, Platt JL. Transient perturbation of endothelial integrity induced by natural antibodies and complement. J Exp Med 1995;181:21–31.
67. Platt JL, Vercelolotti GM, Lindman BJ, Oegema TR Jr, Bach FH, Dalmasso AP. Release of heparan sulphate from endothelial cells: Implications for pathogenesis of hyperacute rejection. J Exp Med 1990;171:1363–1368.
68. Parker W, Saadi S, Lin SS, Holzknecht ZE, Bustos M, Platt JL. Transplantation of discordant xenografts: a challenge revisited. Immunol Today 1996;17:373–378.
69. Alexandre GPJ, Latinne D, Carlier M, et al. Plasmapheresis and splenectomy in experimental renal xenotransplantation. In: Hardy MA, ed. Xenograft 25, 1st ed. Excerpta Medica, New York: 1989, p. 259.
70. Rydberg L, Hallberg E, Samuelsson B, et al. Studies on the removal of anti-pig xenoantibodies in the human by plasmapheresis/immunoadsorption. Xenotransplantation 1995;2:253–263.
71. Gannedahl G, Tufveson G, Sundberg B, Groth CG. The effect of plasmapheresis and deoxyspergualin or cyclophosphamide treatment on an anti-porcine Gal-α(1-3)-Gal antibody levels in humans. Xenotransplantation 1996;3:166–170.
72. Cooper DKC, Human PA, Lexer G, et al. Effects of cyclosporine and antibody adsorption on pig cardiac xenograft survival in the baboon. J Heart Transplant 1988;7:238–246.
73. Taniguchi S, Neethling FA, Korchagina EY, et al. In vivo immunoadsorption of anti-pig antibodies in baboons using a specific Galα1-3Gal column. Transplantation 1996;62:1379–1384.
74. Ye Y, Neethling FA, Niekrasz M, et al. Evidence that intravenously administered alpha-galactosyl carbohydrates reduce baboon serum cytotoxicity to pig kidney cells (PK15) and transplanted pig hearts. Transplantation 1994;58:330–337.
75. Sablinski T, Cooper DKC, Sachs DH. Xenotransplantation. In: Austen KF, Burakoff SJ, Rosen FS, Strom TB, eds. Therapeutic Immunology, 2nd ed. Blackwell Science, Malden, MA: 2001, pp. 535–549.
76. Platt JL. Therapeutic strategies for hyperacute xenograft rejection. In: Platt JL, ed. Hyperacute Xenograft Rejection. RJ Landes, Austin, TX: 1995, pp. 161–187.
77. Cooper DKC, Cairns TDH, Taube DH. Extracorporeal immunoadsorption of anti-pig antibody in baboons using αGal oligosaccharide immunoaffinity columns. Xeno 1996;4:27–29.
78. Simon PM, Neethling FA, Taniguchi S, et al. Intravenous infusion of Galα1–3Gal oligosaccharides in baboons delays hyperacute rejection of porcine heart xenografts. Transplantation 1998;65:346–353.
79. Koren E, Milotic F, Neethling FA, et al. Monoclonal antiidiotypic antibodies neutralize cytotoxic effects of anti-alphaGal antibodies. Transplantation 1996;62:837–843.
80. Koren E, Milotic F, Neethling FA, et al. Murine monoclonal anti-idiotypic antibodies directed against human anti-alpha Gal antibodies prevent rejection of pig cells in culture: implications for pig-to-human organ xenotransplantation. Transplant Proc 1996;28:559.
81. Teranishi K, Gollackner B, Buhler L, et al. Depletion of anti-Gal antibodies in baboons by intravenous therapy with bovine serum albumin conjugated to Gal oligosaccharides. Transplantation 2002;73:129–139.
82. Yang YG, deGoma E, Ohdan H, et al. Tolerization of anti-Galalpha1-3Gal natural antibody-forming B cells by induction of mixed chimerism. J Exp Med 1998;187: 1335–1342.

83. Bracy JL, Sachs DH, Iacomini J. Inhibition of xenoreactive natural antibody production by retroviral gene therapy. Science 1998;281:1845–1847.
84. Ohdan H, Yang YG, Shimizu A, Swenson KG, Sykes M. Mixed chimerism induced without lethal conditioning prevents T cell- and anti-Gal alpha 1,3Gal-mediated graft rejection. J Clin Invest 1999;104:281–290.
85. Leventhal JR, Dalmasso AP, Cromwell JW, et al. Prolongation of cardiac xenograft survival by depletion of complement. Transplantation 1993;55: 857–865.
86. Candinas D, Lesnikoski BA, Robson SC, et al. Effect of repetitive high-dose treatment with soluble complement receptor type 1 and cobra venom factor on discordant xenograft survival. Transplantation 1996;62:336–342.
87. Kobayashi T, Taniguchi S, Ye Y, et al. Delayed xenograft rejection in C3-depleted discordant (pig-to-baboon) cardiac xenografts treated with cobra venom factor. Transplant Proc 1996;28:560.
88. Pruitt SK, Baldwin WD, Marsh HC Jr, Linn SS, Yeh CG, Bollinger RR. The effect of soluble complement receptor type 1 on hyperacute xenograft rejection. Transplantation 1991;52:868–873.
89. Pruitt SK, Kirk AD, Bollinger RR, et al. The effect of soluble complement receptor type 1 on hyperacute rejection of porcine xenografts. Transplantation 1994;57: 363–370.
90. Weisman HF, Bartow T, Leppo MK, et al. Soluble human complement receptor type 1: in vivo inhibitor of complement suppressing post-ischemic myocardial inflammation and necrosis. Science 1990;249:146–151.
91. Cozzi E, White DJG. The generation of transgenic pigs as potential organs donors for humans. Nat Med 1995;1:964–966.
92. McCurry KR, Kooyman DL, Alvarado CG, et al. Human complement regulatory proteins protect swine-to-primate cardiac xenografts from humoral injury. Nat Med 1995;1:423–427.
93. Medof ME, Kinoshita T, Nussenzweig V. Inhibition of complement activation on the surface of cells after incorporation of decay-accelerating factor (DAF) into their membranes. J Exp Med 1984;160:1558–1578.
94. Rosengard AM, Cary NRB, Langford GA, Tucker AW, Wallwork J, White DJG. Tissue expression of human complement inhibitor, decay-accelerating factor, in transgenic pigs. Transplantation 1995;59:1325–1333.
95. Cozzi E, Tucker AW, Langford GA, et al. Characterization of pigs transgenic for human decay-accelerating factor. Transplantation 1997;64:1383–1392.
96. Schmoeckel M, Nollert G, Shahmohammadi M, et al. Prevention of hyperacute rejection by human decay accelerating factor in xenogeneic perfused working hearts. Transplantation 1996;62:729–734.
97. Cozzi E, Yannoutsos N, Langford GA, Pinto-Chavez G, Wallwork J, White DJG. Effect of transgenic expression of human decay-accelerating factor on the inhibition of hyperacute rejection of pig organs. In: Cooper DKC, Kemp E, Platt JL, White DJG, eds. Xenotransplantation. Springer-Verlag, Heidelberg, Germany: 1997, pp. 665–682.
98. Bhatti FN, Schmoeckel M, Zaidi A, et al. Three-month survival of HDAFF transgenic pig hearts transplanted into primates. Transplant Proc 1999;31:958.
99. Kuwaki K, Knosalla C, Dor FJMF, et al. Gal-conjugate anti-CD154 monoclonal antibody, and anticoagulation improve graft survival in pig-to-baboon heart transplantation. Xenotransplantation 2003;10:489.
100. Schmoeckel M, Bhatti FNK, Zaidi A, et al. Orthotopic heart transplantation in a transgenic pig-to-primate model. Transplantation 1998;65:1570–1577.

101. Diamond LE, McCurry KR, Martin MJ, et al. Characterization of transgenic pigs expressing functionally active human CD59 on cardiac endothelium. Transplantation 1996;61:1241–1249.

102. Squinto SP. Genetically modified animal organs for human transplantation. World J Surg 1997;21:939–942.

103. Byrne GW, McCurry KR, Martin MJ, McClellan SM, Platt JL, Logan JS. Transgenic pigs expressing human CD59 and decay-accelerating factor produce an intrinsic barrier to complement-mediated damage. Transplantation 1997;63: 149–155.

104. Chen RH, Naficy S, Logan JS, Diamond LE, Adams DH. Hearts from transgenic pigs constructed with CD59/DAF genomic clones demonstrate improved survival in primates. Xenotransplantation 1999;6:194–200.

105. Sandrin MS, Fodor WL, Mouhtouris E, et al. Enzymatic remodeling of the carbohydrate surface of a xenogeneic cell substantially reduces human antibody binding and complement-mediated cytolysis. Nat Med 1995;1:1261–1267.

106. Sandrin MS, Fodor WL, Cohney S, et al. Reduction of the major porcine xenoantigen Galα(1,3)Gal by expression of α(1,2) fucosyltransferase. Xenotransplantation 1996;3:134–140.

107. Chen C, Fisicaro N, Shinkel TA, et al. Reduction in Gal-α1,3-Gal epitope expression in transgenic mice expressing human H-transferase. Xenotransplantation 1996;3:69–75.

108. Koike C, Kannagi R, Takuma Y, et al. Introduction of α(1,2)-fucosyltransferase and its effect on α-Gal epitopes in transgenic pig. Xenotransplantation 1996;3: 81–86.

109. Cooper DKC, Koren E, Oriol R. Genetically-engineered pigs. Lancet 1993, 342: 682–683.

110. Dai Y, Vaught TD, Boone J, et al. Targeted disruption of the alpha1,3-galactosyltransferase gene in cloned pigs. Nat Biotechnol 2002;20:251–255.

111. Lai L, Kolber-Simonds D, Park KW, et al. Production of alpha-1,3-galactosyltransferase knockout pigs by nuclear transfer cloning. Science 2002;295: 1089–1092.

112. Phelps CJ, Koike C, Vaught TD, et al. Production of alpha 1,3-galactosyltransferase-deficient pigs. Science 2003;299:411–414.

113. Yamada K, Yazawa K, Kamono C, et al. An initial report of alpha-Gal deficient pig-to-baboon renal xenotransplantation: evidence for the benefit of co-transplanting vascularized donor thymic tissue. Xenotransplantation 2003;10:480.

114. Bracy JL, Cretin N, Cooper DK, Iacomini J. Xenoreactive natural antibodies. Cell Mol Life Sci 1999;56:1001–1007.

115. Tearle RG, Tange MJ, Zanettino ZL, et al. The α1,3-galactosyltransferase knockout mouse. Implications for xenotransplantation. Transplantation 1996;61:13–19.

116. Bracy JL, Iacomini J. Induction of B-cell tolerance by retroviral gene therapy. Blood 2000;96:3008–3015.

117. Lin SS, Weidner BC, Byrne GW, et al. The role of antibodies in acute vascular rejection of pig-to-baboon cardiac transplants. J Clin Invest 1998;101:1745–1756.

118. Lin SS, Hanaway MJ, Gonzalez-Stawinski GV, et al. The role of anti-Galalpha1-3Gal antibodies in acute vascular rejection and accommodation of xenografts. Transplantation 2000;70:1667–1674.

119. Goodman DJ, Millan M, Ferran C, Bach FH. Mechanism of delayed xenograft rejection. In: Cooper DKC, Kemp E, Platt JL, White DJG, eds. Xenotransplantation: The Transplantation of Organs and Tissues Between Species. Springer, Heidelberg, Germany: 1997, pp. 77–94.

120. Blakely ML, Van der Werf WJ, Berndt MC, Dalmasso AP, Bach FH, Hancock WW. Activation of intragraft endothelial and mononuclear cells during discordant xenograft rejection. Transplantation 1994;58:1059–1066.

121. Robson SC, Siegel JB, Lesnikoski BA, et al. Aggregation of human platelets induced by porcine endothelial cells is dependent upon both activation of complement and thrombin generation. Xenotransplantation 1996;3:24–34.

122. Robson SC, Kaczmarek E, Siegel JB, et al. Loss of ATP diphosphohydrolase activity with endothelial cell activation. J Exp Med 1997;185:153–163.

123. Bach FH. Genetic engineering as an approach to xenotransplantation. World J Surg 1997;21:913–916.

124. Esmon CT. Cell mediated events that control blood coagulation and vascular injury. Annu Rev Cell Biol 1993;9:1–26.

125. Balla G, Jacob HS, Balla J, et al. Ferritin: a cytoprotective antioxidant stratagem of endothelium. J Biol Chem 1992;267:18,148–18,153.

126. Dong VM, Womer KL, Sayegh MH. Transplantation tolerance: the concept and its applicability. Pediatr Transplant 1999;3:181–192.

127. Platt JL, Dalmasso AP, Lindman BJ, Ihrcke NS, Bach FH. The role of C5a and antibody in the release of heparan sulfate from endothelial cells. Eur J Immunol 1991;21:2287–2890.

128. Whelan J, Ghersa P, van Huijsduijnen RH, et al. An NFκB-like factor is essential but not sufficient for cytokine induction of endothelial leukocyte adhesion molecule 1 (ELAM-1) gene transcription. Nucleic Acids Res 1991;19:2645–2653.

129. deMartin R, Vanhove B, Cheng Q, et al. Cytokine-inducible expression in endothelial cells of an IκBα–like gene is regulated by NFκB. EMBO J 1993;12:2773–2779.

130. Cogswell JP, Godlevski MM, Wisely GB, et al. NF-κB regulates IL-1B transcription through a consensus NF-κB binding site and a nonconsensus CRE-like site. J Immunol 1994;153:712–723.

131. Millan MT, Geczy C, Stuhlmeier KM, Goodman DJ, Ferran C, Bach FH. Human monocytes activate porcine endothelial cells, resulting in increased E-selectin, interleukin-8, monocyte chemotactic protein-1, and plasminogen activator inhibitor-type-1 expression. Transplantation 1997;63:421–429.

132. Buhler L, Awwad M, Basker M, et al. High-dose porcine hematopoietic cell transplantation combined with CD40 ligand blockade in baboons prevents an induced anti-pig humoral response. Transplantation 2000;69:2296–2304.

133. Voraberger G, Schäfer R, Stratowa C. Cloning of the human gene for intercellular adhesion molecule 1 and analysis of its 5′-regulatory region. J Immunol 1991;147:2777–2786.

134. Pescovitz MD, Sakopoulos AG, Gaddy JA, Husmann RJ, Zuckermann FA. Porcine peripheral blood CD4$^+$/CD8$^+$ dual expressing T-cells. Vet Immunol Immunopathol 1994;43:53–62.

135. Siebenlist U, Franzoso G, Brown K. Structure, regulation and function of NF-κB. Annu Rev Cell Biol 1994;10:405–455.

136. Finco TS, Baldwin AS Jr. Mechanistic aspects of NF-κB regulation: the emerging role of phosphorylation and proteolysis. Immunity 1995;3:263–272.

137. DiDonato J, Mercurio F, Rosette C, et al. Mapping of the inducible IκB phosphorylation sites that signal its ubiquitination and degradation. Mol Cell Biol 1996;16:1295–1304.

138. Beg AA, Finco TS, Nantermet PV, Baldwin AS Jr. Tumor necrosis factor and interleukin-1 lead to phosphorylation and loss of IκBα: a mechanism for NF-κB activation. Mol Cell Biol 1993;13:3301–3310.

139. Henkle T, Machieldt T, Alkalay I, Krönke M, Ben-Nerial Y, Baeuerie PA. Rapid proteolysis of IκB-α is necessary for activation of transcription factor NF-κB. Nature 1993;365:182–185.

140. Cooper JT, Stroka DM, Brostjian C, Palmetshofer A, Bach FH, Ferran C. A20 blocks endothelial cell activation through a NF-kappaB-dependent mechanism. J Biol Chem 1996;271:18,068–18,073.

141. Bach FH, Ferran C, Hechenleitner P, et al. Accommodation of vascularized xenografts: expression of "protective genes" by donor endothelial cells in a host Th2 cytokine environment. Nat Med 1997;3:196–204.

142. Soares MP, Lin Y, Anrather J, et al. Expression of heme oxygenase-1 can determine cardiac xenograft survival. Nat Med 1998;4:1073–1077.

143. Sato K, Balla J, Otterbein L, et al. Carbon monoxide generated by heme oxygenase-1 suppresses the rejection of mouse-to-rat cardiac transplants. J Immunol 2001;166:4185–4194.

144. Goodman DJ, von Albertini MA, McShea A, Wrighton CJ, Bach FH. Adenoviral-mediated overexpression of IκBα in endothelial cells inhibits natural killer cell-mediated endothelial cell activation. Transplantation 1996;62:967–972.

145. Dorling A, Lechler RI. T cell-mediated xenograft rejection: specific tolerance is probably required for long term xenograft survival. Xenotransplantation 1998;5:234–245.

146. Chitilian HV, Laufer TM, Stenger K, Shea S, Auchincloss H Jr. The strength of cell-mediated xenograft rejection in the mouse is due to the CD4⁺ indirect response. Xenotransplantation 1998;5:93–98.

147. Rollins SA, Kennedy SP, Chodera AJ, Elliott EA, Zavoico GB, Matis LA. Evidence that activation of human T cells by porcine endothelium involves direct recognition of porcine SLA and costimulation by porcine ligands for LFA-1 and CD2. Transplantation 1994;57:1709–1716.

148. Dorling A, Lombardi G, Binns R, Lechler RI. Detection of primary direct and indirect human anti-porcine T cell responses using a porcine dendritic cell population. Eur J Immunol 1996;26:1378–1387.

149. Murray AG, Khodadoust MM, Pober JS, Bothwell ALM. Porcine aortic endothelial cells activate human T cells: direct presentation of MHC antigens and costimulation by ligands for human CD2 and CD28. Immunity 1994;1:57–63.

150. Zaidi A, Schmoeckel M, Bhatti F, et al. Life-supporting pig-to-primate renal xenotransplantation using genetically modified donors. Transplantation 1998;65:1584–1590.

151. Ildstad ST, Bluestone JA, Barbieri SA, Sachs DH. Characterization of mixed allogeneic chimeras. Immunocompetence, in vitro reactivity, and genetic specificity of tolerance. J Exp Med 1985;162:231.

152. Charlton B, Auchincloss H Jr, Fathman CG. Mechanisms of transplantation tolerance. Annu Rev Immunol 1994;12:707–734.

153. Zinkernagel RM, Althage A, Callahan G, Welsh RM Jr. On the immunocompetence of H-2 incompatible irradiation bone marrow chimeras. J Immunol 1980;124:2356–2365.

154. Wekerle T, Sykes M. Mixed chimerism as an approach for the induction of transplantation tolerance. Transplantation 1999;68:459–467.

155. Ardavin C, Wu L, Li C-L, Shortman K. Thymic dendritic cells and T cells develop simultaneously in the thymus from a common precursor population. Nature 1993;362:761–763.

156. Nikolic B, Sykes M. Clonal deletion as a mechanism of transplantation tolerance. J Heart Lung Transplant 1996;15:1171–1178.

157. Sykes M. Mixed chimerism and transplant tolerance. Immunity 2001;14: 417–424.
158. Alexandre GPJ, Squifflet JP, deBruyere M, et al. Present experiences in a series of 26 ABO-incompatible living donor renal allografts. Transplant Proc 1987;19: 4538.
159. Sachs DH, Sablinski T. Tolerance across discordant xenogeneic barriers. Xeno 1995;2:234–239.
160. Latinne D, Smith CV, Nickeleit V, et al. Xenotransplantation from pig to cynomolgus monkey: approach toward tolerance induction. Transplant Proc 1993; 25:336.
161. Tanaka M, Latinne D, Sablinski T, et al. Xenotransplantation from pig to cynomolgus monkey: the potential for overcoming xenograft rejection through induction of chimerism. Transplant Proc 1994;26:1326.
162. Sachs DH, Sykes M, Greenstein J, Cosimi AB. Tolerance and xenograft survival. Nat Med 1995;1:969.
163. Xu Y, Lorf T, Sablinski T, et al. Removal of anti-porcine natural antibodies from human and nonhuman primate plasma in vitro and in vivo by a Galα1-3Galβ1-4βGlc-X immunoaffinity column. Transplantation 1998;65:172–179.
164. Kozlowski T, Fuchimoto Y, Monroy R, et al. Apheresis and column absorption for specific removal of Gal-alpha-1,3 Gal natural antibodies in a pig-to-baboon model. Transplant Proc 1997;29:961.
165. Buhler L, Awwad M, Treter S, et al. Induction of mixed hematopoietic chimerism in the pig-to-baboon model. Transplant Proc 2000;32:1101.
166. Buhler L, Basker M, Alwayn IP, et al. Coagulation and thrombotic disorders associated with pig organ and hematopoietic cell transplantation in nonhuman primates. Transplantation 2000;70:1323–1331.
167. Tseng YL, Dor FJMF, Kuwaki K, et al. Preliminary results of Gal-knockout porcine bone marrow xenotransplantation in nonhuman primates. Xenotransplantation 2003;10:486.
168. Sachs DH, Smith CV, Emery DW, et al. Induction of specific tolerance to MHC-disparate allografts through genetic engineering. Exp Nephrol 1993;1:128–133.
169. Sykes M, Sachs DH, Nienhuis AW, Pearson DA, Moulton AD, Bodine DM. Specific prolongation of skin graft survival following retroviral transduction of bone marrow with an allogeneic major histocompatibility complex gene. Transplantation 1993;55:197–202.
170. Bagley J, Wu Y, Sachs DH, Iacomini J. Defining the requirements for peptide recognition in gene therapy-induced T cell tolerance. J Immunol 2000;165: 4842–4847.
171. Ierino FL, Gojo S, Banerjee PT, et al. Transfer of swine major histocompatibility complex class II genes into autologous bone marrow cells of baboons for the induction of tolerance across xenogeneic barriers. Transplantation 1999;67: 1119–1128.
172. Lee AL, Gritsch HA, Sergio JJ, et al. Specific tolerance across a discordant xenogeneic transplantation barrier. Proc Natl Acad Sci U S A 1994;91:10,864–10,867.
173. Zhao Y, Fishman JA, Sergio JJ, et al. Immune restoration by fetal pig thymus grafts in T cell-depleted, thymectomized mice. J Immunol 1997;158:1641–1649.
174. Zhao Y, Swenson K, Sergio JJ, Arn JS, Sachs DH, Sykes M. Skin graft tolerance across a discordant xenogeneic barrier. Nat Med 1996;2:1211–1216.
175. Madsen JC, Yamada K, Allan JS, et al. Transplantation tolerance prevents cardiac allograft vasculopathy in major histocompatibility complex class I-disparate miniature swine. Transplantation 1998;65:304–313.

176. Cooper DK, Keogh AM, Brink J, et al. Report of the Xenotransplantation Advisory Committee of the International Society for Heart and Lung Transplantation: the present status of xenotransplantation and its potential role in the treatment of end-stage cardiac and pulmonary diseases. J Heart Lung Transplant 2000;19: 1125–1165.
177. Cooper DK. Xenotransplantation: How far have we come? Graft 2001;4:6–86.
178. Bach FH, Fineberg HV. Call for moratorium on xenotransplants. Nature 1998; 391:326.
179. Stoye JP, Coffin JM. The dangers of xenotransplantation. Nat Med 1995;1:1100.
180. Patience C, Takeuchi Y, Weiss RA. Zoonosis in xenotransplantation. Curr Opin Immunol 1998;10:539–542.
181. Patience C, Takeuchi Y, Weiss RA. Infection of human cells by an endogenous retrovirus of pigs. Nat Med 1997;3:282–286.
182. Paradis K, Langford G, Long Z, et al. Search for cross-species transmission of porcine endogenous retrovirus in patients treated with living pig tissue. The XEN 111 Study Group. Science 1999;285:1236–1241.
183. Onions D, Cooper DK, Alexander TJ, et al. An approach to the control of disease transmission in pig-to-human xenotransplantation. Xenotransplantation 2000;7: 143–155.
184. Fishman JA. Xenosis and xenotransplantation: addressing the infectious risks posed by an emerging technology. Kidney Int Suppl 1997;58:S41–S45.
185. Logan JS. Prospects for xenotransplantation. Curr Opin Immunol 2000;12:563.

12 Left Ventricular Reconstruction for Ischemic Heart Failure

Vincent Dor, MD

INTRODUCTION

Postinfarct ischemic cardiomyopathy is characterized by a variable degree of left ventricular (LV) dyssynergy secondary to dyskinetic and/or akinetic walls. Since 1984, we have surgically repaired such ventricles by inserting a patch inside the ventricle to exclude the nonresectable akinetic/dyskinetic segments and reestablishing the preinfarct ventricular geometry. Left ventricular reconstruction (LVR) using an endoventricular patch is an accepted and efficient technique to treat the dilated, hypocontractile ventricle of ischemic heart disease as both diastolic and systolic function are improved.

From: *Contemporary Cardiology: Surgical Management of Congestive Heart Failure*
Edited by: J. C. Fang and G. S. Couper © Humana Press Inc., Totowa, NJ

THE VENTRICULAR WALL AFTER INFARCTION

In the classic transmural infarct without reperfusion, the infarcted area undergoes necrosis, fibrosis, and sometimes calcification. Although the remaining uninfarcted myocardium is initially normal, the transmural infarction produces increases in load and activates neurohormonal mechanisms that lead to eccentric myocardial hypertrophy and ventricular dilation (i.e., ventricular remodeling) of the myocardium remote to the original infarct. This course of events is most commonly seen in occlusion of the left anterior descending artery (LAD), leading to an antero-apical-septal scar.

However, in the modern era of early reperfusion therapy (i.e., angioplasty and thrombolysis) for myocardial infarction (MI), the classical process of transmural infarction has been modified into nontransmural infarction with necrosis of the subendocardial muscle and sparing of the subepicardial muscle (1). In this situation, the nontransmurally infarcted myocardial wall appears nonviable by echocardiography or ventriculography because of akinesia. Although thallium nuclear imaging may suggest viability, intraoperative findings usually demonstrate a thin rim of subepicardial myocardium of little functional importance, primarily because of the dominant underlying scar. Cardiac magnetic resonance imaging is able to detect these differences between transmural and nontransmural infarction (2,3). Subendocardial scar can induce immediately or progressively an asynergic LV wall.

Pathophysiology

Klein et al. demonstrated in 1967 (4) that if more than 20% of the left ventricle is infarcted, the Starling and Laplace laws will lead to progressive global ventricular hypokinesia. Gaudron et al. (5) showed that 20% of all MIs follow this evolution. The undamaged area is normal at first, then hypertrophied to compensate the lack of contractility of the necrotic wall, and is finally dilated by physical mechanical forces. The dilatation increases the stroke volume and temporarily improves the cardiac index (Starling law), but the increased wall tension has a detrimental effect on the myocardial contractility (Laplace law). This physical and mechanical explanation of the progressive dilatation of the heart—LV remodeling—is based on a complex inflammatory and neurohormonal process, which, in reality, is the result of the reaction of the "organism" against the lack of contractility of a large scar when the remaining nonischemic area is not able to assume and maintain a normal cardiac output. This reaction explains the progressive dilatation (remodeling), but is more a consequence than a cause of it. The real cause of remodeling is anatomical: the extension of the asynergic scarred area of LV wall. Therefore, it is important to detect it early and assess its size precisely. The aim for cardiology would be to analyze the percentage of LV wall circumference, which can be considered a critical trigger of the progressive remodeling. The LV volume is a sensitive marker of ventricular dysfunction, and LV end-systolic volume is an important predictor of prognosis after myocardial infarction *(10)*. If 25 to 30 mL/m^2 for end-systolic volume index (ESVI) and 50 to 60 mL/m^2 for end-diastolic volume index (EDVI) are considered as normal values, doubling these indices can be considered as severe dilatation.

Assessing precisely and regularly the evolving process of remodeling by objective paramaters (LV volumes and performances) by echo or cardiac magnetic resonance (CMR) is mandatory.

The Role of Revascularization

Is the recanalization of the occluded coronary artery able to prevent this process? Immediately after coronary artery occlusion, irreversible cell necrosis can occur within minutes. Prompt reperfusion, when myocytes are in a state of critical ischemia, can reduce cell death, limit infarct size, and thereby increase survival. However, nuclear assessment (sestamibi) after successful recandalization of the culprit artery shows that in more than 80% of cases, a necrotic area exists *(11)*.

Coronary revascularization by percutaneous or surgical techniques during the acute phase of infarct has greatly changed the prognosis of MI and is an essential treatment but, not always sufficient, and the percentage of scarred LV wall must be checked in all cases after MI to avoid or to follow the LV remodeling.

CONVENTIONAL SURGICAL TECHNIQUES

Since Likoff and Bailey's and Cooley et al.'s descriptions in 1955 *(12)* and 1958 *(13)*, respectively, surgery for the LV aneurysm has been well known *(14)*. The classic operation involves resection and exteriorization of scar tissue by a long linear suture on either a beating or an arrested heart. Although this conventional operation is both easy and safe, the classic work of Froelich et al. *(15)* and Cohen et al. *(16)* suggested that the conventional procedure led to disappointing hemodynamics and poor ventricular geometry as a result of resection of only a small part of the dyskinesia. Techniques to improve on the classic linear suture repair of the scarred ventricle are currently referred to as LV "reconstruction" rather than "remodeling" because this term is traditionally reserved for the spontaneous reshaping of the infarcted ventricle.

LVR: CIRCULAR REORGANIZATION OF LEFT VENTRICLE

A more physiological reconstruction of the left ventricle was described in a large study by Jatene in 1985 *(17)*, who used a technique of external circular reconstruction of the LV wall. The akinetic septum is let inside the ventricular cavity and plicated, and either a linear suture or a patch (in 6% of cases) was used to close the reorganized circular defect in the ventricular wall. Coronary revascularization being performed in 20% of cases.

In 1984, we used a patch inserted inside the ventricle on contractile muscle to exclude all akinetic nonresectable areas, to reconstruct the ventricular cavity as it was before the infarct, and to allow for eventual revascularization of all diseased coronary arteries. Our first series of 25 patients using this technique, endoventricular circular patch plasty (EVCPP), was presented in 1985 *(18)*. Following these two pioneering series, other similar techniques were described: the endoaneurysmorrhaphy by Cooley in 1989 *(19)* and a tailored scar incision by Mickleborough et al. in 1994 *(20)*.

Endoventricular Circular Patch Plasty

In EVCPP (Fig. 1), the mitral valve is first examined by transesophageal echocardiography. Surgery is then performed on a totally arrested heart. Coronary revascularization is accomplished first. The left ventricle is then opened at the center of the depression in the myocardium. Thrombi are removed, and the endocardial scar is resected, especially if the scar is calcified or if spontaneous or inducible ventricular tachycardia (VT) exists. In such circumstances, cryoablation is employed at the edges of the resection. If mitral insufficiency is present, the valve is examined by both atrial and ventricular approaches to plan the specific mitral reconstruction (posterior annuloplasty, Goretex neochordae, an Alfieri E-to-E suture, or mitral valve replacement if the posterior papillary muscle is totally diseased).

The rebuilding of the left ventricular cavity is initiated by a continuous 2.0 monofilament suture that follows the border between the fibrous scar and normal muscle (Fig 1B). Tightening of this suture restores the curvature of the LV wall (Fig. 2C), as it was before the

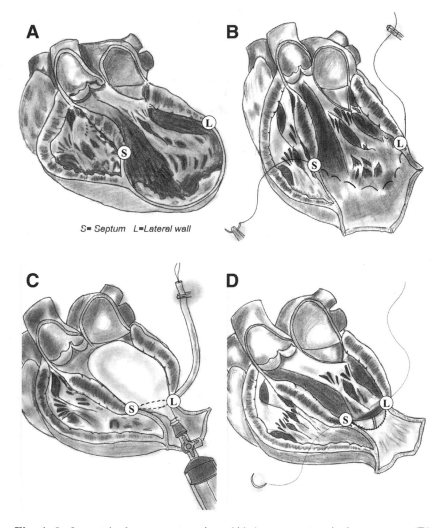

Fig. 1. Left ventricular reconstruction. (**A**) Antero-septoapical aneurysm. (**B**) Endoventricular purse-string suture. (**C**) Curvature restoration and balloon sizing. (**D**) Endoventricular patch reconstruction. S, septum; L, lateral wall.

infarct. To avoid an excessive reduction of volume, with risk of immediate or delayed diastolic incompliance, this suture must be tied with a soft, rubber balloon inside the LV inflated at the patient's theoretical diastolic capacity (i.e., 50 mL/m^2 of body surface area). This maneuver, in addition, gives shape and size of the patch which is anchored on this clothesline inside the LV.

In antero-septo-apical aneurysm, as the septum and apex are more involved than the lateral wall, the patch roughly approximates the direction of the septum (Fig 1D).

Alternatives

Autologous tissue can be used instead of a synthetic patch: Either a semicircle of the fibrous endocardial scar can be mobilized using a septal hinge (if the scar is without calcification or thrombus) or autologous pericardium can be used (autologous tissue patches represent 30% of the cases in our series).

In the case of a posterior or posterolateral infarct (Fig. 2), a triangular patch is used by attaching its base to the posterior or posterolateral mitral annulus and its apex to the base of the posterior or anterolateral papillary muscle. This patch repair reconstructs the normal mitral geometry and a normal posterior wall after large endocardectomy. If resected scar involves the posterior papillary muscle, the mitral valve has to be replaced by a prosthesis, and this can be easily accomplished through a transventricular approach.

If necrotic tissues are encountered during the repair of an acute mechanical complication of a MI (i.e., ventricular septal or free-wall rupture), the patch has to be inserted at the border between viable and necrotic tissue by transmural U stitches reinforced with Teflon pledgets. The patch is anchored above the septal rupture, excluding it from the ventricular cavity.

Concomitant Surgical Problems

Revascularization of all diseased coronary arteries of the contractile area is mandatory. Revascularization of the infarcted area is almost always possible with the left internal mammary artery, even when the left anterior descending artery is thrombosed, and the distal artery is not visualized by collaterals on the preoperative coronary angiogram. In our experience, 97% of our patients underwent coronary revascularization (90% with the internal mammary artery), and at 1 year, more than 80% of these bypassed arteries were patent.

Mitral insufficiency is a common part of the disease and must be looked for carefully both before and during surgery by transesophageal echocardiography. If there is more than grade 2 mitral regurgitation or the mitral annulus is greater 35 mm, a posterior annuloplasty is mandatory. Personally, we prefer the atrial approach with posterior annulus reduction with a Goretex strip, but a transventricular approach is possible (21). Patients with associated degenerative mitral valve disease may require a more complete repair.

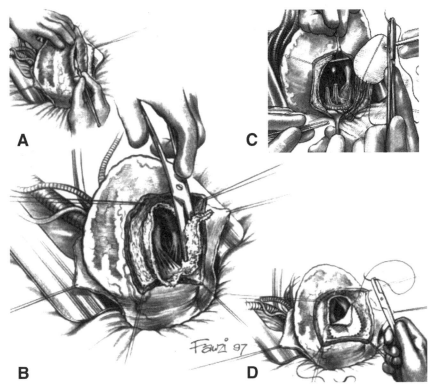

Fig. 2. Technique for posterior and posterolateral localization. (**A**) Primary incision. (**B**) Endocardial resection. (**C**) Mitral valve replacement (as needed). (**D**) Triangular patch repair.

Spontaneous or inducible VT is frequent (13–25% of our patients). In such circumstances, a subtotal nonguided endocardectomy is performed on the endoventricular scar. Cryoablation at the border of this resection completes the surgical excision.

Large Asynergic Ventricles

Large akinetic segments are typically characterized by a congestive heart failure with elevated mean pulmonary artery pressures (>25 mmHg), low ejection fractions (EFs) (<30%), and dilated ventricles (EDVI >150 cc and ESVI >100 cc).

In such cases, the surgery is accomplished with some modifications (Fig. 3). If all of the scarred areas are excluded, an inappropriately small ventricular cavity may result, with a high subsequent risk of immediate or delayed diastolic dysfunction. To avoid this complication, the continuous suture is placed above the limit of the sound muscle in the "transitional" fibrous border zone. The balloon, inside the ventricle inflated to

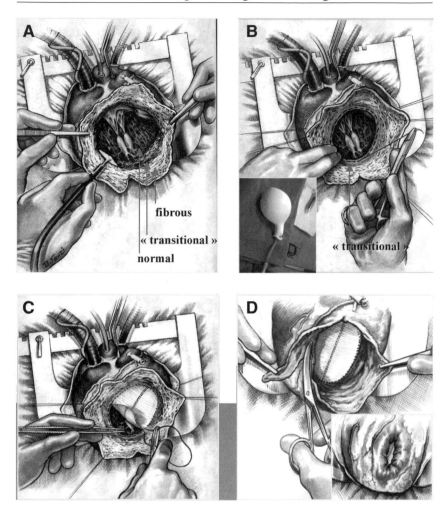

Fig. 3. Technique of left ventricular reconstruction for large akinetic segments. **(A)** Cryoablation at the limit of endocardial resection. **(B)** Endoventricular suture and the balloon to check the diastolic volume. **(C)** Patch anchoring. **(D)** Resection and folding of excluded areas.

the theoretical end diastolic volume, is mandatory before tightening of the circumferential suture. For these reasons, the patch is often larger (3 to 4 cm diameter) than in the usual technique. The excluded septum often cannot be sutured with lateral wall because of potential damage to the revascularized LAD and inappropriate restraint of the right ventricle. In this case, the fibrous tissue is simply folded onto the patch with surgical glue. VT and mitral insufficiences are common in these large asynergia and require attention.

In summary, LVR with EVCPP in combination with coronary revascularization and mitral repair (when needed), improves ventricular performance for several reasons: (1) exclusion of the septal scar promotes more normal ventricular geometry; (2) reconstruction of the ventricular cavity prevents ventricular distortion, decreases wall tension on myocardial segments remote to the area of infarction, and improves regional contractility (demonstrable by pressure volume relationships); and (3) in contrast to a linear repair, the endoaneurysmorrhaphy (patch repair) allows maintenance of reasonably physiological diastolic volume and geometry.

RESULTS

Based on our personal experience of more than 1000 cases and on other published series (23–26), LVR using an endoventricular circular patch works to restore a more normal morphology and physiology to the left ventricle (27,28). This improvement is even apparent by postoperative ventriculography, which demonstrates a return to a normal ventricular cavity, particularly in relationship to the septal exclusion (Fig. 4).

There are also measurable hemodynamic benefits. There is a significant improvement in EF, with a mean increase of 10–15%. In addition, this improvement of EF is apparent whether the abnormal myocardial segment was initially dyskinetic or akinetic (Fig. 5).

Diastolic function is also improved (Fig. 6). The peak filling rate increases from a preoperative baseline of less than 1.8 EDV per second to 3/s EDV/second at 1 month and remains at 2.5/s EDV/second after 1 year, when the time-to-peak-filling rate decreases from 190 ms to respectively 110 ms and 90 ms after 1 year. There is also a shift of the pressure–volume relationship to the left. Finally, ventricular arrhythmias (spontaneous or inducible) are successfully controlled in 90% of cases (29).

Surgical LVR is feasible with acceptable risk. From 1984 to 2001, in our series of 1011 patients (all indications included), there were 76 in-hospital deaths (7.5% operative mortality). With increasing surgical experience, improvements in the management of severely ill patients, larger indication for mitral repair, and greater attention to the remaining postoperative diastolic volume by balloon sizing. The operative mortality in our most recent series since 1998 (more than 400 cases) improved, with an overall mortality of 4.8 and less than 8% in the subgroup with large akinetic segments.

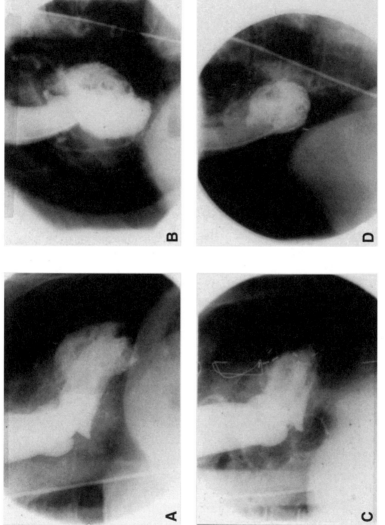

Fig. 4. Ventriculography after EVCPP of antero-septo-apical infarct. (**A**) Preoperative ventriculogram (right anterior oblique). (**B**) Preoperative ventriculogram (left anterior oblique). (**C**) Postoperative ventriculogram (right anterior oblique). (**D**) Postoperative ventriculogram (left anterior oblique). Note: the total disappearance of septal bulging.

288

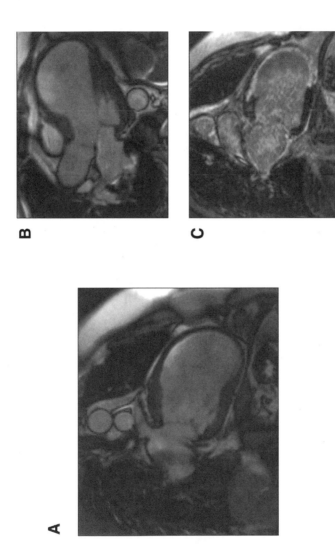

Gadolinium LE>50%

Fig. 5. CMR assessment of an antero-septo-apical aneurysm 4 years after successful stenting of a thrombosed LAD artery (**A,B**) Four chambers and two chambers preoperative view of a large antero-septal dyskinesia LVEF : 23%, EDVI: 180 mL/m², ESVI: 138 mL/m². (**C**) Gadolinium late enhancement shows a transmural apical necrosis and subendocardial necrosis.

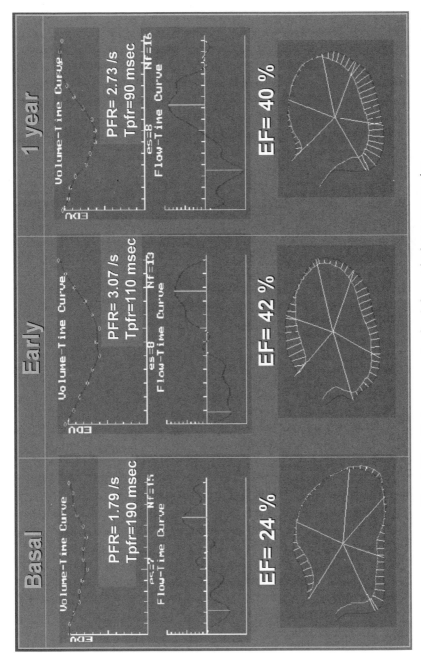

Fig. 6. Diastolic improvements after left ventricular reconstruction.

Table 1
Patients With Preoperative CI <2.0 L/min/m^2 and EF <30% (N = 40)

	Preoperative	Postoperative	1 year postoperative	p
CI (L/min/m^2)	1.7 ± 0.2	2.2 ± 0.5	2.5 ± 1.5	<0.001
EF (%)	22 ± 6	40 ± 7	38 ± 7	<0.001

CI, cardiac index; EF, ejection fraction.

Table 2
Akinetic vs Dyskinetic Postinfarction Segments (N = 245)

	Small dyskinetic (n = 4)	Large dyskinetic (n = 41)	Small akinetic (n = 72)	Large akinetic (n = 48)
Preoperative ejection fraction (EF)	42 ± 11	26 ± 7	41 ± 10	25 ± 9
Postoperative EF	53 ± 11	45 ± 11	49 ± 13	41 ± 12
Hospital death	4.8%	12.2%	0%	12.5%

DISAPPOINTING RESULTS

Some patients with large akinetic ventricular segments and global dilatation who underwent this procedure, developed recurrent mitral insufficiency and secondary pulmonary hypertension months and years after the LVR *(30)*. The mechanism of this process is not clear; continued ventricular remodeling may not be avoidable, especially when the interval between the sentinel infarct and the surgical reconstruction is long (i.e., >40 months) *(31)*. However, since 1998 with "balloon sizing" of the diastolic volume and more liberal use of mitral annuloplasty to keep the annulus smaller than 30 mm became routine, the delayed occurrence of mitral insufficiency and pulmonary hypertension decreased from 25 to 10%. Continued ventricular remodeling also occurs for other reasons than simple mechanical ones (i.e., neurohormonal processes); therefore, patients should be treated medically with β-blockers and angiotensin-converting enzyme inhibitors during the first preoperative year. When delayed hemodynamic control (i.e., essentially CMR) shows stability in terms of ejection fraction and volume, this medical therapy can be discontinued.

Late Survival

Late survival was analyzed in a surgical cohort of 245 consecutive patients operated on between December 1991 and December 1996 *(32)*. There were 20 hospital deaths (8.2%). Eighteen additional patients were lost to follow-up (8% of survivors), 207 patients represented the study cohort. There were no significant differences in baseline characteristics between the excluded patients and the study group. The clinical characteristics of the group are shown in Table 3. There were 163 patients with anterior dyskinesis, 30 with anterior akinesis, and 14 with both anterior abnormalities and severe remote hypokinesis.

During a mean follow-up period of 39 ± 19 months (12–72 months), there were 27 deaths and 3 heart transplants. Event-free survival was 98 ± 1% at 1 year, 95.8 ± 1.4% at 2 years, and 82.1 ± 3.3% at 5 years. Figure 6 shows the Kaplan–Meyer event-free survival curve for the overall population. Late deaths included 16 caused by progressive heart failure, 8 caused by sudden death, and 3 caused by noncardiac causes (2 from strokes and 1 from lung cancer).

Preoperative functional class, EF, and end-systolic volume appeared to predict poor long-term survival. The study population included a significant number of these patients: 57% were New York Heart Association (NYHA) class III–IV; 39% had an EF of 30% or less, and 35% had an ESVI above 120 mL/m^2. For these patient subgroups, the mortality rates were 21, 26, and 28%, respectively. However, it should be noted that these mortality rates are lower than previously reported in patients with reduced LV systolic dysfunction and advanced functional class *(33)*.

The presence of akinesis remote to the anterior wall scar (primarily inferior wall) also identified a high-risk subgroup of patients. Despite surgery, these patients had the worst prognosis, primarily from progressive heart failure. Although the great majority of patients in the study population showed improved regional inferior wall function following LVR, these patients did not. It is reasonable to hypothesize that the lack of recovery in function of these remote inferior segments was related to preoperative nonviability, as reported by Pagley et al. *(34)*. Cardiac transplantation may be more suitable for this patient subgroup.

The postoperative late incidence of malignant arrhythmias was reduced from 46 to 7.1% ($p < 0.0001$; Table 4). Sudden death was the cause of death in 8 of 27 patients. In summary, global life expectancy at 5 years is about 82%. This percentage is above 90% for patients with preoperative ESVI less than 120 mL/m^2 and at 70% for those with ESVI greater than120 mL/m^2. At 10 years, in this last category of very large dilated failing ventricle, the percentage of survival is 50%, whereas it is 80% for patients with ESVI less than 90 mL/m2.

Other clinical, operative, and hemodynamic univariate predictors of survival are reported in Table 5. Patients who died had a worse preoperative functional class (NYHA class 3.4 ± 0.9 vs 2.5 ± 0.9, $p < 0.0001$) and had more clinical signs of heart failure before surgery than did survivors (90 vs 56.5%). Cox regression analysis confirmed preoperative NYHA functional class, EF, ESVI, and remote asynergy were independent predictors of mortality. Actuarial survival curves were also created according to ESVI, EDVI, EF, and NYHA classification (Fig. 7). Although other studies have found the ESVI was the strongest predictor of future cardiac events and mortality in postinfarction patients before or after revascularization (35–38), we found that the preoperative clinical status measured by the NYHA functional class had more predictive power.

In summary, EVCPP improves late survival in postinfarction patients with anterior wall scars, ventricular systolic dysfunction, ventricular dilatation, and significant functional limitation. Survival in this patient population is comparable to cardiac transplantation and much higher than reported in the literature for medical therapy or coronary artery bypass graft alone (33,39).

THE FUTURE

Patient selection remains a critical issue for the success of surgical LVR. Although the clinical assessment of ventricular function is rather sophisticated today, cardiac magnetic resonance imaging may provide a more detailed assessment of viability, ventricular geometry, and hemodynamic performance (40). Such information would allow more precise patient selection and more detailed operative planning.

Other surgical therapies could also be combined with LVR. For example, by combining a ventricular assist device with surgical LVR, the now mechanically unloaded uninfarcted myocardium might "recover" more quickly or more completely and allow for more aggressive pharmacological neurohormonal antagonism, all in the hope of increasing the chances for myocardial recovery. Preliminary data from the Berlin Heart Center (41) and Yacoub et al. (personal communication, 2001) suggest that such a strategy may be possible. In their experience with idiopathic dilated cardiomyopathies, months of ventricular assistance improved ventricular function and morphology to an extent that weaning was possible, a so-called bridge to recovery. In the case of ischemic cardiomyopathies, this type of long-term chronic ventricular unloading may provide similar improvements to the viable but hypocontractile myocardium remote to the areas of infarction. Therefore,

Table 3
Clinical Characteristics

Men/women	183/24
Age (years)	58–8
Time from myocardial infarction (months)	42–52
Urgent operation (%)	20 (9.7)
NYHA I–II (%)	90 (43.4)
NYHA III (%)	69 (33.3)
NYHA IV (%)	48 (23.2)
Angina (%)	133 (64.3)
Congestive heart failure (%)	127 (61.4)
Spontaneous ventricular tachycardia (%)	44 (21.3)
Coronary disease:	
1 vessel (%)	69 (34.8)
2 vessel (%)	73 (35.3)
3 vessel (%)	59 (28.5)
Wall motion	
Dyskinetic (%)	163 (79)
Akinetic (%)	30 (14.5)
Anterior scar and remote asynergy (%)	14 (6.5)

left ventricular surgical reconstruction would improve ventricular geometry by the exclusion of akinetic or dyskinetic segments, and the ventricular assist device would provide mechanical unloading of the viable but hypokinetic segments remote to the area of infarction in those patients suffering from advanced ischemic congestive heart failure. Finally, trials currently in process will inform later if cell transplantation could also be added to the procedure.

SUMMARY

LVR by EVCPP appears useful for pure ventricular dyskinesia (true aneurysm) or akinesia. LVR is performed on the totally arrested heart. Coronary revascularization is completed first. The mitral valve is inspected by transesophageal echocardiography and repaired if necessary. Endocardectomy and cryotherapy can be employed at this time in cases of ventricular tachycardia. At the border between scarred and normal tissue, a continuous suture is placed and tied on a rubber balloon inflated at the patient's theoretical volume in order to avoid diastolic incompliance and to select size and shape of the patch that is anchored on this endoventricular suture. Autologous tissue can also be used. Geometry and performance of the ventricle are improved,

Table 4
Hemodynamic Data for Entire Cohort

	Preoperative	*Postoperative*
CI (L/min/m^2)	2.7–0.6	2.7–0.6
EF (%)	35–13	48–12*
CWP (mmHg)	14–7	12–7
Mean PAP (mmHg)	21–10	18–8
EDVI (mL/m^2)	166–77	86–34*
ESVI (mL/m^2)	112–64	46–26*
Inducible VT (%)	75/163 (46)	13/182 (7.1)*

EDVI, end-diastolic volume index; ESVI, end systolic volume index; EF, ejection fraction; PAP, pulmonary artery pressure; CWP, capillary wedge pressure; CI, cardiac index; VT, ventricular tachycardia.

*$p < 0.0001$.

Table 5
Clinical, Operative, and Hemodynamic Parameters
Associated With Major Events During Follow-Up

	Patients with events (n = 30)	*Patients without events (n = 177)*	*p*
Preoperative*			
NYHA class	3.4–0.9	2.5–0.9	0.0001
EF (%)	27–9	36–13	0.0001
EDVI (mL/m^2)	203–75	159–76	0.006
ESVI (mL/m^2)	150–60	105–63	0.001
Postoperative*			
EF (%)	38–9	50–11	0.0001
EDVI (mL/m^2)	106–42	82–32	0.001
ESVI (mL/m^2)	66–32	42–23	0.0001
Chi-square tests	*N (%)*	*N (%)*	
Preoperative signs of CHF,	27 (90)	96 (57)	0.001
Remote asynergy, *N (%)*	6 (20)	8 (4.8)	.009

Means and standard deviations used.

with a mean increase in the EF between 10 and 15%. The operative mortality on the global series over 1100 cases from 1984 is below 8%. Continued ventricular remodeling, lack of diastolic capacity, or absence of mitral repair may prevent postsurgical improvement.

After myocardial infarction resulting in a large akinetic scar (i.e., >50% of LV circumference), LVR should be considered to prevent pro-

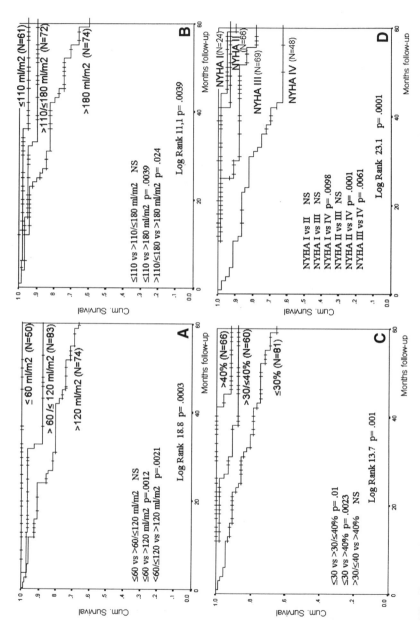

Fig. 7. Actuarial survival curves. **(A)** End-systolic volume index (ESVI). **(B)** End-diastolic volume index (EDVI). **(C)** Left ventricular ejection fraction (LVEF). **(D)** NYHA class.

gressive ventricular dilatation and clinical heart failure. In medically refractory ischemic heart failure, LVR may slow ventricular remodeling and delay the need for heart transplantation. Seventeen years after it was first conceived, LVR is now a good technique to rebuild a scarred and dilated left ventricle after MI. This procedure is easily reproducible, efficient, and safe. It must be considered as one of the major surgical treatments for ischemic cardiomyopathy.

REFERENCES

1. Bogaert J, Maes A, Van de Werf F, et al. Functional recovery of subepicardial myocardial tissue in transmural myocardial infarction after successful reperfusion. Circulation 1999;99:36–43.
2. Fieno DS, Kim RJ, Chen EL, Lomasney JW, Klocke FJ, Judd RM. Contrast-enhanced magnetic resonance imaging of myocardium at risk. Distinction between reversible and irreversible injury throughout infarct healing. J Am Coll Cardiol 2000;36:1985–1991.
3. Rehwald WG, Fieno DS, Chen EL, Kim RJ, Judd RM. Myocardial magnetic resonance imaging contrast agent concentrations after reversible and irreversible ischemic injury. Circulation 2002;105:224–229.
4. Klein MD, Herman MV, Gorlin R. A hemodynamic study of left ventricular aneurysm. Circulation 1967;35:614–630.
5. Gaudron P, Eilles C, Kugler I, et al. Progressive left ventricular dysfunction after myocardial infarction. Circulation 1993;87:755–762.
6. Yousef ZR, Redwood SR, Marber MS. Postinfarction left ventricular remodeling: where are the theories and trials leading us? Heart 2000;83:76–80.
7. Braunwald E, Pfeffer MA. Ventricular enlargement and remodeling following acute myocardial infarction: mechanisms and management. Am J Cardiol 1991; 68(suppl D):1D–6D.
8. McAlpine HM, Morton JJ, Leckie B, et al. Neuroendocrine activation after acute myocardial infarction. Br Heart J 1988;60:117–124.
9. Packer M. The neurohormonal hypothesis: a theory to explain the mechanism of disease progression in heart failure. J Am Coll Cardiol 1992;20:248–254.
10. White HD, Norris RM, Brown MA, et al. Left ventricular end-systolic volume as the major determinant of survival after recovery from myocardial infarction. Circulation 1987;76:44–51.
11. Marber MS, Brown DL, Kloner RA, et al. The open artery hypothesis: to open, or not to open, that is the question. Eur Heart J 1996;17:505–509.
12. Likoff W, Bailey CP. Ventriculoplasty: excision of myocardial aneurysm. JAMA 1955;158:915.
13. Cooley DA, Collins HA, Morris GC, et al. Ventricular aneurysm after myocardial infarction: surgical excision with use of temporary cardiopulmonary bypass. JAMA 1958;167:557.
14. Mills NL, Everson CT, Hockmuth D, et al. Technical advances in the treatment of left ventricular aneurysm. Ann Thorac Surg 1993;55:792–800.
15. Froehlich RT, Falsetti HL, Doty DB, et al. Prospective study of surgery for left ventricular aneurysm. Am J Cardiol 1980;45:923.
16. Cohen M, Packer M, Gorlin R. Indications for left ventricular aneurysmectomy. Circulation 1983;67:717.

17. Jatene AD. Left ventricular aneurysmectomy resection or reconstruction. J Thorac Cardiovasc Surg 1985;89:321–331.

18. Dor V, Kreitmann P, Jourdan J, Acar C, Saab M, Coste P. Interest of "physiological closure (circumferential plasty on contractile areas) of left ventricle after resection and endocardectomy for aneurysm of akinetic zone comparison with classical technique about a series of 209 left ventricular resections [abstract]. J Cardiovasc Surg 1985;26:73.

19. Cooley D. Ventricular endoaneurysmorrhaphy: a simplified repair for extensive postinfarction aneurysm. J Card Surg 1989;4:200–205.

20. Mickleborough L, Maruyama H, Liu P, et al. Results of left ventricular aneurysmectomy with a tailored scar excision and primary closure technique. J Thorac Cardiovasc Surg 1994;107:690–698.

21. Menicanti L, Frigiola A, Buckberg G, et al. Ischemic mitral regurgitation; intraventricular papillary muscle imbrication without mitral ring. Paper presented at: 81st Annual Meeting, American Association for Thoracic Surgery, May 6–9, 2001; San Diego, CA.

22. Di Donato M, Sabatier M, Toso A. Regional myocardial performance of non-ischaemic zones remote form anterior wall left ventricular aneurysm. Effects of aneurysmectomy. Eur Heart J 1995;16:1285–1292.

23. Jakob H, Zˆlch B, Schuster S, et al. Endoventricular patch plasty improves results of LV aneurysmectomy. Eur J Cardiothorac Surg 1993;7:428–436.

24. Grossi E, Chimitz L, Galloway A, et al. Endoventricular remodeling of left ventricular aneurysm: functional, clinical and electrophysiological results. Circulation 1995;92(suppl II):98–100.

25. Shapira O, Davudoff R, Hilkert R, et al. Repair of left ventricular aneurysm: long-term results of linear repair vs endoaneurysmectomorrhaphy. Ann Thorac Surg 1997;63:401–405.

26. Athanasuleas C, Stanley A, Buckberg G, et al. Surgical Anterior Ventricular Endocardial Restoration (SAVER) in the dilated remodeled ventricle after anterior myocardial infarction. J Am Coll Cardiol 2001;37:5.

27. Dor V, Sabatier M, Di Donato, et al. Late hemodynamic results after left ventricular patch repair associated with coronary grafting in patients with postinfarction akinetic or dyskinetic aneurysm of the left ventricle. J Thorac Cardiovasc Surg 1995;110:1291–1301.

28. Di Donato M, Barletta G, Maioli M. Early hemodynamic results of left ventricular reconstructive surgery for anterior wall left ventricular aneurysm. Am J Cardiol 1992;69:886–890.

29. Dor V, Sabatier M, Montiglio F, et al. Results of nonguided subtotal endocardiectomy associated with left ventricular reconstruction in patients with ischemic ventricular arrhythmias. J Thorac Cardiovasc Surg 1994;107:1301–1308.

30. Di Donato M, Sabatier M, Dor V, et al. Effects of the Dor procedure on left ventricular dimension and shape and geometric correlates of mitral regurgitation 1 year after surgery. J Thorac Cardiovasc Surg 2001;121:91–96.

31. Louagie Y, Alouini T, Lesperence J, et al. Left ventricular aneurysm complicated by congestive heart failure: analysis of long term results and risk factors of surgical treatment. J Cardiovasc Surg 1989;30:648–655.

32. Di Donato M, et al. Efficacy of Dor procedure on late survival in patients with post-infarction akinetic or dyskinetic scar and predictors of outcome. Am Coll Cardiol Suppl A 2001:370A.

33. Emond M, Mock MB, Davis KB. Long term survival of medically treated patients in the Coronary Artery Surgery Study (CASS). Circulation 1994;90:2645–2657.

34. Pagley PR, Beller GA, Watson DD, Gimple LW, Ragosta M. Improved outcome after coronary bypass surgery in ischemic cardiomyopathy and residual myocardial viability. Circulation 1997;96:793–800.

35. White HD, Norris RM, Brown MA, Brandt PWT, Whitlock RML, Wild C. Left ventricular end systolic volume as the major determinant of survival after recovery of myocardial infarction. Circulation 1987;76:44–51.

36. Migrino RQ, Young JB, Ellis SG, et al. End-systolic volume index at 90 to 180 minutes into reperfusion therapy for acute myocardial infarction is a strong predictor of early and late mortality. The Global Utilization for Streptokinase and t-PA for Occluded Coronary Arteries (GUSTO)-I Angiographic Investigators. Circulation 1997;96:116–121.

37. Hamer AW, Takaiama M, Abraham RA, et al. End systolic volume and long term survival after coronary artery by pass surgery in patients with impaired left ventricular function. Circulation 1994;90:2899–2904.

38. Yamaguchi A, Ino T, Adachi H, et al. Left ventricular volume predicts postoperative course in patients with ischemic cardiomyopathy. Ann Thorac Surg 1998;65:434–438.

39. Dor V. The endoventricular circular patch plasty ("Dor procedure") in ischemic akinetic dilated ventricles. Heart Failure Rev 2001;6:187–193.

40. Young A, Dougherty A, Bogen D, et al. Validation of tagging with MR imaging to estimate material deformation. Radiology 1993;188:101–108.

41. Hetzer R, Müller J, Weng Y, et al. Midterm follow-up of patients who underwent removal of a left ventricular assist device after cardiac recovery from end-stage dilated cardiomyopathy. AATS April 1999.

13 The Total Artificial Heart in the Surgical Management of Congestive Heart Failure

Jack G. Copeland, MD,
Francisco A. Arabia, MD,
and Richard G. Smith, MSEE, CEE

CONTENTS

INTRODUCTION
DEVICE DESCRIPTION
INDICATIONS
IMPLANTATION
DEVICE MANAGEMENT, PATIENT CONDITION
SURVIVAL, QUALITY OF LIFE, FUTURE USES
REFERENCES

INTRODUCTION

The idea of completely replacing both ventricles of the heart with an orthotopic mechanical substitute for the treatment of severe heat failure is probably as old as the first understanding of cardiac anatomy and function. However, the first clinical use of such a device dates back less than half a century. In 1969, after considerable animal experimentation, Cooley implanted the Liotta heart (Table 1). Twelve years later, he implanted another total artificial heart (TAH), designed by Akutsu *(1)*. Neither of these desperately ill patients survived for more than a

From: *Contemporary Cardiology: Surgical Management of Congestive Heart Failure*
Edited by: J. C. Fang and G. S. Couper © Humana Press Inc., Totowa, NJ

Table 1
World Experience With TAHs as of September 1, 2001

Device	Time frame	Centers	Implants	Transplants	Discharged
Liotta	1969	1	1	1	0
Akutsu	1981	1	1	1	0
Jarvik 7-100	1982–1992	10	44	26	16
Phoenix	1985	1	1	1	0
Penn State	1985–1989	1	4	1	0
Jarvik 7-70	1985–1992	30	159	120	69
Berlin	1986–1990	1	7	2	0
Unger	1986–1990	3	4	2	0
Vienna	1989	1	2	1	1
Brno	1988–1990	3	6	3	0
Poisk	1987–1990	3	16	3	2
CardioWest	1993–2001	10	203	131	115
Phoenix-7	1998	1	2	1	1
Abiomed	2001	1	2	N/A	N/A
Total			452	293	204

N/A, not applicable.

few days. One year later, in 1982, DeVries and his team implanted the Jarvik-100 TAH. This experience with four "permanent" implants demonstrated surprisingly long survivals (2), but was complicated by device endocarditis and subsequent strokes.

Since that experience, 452 TAHs with 11 different names have been implanted. Of the 452 TAHs, 406 have been the basic device that came from Dr. Kolff's laboratory in Salt Lake City, Utah: the Jarvik-7, now renamed the CardioWest TAH. In August 1985, at the University of Arizona, we had the first survival of a bridge-to-transplant patient with a TAH, using this device to support a patient for 9 days prior to cardiac transplantation. He lived for 4.5 years after heart transplantation (3). More than 44 patient-years of implantation have been accumulated with this TAH, 27 with the CardioWest TAH (Tables 2 and 3).

There are currently two types of TAH implanted: the CardioWest TAH and the AbioCor TAH. The CardioWest TAH, a pneumatic device that discussed in detail in this chapter, is approved for commercial distribution in Europe and Canada and is on the verge of such approval in the United States. Marketing of this device has been on hold pending US Food and Drug Administration (FDA) approval. In the interim, experience with this device has been confined to a few centers, which have now accumulated more than 10,000 patient implant days (Tables 2 and 3). In contrast, the AbioCor device, a

Table 2
World Experience With Total Artifical Hearts by Device

Device type	Implants[1]	Days[2]	Years[3]
CardioWest C-70	203	>10,000	27
Symbion J 7-70	159	4000	11
Symbion J 7-100	44	2000	6
Penn State	4	400	1
Poisk	16	100	0.3
AbioCor	2	60	0.2
Berlin	7	60	0.2
Unger	6	50	0.1
Total	441	>16,000	>45

[1]Total number of human implants.
[2]Total duration of implantation in days.
[3]Number of patient-years accumulated.

Table 3
CardioWest Implantation Experience by Center

Center	Implants (on)[1]	Transplants	Discharged[2]	Alive[3]	Average (Range)[4]
Arizona	60 (3)	42 (75%)	38 (91%)	33 (87%)	90 (0–413)
LaPitie	72 (1)	40 (56%)	30 (75%)	26 (87%)	29 (0–268)
Loyola	17	12 (71%)	11 (92%)	9 (82%)	28 (0–123)
Nantes	19 (1)	11 (61%)	11 (100%)	11 (100%)	74 (1–224)
Ottawa	14	14 (100%)	14 (100%)	13 (93%)	16 (1–37)
All centers	203 (7)	131 (67%)	115 (88%)	102 (89%)	47 (0–413)

[1]Number of patients on device support in parentheses.
[2]Discharged to home after transplantation.
[3]Number of patients currently alive.
[4]Average length of implantation in days and range of implant time in days.

totally implantable electrohydraulic TAH, has been implanted in only 10 patients in four centers (Jewish Hospital of Louisville, Kentucky; Texas Heart Institute, Houston; Hahnemann University Hospital, Philadelphia; University of California at Los Angeles).

The extensive experience with the CardioWest TAH provides information on the indications, usefulness, complications, quality of life, and survival that may be helpful in determining the role of a TAH in patients with congestive heart failure (CHF). These data also form the basis for comparison to other circulatory support devices, such as the

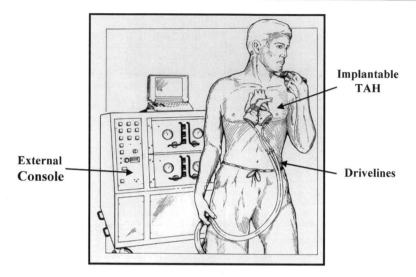

Fig. 1. Drawing to scale of the CardioWest TAH and console.

extracorporeal pulsatile, implantable pulsatile, and continuous flow ventricular assist devices. The remainder of this chapter therefore addresses the use of the CardioWest TAH in CHF.

DEVICE DESCRIPTION

The CardioWest TAH is an orthotopic, biventricular, pneumatic, pulsatile blood pump *(4)*. As shown in Fig. 1, it replaces the native ventricles. It is attached to the left and right atrial cuffs with individual "quick connectors" (elastic polyurethane couplers over rigid ventricular valve mounts) that couple to their respective ventricles. Blood passes through this almost imperceptible junction from the atrium, across a 27-mm Medtronic-Hall valve, to the ventricular chamber. The spherical chamber is lined with segmented polyurethane. The outer chamber is a semirigid polyurethane-lined housing that does not move. The inner chamber contains a four-layer polyurethane diaphragm driven by air pressure. The diaphragm moves toward a rigid plastic wall as the ventricle fills with blood in diastole and toward a 25-mm Medtronic-Hall outflow valve in systole, ejecting about 55 to 60 cc per beat. Blood flows through the outflow valves into woven Dacron conduits to the respective great vessels.

Dacron-covered drivelines exit through tunnels in the left epigastrium and connect to a driver console. This console contains a backup driver, multiple alarms, an internal compressed air supply, and a laptop monitor. The monitor provides beat-to-beat monitoring of ventricular filling, ejection pressure, heart rate, cardiac output on both the left and right sides, and trend monitoring of cardiac output (Fig. 2). The console is mobile within the hospital, allowing patients to attend daily cardiac rehabilitation classes and to ambulate outside. There are at least two portable consoles under development that are compatible with out-of-hospital life. The company plans to use these consoles once commercial approval for the device and large console have been obtained in the United States.

INDICATIONS

Indications that clearly favor the use of an orthotopic TAH in patients with end-stage CHF include incessant malignant arrhythmias, thrombus in the left ventricle, impaired right ventricular (RF) function, acquired ventricular septal defect, the "stone heart," severe rejection of a transplanted heart, diseases of the right ventricle (i.e., arrhythmogenic RF dysplasia), aortic insufficiency, mitral stenosis, and tricuspid stenosis. The TAH has been called the ultimate solution to arrhythmias because both native ventricles are removed and replaced. Situations that result in virtual nonfunction of both ventricles, such as profound rejection and the stone heart, have no better mechanical solution. The niche for TAH use in end-stage heart failure may be quite broad.

Oz and colleagues *(5)* at Columbia University in New York City have reported the influence of preoperative risk factors on postoperative survival in patients with left ventricular assist device (LVAD; Heart-Mate). They found significantly increased risk in those patients with central venous pressure (CVP) above 16 mmHg, urine output less than 30 cc per hour, elevated serum creatinine, and elevated Acute Physiology and Chronic Health Evaluation (APACHE) II scores.

Our own univariate and multivariate stepwise logistic regression analyses of preimplant risk factors comparing the TAH, LVAD, and biventricular assist device supported these findings. In the LVAD group, the predictors of poor outcome were CVP above 20 mmHg, serum creatinine above 2.0 mg/dL, and an APACHE II score of above 28. None of these variables was significant in the TAH group *(6,7)*. CVP in these very sick inotrope-supported heart failure patients seems to be a reasonable way to select those with "right heart failure" (RHF). In addition to the data from Columbia, there seems to be a general consensus among LVAD users that RHF occurs in up to 25% of LVAD cases, and it is associated with a very high mortality rate if present after LVAD implantation.

When we retrospectively compared our LVAD and TAH results *(8)*, we found the mean preimplant CVP for the CardioWest patients was 20 mmHg vs 14 mmHg in the LVAD patients. Thus, the CardioWest recipients had evidence of preimplant RHF, but the LVAD preimplant patients did not; yet, the survival rate was higher in the TAH patients. This observation fits with the experience we have had with LVADs vs TAHs in critically ill patients and the reason that we implant the TAH in all of those with RHF. We reserve LVADs for patients who are "more stable" and lack evidence of RHF *(8)*. Our recommended indications for the TAH in severe congestive heart failure include unstable hemodynamics (rapid decline), failure to wean from cardiopulmonary bypass, cardiac arrest, RHF, pulmonary edema, CVP above16 mmHg, creatinine above 2.0 mg/dL, as well as those conditions mentioned at the beginning of this section. The only qualification is that the TAH must fit in the patient's mediastinum.

Size criteria for the CardioWest TAH include one or more of the following: 70 mm or larger LV end-diastolic dimension by echo, a cardiothoracic ratio above 0.5, a computerized tomographic scan anterior–posterior dimension at T-10 from posterior sternum to anterior vertebral column of 10 cm or more, and a body surface area (BSA) of 1.7 m^2. In general, a combination of BSA over 1.7 m^2 and a "large heart" by one other criterion from this list was a reliable predictor of a "good fit."

Data from the ongoing FDA study of the CardioWest TAH demonstrate that the typical patient has a BSA of 2.0 m^2, a cardiac index of 1.6 L/min/m^2, and a CVP of 19 mmHg. The patient is generally on multiple inotropes (often more than 10 µg/kg/min of dobutamine and/or 3 µg/kg/min dopamine), including milrinone, epinephrine, and/or norepinephrine. Such patients are critically ill and demonstrate high-dose diuretic resistance and hemodynamic instability with minimal patient movement despite escalating degrees of hemodynamic and medical support.

IMPLANTATION

The implantation technique has been previously described in detail *(9)*. Primary considerations include achieving excellent hemostasis,

Fig. 2. *(see facing page)* The console and the laptop screen, which displays driveline pressure (upper left), ventricular filling rate with respect to time (upper right), and, in the second row, heart rate, left fill volume, right fill volume, left cardiac output, and right cardiac output. On the left bottom are average left cardiac output; on the bottom is the average right cardiac output. To the right of these is a trend display of left- and right-sided outputs.

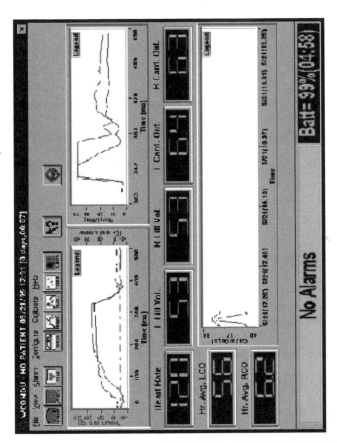

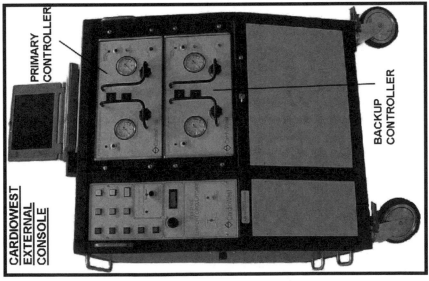

CARDIOWEST
EXTERNAL
CONSOLE

PRIMARY CONTROLLER

BACKUP CONTROLLER

307

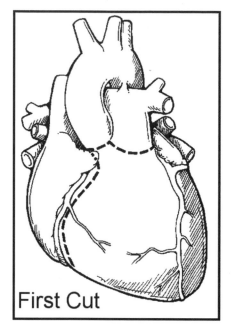
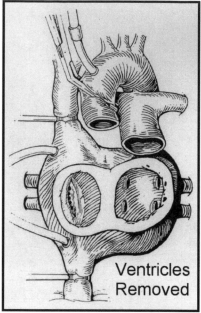

Fig. 3. Lines of resection of the native heart and appearance after ventriculectomy.

good fitting and positioning of the two ventricles, and preparing for explantation.

Briefly, the cardiectomy is made on the ventricular side of the atrioventricular (AV) groove. The great vessels are transected at the sinotubular junctions (Fig. 3). The atrial cuffs are buttressed with an 8-mm Teflon felt band sewn to the free walls (Fig. 4). The gathering stitch includes the Teflon felt, all cut edges that might otherwise bleed, and the endocardium/AV valve remnant on the atrial side. The atrial quick connectors (flanges trimmed to 6 mm) are then sewn to the respective cuffs.

We begin with the elastic connector inverted and then evert them after completing both suture lines. We next anastomose the great vessel conduits. The lengths of the great vessel conduits beyond the connectors are usually 2 to 3 cm for the aorta and 5 to 6 cm for the pulmonary artery. Finally, we check the suture lines for leaks with saline under pressure and then connect the ventricles (Fig. 5). One recent change in

Fig. 4. *(see facing page)* Left: The Teflon felt buttress is sewn in place. Middle: **(A)** The inverted atrial connectors are sewn to the atrial cuffs; **(B)** appearance of the everted connectors after the anastomoses. Right: Appearance of the aortic outflow conduit with proximal connector sewn to the aorta.

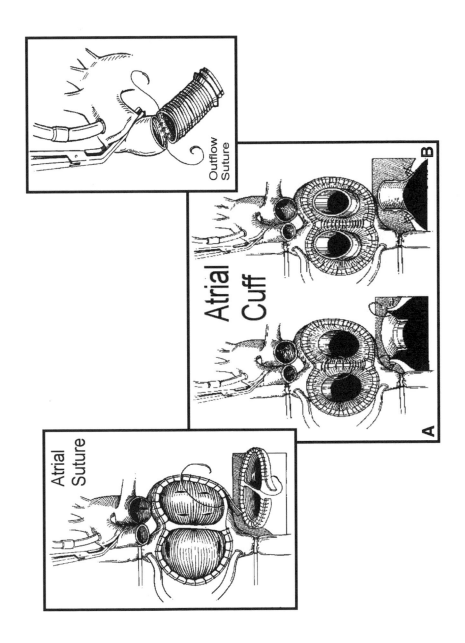

Outflow Suture

Atrial Cuff

B

A

Atrial Suture

309

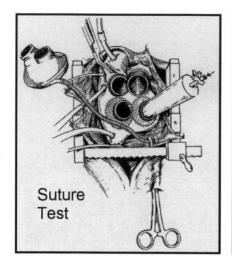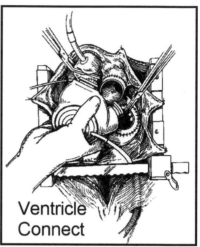

Fig. 5. Left: Testing the suture lines for leaks. Right: connecting the left ventricle.

our technique has been to cover the device, native atrial cuffs, and aorta with 0.1-mm thick extended polytetrafluoroethylene material *(10)*. This creation of a synthetic membrane neopericardium has facilitated explantation and has not, in our early experience with 16 patients, caused clinical infection.

Before cardiopulmonary bypass is discontinued, deairing of the left side is done with a vent in the aorta and the patient in steep Trendelenburg position. After discontinuation of cardiopulmonary bypass, outputs are generally high. Vacuum is not used to facilitate ventricular filling until the chest is closed and chest tubes are placed on suction. As the chest is closed, we look very carefully at the cardiac output and transesophageal echocardiography. The most common problems arise in patients who are too small for the device. Chest closure in this group may cause the right ventricular atrial connector to compress the inferior vena cava and/or the LV atrial connector to compress the left-sided pulmonary veins. Sudden drop in cardiac output and the appearance of flow turbulence by trans-esophageal echo in the inferior vena cava or the left pulmonary veins would indicate the need for device repositioning.

DEVICE MANAGEMENT, PATIENT CONDITION

Most patients have a cardiac output of 6 to 7 L per minutes at the end of the implant procedure, with a CVP in the range of 12 to 15 mmHg.

The systemic vascular resistance is maintained with intravenous vaso-active agents in the range of 700 to 1000 dyne-s-cm^{-5} (e.g., nitroglycerin or nitroprusside for vasodilation and norepinephrine for vasoconstriction). Usually, the vasoactive support is discontinued within 48 hours. Cardiac outputs rise and stay at 7 to 8 L per minute (mean cardiac index of 3.0 L/min/m^2).

Patients are extubated within 3 days, out of bed walking within 3.5 days, able to walk more than 100 feet within 11 days, and discharged from intensive care in 11 days. Within the first week, arterial and central venous lines are removed. Patients participate in cardiac rehabilitation three to five times per week; this includes treadmill walking, use of a stationary bicycle, and upper extremity exercises. They do not have RHF or problems with arrhythmias. They also do not experience symptomatic orthostatic changes in pressure or low output alarms, which are common with LVADs. Finally, they do not have nutritional problems from the presence of a large LVAD compressing the stomach.

In the more than 80 FDA CardioWest study patients, the blood urea nitrogen and creatinine returned to normal and remained normal after postimplant day 25. Total bilirubin fell to normal levels by day 20. Plasma free hemoglobin stayed constant at 8 mg/dL, and the hematocrit was constant over time at 26%. The mean body weight fell by 6 kg in the first 3 weeks, but rose by 4 kg by week 7.

Standard settings on the controller are 200 mmHg LV pressure, 60 mmHg RV pressure, 10 cm H$_2$O vacuum pressure, 50% systole, and beat rate of 120 beats per minute (bpm). Early on, these settings are rarely changed, and after the first week, almost never are changed. The laptop monitor provides continuous assessment of driveline pressure and ventricular diastolic volume (fill volume) as well as cardiac output (the product of the fill volume and the bpm rate).

We try to maintain maximal cardiac outputs based on the concept that high flows discourage thrombus formation. The driveline (ventricular) pressures are set high enough to accommodate sudden rises in peripheral pressures (left driveline pressure is set 60 mmHg higher than the patient's blood pressure; right driveline pressure is set 30 mmHg higher than estimated pulmonary artery pressure). When the ventricular diaphragm has a full excursion (full eject), a small isovolumic pressure rise appears at the end of the pressure curve, indicating full ejection. Vacuum, percentage systole (the percentage of the cardiac cycle taken by systole), and beat rate are set so that ventricular filling is about 85% of the maximal of 70 cc. This allows the device to have reserve to accommodate increased venous return and to exhibit a Starling principle in response to increased filling. In summary, the device is set to provide 85% filling and to eject fully with each beat.

Anticoagulation is based on the prothrombin time, international normalized ratio, partial thromboplastin time, platelet count, hematocrit, platelet activation studies, bleeding time, and thromboelastogram. The anticoagulants used are heparin (generally for the first 1–2 weeks), warfarin (begun just before heparin discontinuation), aspirin, dipyridamole, and pentoxifylline. This strategy has been discussed elsewhere *(4)*. Anticoagulation guidelines include normal coagulability assessed by thromboelastogram, normal reactivity to collagen in platelet aggregometry, and a bleeding time of 17 to 23 min. In 56 patients from September 1994 to September 2001, the incidence of stroke not associated with implant or explant was 1 case (0.08 events/patient-year or 0.007 events/patient-month). There were three additional strokes related to implantation (0.33 events per patient-year). Thus, thromboembolism during device support was extremely rare.

Bleeding, defined as requiring reoperation or requiring 8 or more units of blood within 48 hours, has been almost completely confined to the first postimplant week. The incidence has been 33%. This incidence is attributable to a number of factors. Many of the implant recipients have some element of synthetic liver dysfunction. Many patients have also been anticoagulated as part of their chronic preimplant therapy or for recent operations. Furthermore, balancing heparin therapy early postimplant in the face of ongoing coagulopathies can occasionally lead to excessive bleeding and complications such as atrial tamponade.

Perioperative antibiotic management is the same prophylactic routine as we use in all open heart cases. We do not routinely use any other regimen. As of mid-September 2001, we had seen two clinical infections of the mediastinum (on the basis of positive blood cultures), one bacterial (*Staphylococcus aureus*) and one fungal (*Candida* species). Both infections were treated with continuous intravenous therapy until the time of transplant. Both patients are long-term survivors.

Another theoretical issue is the percutaneous driveline potential for infection. Our experience and those of other investigators suggest that the Dacron covering of the drivelines stimulates marked tissue ingrowth. We have found driveline removal at explant/transplant to be very difficult because of an abundance of healthy adhesions around the Dacron. We have never seen an ascending infection along a driveline. We have seen only superficial infections at the skin level, which are treated topically with antiseptic and cleansing. We do use systemic antibiotics if we find a persistent pathogen.

SURVIVAL, QUALITY OF LIFE, FUTURE USES

The picture of a patient transformed from dying with end-stage CHF to a stable, well-fed individual on the CardioWest TAH who exercises daily and interacts with family and friends within the confines of the hospital and immediate surroundings is at once dramatic and limited. It is a miraculous transition. These patients can reach an oxygen consumption of 12–14 cc/kg per minute on treadmill testing. Renal and hepatic functions return to normal. Pulmonary edema disappears. Serum albumin returns to normal, and the patients start gaining lean body mass. On the other hand, they are bound to a large console and cannot be discharged to home. They await a transplant that represents another brutal hurdle toward a more normal life.

With the CardioWest, 61 to 75% of implanted patients (131 of 203 = 64.5%) have survived for an average of 47 days (range 16 to 90) on device support to receive a transplant (Table 3). Of those who were transplanted, 115 (88%) survived to discharge, and 102 are currently alive. In our national trial, 89% of the bridge-to-transplant patients with CardioWest survived long term compared to 33% ($p < 0.00001$) of matched historical controls transplanted without a mechanical circulatory support device *(11)*. Other subsequent studies have also demonstrated that the TAH as a bridge-to-transplant device prolongs life in very sick patients and is comparable to LVADs and paracorporeal biventricular assist devices in this role. In our own retrospective comparison of these three types of devices, it was clear that the TAH was more effective in sicker patients than the other two devices *(8)*.

What are the prospects for the CardioWest in the future? A portable system (Fig. 6) has been developed and may be used clinically in the near future. A wearable system is also under development. This portability should allow out-of-hospital living, improve the quality of life substantially, and open the possibility for "permanent" implantation. The longest survivor on a TAH (Symbion) lived 603 days, dying in 1988 of a ruptured cerebral aneurysm. There have been 10 other implants of 225 days or longer, 9 of whom survived to transplant. The longest implant time preceding successful heart transplantation was 414 days. These figures suggest that permanent implantation may be reasonable, especially when considering the technical difficulty, morbidity, and mortality (12%) of an explant/transplant operation. This concept is particularly robust in view of the low incidence of stroke (0.08 per year) with the use of multidrug anticoagulation therapy.

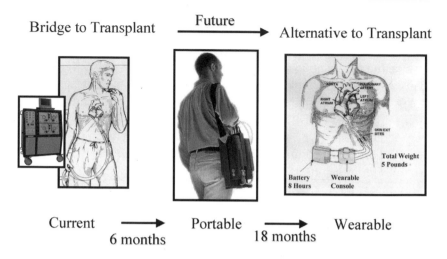

Fig. 6. Consoles for the CardioWest. Current console is on the left. A portable console of the type currently available is in the middle. On the right is a wearable console currently under development.

In summary, the past experience with the TAH has been promising. We have found the implantation of a CardioWest TAH, by providing high cardiac outputs in acutely and chronically ill patients, has led to recovery of vital organs and an improved nutritional status. Simultaneous mechanical support of the left- and right-sided circulations allows for optimal outputs free from the influences encountered with LVADs, such as RHF, low outputs, and recurrent arrhythmias. It also permits optimal transcapillary perfusion pressure (mean systemic pressure, CVP), facilitating vital organ perfusion and recovery. Bridge to transplantation with the TAH has proved effective and reasonably safe in an extremely sick group of patients. Future commercialization, portability, and permanent implantation should provide for extension of life of a good quality in properly selected patients.

REFERENCES

1. Cooley DA, Liotta D, Hallman GL, Bloodwell RD, Leachman RD, Milam JD. Orthotopic cardiac prosthesis for two-staged cardiac replacement. Am J Cardiol 1969;24:723–730.
2. DeVries WC, Anderson JL, Joyce LD, et al. Clinical use of the total artificial heart. N Engl J Med 1984;310:273–278.
3. Copeland JG, Levinson MM, Smith R, et al. The total artificial heart as a bridge to transplantation. JAMA 1986;256:2991–2995.

4. Copeland J, Arabia F, Smith R, Nolan P. Intracorporeal support: the CardioWest total artificial heart. In: Goldstein DJ, Oz MC, eds. Cardiac Assist Devices. Futura, Armonk, NY: 2000, pp. 341–355.

5. Oz MC, Goldstein DJ, Pepino P, et al. Screening scale predicts patients successfully receiving long-term implantable left ventricular assist devices. Circulation 1995;92(9 suppl):II169–II173.

6. Mehta VK, Copeland JG, Arabia FA, Smith RG, Banchy M. Analysis of preoperative comorbid factors associated with biventricular assist device and total artificial heart: a single center experience. J Heart Lung Transplant 2000;19:65.

7. Mehta VK, Copeland JG, Arabia FA, Banchy ME, Smith RG. Mechanical ventricular support as bridge to transplant: risk factor and selection. ASAIO J 2000; 46:192.

8. Copeland JG, Smith RG, Arabia FA, et al. Comparison of the CardioWest total artificial heart, the Novacor left ventricular assist system and the Thoratec ventricular assist system in bridge to transplantation. Ann Thorac Surg 2001;71 (3 suppl):S92–S97.

9. Arabia FA, Copeland JG, Pavie A, Smith RG. Implantation technique for the CardioWest total artificial heart. Ann Thorac Surg 1999;68:698–704.

10. Copeland JG, Arabia FA, Smith RG, Covington D. Synthetic membrane neopericardium facilitates total artificial heart explantation. J Heart Lung Transplant 2001;20:654–656.

11. Copeland JG, Arabia FA, Banchy ME, et al. The CardioWest total artificial heart bridge to transplantation: 1993 to 1996 national trial. Ann Thorac Surg 1998;66: 1662–1669.

INDEX

SENSE OF
EVIL

BANTAM BOOKS BY KAY HOOPER

The Bishop Trilogies
STEALING SHADOWS
HIDING IN THE SHADOWS
OUT OF THE SHADOWS

TOUCHING EVIL
WHISPER OF EVIL
SENSE OF EVIL

The Quinn Novels
ONCE A THIEF
ALWAYS A THIEF

Romantic Suspense
AMANDA
AFTER CAROLINE
FINDING LAURA
HAUNTING RACHEL

Classic Fantasy and Romance
ON WINGS OF MAGIC
THE WIZARD OF SEATTLE
MY GUARDIAN ANGEL
(anthology)
YOURS TO KEEP
(anthology)

KAY HOOPER

SENSE OF
EVIL

BANTAM BOOKS

SENSE OF EVIL
A Bantam Book / August 2003

Published by Bantam Dell
A Division of Random House, Inc.
New York, New York

Book design by Lynn Newmark

Library of Congress Cataloging in Publication Data
Hooper, Kay.
Sense of evil./Kay Hooper.
p. cm.
ISBN 0-553-80300-X
I. Title

PS3558.O587 S46 2003
2003056270
813/.54 21

Manufactured in the United States of America
Published simultaneously in Canada

BVG   10   9   8   7   6   5   4   3   2   1

This one is for Jeff and Tommy,
my shopping buddies.
Mostly because they didn't believe
I'd put them in a book.
Hey, guys!

ACKNOWLEDGMENTS

This time out, Bishop and his Special Crimes Unit owe even greater thanks than usual to the fantastic Team Bantam, whose members worked above and beyond the call of duty to put this story into your hands.

A grateful author wishes to thank Irwyn Applebaum and Nita Taublib, Bill Massey and Andie Nicolay, Kathy Lord, and all the other hardworking professionals in production who made this book possible.

Words aren't enough, but they'll have to do.

Thanks again.

PROLOGUE

THE VOICES WOULDN'T leave him alone.

Neither would the nightmares.

He threw back the covers and stumbled from the bed. A full moon beamed enough light into the house for him to find his way to the sink in the bathroom.

He carefully avoided looking into the mirror but was highly conscious of his shadowy reflection as he fumbled for a drinking cup and turned on the tap. He drank three cups of water, vaguely surprised that he was so thirsty and yet . . . not.

He was usually thirsty these days.

It was part of the change.

He splashed his face with the cold water, again and again, not caring about the mess he was making. By the third splash, he realized he was crying.

Wimp. Spineless coward.

"I'm not," he muttered, sending the next handful of water to wet his aching head.

You're afraid. Pissing-in-your-pants afraid.

Half-consciously, he pressed his thighs together. "I'm not. I can do it. I told you I could do it."

Then do it now.

He froze, bent over the sink, water dribbling from his cupped hands. "Now?"

Now.

"But . . . it's not ready yet. If I do it now—"

Coward. I should have known you couldn't go through with it. I should have known you'd fail me.

He straightened slowly, this time looking deliberately into the dim mirror. Even with moonlight, all he could make out was the shadowy shape of his head, dark blurs of features, faint gleam of eyes. The murky outline of a stranger.

What choice did he have?

Just look at yourself. Wimp. Spineless coward. You'll never be a real man, will you?

He could feel water dripping off his chin. Or maybe it was the last of the tears. He sucked in air, so deep his chest hurt, then let it out slowly.

Maybe you can buy a backbone—

"I'm ready," he said. "I'm ready to do it."

I don't believe you.

He turned off the taps and walked out of the bathroom. Went back to his bedroom, where the moonlight spilled through the big window to spotlight the old steamer trunk set against the wall beneath it. He knelt down and carefully opened it.

The raised lid blocked off some of the moonlight, but he didn't need light for this. He reached inside, let his fingers search gingerly until they felt the cold steel. He lifted the knife and held it in the light, turning it this way and that, fascinated by the gleam of the razor-sharp, serrated edge.

"I'm ready," he murmured. "I'm ready to kill her."

The voices wouldn't leave her alone.

Neither would the nightmares.

She had drawn the drapes before going to bed in an effort to close out the moonlight, but even though the room was dark, she was very conscious of that huge moon painting everything on the other side of her window with the stark, eerie light that made her feel so uneasy.

She hated full moons.

The clock on her nightstand told her it was nearly five in the morning. The hot, sandpapery feel of her eyelids told her she really needed to try to go back to sleep. But the whisper of the voices in her head told her that even trying would be useless, at least for a while.

She pushed back the covers and slid from her bed. She didn't need light to show her the way to the kitchen, but once there she turned on the light over the stove so she wouldn't burn herself. Hot chocolate, that was the ticket.

And if that didn't work, there was an emergency bottle of whiskey in the back of the pantry for just such a night as this. It was probably two-thirds empty by now.

There had been a few nights like this, especially in the last year or so.

She got what she needed and heated the pan of milk slowly, stirring the liquid so it wouldn't stick. Adding in chocolate syrup while the milk heated, because that was the way she liked to make her hot chocolate. In the silence of the house, with no other sounds to distract her, it was difficult to keep her own mind quiet.

She didn't want to listen to the whispering there, but it was like catching a word or two of an overheard conversation and *knowing* you needed to listen more closely because they were talking about you.

Of course, some people would call that paranoia. Had called it. And at least part of the time, maybe they weren't wrong.

But only part of the time.

She was tired. It got harder and harder, as time went on, to bounce back. Harder for her body to recover. Harder for her mind to heal.

Given her druthers, she would put off tuning in to the voices until tomorrow. Or the next day, maybe.

The hot chocolate was ready. She turned off the burner and poured the steaming liquid into a mug. She put the pan in the sink, then picked up her mug and carried it toward the little round table in the breakfast nook.

Almost there, she was stopped in her tracks by a wave of red-hot pain that washed over her body with the suddenness of a blow. Her mug crashed to the floor, landing unbroken but spattering her bare legs with hot chocolate.

She barely felt that pain.

Eyes closed, sucked into the red and screaming maelstrom of someone else's agony, she tried to keep breathing despite the repeated blows that splintered bones and shredded lungs. She could taste blood, feel it bubbling up in her mouth. She could feel the wet heat of it soaking her blouse and running down her arms as she lifted her hands in a pitiful attempt to ward off the attack.

I know what you did. I know. I know. You bitch, I know what you did—

She jerked and cried out as a more powerful thrust than all the rest drove the serrated knife into her chest, penetrating her heart with such force she knew the only thing that stopped it going deeper still was the hilt. Her hands fumbled, touching what felt like blood-wet gloved hands, large and strong. The hands retreated immediately to leave her weakly holding the handle of the knife impaling her heart. She felt a single agonized throb of her heart that forced more blood to bubble, hot and thick, into her mouth, and then it was over.

Almost over.

She opened her eyes and found herself bending over the table, her hands flat on the pale, polished surface. Both hands were covered with blood, and between them, scrawled in her own handwriting across the table, was a single bloody word.

HASTINGS

She straightened slowly, her entire body aching, and held her hands out in front of her, watching as the blood slowly faded until it was gone. Her hands were clean and unmarked. When she looked at the table again, there was no sign, now, of a word written there in blood.

"Hastings," she murmured. "Well, shit."

1

RAFE SULLIVAN ROSE from his crouched position, absently stretching muscles that had begun to cramp, and muttered, "Well, shit," under his breath.

It was already hot and humid even just before noon, the sun burning almost directly overhead in a clear blue sky, and he absently wished he'd had his people put up a tarp to provide some shade. The effort wouldn't be worthwhile now; another half hour, and the coroner's wagon would be here.

The body sprawled at his feet was a bloody mess. She lay on her back, arms wide, legs apart, spread-eagled in a pathetically exposed, vulnerable position that made him want to cover her up—even though she was more or less dressed. Her once-white blouse was dull red, soaked with blood and still mostly wet despite the heat, so that the coppery smell was strong. The thin, springlike floral skirt was eerily undamaged but blood-soaked,

7

spread out around her hips, the hem almost daintily raised to just above her knees.

She had been pretty once. Now, even though her face was virtually untouched, she wasn't pretty anymore. Her delicate features were contorted, eyes wide and staring, mouth open in a scream she probably never had the chance or the breath to utter. From the corners of her parted lips, trails of blood ran down her cheeks, some of it mixing with the golden strands of her long blond hair and a lot of it soaking into the ground around her.

She had been pretty once.

"Looks like he was really pissed this time, Chief. Bit like the first victim, I'd say." Detective Mallory Beck made the observation dryly, seemingly unmoved by the gory scene before them.

Rafe looked at her, reading the truth in her tightened lips and grim eyes. But all he said was, "Am I wrong, or did this one fight him?"

Mallory consulted her notebook. "Doc just did the preliminary, of course, but he says she tried. Defensive injuries on the victim's hands, and one stab wound in her back—which the doc says was probably the first injury."

Shifting his gaze to the body, Rafe said, "In the back? So she was trying to turn—or run—away from him when he stabbed her the first time. And either he turned her around so he could finish her face-to-face or she turned herself trying to fight him."

"Looks like it. And only a few hours ago; we got the call on this one earlier than the others. The doc estimates the time of death as around five-thirty this morning."

"Awfully early to be up and out," Rafe commented. "Caleb opens his office between nine-thirty and ten as a rule. She was still his paralegal, right?"

"Right. Normally went to the office around nine. So she was

out very early. What I don't get is how he was able to lure her this far away from the road. You can see there are no drag marks, and two sets of footprints—we have good casts, by the way—so she walked out here with him. I'm no Daniel Boone, but I'd say from her tracks that she was walking calm and easy, not struggling or hesitating at all."

Rafe had to admit that the ground here looked remarkably calm and undisturbed, for the most part, especially considering the violence of what had been done to the victim. And after last night's rain all the tracks were easily visible. So this murder scene, like the last one, clearly illustrated what had happened here.

From all appearances, twenty-six-year-old Tricia Kane had gotten out of her own car around dawn at an unofficial rest spot off a normally busy two-lane highway and then walked with a companion—male, according to all likelihood as well as an FBI profile—about fifty yards into the woods to this clearing. And then the companion had killed her.

Brutally.

"Maybe he had a gun," Rafe suggested, thinking aloud. "Or maybe the knife was enough to keep her docile until they got this far."

Mallory frowned. "You want my hunch, I say she didn't see that knife until they reached this clearing. The instant she saw it, she tried to run. That's when he got her."

Rafe didn't know why, but that was his hunch too. "And it's the same way he got the other two. Somehow he persuaded these women to leave their cars and walk calmly into the woods with him. Smart, savvy women who, from all accounts, were way too careful to let any stranger get that close."

"Which means they probably knew him."

"Even if, would *you* leave your car and just stroll into the woods with some guy? Especially if you knew two other women had recently died under similar circumstances?"

"No. But I'm a suspicious cop." Mallory shook her head. "Still, it doesn't make sense. And what about the cars? All three women just left their cars on pull-off rest areas beside fairly busy highways and walked away from them. Keys in the ignition, for Christ's sake, and not many do that even in small towns these days. And we don't know whether he was with them when they stopped or somehow flagged them down and *then* persuaded them to come with him. No tracks out at the rest stop to speak of with all that hard dirt and packed gravel."

"Maybe he pulled a Bundy and claimed to need their help."

"Could be. Although I still say that would have worked loads better if they knew who was asking. This guy isn't killing strangers. I think the profilers got that one right, Chief."

With a sigh, Rafe said, "Yeah, me too. I hate like hell the idea that this bastard is local rather than some insane stranger passing through town, but I don't see any other way to explain how he's getting these women to go with him."

"Unless he's some kind of authority figure they'd be inclined to trust and obey on sight. Like a cop."

"Oh, hell, don't even suggest that," Rafe responded so instantly that Mallory knew the possibility had already been in his mind.

She studied him unobtrusively as he scowled down at the body of Tricia Kane. At thirty-six, he was the youngest chief of police ever in Hastings, but with a solid background in law enforcement both in training and experience, nobody doubted Rafe Sullivan's qualifications for the job.

Except maybe Rafe himself, who was a lot smarter than he realized.

Mallory had wondered more than once if his tendency to

doubt himself and his hunches had anything to do with his looks. He wasn't exactly ugly—but she had to admit that his self-described label of "thug" pretty much fit. He had a harsh face, with very sleepy, heavy-lidded eyes so dark they tended to make people uncomfortable. His nose had been broken at least twice, he had a sharp jaw with a stubborn jut to it, and his high cheekbones marked him indelibly with his Celtic ancestry.

He was also a very big man, several inches over six feet tall and unmistakably powerful. The kind of guy you wanted on your side no matter what the fight was about. So he definitely looked the part of a cop, in or out of uniform—and it was mostly out, since he disliked uniforms as a rule and seldom wore his. But anyone, Mallory had long ago discovered, who had him pegged as all brawn and no brain or who expected the stereotypical dense, cud-chewing Southern cop was in for a surprise, sooner or later.

Probably sooner. He didn't suffer fools gladly.

"That's three murders in barely three weeks," he was saying, dark eyes still fixed on the body at their feet. "And we're no closer to catching the bastard. Worse, we've now officially got a serial killer on our hands."

"You thinking what I'm thinking?"

"I'm thinking it's time we yelled for help."

Mallory sighed. "Yeah, that's what I'm thinking."

Quantico

Isabel Adams made her voice as persuasive as she possibly could, and her well-rehearsed arguments sounded damned impressive if she did say so herself, but when she finally fell silent she wasn't surprised that Bishop didn't respond right away.

He stood at the window gazing out, only his profile visible to

Isabel. In deference to the fact that he was actually on FBI terri- tory, he was dressed more formally than was usual, and the dark suit set off his dark good looks and powerful build admirably. Is- abel looked at Miranda, who was sitting on Bishop's desk, idly swinging one foot. Even more of a maverick than her husband and far less deferential to the FBI in any sense, she was wearing her usual jeans and sweater, the casual outfit doing nothing to disguise startling beauty and a centerfold body that turned heads wherever she went.

She gazed at Bishop now, seemingly waiting as Isabel waited for his answer, but her electric-blue eyes were very intent, and Is- abel knew there was communication between the two of them on a level that didn't require speaking aloud. Whatever Bishop's de- cision turned out to be, he would arrive at it only after Miranda's views and recommendations were added to his own; although Bishop had far greater seniority in the Bureau and in the unit he had created and led, no one doubted that his partnership with Miranda was equal in every possible sense of the word.

"It's not a good idea," he said finally.

Isabel said, "I know all the arguments against my going."

"Do you?"

"I've gone over all the material that police chief sent when he requested a profile after the second murder. I even got on-line and read the local newspaper articles. I think I've got a very good feel for the town, for what's happening down there."

Miranda said, "Your basic powder keg, just waiting for a match."

Isabel nodded. "Small town on the teetering edge of panic. They seem to have a lot of faith in their police, especially the chief, and pretty fair medical and forensics facilities for a small town, but this latest murder has everybody jumping at shadows and investing in security systems. And guns."

She paused, then added, "Three murders makes this a serial killer in Hastings. And he's showing no signs of stopping now. Chief Sullivan just officially requested the FBI's help, and he's asking for more than an updated profile. Bishop, I want to go down there."

Bishop turned at last to face them, though instead of returning to his desk he leaned back against the high windowsill. The scar on his left cheek was visible now, and Isabel had been with the unit long enough to recognize, in its whitened appearance, that he was disturbed.

"I know what I'm asking," she said, more quietly than she might otherwise have spoken.

Bishop glanced at Miranda, who immediately looked at Isabel and said, "From all indications, this is the sort of killer that local law enforcement can handle with very little outside help. Maybe a bit more manpower to ask questions, but it'll be inside knowledge that catches this animal, not an outsider's expertise. The profile marks him as nothing out of the ordinary. He's local, he's killing local women he knows, and he's bound to make a mistake sooner rather than later."

"But it wasn't an SCU profile," Isabel pointed out. "None of us developed it."

"Special Crimes Unit can't develop all the requested profiles," Bishop reminded her patiently. "We barely have the manpower to handle the cases we do get."

"We didn't get the call on this one because this killer is so seemingly ordinary, I know that. Around a hundred serial killers active in this country on average at any time, and he's one of them. Nothing raised a red flag to indicate that our special abilities are needed in the investigation. But I'm telling you—there's more to the case than the official profile picked up on. A lot more." She paused, then added, "All I'm asking is that you take a look at the material for yourselves, both of you. Then tell me I'm wrong."

Bishop exchanged another glance with Miranda, then said, "And if you're right? Isabel, even if the SCU took on this investigation, given the circumstances in Hastings you're the last agent I'd want to send down there."

Isabel smiled. "Which is why I have to be the agent you send. I'll go get the file."

She left without waiting for a reply, and as Bishop returned to his desk and sat down, he muttered, "Goddammit."

"She's right," Miranda said. "At least about being the one who has to go."

"Yeah. I know."

We can't protect her.

No. But if this is what I think it is . . . she'll need help.

"Then," Miranda said calmly, "we'll make sure she has help. Whether she likes it or not."

Thursday, June 12, 2:00 PM

"Chief, are you saying we *don't* have a serial killer?" Alan Moore, reporter for the Hastings *Chronicle,* had plenty of practice in making his voice carry without shouting, and his question cut through the noise in the crowded room, silencing everyone else. More than thirty pairs of expectant eyes fixed on Rafe.

Who could cheerfully have strangled his boyhood chum. With no particular inflection in his voice, Rafe answered simply, "We don't know what we have as yet, except for three murdered women. Which is why I'm asking you ladies and gentlemen of the press not to add unnecessarily to the natural anxiety of our citizens."

"In this situation, don't you think they should be anxious?" Alan glanced around to make certain all attention was on him, then added, "Hey, I'm blond, and even I'm nervous. If I were a twenty-something blond *woman*, I'd be totally freaked out."

"If you were a twenty-something blond woman we'd all be freaked out," Rafe said dryly. He waited for the laughter to subside, fully aware of the fact that it was as much nervous as amused. He was good at taking the pulse of his town, but it didn't take any particular skill to feel the tension in this room. In the town.

Everybody was scared.

"Look," he said, "I know very well that the women here in Hastings are worried—whether they're blond, brunette, redhead, or any shade in between—and I don't blame them a bit. I know the men in their lives are worried. But I also know that uncontrolled speculation in the newspaper and on the radio and other media will only feed the panic."

"Uncontrolled?"

"Don't start yelling censorship, Alan. I'm not telling you what to print. Or what not to print. I'm asking you to be responsible, because there is a very fine line between warning people to be concerned and take precautions, and yelling fire in a crowded theater."

"Do we have a serial killer?" Alan demanded.

Rafe didn't hesitate. "We have three murders we believe were committed by the same person, fitting the established criteria for a serial killer."

"In other words, we have a lunatic in Hastings," somebody he didn't recognize muttered just loud enough to be heard.

Rafe responded to that as well, still calm. "By definition a serial killer is judged conventionally if not clinically to be insane, yes. That doesn't mean he'll be visibly any different from you or me. And they seldom wear horns or a tail."

The reporter who'd made the lunatic comment grimaced. "Okay, point taken. Nobody is above suspicion and let's all freak out." She was blond.

"Let's all take care, not freak out," Rafe corrected. "Obviously, we would advise blond women in their mid to late twenties to take special care, but we have no way of knowing for certain if age and hair color are factors or merely a coincidence."

"I say err on the side of factor," she offered wryly.

"And I can't say I'd blame you for that. Just keep in mind that at this point there is very little we can be sure of—except that we have a serious problem in Hastings. Now, since a small-town police department is hardly trained or equipped to deal with this type of crime, we have requested the involvement of the FBI."

"Have they provided a profile?" This question came from Paige Gilbert, a reporter with one of the local radio stations. She was more brisk and matter-of-fact than some of the other women in the room had been, less visibly uneasy, possibly because she was brunette.

"Preliminary. And before you ask, Alan, we won't be sharing the details of that profile unless and until the knowledge can help our citizens. At this stage of the investigation, all we can realistically do is advise them to take sensible precautions."

"That's not much, Rafe," Alan complained.

"It's all we've got. For now."

"So what's the FBI bringing to the table?"

"Expertise: the Special Crimes Unit is sending agents trained and experienced in tracking and capturing serial killers. Information: we will have access to FBI databases. Technical support: medical and forensics experts will study and evaluate evidence we gather."

"Who'll be in charge of the investigation?" Alan asked. "Doesn't the FBI usually take over?"

"I'll continue to head the investigation. The FBI's role is assistance and support, no more. So I don't want to read or hear any BS about federal officials superceding states' rights, Alan. Clear?"

Alan grimaced slightly. He was a good reporter and tended to be both fair and even-handed, but he was close to phobic about governmental "interference," especially from the federal level, and was always loud in protest whenever he suspected it.

Rafe took a few more questions from the assembled reporters, resigned rather than surprised to find that several of the people were from TV stations in nearby Columbia. If the investigation was getting major state coverage now, it was only a matter of time before it went national.

Great. That was just great. The last thing he wanted was to have the national press looking over his shoulder and second-guessing every decision he made.

Bad enough he had Alan.

"Chief, do you believe this killer is local?"

"Chief, has anything else turned up linking the victims?"

"Chief . . ."

He answered the questions almost automatically, using variations of "no comment" or "we have no reliable information on that" whenever possible. Even though he had called the press conference himself, it was only because he'd gotten wind of some pretty wild speculation going on and hoped to head off the worst of it before it was in print or other media, not because he had any real progress to report.

He was concentrating on the crowd in front of him as he answered their questions, but even as he did, he felt an odd change in the room, as if the very air had somehow sharpened, freshened. Cleared. It was a weird feeling, like waking suddenly from a dream thinking, *Oh, that wasn't real. This is real.*

Something had changed, and he had no idea if it was for better or worse.

From the corner of his eye, he caught a glimpse of movement and was able to turn his head just a bit, casually, so that none of the reporters picked up on his suddenly diverted attention.

Still, he was surprised that no one else seemed to have observed her entrance, even though she came into the room from the hallway, behind the flock of reporters. Rafe doubted she went unnoticed very often. He saw her pause to speak briefly to one of his officers, producing what appeared to be an I.D. folder, saw Travis's visible surprise and undoubtedly stuttering response, then saw her move past him and take up a position near the door. She scanned the crowd of reporters and their tangle of cameras, a small half smile that was not so much amused as it was rueful playing around her mouth. She was dressed casually and for the weather in jeans and a sleeveless top, her hair pulled up into a neat ponytail. She could easily have been one of the reporters.

She wasn't.

When her gaze met his fleetingly across the crowded room, Rafe was conscious of an instant certainty that made him go cold to his bones.

No. The universe couldn't hate him that much.

"Chief, could you—"

He cut off the question abruptly. "Thank you all very much for coming today. When there are further developments, you'll be notified. Good afternoon."

He stepped away from the podium and went straight through the crowd to the other side of the room, ignoring the questions flung after him. When he reached her, his statement was brief and to the point.

"My office is across the street."

"Lead the way, Chief." Her voice was as extraordinary as the rest of her, one of those smoky, husky bedroom voices a man would expect to hear if he called a 900 sex-talk line.

Rafe wasted no time in leading the way past his still-goggling officer, saying merely, "Travis, make sure nobody bothers the mayor on their way out."

"Yeah. Okay. Right, Chief."

Rafe started to ask him if he'd never seen a woman before, but since that would have resulted in either stuttering incoherence or else a lengthy explanation that would have boiled down to "Not a woman like this one," he didn't bother.

He also didn't say a word as they left the town-hall building and walked across Main Street to the police department, although he did notice that she was a tall woman; wearing flat sandals she was only a few inches shorter than he was, which would put her at about five-ten.

And her toenails were polished red.

With most of his people out on patrol, the station wasn't very busy; Mallory was the only detective at her desk in the bullpen, and though she looked up with interest as they passed, she was on the phone, and Rafe didn't pause or greet her except with a nod.

His office looked out onto Main Street, and as he went around behind his desk he couldn't help a quick glance to see whether the reporters had left the town hall. Most were still clustered out in front, some obviously recording spots for today's evening news and others speaking to each other—speculating, he knew. It didn't bode well for his hopes of keeping things calm in Hastings.

An I.D. folder dropped onto his blotter as he sat down, his visitor taking one of the chairs in front of his desk.

"Isabel Adams," she said. "Call me Isabel, please. We're pretty informal. Nice to meet you, Chief Sullivan."

He picked up the folder, studied the I.D. and federal badge inside, then closed it and pushed it across the desk toward her. "Rafe. Your boss saw the profile, right?" was his terse response.

"My boss," she answered, "wrote the profile. The updated one, that is, the one I brought with me. Why?"

"You know goddamned well why. Is he out of his mind, sending *you* down here?"

"Bishop has been called crazy on occasion," she said in the same pleasant, almost careless tone, not visibly disturbed by his anger. "But only by those who don't know him. He's the sanest man I've ever met."

Rafe leaned back in his chair and stared across the desk at the special agent sent by the FBI to help him track and capture a serial killer. She was beautiful. Breath-catching, jaw-dropping gorgeous. Flawless skin, delicate features, stunning green eyes, and the kind of voluptuous body most men could expect to encounter only in their dreams.

Or in their nightmares.

In Rafe's nightmares.

Because Isabel Adams was also something else.

She was blond.

The voices were giving him a pounding headache. It was something else he was getting used to. He managed to unobtrusively swallow a handful of aspirin but knew from experience it would only take the worst edge off the pain.

It would have to be enough.

Have to.

Still exhausted from the morning's activities, he managed to do his work as usual, speak to people as though nothing out of the ordinary had happened. Nobody guessed, he was certain of that.

20

He'd gotten very good at making sure nobody noticed anything out of the ordinary.

You think they don't all see? Don't all know?

That was the sneering voice, the dominant one, the one he hated most and heard most often. He ignored it. It was easier to do that now, when he was drained and oddly distant from himself, when the only thing for him to do, really, was wait for his next opportunity.

They know who you are. They know what you did.

That was more difficult to ignore, but he managed. He went about his business, listening whenever possible to the nervous gossip. Everybody was talking about the same thing, of course. The murders.

Nobody talked of anything else these days.

He didn't hear much he hadn't already known, although the speculation was amusing. Theories, most of them absurd, abounded as to why the killer was targeting blondes.

A hatred of his mother, for Christ's sake.

Rejection by a blond girlfriend.

Idiots.

The pharmacist downtown told him there'd been a run on hair color, that those women trying blond as an option were going back to their natural colors.

He wondered if the natural blondes were considering changing, but thought probably not. They liked the effect, liked knowing men were watching them. It gave them a sense of power, of . . . superiority.

None of them could imagine dying because of it.

He thought that was funny.

He thought that was funny as hell.

2

RAFE SAID, "Please don't tell me the general idea is for you to be bait."

"Oh, I'm probably too old to tempt him."

"If you're past thirty, I'll eat my hat."

"Salt and pepper?"

Rafe stared at her, and she chuckled.

"I'm thirty-one. And, no, that isn't the idea. I'll do a lot for king and country, but I don't have a death wish."

"Done anything to piss off this Bishop of yours?"

"Not lately."

"Has the profile changed?"

"Not as far as this animal's fixations go. He's still after white females with blond hair, and he's likely to stay within the age range of twenty-five to thirty-five. He apparently likes them smart and savvy as well as strong, which is an interesting twist on the stereotypical image of helpless dumb blondes as victims."

Rafe said something profane under his breath.

Ignoring that, Isabel went on briskly, completely professional now. "He's someone they know or at least obviously believe they can trust. Possibly an authority figure, maybe even a cop—or impersonating one. He's physically strong, though he won't necessarily look it; he might even appear effeminate."

"Why effeminate?" Rafe was listening intently, his eyes narrowed.

"These women were killed brutally, with a viciousness that suggests both a hatred of women and doubts or fears about his own sexuality. All three were sexual crimes—deep, penetrating wounds and targeting the breasts and genitals are classic signs of a sexual obsession—and yet none of the women was raped. That, by the way, will probably be his next escalation, raping as well as killing."

"And if he's impotent? This sort of killer often is, right?"

Isabel didn't hesitate. "Right. In that case, an object rape, possibly even with the murder weapon. And it will be postmortem; he doesn't want his victim to see his possible sexual failure. In fact, he'll probably cover her face, even after he kills her."

"So he's a necrophiliac as well."

"The whole nasty bag of tricks, yeah. And he will be escalating, count on it. He's got the taste for it now. He's enjoying himself. And he's feeling invulnerable, maybe even invincible. He's likely to begin mocking us—the police—in some way."

Rafe thought about all that for a moment, then asked, "Why blondes?"

"We don't know. Not yet. But it's very possible that his first victim—Jamie Brower, right?"

"Right."

"Twenty-eight-year-old real-estate broker. It's very likely, we believe, that something about her was the trigger. Maybe something she did to him, that's possible. An emotional or psychological rejection of some kind. Or something he saw, something she made him feel, whether or not she was aware of doing so. We believe she was a deliberate choice, not merely a random blonde."

"Because she was the first victim?"

"That, plus the uncontrolled violence of the attack. According to the crime-scene photos and ME's report you sent us, she was riddled with stab wounds."

"Yes." Rafe's lips tightened as he remembered.

"The wounds were ragged, multiple angles, but virtually all of them so deep the hilt or handle of the knife left bruises and imprints in her skin. He was in a frenzy when he killed her. With the second and third victims, except for some minor defensive injuries, most of the wounds were concentrated in the breast and genital areas; Jamie Brower had injuries to her face and wounds from her neck to her lower thighs."

"It was a bloodbath."

"Yes. That sort of fury usually means hatred, very specific, very personal hatred. He wanted to kill *her*. Not just a blonde, not just a representation of his killing fantasy. Her. We believe that by focusing the investigation on the life and death of Jamie Brower, we're likely to uncover facts or evidence that will help us to identify her killer."

"Focusing on her how? We've accounted for all her movements the week before she was killed."

"We'll have to go further back than that. Months, maybe even years; the pressure built inside him for a while before he acted, and during that time their paths crossed."

"If she was the trigger."

Isabel nodded. "If she was the trigger."

"And if she wasn't?"

Isabel shrugged. "Still a valid, even critical, investigative approach, knowing who the victim was. Who all of them were. We won't understand him until we understand the women he's killing. Something more than superficial appearance connects them."

"They were all unusually successful at their jobs," Rafe said, relaying the information without the need to consult any file or notes. "Jamie had been Broker of the Year with her company the past three years; Allison Carroll had been recognized both locally and statewide as an outstanding teacher; and Tricia Kane not only had a very good job as a paralegal to one of our most successful attorneys but also was a very talented artist gaining regional recognition."

"It might be the public recognition of their abilities as much as their success that drew his interest," Isabel mused. "They stood in a spotlight, lauded for their achievements. Maybe that's what he likes. Or doesn't like."

"You mean he could be punishing them for their success?"

"It's a possibility. Also a possibility that he was attracted to them because of their success and was rejected by them when he expressed his interest."

"Men get rejected all the time. They don't turn to butchery."

"No. The vast majority don't. Which is a good thing, don't you think?"

Rafe frowned slightly, but she was going on before he could comment.

"It means this particular man has some serious, deep-seated emotional and psychological problems, which have apparently lain dormant or at least were hidden here in Hastings until about three weeks ago."

25

"Hence the trigger."

Isabel nodded. "There's no question about that, not as far as we're concerned. Something *happened*. To him, in his life. A change. Whether it was an actual event or a paranoid delusion on his part remains to be seen. But something set him off. Something definitive."

Rafe glanced at his watch, wondering if there was time today to visit all three crime scenes.

"Starting with the actual crime scenes," Isabel said, "would probably be the best way to go. According to the map I studied, they're within a five-mile area. And it's still hours till sunset, so we have time."

"Where's your partner?" Rafe asked. "I was told there'd be at least two of you."

"She's settling in. Wandering around, getting a feel for the town."

"Please tell me she isn't blond."

"She isn't." Isabel smiled. "But if you're wondering, she doesn't resemble the conventional FBI *suit* any more than I do. The SCU really is an unusual unit within the Bureau, and few of us conform to any sort of dress code unless we're actually on FBI grounds. Casual and understated are sort of our watchwords."

Rafe eyed her but decided not to comment on that. "And do you normally show up unarmed?"

"Who says I'm unarmed?" She lifted one hand and gently wiggled her fingers, each one adorned with a neat, but hardly understated, red-polished oval nail.

Hearing the faint note of mockery in her voice, Rafe sighed and said, "Let me guess. Martial-arts expert?"

"I've trained," she admitted.

"Black belt?"

"Got that when I was twelve." She smiled again. "But if it

makes you feel better, I'm also wearing a calf holster—usually my backup, since my service automatic is worn in a belt holster. Our unit doesn't break all the rules, just some of them; on duty, we're expected to be armed. Since I was taking a casual look around town, a visible weapon would have been a bit conspicuous, I thought."

Rafe had noticed that her jeans were very close-fitting from waist to knees, so he couldn't help asking, "Can you get to that weapon in a hurry if you have to?"

"You'd be surprised."

He wanted to tell her he wasn't sure he could take too many more surprises but instead said only, "We've set up a conference room here as a base of operations, so all the reports, evidence, and statements are there. Couple of good computers with high-speed Internet access, plenty of phones. Standard supplies. Anything else that's needed, I'll get."

"In a situation like this, the city fathers generally say to hell with the budget."

"Which they pretty much did."

"Still, you and I both know it'll come down to basic police work, so the budget is likely to go toward overtime rather than anything fancier. As for the crime scenes, I really would like to take a look at them today. And it would help if it's just you and me out there this time. The fewer people around me when I'm studying a crime scene, the better."

"Fewer distractions?"

"Exactly."

"We've kept the scenes roped off," Rafe said, "but I'd bet my pension that at least a dozen kids have tramped all over them despite the warnings. Or because of them."

"Yeah, kids tend to be curious about crime scenes, so that's to be expected."

More than a little curious himself, Rafe said, "It's rained since we found Tricia Kane's body on Monday; what do you expect to find?"

"I'm not likely to find anything you and your people missed," Isabel replied, her matter-of-fact tone making it an acknowledgment rather than a compliment. "I just want to get a sense of the places, a feel for them. It's difficult to do that with only photographs and diagrams."

It made sense. Rafe nodded and rose to his feet, asking, "What about your partner?"

"She may want to take a look at the scenes later," Isabel said, getting up as well. "Or maybe not. We tend to come at things from different angles."

"Probably why your boss teamed you up."

"Yes," Isabel said. "Probably."

Caleb Powell wasn't a happy man. Not only had he lost his efficient paralegal to the killer stalking Hastings, he had also lost a friend. There hadn't been the slightest romantic spark between Tricia and him, particularly since she was almost young enough to be his daughter, but there had been an immediate liking and respect from the day she first began working for him almost two years before.

He missed her. He missed her a lot.

And since the temp he had hired was still trying to figure out Tricia's filing system—and kept coming to him with questions about it—his office wasn't exactly his favorite place to be right now. All of which explained why he was sitting in the downtown coffee shop sipping an iced mocha and staring grimly through the front window at the media-fest still going on across the street at the town hall.

"Vultures," he muttered.

"They have their jobs to do."

He looked at the woman seated at the next table, not really surprised she had responded to his comment because people did that in small towns. Especially when there were only two customers in the place at the time. He didn't recognize her, but that didn't surprise him either; Hastings wasn't *that* small.

"Their jobs stop when they cross the line between informing the public and sensationalizing a tragedy," he said.

"In a perfect world," she agreed. "Last time I checked, we didn't live in a perfect world."

"No, that's true."

"So we have to cope with less than the ideal." She smiled faintly. "I've even heard it said that the world would be better off without lawyers, Mr. Powell."

Just a bit wary now, he said, "You have me at a disadvantage."

"Sorry. My name is Hollis Templeton. I'm with the FBI."

That did surprise him. An attractive brunette with a short, no-fuss hairstyle and disconcertingly clear blue eyes, she looked nothing at all like a tough federal cop. Slender almost to the point of thinness, she was wearing a lightweight summer blouse and floral skirt, an outfit eerily like the one Tricia had reportedly worn the day she was killed.

His disbelief must have been obvious; with another faint smile, she drew a small I.D. folder from her purse and handed it across to him.

He had seen a federal I.D. before. This one was genuine. Hollis Templeton was a Special Investigator for the FBI.

He returned the folder to her. "So this isn't a coincidental meeting," he said.

"Actually, it is." She shrugged. "It was hot as hell outside, so I came in for iced coffee. And to watch the circus across the street. I recognized you, though. They ran your photo in the local paper Tuesday after Tricia Kane was killed."

"As you noted, Agent Templeton, I'm a lawyer. I don't really appreciate impromptu interviews with federal officials."

"But you do want to find out who killed Tricia."

He noticed that she didn't deny it was an interview. "I also don't appreciate typical law-enforcement tactics and questions designed to *encourage* me to talk carelessly to a cop."

"Take all the care you like. If a lawyer doesn't know how much is . . . safe . . . to disclose, nobody does."

"I think I find that offensive, Agent Templeton."

"And I think you're awfully touchy for a man with nothing to hide, Mr. Powell. You know the drill better than most. We'll be talking to everyone who knew Tricia Kane. You were her employer and her friend, and that puts you pretty high up on our list."

"Of suspects?"

"Of people to talk to. Something you know, something you saw or heard, may be the key we'll need to find her killer."

"Then call me in to the police station for a formal interview or come see me at my office," he said, getting to his feet. "Make an appointment." He left a couple of dollars on the table and turned away.

"She liked tea instead of coffee, and took it with milk. You always thought that was odd."

Caleb turned back, staring at the agent.

"She always felt she had disappointed her father by not becoming a lawyer, so being a paralegal was a compromise. It gave her more time for her art. She had asked you to pose for her, but you kept putting her off. And about six months ago, you offered her a shoulder to cry on when her relationship with her boyfriend ended badly. You were working late at the office when she broke down, and afterward you drove her home. She fell asleep on the couch. You covered her with an afghan and left."

Slowly, he said, "None of that was in the police report."

"No. It wasn't."

"Then how the hell do you know?"

"I just do."

"How?" he demanded.

Instead of replying to that, Hollis said, "I saw some of her work. Tricia's. She was talented. She might have become very well known if she'd lived."

"Something else you *just* know?"

"My partner and I got into town last night. We've checked out a few things. Tricia's apartment, for one. Nice place. Really good studio. And some of the paintings she'd finished were there. I . . . used to be an artist myself, so I know quality work when I see it. She did quality work."

"And you read her diary."

"She didn't keep one. Most of the artists I know don't. Something about images as opposed to words, I guess."

"Are you going to tell me how you know what you know?"

"I thought you didn't want to talk to me, Mr. Powell."

His mouth tightened. "What I think is that alienating me is not at all a good idea, Agent Templeton."

"It's a risk," she admitted, not noticeably disturbed by that. "But one I'm willing to take if I have to. You're smart, Mr. Powell. You're very, very smart. Too smart to play dumb games. And at the end of the day I'd really rather not have you as an enemy, never mind the fact that you know all the legal angles and could keep us at arm's length for a long time."

"You think I'd do that? Potentially put other lives in danger by withholding information?"

"You tell me."

After a moment, Caleb crossed the few feet separating them and sat down in the second chair at her table. "No. I wouldn't. And not only because I'm an officer of the court. But I don't know anything that could help you find this killer."

"How can you be so sure of that? You don't even know what questions we want to ask you." She shook her head slightly. "You aren't a suspect. According to Chief Sullivan's report, you have a verifiable alibi for the twenty-four hours surrounding Tricia Kane's murder."

"What the thrillers like to call a cast-iron alibi. I spent the weekend in New Orleans for a family wedding and didn't fly back here until Monday afternoon. I got the news about Tricia when Rafe called me at my hotel around noon."

"And a companion places you in your hotel room from just before midnight until after eight that morning," Hollis said matter-of-factly. "She's positive you never left the room."

Without at all planning to, Caleb heard himself say, "A former girlfriend."

"Former?" Her voice was wry.

A bit defensive despite himself, he said, "We also happen to be old friends, what my father used to call scratch-and-sniff buddies. We see each other, we end up in bed. Happens about twice a year, since she lives in New Orleans. Where we both grew up, and where she practices law, which makes her highly unlikely to per-jure herself. Any other nuggets you want to mine from my per-sonal life, Agent Templeton?"

"Not at the moment."

"Too kind."

She didn't react to his sarcasm except with another of those little smiles as she said, "About Tricia Kane. Do you think her ex-boyfriend might have wanted to hurt her?"

"I doubt it. She never said he was violent or in any way abusive, and I never saw any signs of it. Besides, unless he slipped back into town in the last three weeks, he's out of the picture. They broke up because he thought his pretty face could earn him screen time in Hollywood and he didn't want Tricia along for what he was convinced was going to be a wild and award-winning ride."

"Sounds painful for her."

"It was. Emotionally. She went home for lunch that day and found him packing to leave. That's when he told her he was going. Until that moment, she'd believed they would end up married."

"Since then had she ever talked about a particular man?"

"I don't think she was even dating. If so, she never mentioned it. She was concentrating on her painting when she wasn't at the office."

"Do you know if anything unusual had happened lately? Strange phone calls or messages, someone she'd noticed turning up wherever she went, that sort of thing?"

"No. She seemed fine. Not worried, not stressed, not upset by anything. She seemed fine."

"There was nothing you could have done," Hollis said.

Caleb drew a deep breath and let it out slowly. "Oh, I have no illusions, Agent Templeton. I know how quickly random acts of violence can snuff out lives, no matter how careful we think we are. But those acts tend to be committed by stupid or brutal people, for stupid and brutal reasons. This is different. This bastard is pure evil."

"I know."

"Do you?"

She smiled an odd, twisted smile, and her blue eyes had an equally strange, flat shine to them that made Caleb feel suddenly uneasy. "I know all about evil, Mr. Powell, believe me. I met it up close and personal."

Thursday, 3:30 PM

Isabel stood gazing around the clearing where Tricia Kane's body had been found. It was mostly in shade now that the sun was no longer directly overhead, which she appreciated since the day was hot and humid. She was conscious of Rafe Sullivan's scrutiny, but she had been at this too long to allow him to distract her.

Much.

Both the blood and the chalk used to mark body position and location had been washed away by the rain, but she didn't need either to know exactly where Tricia Kane had suffered and died. She looked down just inches from her feet, her gaze absently tracing the shape of something—someone—that was no longer there.

She had been here, in this sort of place, so many times, Isabel thought. But it never got any easier. Never.

"He got her in the back," she said, "then jerked her around by the wrist and began driving the knife into her chest. The first blow to her chest staggered her backward, the second put her on the ground. She was losing blood so fast she didn't have the strength to fight him off. She was all but gone when he began stabbing her in the genital area. And either her skirt came up when she fell, or else he jerked it out of the way when he began stabbing her, since the material wasn't slashed. He pulled the skirt back down when he was done. Odd, that. Protecting her modesty, or veiling his own desires and needs?"

Rafe was frowning. "The ME says she died too fast to leave any bruises, but he told me privately he felt she'd been jerked around and held by one wrist. It wasn't in his report."

Isabel looked at him, weighing him for a moment, then smiled. "I get hunches."

"Yeah?" He crossed powerful arms over his chest and lifted both eyebrows inquiringly.

"Okay, they're a little more than hunches."

"Is this where the *special* in Special Crimes Unit comes in?"

"Sort of. You read the Bureau's brief on our unit, right?"

"I did. It was nicely murky, but the gist I got is that the unit is called in when a judgment is made that the crimes committed are unusually challenging for local law enforcement. That SCU agents use traditional as well as *intuitive* investigative methods to solve said crimes. By *intuitive* I gather they mean these *hunches* of yours?"

"Well, they couldn't very well announce that the SCU is made up mostly of psychics. Wouldn't go over very well with the majority of cops, considering how . . . um . . . levelheaded you guys tend to be. We've discovered through bitter experience that proving what we can do is a lot more effective with you guys than just claiming our abilities are real."

"So why're you telling me?"

"I thought you could take it." She lifted an eyebrow at him. "Was I wrong?"

"I'll let you know when I make up my mind."

"Fair enough."

"So I gather you don't normally inform local law enforcement of this?"

"Depends. It's pretty much left up to our judgment. The assigned team, I mean. Bishop says you can't plan some things in advance, and whether or not to spill the beans—and when—is one of them. I've been on assignments where the local cops didn't have a clue, and others where they were convinced, by the time we left, that it was some kind of magic."

35

"But it isn't." He didn't quite make it a question.

"Oh, no. Perfectly human abilities that simply don't happen to be shared by everyone. It's like math."

"Math?"

"Yeah. I don't get math. Never have. Balancing my checkbook stresses me out like you wouldn't believe. But I always liked science, history, English. Those I was good at. I bet you're good at math."

"It doesn't stress me out," he admitted.

"Different strokes. People have strengths and weaknesses, and some have abilities that can look amazing because they're uncommon. There aren't a lot of Mozarts or Einsteins, so people marvel at their abilities. Guy throws a hundred-mile-an-hour fastball and puts it over the plate three out of five pitches, and he's likely to be set for life, because very few people can do what he does. Gifts. Rare, but all perfectly human."

"And your gift is?"

"Clairvoyance. The faculty of perceiving things or events beyond normal sensory contact. Simply put, I know things. Things I shouldn't be able to know—according to all the laws of conventional science. Facts and other bits of information. Conversations. Thoughts. Events. The past as well as the present."

"All that?"

"All that. But more often than not it's a random jumble of stuff, like the clutter in an attic. Or like the chatter of voices in the next room: you hear everything but really catch only a word or two, maybe a phrase. That's where practice and training come in, helping make sense of the confusion. Learning to see the important objects in that cluttered attic or isolate that one important voice speaking in the next room."

"And you use this . . . ability? In investigating crimes, I mean."

"Yes. The Special Crimes Unit was formed to do just that. For most of us, becoming a part of the unit was the first time in our lives that we didn't feel like freaks."

Rafe thought that much, at least, made sense. He could understand how people with senses beyond the "normal" five might feel more than a little alienated from society. Having a useful and rewarding job and a place where they were considered entirely normal had probably changed their lives.

Isabel didn't wait for his response, just went on in that slightly absentminded tone. "There's been very little study into the paranormal, really, but we've built on that with our own studies and field experience. We've developed our own definitions and classifications within the SCU, as well as defined degrees of ability and skill. I'm a seventh-degree clairvoyant, which means I have a fair amount of ability and control."

Rafe watched as she knelt down and touched the ground, no more than an inch or so from where Tricia Kane's blond hair had lain. "Touching the ground helps?" he asked warily.

"Touching things sometimes helps, yeah. Objects, people. It's better when the area is contained, enclosed, but you work with what you've got. The ground is pretty much the only thing left out here, so . . ." She looked up at him and smiled, though her eyes held a slightly abstracted expression. "Not magic. Maybe we're just a lot more connected to this world and to one another than we think."

It was hot, the way it is now. But barely light. She could smell the honeysuckle. But that's all . . . all she could get about the murder, at least. That and her certain sense of something dark and evil crouching, springing . . . But only that. Isabel wasn't really surprised. This place was wide open, and they were always the toughest.

He watched her intently. "What do you mean?"

He had very dark eyes, she thought. "We leave footprints when we pass. Skin cells, stray hairs. The scent of our cologne lingering in the air. Maybe we leave more than that. Maybe we leave energy. Even our thoughts have energy. Measurable electromagnetic energy. Today's science admits that much."

"Yeah. And so?"

"Our theory is that psychics are able to tap into electromagnetic fields. The earth has them, every living thing has them, and many objects seem to absorb and hold them. Think of it as a kind of static electricity. Some people get shocked more often than others. I get shocked a lot."

"Are you getting shocked now?"

Isabel straightened and brushed the dirt off her hand. She was frowning slightly. "It'd be easier if the clairvoyant bits came in neon, but they don't. That cluttered attic. That noisy party in the next room. In the end it's usually just a jumble of information, stuff I could have read or heard or been told."

Rafe waited for a moment, then said, "Except?"

"Except . . . when the information comes in the form of a vision. That *is* in neon. Sometimes in blood."

"Not literally?"

"Afraid so. It's rare for me, but it does happen from time to time. In the case of a murder, it's as if I become the victim. I see or hear—or sometimes feel—what they do. While they're being killed. I'm told it's a bit startling to watch. Don't freak out if it happens, okay?"

"You're telling me you actually *bleed*?"

"Sometimes. It fades away pretty fast, though. Like I said, don't let it bother you."

"Don't let it bother me? Cops see blood, Isabel, we tend to freak out. In a controlled, professional manner, of course. We take it as a signal that it's time to do our job."

Her eyes sharpened abruptly, and she smiled. "Well, if you see blood on me, resist your instincts. Chances are, it'll belong to somebody else."

"In Hastings, chances are it'll be yours. Unless you want to color your hair for the duration."

"Wouldn't help. He already knows."

"Knows what?"

"He's already seen me, Rafe. One of the clairvoyant bits I've picked up. I'm on his A-list."

3

GODDAMMIT, YOU TOLD ME being bait for this bastard wasn't the idea."

"It wasn't the plan. It was always a possibility, of course, but it wasn't the plan."

"Isabel—"

"Besides, it isn't that clear-cut. I said I was on his A-list, but I'm not next. He gets to know his victims before he kills them, Rafe. He doesn't know me. Not yet. And he won't come after me until he does. Or thinks he does."

"Are you willing to bet your life on that?"

She didn't hesitate. "To catch this bastard? Yes."

Rafe took a step toward her. "Have you reported it to your boss? Does he know you're on the A-list?"

"Not yet. I'm scheduled to report in later today. I'll tell him then."

"Will you?" His doubt was obvious.

Isabel chuckled. "Rafe, our unit is made up of psychics. You don't keep secrets, or withhold vital bits of information, when half the team can read your mind. Very few of us have been able to keep anything important from Bishop no matter how far away we were."

"Have you?"

Isabel took a last look down at the ground where Tricia Kane had died, then started toward him with a slight gesture to indicate they might as well walk back to his Jeep. "I thought so once. Just after I first joined the unit. I thought I was being very clever. Turned out he'd known all along. He usually does."

Rafe didn't say anything else until they were in the Jeep and he had turned the air-conditioning on full-blast. "The simplest thing to do," he said, "is to have you recalled and somebody else sent down here. Somebody who won't draw this bastard's attention."

"The simplest thing," Isabel said, "is not always the smartest thing."

"I am not going to stand by while you're dangled on a god-damned hook."

"I told you, I'm not next on his hit parade. But somebody else is. Some woman is walking around in your town right now, Rafe, and a killer is stalking her. My partner and I are up to speed on this investigation. Bishop thought we were the best team to send down here, and his success rate, *our* success rate as a unit, is over ninety percent. We can help you catch him. Send me back, and the next team has to start from scratch. Do you really want to waste that time, especially when this killer is averaging a victim a week so far?"

"Shit." He stared at her grimly. "I'm taking a hell of a lot on faith here. This psychic stuff."

"At least you didn't call it bullshit," she murmured. "That's usually the first reaction."

Ignoring that, he said, "I'm supposed to be okay with you being on our killer's list because you assure me you aren't *next*. That we have time while he stalks his next victim and, not incidentally, finds out enough about you to feel that he knows you. So he can kill you."

"That pretty much sums it up, yeah."

"Convince me. Convince me that this *clairvoyant* knowledge you have is genuine. That it's something I can trust."

"Parlor tricks. It always comes down to parlor tricks."

"I'm serious, Isabel."

"I know you are." She sighed. "You sure you want to do this?"

Suddenly wary again, he asked, "Why wouldn't I be?"

"Because the best way for me to convince you is to open up a connection between us and tell you things about yourself, your life, your past. Things I couldn't possibly know any other way. You might not find that very comfortable. Most people don't."

"Women are dying, Isabel. I think I can endure a little psychic reading."

"Okay. But when we speak of this later—and we will—just remember that I tried to warn you. I get bonus points for that."

"Fine."

She held out a hand, palm up, and Rafe hesitated only an instant before placing his hand on hers. He nearly jerked away when their flesh touched, because there was a literal, visible spark and a definite, if faint, shock. But her fingers closed over his strongly.

Matter-of-factly, she said, "Well, that's new."

Rafe wanted to say something about static, but he was busy having another of those strange feelings, just as he'd had when she walked into the press conference, but much, much stronger.

That a door had opened and a fresh breeze was blowing through. That everything around him was in sharper focus, more real than it had been before. That something had changed.

And he still didn't know if it was a good change or a bad one.

Isabel didn't go into some kind of trance or even close her eyes. But her eyes did take on that abstracted expression he had noticed before, as if she were listening to some distant sound. Her voice remained calm.

"You have an unusual paperweight on your desk at home, some kind of car part encased in acrylic. You prefer cats over dogs, though you don't have either because of your long working hours. You're allergic to alcohol, which is why you don't drink. You're fascinated by the Internet, by the instant communication of people all over the world. You're a movie buff, especially interested in science fiction and horror."

Isabel smiled suddenly. "And you wear a particular style of jockey shorts because of a commercial you saw on TV."

Rafe jerked his hand away. "Jesus," he muttered. Then, getting back on balance, he added somewhat defensively, "You could have found out any of that. All of it."

"Even the jockey shorts?"

"Jesus," he repeated.

She was looking at him steadily, her eyes still faintly abstracted, distant. "Ah, now I understand why the idea of an FBI unit made up of psychics didn't throw you. Your grandmother had what she called 'the sight.' She knew things before they happened."

Rafe looked at his hand, which he had been unconsciously rubbing with the other one, then at her. "You aren't touching me," he noted in a careful tone.

"Yeah, well. Once a connection is made, I tend to pick up stuff from then on."

"Jesus Christ," he said, varying the oath somewhat.

"I tried to warn you. Remember, bonus points."

"I still don't— You could have found out most of that some other way."

"Maybe. But could I have found out that your grandmother told you on your fifteenth birthday that your destiny was to be a cop? It was just the two of you there at the time, so nobody else knew. You believed it was weird, she was weird, because you hadn't thought of being a cop. The family business was construction. That's what you were going to do, especially as you'd been swinging a hammer since you were twelve."

Rafe was silent, frowning slightly.

"She also told you . . . there would come a point in your life when you would have to be very, very careful." Isabel was frowning herself now, head slightly tilted, clearly concentrating. "That there was something important you were meant to do as part of the destiny she saw for you, but it would be dangerous. Deadly dangerous. Something about . . . a storm . . . a woman with green eyes . . . a black-gloved hand reaching . . . and glass shattering."

He drew a breath. "Vague enough."

Isabel blinked, and her green eyes cleared. "According to what our seers have told me, visions often come that way, as a series of images. Sometimes they prove to be literal, other times it's all symbolic. The green-eyed woman could be a jealous woman or someone who resents you or someone else. The black-gloved hand a threat. The storm, violence. Like that."

"Still vague," he insisted. "Any of that is something a cop deals with regularly."

"Well, we'll see. Because I have more than a hunch that what your grandmother saw was this point in your life—otherwise I probably wouldn't have picked up her prediction."

"What do you mean?"

"Patterns are everywhere, Rafe. Events touch other events like a honeycomb, connecting to one another. And seeming coincidences usually aren't. I may pick up some trivial information unrelated to what's going on at present, and not all the stuff I get could even be called hits, but I'm focused on this investigation, this killer—and when that's the case it almost always turns out that most of what I get is relevant to what's going on around me at the time."

"Want to use a few more qualifiers?"

She smiled at his exasperation, though it was more rueful than amused. "Sorry, but you've got to understand we're in frontier territory here. There aren't a whole lot of absolute certainties. Conventional science pretty much sneers at psychic ability, and those who were brave enough to test and experiment found themselves dealing with an unfortunate commonality among psychics."

"Which is?"

"Very few of us perform well under laboratory conditions. Nobody really knows why, that's just the way it is." Isabel shrugged. "Plus, the tests tended to be poorly designed because, to begin with, they didn't know what they were dealing with. How can you effectively measure and analyze something without even knowing how it works? And how do you figure out how it works when you can't *make* it work within a controlled situation?"

"Somebody must have known, or you wouldn't be here. Would you?"

"The SCU wouldn't exist if Bishop hadn't been highly motivated and exceptionally driven to figure out how to use his own abilities to track and capture a serial killer years ago. Once he was able to do that, he believed other psychics could be trained, that we could learn to use our abilities as investigative tools. And that those tools would give us an edge. We're proving it works.

45

Slowly, carefully—and with setbacks now and then. We're also learning as we go.

"What we've found through sheer trial and error in the field is that our abilities function best when we're focused on something compelling—such as a murder investigation. But that doesn't mean we can flip a switch and get exactly the piece of information we need. As with everything else in life, we have to work for it. It's still trial and error."

"So, bottom line, your best guess is that because you *picked up* what my grandmother told me over twenty years ago it means what she saw has something to do with what's happening in my life today. This investigation."

"It's a good bet, based on how my abilities have worked so far. Plus, logically this'll probably be the toughest case of your career, assuming you don't move to a big city and deal often with violent killers. And though I can't speak to the specifics of your grandmother's vision—yet—I can tell you it's going to be dangerous as hell tracking and catching this killer."

Listening to her tone as well as the words, Rafe said, "You picked up something else out there where Tricia Kane was killed, didn't you? What was it?"

She hesitated just long enough to make the internal debate obvious, then said, "What I picked up out there confirmed something I suspected even before I came to Hastings. This town is just his latest hunting ground."

"He's killed before?"

"In at least two previous locations. Ten years ago, he butchered six women in Florida. And five years ago, six women in Alabama."

"Blondes?" Rafe asked.

"No. Redheads in Florida. Brunettes in Alabama. We have no idea why."

"And nobody caught him then."

"Lots tried. But he hit quick—one victim every week, just like here—and then he vanished. Typical serial killer cases, if there is such a thing, usually drag on months, years, and it takes time to get law enforcement organized once a pattern is even noticed. But this monster hit and vanished before the task forces could even get up and running. And he didn't leave so much as a hair behind to help I.D. him, so they had almost nothing to work with."

"Then how do you know it's the same killer?"

"The M.O. The profile. The fact that Bishop himself worked on the second set of murders—one of his very few unsuccessful cases."

"I wasn't told about any of this in the initial profile."

"No. The first profiler wasn't a member of the SCU. And even though the two earlier sets of murders came up on the computer as possibly connected, he discounted them because it was believed at the time that the most likely suspect was killed trying to escape police in Alabama. His car went off a bridge. But they never found the body."

"So do you and Bishop believe he didn't die—or that the suspect the police were chasing wasn't the killer?"

"We believe the latter, actually. The man the police were after had a few violent crimes on his rap sheet, but neither Bishop nor I was convinced he had the right psychological makeup to be the clever serial killer we were after."

"So he kills his six victims, lays low for five years, and then starts up all over again. That's a hell of a cooling-off period."

"And unusual. We believe he uses the time to relocate and get to know the people around him. We also believe there's always a trigger, as I said. Something sets him off. Something *always* sets him off."

47

Again, Rafe heard a note in her voice that made him wary. "There's another reason you believe this is the same killer. What is it?"

Isabel answered without hesitation. "Standing where Tricia Kane was murdered, I felt him. Just the way I felt him five years ago when I first encountered Bishop and joined the team. And the way I felt him ten years ago when he killed a good friend of mine."

It was nearly midnight when Mallory Beck pulled herself reluctantly from bed and began getting dressed. "Dammit. Where on earth did my bra get to?"

"Over there by the bookcase. You could stay, you know. Spend the night."

"I'm back on duty at seven," she said. "First big meeting of our task force, FBI agents included, starts at eight. That's off the record, Alan."

"Mal, I've told you before, anything you say to me privately is off the record." His voice was patient. He propped himself up on an elbow and watched her dress. "I'm not going to cross that line."

She was reasonably sure he wouldn't. But only reasonably sure.

"Okay. But I still need to go home. I won't sleep much if I stay here, and I want to be rested tomorrow."

"You don't have anything to prove, you know. To these FBI agents, I mean. Or to Rafe. You're a damned good cop, everybody knows that."

"Yeah, well, being a good cop hasn't been enough so far, has it?"

He frowned a little as he watched her, wondering as he so often had in the last few months if he would ever really know her. It was undoubtedly part of the attraction as far as he was concerned, he knew that very well; there was so much of her beneath the surface, and his instinct was to dig, to explore and understand.

She wasn't making it easy for him.

Maybe that was part of the attraction as well. Plus the mind-blowing sex, of course. Either it was sheer natural talent, or else Alan had to take his hat off to the men in her past, because Mallory was something else in bed.

Addictive was the word that came to mind.

"You can't blame yourself," he said finally.

"*To Protect and Serve*. It says that on the sides of our cruisers and Jeeps. It's what we get paid for. Our entire reason for being, so to speak."

"It's not a one-woman police force, Mal. Let some of the others carry the weight."

"They do. Especially Rafe."

"Yeah, give him his due. He wasn't too proud to yell for help."

Mallory sat down on the bed to put her socks and shoes on, eyeing her lover. "We've both known him a long time. Pride is never going to be his downfall."

"No. But failing to trust himself might be."

Since she'd had the same thought herself, Mallory could hardly disagree. But she felt uncomfortable on several levels discussing her boss with Alan, so she simply changed the subject. "I'm sorry I missed the press conference today. I hear you cracked up the room."

"Rafe did—with a joke at my expense. I gather that gorgeous blonde he left with is one of the FBI agents?"

"Mmm. Isabel Adams—and I better not see that name printed in the paper unless and until it's released officially."

"You won't, dammit." Still, Alan couldn't stop asking questions. "She's not down here alone?"

"No, she has a partner. Another woman. I haven't met her yet."

"Did it occur to anybody at the Bureau that sending a blond female agent down here at this particular time might be a little dicey?"

Mallory shrugged. "They wrote the profile. I have to assume they know what they're doing."

"I bet Rafe is pissed."

"You'll have to ask him about that."

"Jesus, you're pigheaded."

"It'd be more polite to call me stubborn."

"And less accurate. Mal"—he leaned over to grasp her wrist before she stood up—"is something wrong? I mean, aside from the obvious maniacal-killer-stalking-Hastings thing."

"No."

That mild syllable didn't give him much room to maneuver, but he tried. "I know you're preoccupied. Hell, we all are. But sometimes I get the feeling you're not even here."

"I didn't hear you complaining a little while ago. Even though I always wonder when a guy calls out God's name instead of mine."

Refusing to be sidetracked, Alan said, "You barely caught your breath before you were up and dressing."

"I told you. I have to go to work early."

"If you'd leave some stuff here, you could spend the night occasionally and still get to work early." He heard the note of frustration in his own voice, and the familiar resentment prickled inside him. *Why does she make me do this?*

"Alan, we've been over this. I like my own space. I never leave any of my stuff at a man's apartment. I don't like sleepovers except for vacation trips out of town. And I'm not *real* comfortable being in bed with a reporter in the first place. *Conflict of interest* rings a rather ugly bell."

Her patient tone grated, but he managed to keep his own voice calm. Even careless, around the edges. "It's that last that really bugs you, and don't think I don't know it. You don't trust me, Mal. You don't believe I can separate my work from my personal life."

"Why should you be different from the rest of us?" she asked dryly, pulling away from him and rising to her feet. "My job is in my head twenty-four seven. And so is yours. We're both career people. We live on takeout and caffeine. Half the time our socks don't match, and when we realize it we just buy new socks. We do our laundry when we run out of clean clothes. And when the biggest, baddest bad to ever hit Hastings rears its ugly head, both our careers kick into high gear. Right?"

"Right," he agreed reluctantly.

"Besides, let's not kid ourselves. Neither one of us is looking for anything more than a few hours of stress-busting sex every week." She smiled down at him. "Don't get up. I'll let myself out. See you."

"Good night, Mal." He remained where he was until he heard the front door of his apartment close. Then he fell back against the pillows and muttered a heartfelt "Shit."

Outside Alan's apartment building, Mallory stood on the sidewalk for a moment breathing in the slightly breezy but otherwise mild night air. It was a well-lighted sidewalk close to downtown Hastings, and Mallory shouldn't have felt particularly threatened.

The breeze intensified suddenly, blowing an empty soft drink can across the sidewalk a few feet away, and Mallory nearly jumped out of her skin.

"Shit," she muttered.

51

She could hear the trees whispering softly as the wind stirred their leaves. Hear the occasional swish of a car passing a block or so away. Crickets. Bullfrogs.

Her name.

Not that she really heard that, of course. It was just that she had the uneasy feeling she was being watched. Even followed sometimes.

She'd been conscious of it for some time now, days at least. At odd moments, usually but not always when she was outside, like now. If she were a blonde, she would have been getting really nervous about it; as it was, the sensation just made her wary and a lot more careful.

And jumpy as hell.

She had to wonder if this killer, like so many she'd read about in the police manuals, kept an eye on the cops as they investigated his crimes. Was that it? Was some wacko watching gleefully from behind the bushes, congratulating himself on his cleverness and their incompetence?

If so, maybe it made sense that he'd concentrate on one—or more—of the female officers rather than the guys. She made a mental note to herself to ask some of the other women in the department if any of them had been aware of this creepy feeling. And if they had, or maybe especially if they hadn't, she'd have to ask the FBI profiler about it.

The gorgeous female blond FBI profiler.

Mallory knew Rafe was pissed and unhappy about that; he'd never been a man to hide his feelings. But she also knew that Isabel Adams had somehow managed to persuade him to accept her presence in the investigation.

And it hadn't been by batting her baby greens at him either.

No, there was a lot more to this than sex appeal; she knew Rafe too well not to feel sure that his reasons for accepting Isabel were logical and completely professional. She was still here because he believed she was an asset to the investigation. Period.

Which wasn't to say he was immune to the effects of a beautiful face, green eyes, and a body that looked really good in clingy summery clothing. He was a man, after all.

She half laughed under her breath but kept a wary eye on her surroundings as she unlocked her car and got in. Then again, she thought, maybe she wasn't being quite fair to Rafe. Maybe having her own man problems at the moment made her overly sensitive to undercurrents.

Not that Alan was being particularly subtle. Mallory was somewhat bemused to find herself, for the first time in her adult life, on the traditionally male side of things in their relationship: she was the one who was perfectly happy with casual sex a couple of times a week, no strings or promises.

Alan wanted more.

Sighing, Mallory started the car and headed off toward her own apartment on the other side of town. It was relatively easy to push Alan and the various problems he presented to the back of her mind, at least for the moment, because in the forefront there was still the vague but persistent feeling that she was being watched.

All the way home, she couldn't shake the feeling, even though she didn't see anyone following her. Or anyone in the vicinity of her apartment building. She parked her car carefully in its slot in a well-lighted area and locked it up, then kept her key-chain pepper spray in one hand and her other hand resting on or near her weapon all the way inside and up to her apartment.

Nothing.

No one.

Just this nagging feeling that someone was watching every move she made.

Once inside, Mallory leaned back against her locked apartment door and softly muttered, "Shit."

"Let me get this straight." Isabel rubbed the nape of her neck, staring at her partner. "You met Caleb Powell in that coffee shop on Main Street, and you spilled all that stuff I picked up at Tricia Kane's apartment?"

"Not all of it." Hollis shrugged. "Just some . . . selected bits. I told you, he didn't want to talk to me. And from the jut of his jaw, I'd say he wouldn't have been willing to talk to any of us. So I got his attention. What's wrong with that?"

"Did he ask you how you obtained this information?"

"Yeah, but I distracted him. More or less."

"Hollis, he's a *lawyer*. They don't get distracted, as a rule. Not for long, anyway. What happens when he starts asking questions?"

"I don't think he will. He wants to find out who killed Tricia Kane. Besides, you told Chief Sullivan."

"As closely as we'll have to work with Rafe and his lead investigator on this case, he had to know. So will she. But a civilian?"

Hollis sighed, clearly impatient with the discussion. "Somehow I don't think a lawyer finding out we're psychics is going to be our major problem. I'm new at this whole thing, and you might as well have a bull's-eye target on your back. In neon." She stood up. "Since we have that early meeting in the morning, I think I'll go back to my own room and get some sleep, if you don't mind."

Without protest, Isabel merely said, "I'll be up and ready for breakfast at seven if you want to meet me here." The small inn where they were staying didn't provide room service, but there was a restaurant nearby.

"Okay. See you then."

"Good night, Hollis."

When she was alone in her room again, Isabel got ready for bed, brooding. Just as the night before, she barely noticed the uninspired, any-hotel-in-any-town-U.S.A. decor, and out of habit she filled the silence by having the air-conditioning on high and the TV tuned to an all-news network.

She hated silence when she was in an unfamiliar place.

She had put off calling Bishop, undecided despite what she'd told Rafe as to what she intended to report. So when her cell phone rang, she knew who it was even without the caller I.D. and answered by saying, "This is supposed to be one of those lessons you're always saying we have to learn, right? A reminder from the universe that we don't control anything except our own actions? When we're able to control them, that is."

"I don't know what you're talking about," Bishop replied, calm and transparently unconvincing.

"Yeah, yeah. Why team me with Hollis? Answer that."

"Because you're the one most likely to help her through this first real test of her abilities."

"I'm not a medium."

"No, but you understand how it feels to be forced suddenly to cope with abilities you never even dreamed were possible."

"I'm not the only other team member who wasn't born a psychic."

"You're the best adjusted."

"That's an arguable statement. Just because this stuff no longer scares the hell out of me doesn't necessarily mean I'm all that well adjusted."

"I didn't say well adjusted. I said best adjusted."

"Which only proves my point. I would think you'd want somebody well adjusted to help Hollis."

"You're going to keep arguing about this, aren't you?" Bishop said.

"I thought I might."

"Are you asking me to recall Hollis?"

Isabel hesitated, then said, "No. Dammit."

"You can help her. Just listen to your instincts."

"Bishop, we both know mediums are fragile."

"And we both know how difficult it's been for us to find a medium for the unit. They're rare, for one thing. And, yes, they're emotionally fragile. Most can't handle the job, and those who can tend to burn out quickly."

"So far," she reminded him, "we haven't found a single one who was able to gain information for us by contacting murder victims. I mean an agent. Bonnie did it, but she wasn't an agent. When she grows up, though—"

"She still has a lot of growing to do. Right now, she's preoccupied with being a teenager. It's not the easiest time of life, remember? Especially when you're gifted."

"Or cursed. Yeah, I remember. Bonnie aside, the few mediums we've found and tried to bring into murder investigations have either been terrified of opening that particular door or else didn't have enough strength or control to do it in any way helpful to us."

"Which is another reason you're teamed with Hollis and why she's in Hastings. She's strong enough to handle the work, and her control has been steadily improving."

"Maybe, but her field experience is zilch. And she's not ready to open that door, not yet. Strong or not, she's one of the scared ones. She doesn't show it, unless you count the chip on her shoulder, but she's terrified of facing death."

"Can you blame her? She fought like hell to keep death at bay on her own account hardly more than six months ago. Willingly opening that door and confronting what's on the other side is going to be the hardest thing she'll ever have to do."

"Yeah, which is one reason I don't think she's ready for this job, not yet. Look, I'm as sympathetic as anyone about what Hollis has been through, but—"

"She doesn't need sympathy. She needs to work."

"She isn't ready to work, if my opinion counts for anything."

"She believes she is ready."

"And what do you believe?" Isabel challenged.

"I believe she needs to work."

Isabel sighed. "This killer is vicious. The attacks have been vicious. If Hollis is even able to nerve herself to open the door, she's going to find a hell of a lot of terror and pain barreling through at her."

"I know."

"I can't push her, Bishop."

"I don't want you to."

"Just be here to catch her when she falls?"

"No. Don't focus on that. It's not what this is about. You investigate your case. Hollis is intelligent, curious, intuitive, and observant, and that plus the training we've given her means she'll be an asset to the investigation. If she's able to use her psychic abilities, we'll find out in a hurry whether she can handle the fallout."

"And whether I can. She could end up a basket case."

"Possibly, but don't count her out. She's exceptionally strong." Bishop paused, then added dryly, "The more imperative problem, I'd say, is that this killer you and I are both all too familiar with has noticed you this time around. For all we know, he may remember you. In any case, you're on his hit list."

"Damn," Isabel said.

4

H E WOKE UP with blood on his hands.
It wasn't an instant realization. The alarm was droning on and on, and he had the vague notion that he had overslept. Again. He'd been doing that a lot lately. The bed-clothes were tumbled, tangled around him, and it took a consider-able amount of effort just to roll himself over and slap at the irritating alarm clock to stop the damned noise.

He froze, hand on the now-silent clock.

His hand was . . . there was blood.

He pushed himself slowly up on an elbow and looked at his hand, at both hands. Reddish stains covered the palms. Dried stains, not wet. But now that they were close to his face, he could smell the blood, sharp and metallic, so strong it made his stomach heave.

The blood.

Again.

He fought his way out of bed and hurried to the bathroom. He stood at the sink, washing his hands over and over until there was no sign of the red. He splashed water on his face, rinsed his mouth, trying to get rid of the sour taste of fear.

He raised his head and stared into the mirror, hands braced on the sink.

A white, haggard face stared back at him.

"Oh, Christ," he whispered.

8:00 AM

Isabel wasted no time, at the first meeting of the four lead investigators of their combined police and FBI task force, in explaining to Detective Mallory Beck what made the SCU team "special."

Mallory, like Rafe the previous day, took the news quite calmly, saying only, "I'd call that a pretty unusual sort of unit for the FBI."

Isabel nodded. "Definitely. And we exist as a unit only as long as we're successful."

"Like that, is it? Politics?"

"More or less. Not only are we unconventional in too many ways to count, but the Bureau can't use us and our success to improve their own image; what we do too often looks like magic or some kind of witchcraft rather than science, and that is *not* something the FBI wants to publicize no matter how high our success rate is. We're becoming quietly well known within other law-enforcement organizations because of our successes, but there are still plenty of people inside the Bureau who'd love it if we failed."

"So you haven't yet?"

"Debatable point, I suppose." Isabel pursed her lips. "A few got away. But the successes have far exceeded the failures. If you call them failures."

"You don't?"

"We don't give up easily. Bishop doesn't give up easily. So . . . just because a case goes cold doesn't mean we forget about it or stop working on it. Which brings me back to this case." She explained their belief that they were dealing with a killer who had terrorized two previous towns and had a dozen murders under his belt even before he came to Hastings.

"I think we're gonna need a bigger task force," Mallory said dryly.

Even though he smiled faintly, Rafe's response was matter-of-fact. "Technically, we have one. Every officer and detective we have will be working on some aspect of the investigation. Overtime, more people to handle the phones, whatever it takes. But only you and I know about Hollis's and Isabel's psychic abilities. That's the way it stays. The last thing I want is for the press to turn this thing into a carnival sideshow."

"And they will, given the chance," Isabel said. "We've seen it happen before."

Great, Mallory thought, *one more thing I have to hide from Alan.* Out loud, she said, "I don't know much about ESP, unless you count commercials from those psychic hotlines, but I gather neither of you can just I.D. our perp for us like snapping your fingers?"

"Our abilities are just another tool," Isabel told her. "We use standard investigative techniques like every other cop, at least as much as possible."

Mallory was more resigned than scornful. "Yeah, I figured that would be the deal."

"It can't be too easy," Hollis said. "The universe has to make us work for everything."

"So how will your abilities help us, assuming they do?" Mallory asked. "I mean, what specifically is it that you're able to do?"

"I'm clairvoyant," Isabel said, explaining the SCU's definition of the term.

"So you have to touch something or someone to pick up information about them?"

"Touching helps, usually, because it establishes the strongest connection. But I also get information randomly sometimes. That tends to be trivia."

"For instance?" Mallory was clearly curious.

Without hesitation, Isabel said, "You had a cinnamon bun for breakfast at home this morning and you feel guilty about it."

Mallory blinked, then looked at Rafe.

"Spooky, isn't it?" he said.

Mallory cleared her throat and, without commenting on Isabel's statement, looked at Hollis. "And you?"

"I talk to dead people," she replied with a wry smile. "Technically, I'm a medium."

"No shit? That must be . . . disconcerting."

"I'm told you get used to it," Hollis murmured.

"You're told?"

"I'm new at this."

Rafe frowned. "You weren't born with it?"

"Not exactly." Hollis looked at Isabel, who explained.

"Some people possess latent—inactive—paranormal abilities. For most of those people, the abilities remain unknown and unused their entire lives. They may get hunches, flashes of knowledge they can't logically explain, but they generally ignore it or dismiss it as coincidence."

"Until something changes," Rafe guessed.

"Exactly. Every once in a while, something happens that

causes latent psychics either consciously or subconsciously to tap into the previously dormant ability and actually begin using it."

"What could do that?" Mallory asked warily.

"The most common, and most likely, scenario is that a latent becomes an adept—our term for a functional psychic—due to a physical, emotional, or psychological injury. A head injury is the most common, but almost any severe trauma can do it. Generally speaking, the greater the shock of the awakening, the stronger the abilities tend to be."

"So Hollis—"

"Both of us. Both of us survived a traumatic event," Isabel said matter-of-factly. "And became functional psychics because of it."

9:00 AM

Officer Ginny McBrayer hung up the phone and frowned down at the message pad for a moment, debating. Then she got up and went around the corner to Travis's desk. "Hey. Is the chief still in that meeting?"

On the phone himself, but obviously on hold judging by his propped-up feet, bored expression, and only semicontact between the receiver and his ear, Travis replied, "Yeah. Not to be disturbed unless it's an emergency. Or 'relevant,' I think he said."

"This might be." Ginny handed over the message slip. "What do you think?"

Travis studied the slip, then searched his cluttered desk for a minute, finally producing a clipboard. "Here's the list we already have going. Women of the right general age reported missing within a fifty-mile radius of Hastings. We're up to ten in the last three weeks. It was twelve, but two of them came home."

Ginny looked over the list, then picked up her message slip again and frowned. "Yeah, but the one I just got the call about is local, from that dairy farm just outside town. Her husband really sounded upset."

"Okay, then tell the chief." Travis shrugged. "I'm waiting for the clerk at the courthouse to get back to me about all that property Jamie Brower owned. She's got me on hold. Remind me to tell them they need some new canned music, okay? This shit is giving me a headache."

"I don't want to interrupt the chief's meeting," Ginny said, ignoring the irrelevant information he'd offered. "What if this is nothing?"

"And what if it's something? Go knock on the door and report the call. Better for him to be mad at an interruption than to be mad because he wasn't told something he should have been."

"Easy for you to say," Ginny muttered. But she turned away from the other cop's desk and headed for the conference room.

"Neither of you was born psychic?" Mallory said in surprise. "But—"

Isabel smiled, but said, "Understandably, neither one of us is all that eager to talk about what happened to us, so if you two don't mind, we won't. We're both trained investigators, of course, and I'm a profiler. Plus we have the full backing of the SCU and the resources of Quantico. But anything Hollis and I are able to glean from our abilities or spider sense will have to be considered a bonus, not something we can count on."

Rafe eyed her. "Spider sense?"

"It's not as out there as it sounds." She smiled. "Just our informal term for enhanced normal senses—the traditional five. Something Bishop discovered and has been able to teach most of us is how to concentrate and amplify our sight, hearing, and other senses. Like everything else, it varies from agent to agent in terms of strength, accuracy, and control. Even at its best it isn't a huge edge, but it has been known to help us out from time to time."

"I have a question," Mallory said.

"Only one?" Rafe murmured.

"Shoot," Isabel invited.

"Why you? I mean, why did this Bishop of yours pick you to come down here? You fit the victim profile to a T, unless there's been a change I don't know about."

"It gets worse," Rafe told his detective, his voice grim. "Isabel believes our killer has already spotted her. And added her to his list of must-kill blondes."

"Well, I can't say I'm all that surprised." Mallory lifted a brow at the blond agent. "So why're you still here? Bait?"

"No," Rafe said immediately.

Isabel said, "We have some time before it becomes an issue. This bastard gets to know his victims before he kills them, or at least has to feel that he knows them, and he doesn't know me. In any case, the reason why I'm here is much more compelling than any risk I face as a possible target."

"And that reason is?"

"As I told Rafe yesterday, patterns and connections are everywhere, if we only know how to look for them." Isabel spoke slowly. "I have a connection with this killer. He killed a friend of mine ten years ago, and five years ago I was involved in the investigation in Alabama of the second series of murders."

Mallory was frowning, intent. "Are you saying you know him? But if you know him, doesn't that mean he knows you? Knows you the way he has to know his victims? That thing that's rapidly becoming an issue?"

"No. I wasn't in law enforcement when my friend was killed,

I was just another shocked and grieving part of her life—and her death. And I was on the fringes of the official investigation in Alabama; by the time I was officially involved, he'd already murdered his sixth victim and moved on. So it's at least as likely as not that he won't even know I was involved in the previous investigations."

"But you're on his hit list."

"On it, but I'm not next in line. I'm not local, so it won't be easy for him to find information about me, especially since I don't plan to become too chatty with anyone outside our investigation."

"What about inside?" Mallory asked. "We've had at least the suspicion that the perp could be a cop. Has that been ruled out?"

"Unfortunately, no. Our feeling is that we're not dealing with a cop, but there are some elements of the M.O. that make it at least possible."

"For instance?" Rafe was frowning slightly. "We haven't seen the updated profile," he reminded her.

"I have copies here for both of you," Isabel replied. "Not a lot has changed from the first profile as far as the description of our unknown subject is concerned. We have revised his probable age range upward a bit, given the time frame of at least ten years as an active killer. So, he's a white male, thirty to forty-five years old, above-average intelligence. He has a steady job and possibly a family or significant other, and he copes well with day-to-day life. In other words, this is not a man who's obviously stressed or appears in any way at odds with himself.

"Blondes are only his latest targets; in the earlier murders, he killed first redheads in Florida ten years ago, and then, five years ago, brunettes in Alabama. Which, by the way, is another reason he wouldn't have noticed me then even if he'd seen me; he's always very focused on his targets and potential targets, and I had the wrong hair color for him both times before."

"What about the elements that could indicate he's a cop?" Rafe asked.

"The central question of this investigation—and the two before this one—is how he's been able to persuade these women to calmly and quietly accompany him to lonely spots. These are highly intelligent, very savvy women, in several cases trained in self-defense. None of them was stupid. So how did he get them to go with him?"

"Authority figure," Rafe said. "Has to be."

"That's what we're thinking. So we can't rule out cops. We also can't rule out someone who appears to be a member of the clergy, or any other trustworthy authority figure. Someone in politics, someone well known within the community. Whoever he is, these women trusted him, at least for the five or ten minutes it took him to get them alone and vulnerable. He looks safe to them. He looks unthreatening."

Mallory said, "You said earlier that he'd killed a dozen women before coming to Hastings. Exactly twelve?"

"Six women in six weeks, both times."

"So it is just women," Mallory said. "Bottom line, he hates women."

"Hates, loves, wants, needs—it's probably a tangle. He hates them for what they are, either because they represent what he wants and can't have or because he feels somehow emasculated by them. Killing them gives him power over them, gives him control. He needs that, needs to feel he's stronger than they are, that he can master them."

"A manly man," Hollis said, her mockery both obvious and hollow.

Isabel nodded. "Or, at least, so he wants to believe. And wants us to believe."

———

Alan Moore had always thought that calling the central work area of the *Chronicle* offices "the newsroom" must have been someone's idea of irony. Because nothing newsworthy ever happened in Hastings.

Or hadn't, until the first murder.

Not that there hadn't been killings in Hastings before, of course; when a town had been in existence for nearly two hundred years, there were bound to be killings every now and then. People had died out of greed, out of jealousy, out of spite, out of rage.

But until the murder of Jamie Brower, no one had been killed by pure evil.

Alan hadn't hesitated to point that out in his coverage of the murders and their investigation. And not even Rafe had accused him—publicly or privately—of sensationalizing the tragedies of those murders.

Some things damned well couldn't be denied.

There was something evil in Hastings, and the fact that it was walking around on two legs passing itself off as human didn't change that fact.

"How many times have I told you to pick up your own damned mail, Alan?" Callie Rosier, the *Chronicle*'s only full-time photographer, dumped several envelopes on his already cluttered desk. "It's in a little box with your name on it right on the other side of that wall. You can't miss it."

"I just said you could pick up mine while you were getting yours, what's wrong with that?" Alan retorted.

"What is this 'while you're up' thing with you men?" She continued to her own desk, shaking her head as she sat down. "You sweat your brains out running miles every morning and lifting weights in the gym so you'll look good in your jeans but pester other people to get stuff for you when it's in the same damned room. Jesus."

"Don't you have film to develop?" The question was more habit than curiosity, and absentminded to boot since he was leafing through his mail.

"No. Why are all these places offering me credit cards?"

"The same reason they're offering them to me," Alan replied, tossing several into his overflowing trash can. "Because they haven't checked our credit records." He eyed his final bit of mail, a large manila envelope with no return address, and hesitated only an instant before tearing it open.

"I think these telemarketers are morons," Callie said, studying the contents of one envelope marked URGENT! "They don't even bother to be accurate in who they're sending this stuff to anymore. I ask you, does the name Callie sound like it belongs to a man? This one should have been addressed to you. Take a little blue pill and get another inch or two. I'm sure you'd like another inch or two. And more staying power, says here."

"I'll be a son of a bitch," Alan said.

"Aren't you usually?"

He looked at her, saw that she was focused on her own mail and not even paying attention to the conversation. With only an instant's pause, Alan said casually, "Oh, yeah, always." Then he looked back down at his mail and, this time under his breath, repeated, "I'll be a son of a bitch."

Rafe accepted the message slip, absently introduced Officer McBrayer to the federal agents, then read the information she had offered. "Her husband says she's been gone since Monday?"

"He thinks since Monday." Ginny made an effort to sound as brisk and professional as she could, even though she was nervous and knew it showed. "He didn't see her that afternoon, and with two cows calving he was out in his barns all night. He says it could have been Tuesday; that's when he realized she wasn't in the house. He thought she'd gone to visit a friend in town, since it's something she often does, but when she didn't come home, he checked. She wasn't there. Isn't anywhere he could think to check. I think it only slowly dawned on him that maybe he should be worried."

"Yeah," Rafe muttered, "Tim Helton isn't the sharpest pencil in the box."

"Understatement," Mallory offered. "The way I heard it, he once decided that moonshine would work just as well as fuel in his tractor. Dunno if he got a bad batch or what, but it blew the sucker all to hell and nearly took him with it."

"Moonshine?" Isabel asked curiously. "They still make that stuff?"

"Believe it or not. We've had the ATF out here a few times over the years because of illegal brew. Seems like a lot of trouble to go to, if you ask me, but the bootleggers seem to feel it's worth it. Either that or they just don't want to pay The Government a cent more than they have to."

Rafe said, "And there's at least one survivalist group in the area. They consider it the norm to make everything they need themselves. Including booze." He made a note on the pad before him, then handed the message slip back to his officer. "Okay, standard procedure, Ginny. I want a detective out there to talk to Tim, and let's get a list of places she might possibly be. Friends, relatives, anybody she might be visiting. From now on, we treat every missing person, man or woman, as if he or she could be a murder victim."

69

"Yes, sir."

When the young officer had hurried from the room, Isabel said, "Is this people starting to panic? I mean, is this an unusual increase in women reported missing?"

He nodded. "Oh, yeah. In the past three weeks, we've seen the reports jump tenfold. Most come home within twenty-four hours or are discovered visiting relatives or talking to divorce attorneys, or just at the grocery store."

"Most. But not all."

"We still have a few missing in the general area, but we haven't yet been able to rule out a voluntary absence in any of the cases."

"We'll probably see even more of this," Isabel commented.

"Problem is," Mallory said, "we have to treat every report seriously, just as Rafe said. So we'll waste a lot of manpower searching for women who aren't really missing or who ran off and don't want to be found. Lady last week cussed me out good for *finding* her."

"Motel?" Isabel inquired sapiently.

"Uh-huh. Not alone, needless to say."

"Still, we have to look for them," Hollis said.

Rafe nodded. "No question. I'm just hoping it won't muddy the water too much. Or deplete resources needed elsewhere."

"In the meantime," Isabel said, "those of us in this room at least have to focus on what we know we've got. Three murdered women."

Rafe said, "You told me there's always a trigger. Always something specific that sets him off."

"There has to be," Isabel responded. "You said yourself that five years is a hell of a long cooling-off period for a serial killer; it is, especially after a fairly frenzied six-week killing spree. A gap that long usually means either that murders in another location have gone unnoticed or at least weren't connected to him, or that he's in prison somewhere or otherwise unable to keep killing."

"I gather you're certain that isn't the case here."

"When he hit in Alabama five years ago, we combed through police files of unsolved murders from coast to coast. Nothing matched his M.O. except for the series of murders five years before that. We were convinced he had been inactive during that five-year gap, yet there was also no even remotely likely suspect we could find who had been in prison for exactly that length of time. And according to all the information gleaned from databases we had Quantico double-check yesterday, he's also been inactive in the five years since Alabama. Until he started killing in Hastings a little over three weeks ago."

Mallory rubbed her temple, scowling. "So something sets him off and he kills six women in six weeks. Then, apparently sated for the time being, vanishes before the cops can even get close to catching him. Why six women?"

"We don't know," Isabel replied. "The number has to be important, since it's been exactly the same twice before, but we don't know how or why. We can't even be absolutely positive he'll stop at six this time. He could be escalating. Most killers of this sort do sooner or later kill more or get more viciously creative in the killing itself."

Mallory shook her head. "Great. Because we didn't have enough to look forward to. So he kills at least six women. Moves on to a new location. Then waits five years—it's not exact, is it?" she interrupted herself to ask.

Isabel shook her head. "Not to the day, no. The gap between the first and second set of murders was actually four years and ten months. The gap between the last set and this one was five years and one month. Give or take a few days."

"Okay. But he moves somewhere new after his six-week

71

killing spree, settles down, settles in. Which has to mean we're looking for someone who's been in Hastings no more than five years, right?"

"Or someone who used to live in the area and has moved back. Or someone who works in Hastings but lives outside the town—or the other way around. Or someone who takes long vacations every few years; that's at least possible."

"Goes on vacation to kill people?"

"We've encountered stranger things. He could scout out his hunting grounds in advance, maybe start picking his victims, and return later for the actual kill." Isabel shook her head. "Honestly, if you look at a map, the two previous hunting grounds and Hastings are all within a day's drive, despite being in three different states. So we can't even rule out the idea that he lives in an area central to his hunting grounds and has just somehow managed to spend enough time in each to get to know his victims."

"Oh, hell, I was hoping we could narrow down the possibles at least a little bit."

Hollis said, "The universe never makes it easy, remember? Probably the only people we can even begin to rule out are those who have lived continuously in Hastings during the last fifteen years at least. And I mean continuously: no vacations longer than, say, two weeks; no going away to college; no out-of-town visits, no day trips fitting the right time periods."

Mallory grimaced. "Which is just not possible. Even those of us who've lived here our whole lives tend to go away to school or travel or something. And day trips? Lots of good shopping in Columbia, Atlanta, other places within a day's drive."

"I was afraid of that," Isabel said with a sigh.

With a nod, Mallory said, "That sort of thing is so common I doubt we could find anybody who was absent or took weekly day trips out of town during those six-week stretches specifically, not without questioning every soul in town and probably not then. Who remembers specific dates from years ago? And like I said, people travel on vacations or for business, go away to school. I was away in Georgia three years finishing college. It was four for you, wasn't it, Rafe?"

"Yeah. And I went to Duke, in North Carolina." He sighed. "It's like Mal said, we've all traveled, been away from Hastings, most of us more than once. And people do take regular day trips, even out of state, for shopping or business. I get the feeling this isn't going to help us narrow the list all that much."

"Probably not," Isabel agreed. "Although if we get lucky enough to find a suspect or two, we have some concrete questions to ask . . ."

Hollis didn't intentionally tune out the discussion. She didn't want to; despite the repetition of details she already knew, she was still new enough to the investigative process itself to find it interesting, even fascinating.

She wasn't even aware at first that Isabel's voice had faded into a peculiar hollow silence. But then she realized the discussion around her had gone distant, deadened. She felt the fine hairs on her body rise, her flesh tingle.

It was not a pleasant sensation.

She looked around the table at the others, watching their mouths move and hearing only a word now and then, muffled and indistinct. And they themselves appeared different to her. Dim, almost faded. They seemed to be growing ever more distant moment by moment, and that frightened her.

Hell, it terrified her.

She opened her mouth to say something, or try to, but even as she did, a new and unfamiliar instinct urged her to turn her head toward the doorway. Again without meaning to, without wanting to, she looked.

Standing near the doorway was a woman.

A blond woman.

She was clearer than the people around Hollis, brighter somehow, and more distinct. She was beautiful, with perfect, delicate features. Her hair was burnished gold, her eyes a clear, piercing blue.

Eyes fixed on Hollis.

Her lips parted, and she started to speak.

A chill swept through Hollis and she quickly looked away, instinctively trying to close the door, to disconnect herself from the place from which this woman had emerged.

It was a cold, dark place, and it terrified Hollis.

Because it was death.

Mallory rubbed her temple again. "Okay, back to what sets him off. What sets him off?"

Isabel answered readily, if not too informatively. "Something specific, but we don't know what that is, at least not yet. The gaps between his killing sprees can and might be explained by his need to get to know these women."

"Might," Rafe said. "But you aren't sure?"

"I'm sure he has to feel he knows them. For whatever reason, they can't be total strangers to him. Maybe in getting to know them, he discovers something about them—at least the initial victim—that sets him off, something that pushes his button. Or maybe he has to win their trust; that could be part of his ritual, especially since these women appear to be leaving their cars and going willingly with him."

"He doesn't pick out all six women before he starts killing, right? Otherwise you wouldn't have made his list."

"Good point." Isabel nodded. "It's also a point that he is able to look beyond the woman he's currently stalking in order to take note of, and even choose as a future victim, another woman. Even though this guy's actual killings are frenzied, it's becoming clear that he's quite able to think coolly and calmly right up until the moment he kills them."

"We have to find her."

They all looked at Hollis. Her voice had been tight, and her face showed visible tension. She was chewing on a thumbnail, which, Rafe noticed, was already bitten short.

"He's stalking her even now. Watching her. Thinking about what he's going to do to her. We have to—"

"Hollis." Isabel spoke quietly. "We'll do all we can to find her before he gets to her. But the only way we have of doing that is by starting with the women he's already killed. We have to find out what they all have in common besides the color of their hair. What connects them to each other. And to him."

Hollis looked at her partner almost blindly. "How can you be so calm about it? You know what's going to happen to her. We both know. We both know how it feels. The helpless terror, the agony—"

"*Hollis.*" Isabel's voice was still quiet, but something in it caused her partner to blink and stiffen in her chair.

"I'm sorry," Hollis said. She pressed her fingertips briefly to her closed eyes, then looked at them again. "It's just that—" This time, no one interrupted her.

But something did.

She turned her head abruptly as if someone had called her name, staring toward the closed door of the room. Her eyes dilated until only a thin rim of blue circled the enormous pupils.

Rafe sent a quick glance toward Isabel and found her watching her partner intently, eyes narrowed. When he looked back at Hollis, he saw that she was even more pale than she had been before, and trembling visibly.

"Why are you here?" she whispered, looking at nothing the others could see. "Wait, I can't hear you. I want to. I want to help you. But—"

Softly, Isabel said, "Who is it, Hollis? Who do you see?"

"I can't hear her. She's trying to tell me something, but I can't hear her."

"Listen. Concentrate."

"I'm trying. I see her, but . . . She's shaking her head. She's giving up. No, wait—"

Rafe was a bit startled to feel his ears pop just an instant before Hollis slumped in her chair. He told himself it was his imagination, even as he heard himself ask, "Who was it? Who did you see?"

Hollis looked at him blankly for a moment, then past him at the bulletin board where they had posted photos and other information about the victims.

"Her. The first victim. Jamie Brower."

MILY BROWER WOULDN'T have admitted it to a soul, but she was a horrible person. A horrible daughter. A really horrible sister. People kept coming up to her with shocked eyes and hushed voices, telling her how sorry they were about Jamie, asking her how she was holding up.

"Fine, I'm fine," Emily always replied.

Fine. Doing okay. Holding up. Getting on with her life.

"I'm okay, really."

Being there for her grieving parents. Allowing people she barely knew or didn't know at all to hug her while they whispered their condolences. Writing all the thank-you cards to people for their cards and flowers, because her mother couldn't do anything except cry. Dealing with all the phone calls from Jamie's college friends as the news rippled out.

"I'm getting through it."

I'm a hypocrite.

They had never been close, she and Jamie, but they had been sisters. So Emily knew she should feel something about Jamie being dead, being horribly *murdered,* something besides this slightly impatient resentment.

She didn't.

"I don't know what she was doing those last few weeks," Emily told Detective Mallory Beck in response to the question she'd asked. "Jamie had her own place, a job that kept her busy, and she liked to travel. She came to Sunday dinner a couple of times a month, but other than that . . ."

"You didn't see much of her."

"No. She was six years older. We didn't really have anything in common." Emily tried not to sound as impatient as she felt, even as she stole glances at the tall blond FBI agent who was across the living room standing before the shrine.

"So you don't know who she might have been dating?"

"No, I already told you that." Emily wondered what the FBI agent found so fascinating in all the photos and trophies and awards littering the built-in shelves on either side of the fireplace. Hadn't she ever seen a shrine before?

"Do you know if she had an address book?"

Emily frowned at Detective Beck. "Everybody has an address book."

"We didn't find one in her apartment."

"Then she must have kept it at her work."

"The one in her office held business information and contacts only."

"Well, then I don't know."

"She had a good memory," Agent Adams said suddenly. She looked back over her shoulder and smiled at Emily. "There are awards here for spelling and science—chemistry. Jamie didn't have to write things down, did she?"

"Not usually," Emily admitted grudgingly. "Especially numbers. Phone numbers. And math. She was good at math."

Agent Adams chuckled. "One of those, huh? My sister was good at math. I hated it. Used to turn numbers into little cartoons. My teachers were never amused by that."

Emily couldn't help but laugh. "I always tried to make faces out of the numbers. My teachers didn't like it either."

"Ah, well, I've found there are numbers people and words people. Not a lot who do well with both." She reached out and lightly touched a framed certificate that was part of the shrine. "Looks like Jamie was one of the rare ones, though. Here's an award for a short story she wrote in college."

"She liked telling stories," Emily said. "Made-up ones, but stuff that happened to her too."

"You said she traveled; did she tell you any stories about that?"

"She talked about it sometimes at Sunday dinner. But with Mom and Dad there, she only talked about the boring parts. Museums, shows, sightseeing."

"Never talked about any of the men she met?"

"Nah, to hear her tell it she was a nun."

"But you knew the truth, naturally. Was she seeing anybody, locally?"

"She didn't talk to me about her private life."

Agent Adams smiled again at Emily. "Sisters don't have to talk to know, do they? Sisters always see what's there, far more than anybody else ever does."

Emily wavered for a moment, but that understanding, conspiratorial smile combined with the stresses and strains of the last few weeks finally caused her resentment to escape.

"Everybody thought she was so perfect, you know? It all came so easy to her. She was good at everything she tried, everybody loved her, she made loads of money. But underneath all that, she was scared. It really showed in the last few weeks before she died. To me, anyway. Nervous, jumpy, rushing around like she had too much to do and not enough time. She was scared shitless."

"Why?" Detective Beck asked quietly.

"Because of her big secret. Because she knew how upset and disappointed our parents would be, other people would be, how horrified. It's just not something you do in a little town like Hastings, not something people could accept. And she was always scared they'd find out. Always."

"Scared they'd find what out, Emily?" Agent Adams asked.

"That she was gay." Emily laughed. "A lesbian. But not just any sort of lesbian, mind you, that's not the part she was terrified people would find out. Lovely, sweet, talented, good-at-anything-and-everything Jamie was a dominatrix. She dressed in shiny black leather and stiletto heels with fishnet stockings, and she made other women crawl and fawn and do whatever she wanted them to."

Agent Adams didn't seem in the least surprised. "Are you sure about that, Emily?"

"You bet I'm sure. I've got pictures."

As they got into Mallory's Jeep a few minutes later, she said, "Did you know about Jamie Brower going in or pick up something there in the room?"

"Picked it up while I was there. That house was practically screaming at me."

"Really? Amazing how much people can keep hidden. Because we didn't get any of this before, and both Rafe and I talked to Emily several times. And Jamie's parents, friends, coworkers. Not so much as a hint that Jamie led any kind of unconventional life sexually."

"Yeah, I read the statements you guys collected. Jamie even dated local men, and at least two claimed fairly recent sexual relationships."

Mallory started the Jeep but didn't put it in gear, turning her head to frown at Isabel. "They weren't lying about that. I'd bet my pension on it."

"I think you're right. Just the fact that they were willing to admit to intimate relationships and put themselves in that police spotlight makes it fairly certain they were telling the truth. But I don't believe Jamie was truly bisexual, that she enjoyed sex with men *and* women."

"Then why sleep with the men? Just to keep her secret life secret?"

"I'd say so. Emily was right; in a small town like Hastings, any successful woman like Jamie would hesitate to come out of the closet. Especially if that closet contained whips, chains, and black leather. She wouldn't have wanted that image in a client's mind while she was trying to sell them real estate."

"Hell, I don't want the image in my head. But it's there now."

Isabel smiled wryly. "I know. The question is, how important is this information? Is it what triggered our killer's compulsion? Did he find out he could never possess Jamie Brower the way he needed to? Did he discover her secret and find himself unable to bear it for some other reason?"

"Or," Mallory finished, "is it just an extraneous fact completely unconnected with Jamie's murder."

"Exactly."

Mallory put the Jeep in gear and headed toward the end of

81

the Browers' circular driveway. "Well, it's a new fact for us, at any rate. Lucky you could get chummy with Emily about the trials of sisterhood."

"I never had a sister," Isabel said.

After a beat, Mallory said, "Ah. You used what you picked up psychically from Emily to encourage her to talk. The cartoon numbers she drew in school. Being lousy at math when her sister was so good at it. You used the knowledge to be sympathetic, be on her side so she'd feel comfortable talking to you. So that's how your abilities can be used as investigative tools."

"That's how," Isabel said. "An edge that sometimes makes all the difference. But something else I learned in there is that Emily was all but invisible in that family. Which is why she knew about Jamie's secret life. Why she saw more than anyone else realized. And why there's a good chance she saw something that could get her killed."

"What?"

"Her sister's murderer."

3:30 PM

Isabel closed the folder and looked at Rafe with a sigh. "Just like I remembered. As far as we could determine both times, the twelve women killed before he came to Hastings were all straight. No secret sexual closet, with or without whips and chains. And the second and third victims here, Allison Carroll and Tricia Kane, were straight as well, according to the information you got. Right?"

"Right."

"Still, I'm going to ask Quantico to reopen those old files, maybe send an agent to the towns in Florida and Alabama to double-check, particularly the lives of the primary victims just

82

before they were killed. With Jamie's secret life staring us in the face, we have to be sure whether or not it has anything to do with what triggers his killing rage."

"Makes sense to me. Could be, he got the kind of rejection he couldn't take. Rejection as a man, for being a man."

"That is entirely possible."

Rafe looked down at the three small in-living-color photographs of Jamie Brower in full dominatrix gear: a silver-studded, black leather bustier, fishnet stockings held up by garters, stiletto heels—and a whip. In each shot, there was another woman, crawling, fawning, or in some clearly submissive pose, just as Emily had said.

And while Jamie's face was unmasked and highly visible, her companion was completely unidentifiable due to a black leather hood and mask.

He lined up the photos on the table and studied them intently. "I'd say this is the same woman in all three shots."

Isabel nodded. "And I'd guess all three shots were taken on the same day. Same . . . session. Though all the details of costume and . . . um . . . accessories being exactly the same could be part of their whole ritual, so we can't assume too much."

"Can I assume the second woman is nobody I know personally? Please?"

Isabel smiled wryly. "It is unsettling, isn't it? Other people's secrets."

"This sort of secret, at least. I guess you never really know about people."

"No. You don't." There was something oddly flat about Isabel's response, but she went on before Rafe could question it. And her voice was easy once again. "That outfit the other woman is wearing shows a lot of skin, but considering how tight and rigid it is, it's also doing a dandy job of disguising her true body shape.

So are her positions; we can't even realistically estimate how tall she is. Her face is never turned to the camera, so not even her eyes are visible. And her hair's caught up under that hood."

Rafe cleared his throat. "And since she's shaved . . ."

Isabel didn't seem at all embarrassed or disturbed, and nodded matter-of-factly. "Not uncommon in S&M scenarios, according to the list Quantico sent us, but pubic hair would at least have given us a hair color, and probably natural. I didn't see a birthmark, tattoo, even a blemish that might help us I.D. her."

She paused, then added, "Several things interest me about this little twist. We don't know if any or all of Jamie's playmates lived here in Hastings, though my guess is that more than one isn't very likely."

"A few weeks ago," Rafe said, "I would have said investigating a serial killer in Hastings would be the next thing to impossible. A few S&M games seem fairly tame by comparison. Hell, almost innocent."

"Yeah, but not innocent to Jamie. If she was so afraid of discovery, it could well have been because her partner—at least the most recent one—lives here and maybe isn't as good at keeping secrets as Jamie was. That might explain what Emily saw as Jamie's increasing worry and fear. Another thing is that we don't know where these photographs were taken, and though Emily claims she *borrowed* these three from a photo box full of them, your people found no sign of the box at Jamie's apartment when they did an intensive search."

"I'm surprised Emily found it," Rafe said. "This is not the sort of thing you'd leave lying around, I'm thinking."

"Oh, you can bet Emily snooped. She said she caught a glimpse of the corner of the box under her sister's bed and was curious, but she had to be looking for secrets. She knew her sister was afraid of something, and she wanted to know what that was. It was the first chink she'd seen in Jamie's armor."

"Why take these?" Rafe wondered.

"Proof. Even if she never planned to show them to anyone—including Jamie—she had something that proved to her that Jamie wasn't as perfect as her family believed she was. That was probably enough for Emily; she doesn't strike me as a black-mailer or the vindictive type."

"Yeah," Rafe said, "I'd agree with you there."

Isabel shrugged. "I'm also willing to bet that she left the box just enough out of place to make Jamie uneasy about it. If it really was filled with photos, then she couldn't be sure any were missing. But she had to wonder if her sister found the box. That's probably why we haven't found it."

"Because she hid it somewhere safer."

"I would have. The question is, where? Your people checked her office thoroughly, but I wouldn't have expected to find something like those photographs there anyway. Did she have a safe-deposit box?"

"Yeah, but the only items in it were legal documents. Insurance policies, deeds to some property she owned, stuff like that. I've got some people putting together a list of the properties, what they are, where they are, but nothing else in the box provided anything in the way of a lead."

Mallory came into the room in time to hear that, and said, "Jamie's lockbox? I just double-checked, and that's the only one she had. No other bank has her on their customer list."

"At least not under her real name," Rafe said.

Mallory sighed. "I can go around to all the area banks and show them a picture of her. Or, better yet, send a few of the guys out on Monday to do that, since it's too late to get a decent start today. Although you'd think someone would have come forward after seeing all the pictures of her in the newspapers."

"People generally don't," Isabel said. "Don't want to get involved, or honestly don't believe they have any knowledge of value."

"And secrets of their own to protect," Rafe noted.

"Definitely. It's amazing how many people get nervous about some little transgression they're afraid we'll be interested in."

"Transgressions can be entertaining," Mallory noted.

Isabel grinned, and said, "True enough. But in this case, we hardly have time for them. Pity we can't make that announcement publicly. It'd probably save us time."

"And trouble," Rafe agreed.

"Yeah. Anyway, if Jamie had a lockbox under another name, she may well have worn a disguise of some kind when she visited. Just a wig, most likely, something that wouldn't have looked too phony. You probably won't have much luck showing her photo, but it's something that needs to be done. And we might get lucky."

Rafe nodded. "We do need to do whatever we can to make sure we've covered all the bases. But I'm not holding out much hope either. Especially after finding out she was pretty good at keeping secrets."

"Maybe a lot more secrets than we've yet discovered," Isabel said. "I know she made very good money, but she's also invested quite a bit in properties in the area, and she lived very well. I'm thinking that maybe the S&M stuff wasn't all fun and games for Jamie."

"Shit," Rafe said. "Mistress for hire?"

"Lots of people, apparently, willing to pay to be humiliated. Jamie was a smart businesswoman, so why wouldn't she charge for *all* her talents?"

———

Cheryl Bayne had been working hard on her career, doing all the frequently boring and certainly fluffy junk demanded of baby reporters—and female reporters. Especially when they worked for fourth-place TV stations. Dumb filler pieces on what the society ladies were wearing this season, or the mayor's daughter's birthday party, or the baby lion cub born at the zoo.

She was really sick of fluff.

So when her producer had offered her the chance to come to Hastings and cover this story—because a woman would play better, he'd said, and she was brunette, after all—Cheryl had jumped at it.

Now she was mostly just jumping at shadows.

Presently, on this Friday afternoon, she felt relatively safe standing in front of the town hall under the shade of a big oak tree. Her cameraperson was off getting background shots of the town, but she wasn't really alone, since the area was crawling with media.

"This is getting old." Dana Earley, a more experienced reporter for a rival Columbia station, sidled closer, studying the police department across Main Street with a slightly jaundiced eye. "Whatever they know over there, they aren't anxious to share."

"At least the chief called that press conference yesterday," Cheryl offered.

"Yeah, and told us squat." Dana reached up to tuck a strand of blond hair behind one ear. She looked at Cheryl, hesitated, then asked, "Have you had the feeling you were being followed, watched, especially at night? Or it is just us blondes?"

A little relieved to be able to talk about it, Cheryl said, "Actually, yeah. I thought it was my imagination."

"Umm. I've been asking around, and so far every woman I've

talked to has had the same feeling. Including, by the way, a couple of female cops who refused to speak on the record. I'd say it was just paranoia if it was only one or two of us, but all of us?"

"Maybe it's just . . . nerves."

Bluntly, Dana said, "I think he's watching us. And I have a very bad feeling about it."

"Well, you're blond—"

Dana shook her head. "I just got a peek at a list of women missing in the general area. And very few of them are blondes. Watch your back, Cheryl."

"I will. Thanks." She watched the blond reporter walk away, hearing the hollowness in her own voice when she added half under her breath, "Thanks a lot."

"Jesus," Mallory muttered.

"She wouldn't have considered it prostitution," Isabel pointed out. "Merely a fee-for-services-provided arrangement. Especially since she was the one in charge, the one making all the rules. No emotional involvement to clutter up her life, yet she gets the satisfaction of dominating other women. Maybe men as well. We don't *know* all her lovers—or clients—were women, after all. We only have Emily's word for it, and even she claims she didn't look through all the photos in that box."

"Do you believe her on that point?" Rafe asked.

"I think she saw more than she's admitted, but I didn't get a good sense of just how much."

"Every answer we get just opens up more questions," he said with a sigh.

Isabel, who was sitting at the end of the conference table near him, reached over and turned one of the photos so that she could study it. "Par for the course in serial-murder investigations, I'm afraid. In the meantime, does either of you have a clue where this room might be? It doesn't look like a room at the inn, and I doubt it's any other local hotel or motel. Anything about it look familiar to either of you?"

Mallory sat down on the other side of Rafe and leaned an elbow on the table, staring at the photos. "Not to me. There's not a lot there to go by. Bare paneled walls, what looks like an old vinyl floor, and a—yuck—stained mattress on a plain wooden platform. I guess comfort wasn't the point."

"The opposite, if anything," Isabel said with a grimace. "Have you *tried* stilettos? I have. It's a hideous thing to do to a foot."

Rafe looked at her with interest. "Stilettos? My God, how tall are you in them?"

"The ones I was wearing put me at about six-four. Note the past tense. I will never wear them again."

Curious, Mallory said, "Why did you wear them once? Or would that be sharing too much?"

Isabel chuckled. "Business, not pleasure, I promise you. Bishop believes our law-enforcement training should be varied and extensive, so at one point I worked for a while with a narc squad. Naturally, when they needed somebody to pose as a hooker . . ."

"You got the call."

"And the makeup and big hair and skanky outfit—and the stilettos. I gained a whole new respect for hookers. Their job is *hard*. And I mean just the walking around on the streets part."

Rafe cleared his throat again and tried to clear his mind of the image of Isabel dressed as a hooker. He tapped one of the photos in front of him. "Getting back to this room . . ."

Mallory grinned, but then sobered and said, "Maybe it's a

basement, but look at the shaft of light on the floor; that doesn't look like it's artificial light. There's a window in that room, and not a little basement window, I'm thinking. High, though."

"A walk-out basement could have full-size windows," Rafe noted almost absently. "I don't know, though, it doesn't look like a basement to me. The angle of the camera gives us a floor-to-ceiling view, and that ceiling's too high for most basements I've seen. Might even be something like a warehouse."

"Could be. And, judging by how fixed the positioning is, I'm guessing the camera was on a tripod and taking timed shots; neither woman is paying particular attention to it. So no third person was present. Probably."

"Maybe the submissive isn't even aware there is a camera," Rafe suggested.

"The submissive?" Mallory eyed him with faint amusement. "Did you take a crash course in S&M, or is the lingo a lot more standard than I thought it was?"

"I should refuse to answer that," Rafe said, "but in my defense I have to say we spent time about half an hour ago gathering and downloading information on the S&M scene from Quantico. Your tax dollars at work. I am now much more informed on the subject."

"I'll just bet you are."

"They sent plain facts, Mal, not pages from a magazine or some how-to manual."

"Ah. Learn anything interesting?"

"Nothing helpful."

"That wasn't what I asked."

"That's what I answered."

"Do you two do parties?" Isabel asked.

Rafe sighed. "Sorry."

"Oh, don't apologize. In a case like this one, I'd much rather laugh when I can. The chuckles tend to be few and far between."

Mallory said, "We've already had a few moments of gallows humor here and there. And I have a feeling this dominatrix stuff is going to provide a few more. Hard to take it seriously, you know? I mean, hard to imagine somebody you knew dressing up and making another woman lick her foot. What's *that* about?"

"In this context, a need to be in control and a high level of insecurity. Or, at least, that's my reading of Jamie Brower."

"Your psychic reading?" Rafe asked.

"From what I picked up at her parents' home and from Emily, yeah. Also a fair psychological stab in the dark. I'd like to check out her apartment, though, and try to get a better sense of her."

"I'd rather do that than keep staring at these damned pictures," Rafe said frankly. "I'd also rather not post them on the board, if it's all the same to you."

Knowing that virtually every cop in the place had access to the conference room and the boards set up with victim information, Isabel agreed with a nod. "We'll keep them in the Eyes Only file."

"We have one of those?" Mallory asked.

"We do now. I have a feeling there'll be more stuff for it as we go along, but for now I'd just as soon keep these photos and Jamie's secret between us. If this particular avenue of pursuit turns out to be a dead end, I don't see any reason for us to be the ones to out Jamie. Especially posthumously."

"Emily will probably take care of that," Mallory said.

"Or," Isabel said, "she'll keep it to herself and feel superior knowing her sister's dirty little secret. Could go either way, I'd say."

Mallory said, "You suggested to me that Emily might have caught the attention of her sister's killer; how serious were you about that?"

Isabel leaned back in her chair, absently rubbing the nape of her neck. "I don't have anything concrete, no evidence to support it. Not even a clairvoyant sense, really. Emily just barely fits the victim profile; she's blond, but on the young side for our killer. Not especially successful in any career, since she's still in school, but she's smart and observant."

"But?" Rafe said.

"It's just . . . a feeling I got in that house. Emily was actively snooping in Jamie's life during the weeks before she was killed, and we can be reasonably sure that during that period our killer was involved in Jamie's life, that he crossed her path. Which means he probably crossed Emily's path as well."

"And maybe she noticed him," Rafe said.

"Maybe. It's just a theory, but . . . it might not be such a bad idea to have your people keep an eye on Emily, at least when she's out of the house."

"Done. I'll assign a patrol. Plainclothes or uniformed?"

Isabel debated silently for a moment. "Let's not try to be subtle. Uniformed. Tell them to be casual but stay alert. If nothing else, focusing on the family member of a victim may lead the killer to think we're on the wrong track."

"Or on the right one," Mallory murmured.

"If he is after her, yeah. And, if so, a police escort may cause him to think twice. Worth the risk, I think."

Rafe nodded. "I agree. I'll assign the patrol on our way out and then go with you to check out Jamie's apartment. Mal, Hollis is at Tricia Kane's office; why don't you go over Jamie's office one more time? Just to make sure."

"Her boss is already pissed that we've taped the door to her office so none of his other agents can use it. Can I release it to him if I don't find anything this time?"

"Yeah, might as well. Unless the FBI has an objection?"

"Nope." Isabel shook her head. "But if you find anything at all that seems out of place to you, bring it back here."

"Gotcha."

Rafe watched as Isabel opened her briefcase and pulled out a bottle of ibuprofen. She swallowed several pills with the last of her coffee, then added cheerfully, "I'm ready when you are."

"Headache?"

"Usually," she confirmed, still cheerful. "Shall we?"

"It's getting late," Caleb Powell said.

Hollis looked up from her position behind what had been Tricia Kane's desk and nodded. "Yeah. I do appreciate you pretty much shutting down the office for a couple of hours today so I could go through her desk."

"Not a problem. I haven't felt much like working this week anyway. Find anything?"

"Nothing useful, as far as I can tell." Hollis pressed slender fingers to her closed eyes briefly in what he was beginning to recognize as a characteristic gesture, then studied the small pile of items on the neat blotter.

"Nothing new, I'd say," Caleb observed, wondering if she was as tired as she seemed. Telling himself he shouldn't take advantage.

Hollis agreed with a nod. "The police have already photocopied and gone through every page of the day planner: everything in it is purely work related. What few personal effects she kept in the desk are the usual, innocuous sort of thing any woman would keep at work. Extra compact and lipstick, small bottle of perfume, emery board and nail clippers, a ripped-in-half photo of the ex-boyfriend she clearly wasn't quite ready to throw away."

Caleb grimaced. "I caught her looking at that once or twice. She said just what you did, that she wasn't quite ready to toss it."

"It takes time for some people to let go."

He decided not to comment on that. "So there's nothing helpful here in the office."

"Nothing I can see." Hollis rose to her feet. She glanced past Caleb toward the front door and for an instant went still, eyes widening.

Caleb looked back over his shoulder, then at her. His first, instinctive reading of her posture and expression was that she had received a shock but was almost immediately back in control of whatever emotions that shock had caused.

"What?" he asked.

She blinked, her gaze returning to him. "Hmm? Nothing. It's nothing. Listen, Mr. Powell, confidentially, the focus of the investigation is going to shift back to the first victim. We believe something about that victim or that murder is most likely to help us identify the killer."

He thought she was a little pale, but what she'd told him pushed that awareness out of his mind. "So Tricia's murder goes on the back burner."

Gravely, Hollis said, "In the conference room at the police department where we'll work every day, there are bulletin boards sectioned, so far, into thirds. Each third is filled with photos and information on each victim. Time lines of the last weeks of their lives. Habits, haunts, events that might or might not have been important. Every day, we look at those boards. Every day, we look at the pictures of those women. And every day, we'll discuss their lives and the people who knew them and try to figure out who killed them. Every day."

Caleb drew a breath and let it out slowly. "Sorry. It's just that . . . she was my friend."

"I know. I'm sorry." Her blue eyes gazed past him for another moment, briefly. "Just know that nobody is going to forget Tricia. And that we'll get her killer."

"You seem so certain of that."

Hollis looked faintly surprised. "We won't give up until we do get him. It's only a matter of time, Mr. Powell."

"Caleb," he said, "please. And thank you for your efforts, Agent Templeton."

She smiled wryly. "Hollis. Especially since I'm not a full agent yet. *Special Investigator* is a title the SCU gives its members who lack a background in law or law enforcement. I've only been with the unit a few months."

"But you're a trained investigator?"

"Recently trained, yeah. In my . . . previous life . . . I did something else." Hollis came out from behind the desk, adding in a slightly preoccupied tone, "My partner, on the other hand, has a solid background in law and law enforcement, as well as years of experience, so you don't have to worry that the Bureau sent two rookies down here."

"I wasn't worried, actually." Realizing she was about to leave, and reluctant to let her go, he said quickly, "I remember you saying something about being an artist."

"Used to be."

"Used to be? Does a creative person ever stop being creative?"

For the first time, Hollis was clearly uncomfortable. "Sometimes things happen that change your whole life. I—uh—need to get back to the police station. Thank you very much for your cooperation, Mr.—Caleb. I'll be in touch."

"I'll be here."

"Thanks again. Bye."

He didn't try to stop her, but for several minutes after she left, Caleb gazed after her, frowning, wondering what had happened to change Hollis Templeton's entire life.

"I know all about evil, Mr. Powell, believe me. I met it up close and personal."

He hadn't thought she'd been speaking literally.

Now he was very much afraid she had been.

When Rafe and Isabel were in one of the department Jeeps and on their way to Jamie Brower's apartment, he said, "I notice you haven't suggested that Hollis visit any of the crime scenes."

"Since what happened earlier, you mean?" Isabel shrugged. "You've obviously also noticed Hollis is a bit . . . fragile."

"It's a little hard to miss."

"She has a lot of potential. But becoming a medium cost her a trip to hell you wouldn't believe, and she hasn't completely dealt with that yet.

"But despite being afraid, despite her not reaching out, not trying to make contact—she did. Which is an indication of just how much potential she has."

Rafe sent his companion a glance. "You really believe there was a ghost in the room with us?"

"I believe the spirit of Jamie Brower was there, yes."

"But you didn't see her? It?"

"No, I can't see the dead." Isabel's voice was utterly matter-of-fact. "Or hear them, for that matter. But I can sometimes feel them near me. The very air in the room changes, maybe because they aren't supposed to be a part of this dimensional plane. You felt it yourself."

This time, Rafe kept his eyes on the road. "My ears popped. It happens."

"All the time," she agreed mildly.

"Look, if Jamie was really there, why didn't she say or do something to help us find her killer?"

"She was trying. Trying to speak to Hollis, the only one in the room with the ability to hear her. Unfortunately, Hollis isn't ready to listen."

"I don't suppose Jamie could just scribble us a note, huh? *X killed me.*"

Isabel answered the question seriously. "So far, none of us has encountered a spirit or noncorporeal force with enough focus and power to physically touch or move objects. Unless they were inside a host, of course. Or controlling one."

6

SHE'LL TELL. *You know she'll tell.*
He listened to the voice this time because he wanted to. Because he enjoyed this part of it so much. Watching them. Following. Learning their routines.

Hunting.

Like the others. Just like them.

The voice was right about that. She was just like all the rest. Laughing behind his back. So eager to tell his secrets. He had to stop her before she could do that.

You've done three. Only three more. And then you can rest. Then you can be.

"I'm tired," he murmured, still watching her. "This time, I'm tired."

That's because you're changing.

"I know." He moved carefully, staying in the shadows as he

followed her. This one was tricky; she was aware of her surroundings, watchful. Uneasy. They were all beginning to act that way, he'd noticed. Part of him loved that, that he made them so uneasy.

But it made things more difficult.

You can do this. You have to. Or she'll tell. She'll tell them all about you.

"Yes," he murmured, easing a little closer despite the risk that she would see him. "I have to. I can't let her tell. I can't let any of them tell."

Rafe pulled the Jeep abruptly to the curb and parked. They were still in the downtown area, not even halfway to Jamie's apartment. He continued to stare through the windshield, his rugged face completely unreadable. "A host."

Isabel didn't have to be clairvoyant to know he had just about reached the end of his willingness to believe in the paranormal. Or even to accept that it might be possible.

Or possibly he had simply reached the end of his rope.

Hard to blame him for that.

"A host," he repeated, his deep voice still extremely calm. "You want to explain that?"

Matching his tone, Isabel replied, "When it's a spirit, the simple truth is that some of them refuse to accept what's happened to them when they die. Whether it's unfinished business or simply an unwillingness to move on, they want to stay here."

"I guess that explains haunted houses." He was trying hard to keep his voice matter-of-fact.

"Well, only partly. Some houses really do contain the spirit or spirits of people who didn't want to move on. But some of what people call hauntings are just place memories."

"Place memories?"

"Yeah. When people report seeing the same *ghost* repeat the same actions again and again, that's likely a place memory. A good example is the Roman soldiers so many people have seen marching on their battlefield, endlessly. Or other battlefields, like Gettysburg. We don't believe those poor men keep reenacting the battles that killed them; we believe the places remember what happened there."

"How?"

"We can only theorize. Either because those particular areas have a specific energy of their own or possibly just the ability geographically or topographically to contain energy better than other places do. We believe that the extreme psychic—electromagnetic—energy of such horrific, tragic events literally soaked into the earth at places like that.

"And sometimes there's a buildup of pressure and those 'memories' are discharged in the form of energy, like static. If anybody happens to be around, especially a functional or latent psychic, what's seen is what that place remembers. An image of what happened there."

"That actually makes a kind of sense," Rafe said, sounding both reluctant and bemused.

"Yeah, most of this does, if you consider possible scientific explanations. Which we always do. All based on some form of energy."

"So explain this host thing."

"Well, like I said, some people who die don't want to be dead. If they're desperate enough, or angry enough, sometimes they're able to muster enough power to . . . find and inhabit a physical host. Another person."

"Possession. You're talking about possession?" He was beginning to sound incredulous again.

Isabel waited until he finally looked at her, then said, "Not in the . . . Hollywood . . . sense of the word. This isn't some pea-soup-spewing demon a priest could exorcise. Often, they aren't even negative, or bad, spirits. They just want to live. It's a case of a stronger mind and spirit overpowering a weaker or otherwise vulnerable one."

"You're telling me this has actually happened?"

"We believe it has, although I can't offer you any proof. Bishop and Miranda actually fought the spirit of an insanely determined serial killer once. Quite a story there."

Rafe blinked, but said only, "Who's Miranda?"

"Sorry. Bishop's wife and partner. Years ago, Miranda touched several mental patients who were being treated for severe schizophrenia. She definitely felt, in each case, that there were two distinct and separate souls fighting for possession of those people. It convinced her. It convinced us, even before we duplicated the experiment and got the same results in three out of the five diagnosed schizophrenic mental patients we tested."

"This is a little hard to swallow," Rafe said finally.

"I know. Sorry about that." She might have been apologizing for bumping him in a crowd.

He stared at her, then pulled the Jeep away from the curb and continued on their way. "So, worst-case scenario in a situation like that, the host goes nuts and ends up in a mental institution being *treated* for a mental disease he doesn't have."

"I can think of worse things that might happen, but, yeah, we do believe that has happened. Theoretically, if the host mind and spirit were really weak, the invading spirit would just take over. You'd have a person who appeared to suddenly develop a whole new personality." Isabel reflected, then said, "Which, I suppose, could explain teenagers."

Rafe didn't smile. "What happens to the host's spirit?"

101

"I don't know. We don't know. Withers away, maybe, like an unused limb. Gets booted out and passes on to whatever awaits all of us when we leave this mortal coil." Isabel sighed. "Frontier territory, remember? We have a lot of theories, Rafe. We have some personal experiences, war stories we can tell. Even a few nonpsychic if not unbiased witnesses to testify to things they've seen and heard. But scientific data to back us up? Not so much. For most of us, we believe because we have to. Because it's us experiencing the paranormal. Hard to deny something when it's part of your everyday life."

"And the rest of us have to take it on faith."

"Unfortunately. Unless and until you have your own close encounter with the paranormal."

"I'd rather not."

Isabel's smile twisted a bit. "Yeah. Well, let's hope you get your wish. But don't count on it. Maybe it's just because we psychics are present to pull in and focus the energy, but people around us do tend to experience things they never would have imagined before. Fair warning."

"You keep warning me."

"I keep trying."

It was Rafe's turn to sigh, but all he said was, "You made a distinction earlier between a spirit and a—what did you call it?— a noncorporeal force? What the hell is that supposed to be?"

"Evil."

He waited a moment, then said, "Evil as in . . . ?"

"As in the force opposing good, the negative to offset the positive. As in the precarious balance of nature, of the universe itself. As in worse than you can imagine, breath smelling like brimstone, glowing red eyes, straight-out-of-a-fiery-hell evil."

"You're not serious?"

When he glanced over at her, he found something in her green eyes older and wiser than any woman's eyes should ever have held. Than any human eyes should ever have held.

"Didn't you know, Rafe? Hadn't you even considered the possibility? Evil is real. It's a tangible, visible presence when it wants to be. It even has a face. Believe me, I know. I've seen it."

Alan had every intention of taking the note to Rafe and the federal agents. Just not right away.

He wasn't stupid about it, of course. He made a copy and put the original in a clear plastic sleeve to protect it. And then he spent a lot of time staring at the note. The words. Trying to figure out what the author was trying to tell him.

And trying to decide if the author was the killer.

Despite his sometimes provocative attitude in print, Alan wasn't a big fan of conspiracy theories, so his natural inclination was to believe that the note had been written by the killer. It was the simplest explanation, and it made sense to him. What didn't make sense was that someone in town knew who the killer was and had done nothing to stop him.

Unless that someone was very, very afraid.

And if that was the case . . . how could Alan flush him or her out of hiding?

It would be such a coup. And stop the killings, of course.

But how to bring that person, if he or she existed, out of the woodwork?

Musing over that question, Alan left the original of the note securely locked in his desk, but took the copy with him when he left the office—a bit early—for the day. He didn't go straight home but stopped by the town-hall building, which had become the unofficial hangout for most members of the media.

There were quite a few hanging around, but most were

talking companionably, with the relaxed posture that came of having passed the deadline for the six o'clock news. The pressure was off, at least for most of them and for the moment.

Dana Earley, the only blond female in the bunch, was also the most obviously tense. Understandably. She was also the only TV reporter still present today, and kept her cameraman close.

Alan doubted it was because she liked the guy, who was skinny, clearly bored, and appeared to be about seventeen.

Some protection he'd be, Alan thought.

"You," Dana said to him, "are looking far too smug. What do you know that the rest of us don't?"

"Oh, come on, Dana. You think I want a Columbia TV station to scoop me?"

Her brows disappeared up under her bangs. "Scoop you? What old movies have you been watching?"

Refusing the bait, Alan merely said, "It'll be dark soon. I think if I were a blond TV reporter, I'd want to be inside. Behind a locked door. With a gun. Or at least some muscle." He eyed the cameraman sardonically.

"I hear you have some muscle of your own," she retorted. "Police muscle. Sleeping with a cop, Alan?"

"If I am, it's hardly newsworthy," he said dryly, showing no outward sign of an inward flinch. Mallory was not going to like it if this *news* was common knowledge, dammit. "Unless your station prefers tabloid gossip over substantive news."

"Don't sound so superior. You were the first print journalist to use the phrase *serial killer,* and however you intended it, it sounded gleeful and excited in your article."

"It did not," he found himself countering irritably.

"Go back and read it again." She tucked an errant strand of blond hair behind her ear, smiled at him gently, and wandered off toward a magazine journalist here to research serial killers.

"Here you go, Alan."

He jumped, and frowned at Paige Gilbert, who was holding out a tissue to him.

"Jesus, don't sneak up on people. And what's that?"

"I thought you might need it. For the spit in your eye."

For just an instant, he was blank, but then he glanced after Dana and scowled as he looked back at the radio reporter. "Ha ha. She was just being all superior because she's a talking head on the six o'clock news."

"Not today she wasn't," Paige murmured.

"None of us has had much to report today," he reminded her.

"True. But you might as well have canary feathers smeared all around your mouth. Come on, Alan, give it up. You know we'll find out sooner or later."

Alan made a mental note to stop playing poker with Rafe and a few other of their friends; obviously, his serious lack of a poker face was why he had lost so much imaginary money to them.

"I'm done for the day," he informed Paige. "And even though this is your first really big story, if you want some advice from a veteran, you should go home and get some sleep as well. You never know when you'll get that call that pulls you out of bed at two in the morning."

Paige gazed after him, then jumped slightly herself when Dana said at her elbow, "He knows something."

"Yeah," Paige said. "But what?"

The rented car she and Isabel were sharing was parked near Caleb Powell's law office, so Hollis was able to make it that far. Once locked inside, though, engine and air-conditioning running, she sat behind the wheel and watched her hands shake.

Bishop had warned her that until she learned to fully control

105

her abilities, the door that devastating trauma had created or ac-tivated in her mind was likely to open up unexpectedly. And that the experiences were apt to be particularly powerful ones in the midst of a murder investigation when several people had died re-cently and violently.

But all the months spent in the relative peace of Quantico, learning how to be an investigator, learning about the SCU, plus learning all the exercises in concentration, meditation, and con-trol, had given her a false sense of security.

She had thought she was ready for this.

She wasn't.

First seeing Jamie Brower in the conference room, and now this. Seeing Tricia Kane standing near the desk where she had worked in life, less clearly visible than Jamie had been, oddly dreamlike but obviously trying to say something Hollis hadn't been able to hear.

Why couldn't she hear them? Before, it had been a voice in her head and only the sense of a presence, at least until the very end. Not . . . this. Not these misty images of people—souls—trapped between worlds. No longer alive, but not yet gone, stand-ing in the doorway between this life and the next, the doorway Hollis's own traitorous mind kept opening for them. Talking to her.

Trying to talk to her.

Hollis hadn't expected this.

Not this.

She didn't know how to cope with this. She didn't know if she wanted to even try to learn to cope.

She wanted to run, that's what she wanted to do. Run and hide, from the dead and from—

The ringing demand of her cell phone jarred her from the

panic, and she took a deep breath to try and steady her voice before she answered it. "Templeton."

"What happened?" Isabel asked without preamble.

"I checked out Tricia Kane's office, but—"

"No, Hollis. What happened?"

She'd already had a few unsettling experiences with other SCU members and their easy connections with one another, so Isabel's obvious awareness of Hollis's state of mind didn't surprise her all that much. It still unsettled her, however.

"I saw Tricia Kane," she said finally, baldly.

"Did she tell you anything?" Isabel's voice was calm.

"She tried. I couldn't hear her. Like before."

"How long did it last?"

Hollis had to stop and think about that. "Not long. Not as long as in the conference room. And not as clear. She was . . . the image was fainter. Wispy. And it didn't feel as spooky."

"Powell didn't notice anything?"

"I don't think so."

"You're out of the office now?"

"Yeah."

"Okay. It's getting late. Why don't you go back to the inn and soak in the tub, have a hot shower, something like that. Relax. Order a pizza. Watch something mind-numbing on TV for a while."

"Isabel—"

"Hollis, trust me. Take the time while you can, and chill. Just chill. Sleep if you can. Don't think too much. We're just getting started here, and it's only going to get harder."

"I have to learn how to handle this."

"Yes. But you don't have to learn everything today. Today you just have to get some rest and get centered again. That's all. I'll be back at the inn myself in a couple of hours. I'll check, see if you feel like company. If not, that's cool, I'll see you at breakfast. But if you want to talk, I'll be there. Okay?"

"Okay. Thanks."

"Don't mention it, partner."

Rafe watched Isabel close her cell phone and return it to the belt pack she wore in lieu of a purse. They were standing in the living room of Jamie Brower's apartment, but they had barely arrived before Isabel reached for her phone, saying without explanation that she had to call Hollis.

"She was in trouble," Rafe guessed, watching Isabel.

"She saw another of the victims. Tricia Kane. It freaked her out a bit." Isabel shrugged, frowning slightly. "Still couldn't hear what Tricia was trying to tell her, so no help for us."

"You knew she was in trouble before you called her. How?" Before Isabel could answer, Rafe did himself. "Connections. A psychic connection. She's your partner."

"A connection she finds more unnerving than reassuring at this point," Isabel said wryly. "I'm sure you can relate." She began walking through the very nice apartment, looking around her with interest.

Rafe followed. "What do you mean by that?"

"I make you nervous. Admit it."

"I've known you barely twenty-four hours," Rafe retorted. "That isn't enough time to get used to a woman's perfume, let alone the fact that she knows without looking what kind of shorts you happen to be wearing."

Isabel chuckled. "Okay, you win that round."

Rafe thought it was about time he won one. "Is Hollis all right?"

"She will be, I think. This time. But if she doesn't get a handle on her abilities pretty fast, things are just going to get harder for her."

"I'd think talking to dead people would never get easier."

"No, from all I'm told, that part doesn't. It takes an exceptionally powerful medium with a strong sense of self to open that door and yet remain detached—and protected—from all the emotional and spiritual energy pouring through."

"Protected?"

Isabel paused in the kitchen, running a hand lightly along the immaculate granite countertops. The usual small appliances were scattered about: toaster, blender, coffeemaker. "She didn't cook much."

"Not according to what her family and friends said, no. A lot of takeout. What do you mean about a medium needing to protect herself?"

"Or himself. It's not a gender-specific ability, you know."

"I stand corrected. *Are* there any gender-specific abilities?"

"Not as far as we know."

"Okay. What did you mean about the medium protecting him- or herself?"

Isabel left the kitchen and went down the short hallway to the bedroom. She stood in the center, looking around. "A medium is the most vulnerable of all psychics to what you called possession. They're the ones who open the doors angry or desperate spirits usually need in order to return to this plane of existence. And the nearest potential host when the spirit comes through."

"*Usually* need?"

"We've theorized that an unusually powerful spirit could make its own doorway, if it were determined enough. So far, though, our experience has been that mediums or latent mediums provide the doorways."

"I can't believe I'm talking about this. Listening to this."

She looked at him, smiling faintly. "This stuff has always been with us, always been a part of our lives. For most of us, it was simply a case of not seeing what was there. Who knew there were protons and electrons until we found them? Who knew germs were responsible for illnesses until somebody figured it out? Who knew even fifty years ago that we had a chance in hell of mapping the human genome?"

"I get the point," Rafe said. "Still, this is—or at least feels—different."

"It's human. And one day, eventually, science will catch up, figure out a way to define, measure, and analyze, and make us legit."

"It's just . . . it's difficult to wrap my mind around it."

"I know, but you have to." Isabel walked over to the bed and rested a hand on it, frowning. "There are more things in heaven and earth, Horatio. Get used to it. Here endeth the lesson."

Rafe accepted the mild rebuke with a nod. "Okay. Though I do reserve the right to ask questions if anything unusual happens right in front of me."

"I wouldn't expect anything else."

He had to smile a little at her dry tone. "Picking up anything useful here?"

Touch me there . . . like that . . .

Harder . . .

Christ, you feel good . . .

Years of practice enabled Isabel to keep her face expressionless, but it was unexpectedly difficult with Rafe's eyes on her. He had very dark eyes, and there was something very compelling in them. She hadn't expected that.

Hadn't expected him.

"This is where she kept her sex straight. A few male lovers over the years. No women."

"So you think the room in the pictures was hers? One of the

110

properties she owned? A place she kept separate and secret for those . . . encounters?"

"Seems likely. She led a very traditional life here, so obviously her secret life was kept a thing apart. Really a thing apart; there are no secrets at all here. In fact, I'm more than a little surprised Emily found the photo box in this apartment."

"Unless Jamie had lost her most recent lover and hadn't yet found another. In that case, she might have needed to look at those pictures."

Isabel smiled. "You'd make a fair profiler, know that?"

Rafe was more than a little startled. "I was just guessing, that's all."

"What do you think profilers do? We make guesses. Mostly educated guesses, and for some of us occasionally psychic ones, but at the end of the day they're still guesses. Speculation based on experience, knowledge of criminals and how their minds work, that sort of thing. A good profiler probably gets sixty to seventy-five percent right if he or she is especially tuned in to a particular subject. A good psychic with solid control gets, maybe, forty to sixty percent in hits."

"Is that your percentage?"

She shrugged. "More or less."

He decided not to try to pin her down on that; he had a feeling it was one he wouldn't win. He hadn't known Isabel Adams an hour before reaching the conclusion that she was extremely unlikely to let slip by accident anything she didn't want him to know.

Isabel said, "We have to find the box or that room. Both, preferably. I need to know how Jamie felt about her secret life, really felt about it. And I'm getting nothing about that here."

"So you're getting no sense of a secret hiding place my people missed?"

"No sense of anything secret. I mean at all; this lady obviously knew how to compartmentalize her life. This was her public self, what the world was allowed to see. All bright and shiny and picture-perfect. We know her public self. We need to know her private self."

Rafe frowned as he followed her from the room. "Do you believe Jamie was targeted because of her sexual preferences? Because she was a dominatrix?"

"I don't know. It's about relationships, I'm sure of that. Somehow, it's about relationships. I'm having a hard time seeing Jamie's sexuality, or even the S&M games, as the trigger, that's all. Given his history. But it's the only thing hidden in Jamie's day-to-day life, and that means we have to be sure how much it means."

"Makes sense."

"So we need to find that room. And we need to find it quickly. It's been four days since he killed Tricia Kane; even if he waits a full week between murders, we only have three days to find him and stop him before another woman dies."

And before Isabel moved up on the hit list, Rafe thought but didn't say.

"You think he's stalking her now?" he asked instead.

"He's watching her. Thinking about what he's going to do to her. Imagining how it's going to feel. Anticipating." She was surprised that after all these years and so many similar investigations, it could still make her skin crawl.

But it wasn't just the fact of this killer, she knew that. It wasn't even what he had done to his victims. It was him. What she felt in him. Something twisted and evil crouching in the shadows, waiting to spring forward.

She could almost smell the brimstone.

Almost.

"Isabel—"

"Not now, Rafe." For the first time, there was a hint of vulnerability in her slightly twisted smile. "I'm not ready to talk about that evil face I saw. Not to you. Not yet."

"Just tell me this much. Does it have something to do with you becoming psychic?"

"It had everything to do with it." Her smile twisted even more. "The universe has an ironic sense of humor, I've noticed. Or maybe just an innate sense of justice. Because sometimes evil creates the tool that will help destroy it."

Cheryl had planned to drive back to Columbia for the night, especially after Dana's warning, but something was bugging her. It had been bugging her all day, ever since she'd noticed it early this morning.

She had her cameraman wait for her in the van and went to check it out, telling herself she'd be safe; it wasn't even dark yet, for God's sake. Of course, telling herself was one thing, and feeling it something else entirely.

Every time the breeze stirred it felt like somebody touching her with a ghostly hand, and she caught herself looking back over her shoulder more than once.

Nothing there, naturally. No one there.

The whole thing was just her imagination, probably. Because it didn't make sense, not if she'd seen what she thought she had. Not if it meant—

A hand touched her shoulder, and Cheryl whirled around with a gasp. "Oh, Jesus. Scare a person, why don't you?"

"Did I? Sorry about that."

"You of all people should know—"

"I do. Like I said, sorry. What're you doing out here?"

"Just following up a hunch. I'm sure the rest of you saw it, but it's been bugging me, so . . . here I am."

"You really shouldn't be out by yourself."

"I know, I know. But I'm not a blonde. And I hate it when something bugs me. So it seemed like a risk worth taking."

"Just for a story?"

"Well," Cheryl said self-consciously, "that's part of it, sure. The story. And maybe to stop him. I mean, it would be so cool if I could help stop him."

"Do you really believe your hunch could do that?"

"You never know. I could get lucky."

"Or unlucky."

"What're you—"

"Not a blonde. But nosy just like they are. And you'll tell. I really can't let that happen."

Cheryl saw the knife, but by the time understanding clicked into place in her head, it was too late to scream.

Too late to do anything at all.

Friday, 11:30 PM

Just occasionally, whenever her day had been particularly stressful, Mallory was so wild in bed that it took everything Alan had just to keep up with her.

Friday night was like that.

She held him with her arms, her legs, her body, as though he might escape her. The pillows were shoved off the bed, and the sheets tangled around them, and still they wrestled and rolled and held on to each other. They finished, finally, with Mallory on top, riding him fiercely, one hand on his chest and the other

114

braced behind her on his leg, grinding her loins to his in a hard, hungry, rhythmic dance.

He held her hips, surging up to meet her, his gaze fixed on the magnificence of her face taut in primitive need, her eyes darkened, her lithe, toned body glowing with life and exertion.

When she finally came with a cry, shuddering, he spent in almost the same instant, feeling her inner muscles spasming, milking him dry.

Usually, at that point Mallory rolled off him to lie at his side, however briefly, but this time he held on and shifted their bodies himself so that they lay on their sides, facing each other. He kept his arms around her.

"Good," she murmured, relaxed at least for the moment. "That was . . . good."

Drained himself, Alan nevertheless consciously tried to control the moment, his hand stroking her back in a soothing motion, enjoying the sensation of her warm breath against his neck. "More than good." He knew better than to comment on her passion, knowing from experience that it would only cause her to draw away, to start making excuses for leaving.

He had never figured out if it was the intimacy of the act that bothered Mallory when she allowed herself to think about it, or was reminded of it, or if it was her own lack of control that disturbed her. Either way, he was careful not to push that particular button.

He had learned.

"Long day," he murmured finally, intentionally keeping his voice as easy and soothing as his hands.

"Very long." She sounded a little sleepy. She moved just a bit against him, but closer, and sighed. "And a longer one tomorrow. God, I'm tired."

He didn't say anything, but continued to stroke her back gently even after he knew she had fallen asleep. He held her close and caressed her warm, silky skin, and felt her heart beat against his. And it was enough. For now.

A storm woke him before dawn, and Mallory was gone.

She hadn't even left a note on the fucking pillow.

Saturday, June 14, 6:30 AM

HE WOKE UP with blood on his hands.
Wet blood.
Fresh blood.

The pungent, coppery smell of it was thick and heavy in the room, and he gagged as he stumbled from the bed and into the bathroom. He didn't bother to turn on the light even though the room was dim, just turned on the taps and fumbled for soap, washing his hands in the hottest water he could stand, soaping again and again.

The water, first bright red and then rusty-colored, swirled around the drain and slowly, so slowly, grew fainter and fainter. Like the smell.

When the water ran clear and he couldn't smell the blood anymore, he turned off the taps. For a long moment he stood there, hands braced on the sink, staring at his shadowy reflection in the mirror. Finally, he went back into the bedroom and sat on the side of the tumbled bed, staring at nothing.

Again.

It had happened again.

He could still smell the blood, though there was no sign of any on the sheets. There hadn't been before either. There never was, on anything he touched.

Just his hands.

He leaned forward, his elbows on his knees, and stared at his hands. Strong hands. Clean hands. Now.

No blood. Now.

"What have I done?" he whispered. "Oh, Christ, what have I done?"

Travis Keech yawned widely as he sat up in bed and vigorously rubbed his head with both hands. "Jesus. It's after eight."

"It's dawn," Alyssa Taylor said sleepily. "And it's Saturday, so who cares?"

"I care. I have to. I'm supposed to work. The chief said we could come in later if we've worked late—which I did last night—but we're all working overtime."

"I suppose it's taking all of you to investigate these murders."

"You can say that again."

"And I suppose you've got leads to follow."

Her voice still sounded sleepy, but Travis looked down at her with a tolerant smile. "You know, just because you're convinced I'm a yokel with straw in my hair doesn't mean you're right."

"I don't know what you're talking about." Sounding less sleepy now, she stretched like an elegant cat. The position showed him a nice expanse of bare skin already wearing a light summer tan, which really set off her gleaming dark hair and pale eyes.

"Oh, come on, Ally. I don't normally end up in bed with gorgeous women just hours after meeting them in our one little excuse for a bar. Unless, of course, they happen to be TV reporters from the big city and I happen to be involved in a serial-killer investigation."

"Don't underrate yourself," Alyssa told him. "And don't measure my morals with your yardstick, if you don't mind. I didn't set out to sleep with a cop, and I don't go after stories on my back."

"A lot of reporters do, I hear."

"I'm not one of them."

The sheet had slipped to show him most of one generous breast, and Travis decided he didn't want to offend her. "I never said you were," he protested, lying back down beside her and reaching underneath the covers. "But you could have had any guy in that bar and you came home with me. What else was I supposed to think?"

"That I thought you were sexy?" She didn't exactly pout, but her body was just the slightest bit stiff when he pulled her into his arms. "That I was bored and didn't want to go back to my hotel room alone? That I like guys in uniform?"

"Which was it?" he asked, nuzzling her neck.

"All of the above." She sighed and relaxed in his embrace, her arms slipping around his middle and her hands sliding downward. "And you've got a cute ass too."

He made an urgent sound, his body responding instantly to her caress, and she thought with faint, fleeting amusement that there was a lot to be said for catching a guy in his early twenties and at the peak of his sexuality.

A lot to be said.

She murmured, "I thought you had to go in to work."

"Later," Travis said.

It was nearly half an hour later when he finally, reluctantly pulled himself out of the bed. "I've gotta get to work. Want to join me in the shower?"

Alyssa stretched languidly. "Are you kidding? That tiny stall isn't even big enough for you. I'll wait my turn, thanks. I can shower while you're shaving."

"Okay, suit yourself."

Alyssa waited until she heard the water running, then slipped from the bed and gathered her scattered clothing from the floor. She had to follow a trail halfway to the front door to get it all, which amused her yet again. Her purse had been left carelessly on a chair near the front door, something that made her shake her head.

Not smart. Not at all smart.

Could be she was slipping.

"Nah," she murmured in response to that idea.

Returning to the bedroom, she laid the clothing out on the bed and then got her cell phone from the purse. She turned it on and punched in a number, keeping her gaze fixed on the half-open bathroom door.

"Hey, it's Ally." She kept her voice low. "I've found that source we talked about. A pretty good one. He's already told me more than he realizes. He must have had half a dozen strong drinks last night, and no hangover this morning. Oh, to be twenty-four again."

She listened for a moment, then said, "Yes, *my* head hurts. Well, I had to at least seem to keep up with him, didn't I? Never mind. He's going in to work, and the plan is to get him to meet me for lunch."

A question made her laugh under her breath. "No, I don't

think there'll be any problem persuading him to meet me. And I have a . . . hunch . . . that he'll be perfectly happy to have me sticking close for the duration. So I should have a fair idea of what's going on inside the department. Yeah. Yeah, I'll check in at least twice a day, as arranged."

10:05 AM

The third property they checked turned out to be an old commercial building off what had once been a busy two-lane highway until the bypass opened years before. Several companies had lost most of their customers, and more than one derelict office building or small store now stood abandoned and slowly falling into ruin. But a few, like the one Jamie Brower had owned, had been converted to have some kind of a useful life not dependent on passing customers.

"She was ostensibly using it for storage," Rafe noted as they stood just inside the front door. The early sunlight slanted through the dusty front windows so that the interior of the front part of the building was easily visible to them.

"Just barely ostensibly," Isabel agreed, looking around at a half dozen or so large pieces of old furniture in obvious need of restoration or repair, and a few crates labeled STORAGE. "Only enough stuff so that anybody looking in the front window would assume that was what she was using it for."

"The real story is in the back," Mallory called from a doorway about thirty feet from the front door and roughly halfway down the length of the building, where a wall divided the space. "The tools the locksmith gave us worked on this door and the rear entrance—which is conveniently hidden from the road. Great place to park your car if you don't want anybody to know you're here. And there are signs quite a few cars have been parked back there in recent months."

"Why does that not surprise me?" Hollis wondered aloud.

"It's about time we got lucky," Rafe said as he, Isabel, and Hollis joined Mallory, all of them stepping into the half of the building that was quite obviously the reason Jamie had bought this place.

It was the room in the photographs.

"The submissive did know she was being photographed," Rafe said, gesturing toward the camera set up on a tripod several yards from the bed platform. "There's no place in here to hide that thing. The distance and angle look just right."

Hollis, wearing latex gloves, as they all were, went to examine the camera. "Yeah, it's set up to work on a timer. No cartridge or disk," she said. "Whatever last photos she took weren't left in the camera."

"No, I'd expect her to be more cautious than that," Isabel said, looking slowly around. "The really interesting thing is the question of whether the camera was part of the ritual. If she really does have a box full of photos, as Emily said, then it's likely most if not all of her partners were photographed."

Rafe kept watching her instead of studying the room, bothered by something he couldn't quite put a finger on. He thought Isabel was somehow uncomfortable or uneasy here. Her posture seemed a bit stiffer than usual, and something about the very calm of her features was almost masklike.

So when he spoke, it was absently. "It's all about control. And submission. Being photographed probably was part of the ritual, one of Jamie's rules. Her partners had to submit completely to her and her rules, even to the extent of having their secret needs and desires, their humiliation, recorded on film—and left in the hands of the dominant."

Mallory had located a large built-in closet or storage area on the right-hand wall and was working on the padlocked double doors with the ring of all-purpose tools provided by the locksmith. "Just for the record," she said, "I don't ever want to want anything that much."

"I'll second that," Rafe said. He was still watching Isabel, and directed his question to her. "Picking up anything?"

"Lots," she answered. "I don't know yet how much of it will be important, though. Or even relevant."

Her voice had been completely serene, but Rafe found himself frowning nevertheless. He glanced at Hollis and saw that she was also watching her partner intently, a crease between her brows indicating worry or unease.

Isabel walked over to the bed platform and bent slightly to place her gloved hand on the bare, stained mattress. Her face remained expressionless, though her mouth seemed to firm.

"I guess the latex doesn't interfere with psychic contact," Rafe said.

It was Hollis who replied, "No, it doesn't seem to. Although some of the SCU psychics say it has a slight muffling quality. Like everything else, it varies from person to person."

"Got it," Mallory announced suddenly. She unfastened the padlock and opened the two doors. "Christ."

"The toy box," Hollis murmured.

Dana Earley would have been the first to admit that being in Hastings at this particular time was making her extremely nervous. It had always been easy in the past for her to blend in, become a part of the background until she was ready to step in front of the camera and report the news.

This time, she was afraid of *becoming* the news.

"You shouldn't be out here," one male citizen of the small town scolded her in front of the coffee shop when she attempted to interview him about his feelings.

"I'm not alone," Dana said, gesturing toward Joey.

The man gave her cameraman the same scornful look Alan had offered the previous day. "Yeah, well, he might drop his camera on the killer's toe before he cuts and runs, but I wouldn't count on it if I were you."

"I resent that," Joey said sullenly.

They both ignored him.

"You should at least protect yourself," the man told Dana earnestly. "The police department is offering pepper spray to any woman who asks. I got some for my wife. You need to go get some for yourself."

"What about you?" Dana asked, making a mental note about the pepper spray. "Aren't you worried the killer might start going after men?"

He glanced from side to side warily, then opened his lightweight windbreaker to show her a pistol tucked into his belt. "I hope the bastard does come after me. I'm ready. A lot of us are ready."

"Looks like," she offered brightly, trying not to show him how much it frightened her to see guns in the hands of people other than the police. Especially angry and very nervous people. "Thank you very much, sir."

"No problem. And you watch it, you hear? Stay off the streets as much as you can."

"Yes. I will." She watched him walk away, then stood gazing around at Main Street, where there was less than normal activity for a lovely Saturday morning in June. And where there were far too many men just like the one she'd interviewed, walking

around with windbreakers half-zipped and wary, watchful expressions on their faces.

"Can we go now?" Joey whined.

"I wish we could," Dana said, half-consciously reaching up to
touch her hair. "I really wish we could. Hey—have you seen
Cheryl?"

"Nah. Saw their van parked near the town hall this morning.
Why?"

Dana bit her lip, hesitated, then said, "Let's head back
toward the town hall."

"Ah, jeez."

"You're getting paid," she reminded her cameraman.

"Not enough," he muttered, following behind her.

"It could be a lot worse," she told him irritably. "You could be
a blond woman. The way I hear it, the surgeon wouldn't have to
cut off much to make that happen."

"Bitch," he grunted under his breath.

"I heard that."

He gave her the finger silently, reasonably sure she didn't
have eyes in the back of her head.

"And I saw that," she said.

"Shit."

Inside the large storage closet of Jamie's playroom was, neatly
arranged on shelves and hanging on hooks, all the paraphernalia
necessary for sadomasochistic games. Whips, masks, padded and
unpadded handcuffs, an extremely varied selection of dildos and
vibrators, ropes, chains, and a number of unidentifiable objects,
some quite elaborate.

Also a tasteful selection of leather bustiers, garters, and

stockings, including, seemingly, the outfits Jamie and her partner had worn in the photographs.

"I'm no expert," Hollis said, "but I'm thinking at least a few of those gadgets are meant to be used on a man."

Rafe could see the ones she meant. "I'd say so. And given that, it's beginning to look more and more like Jamie was . . . an equal-opportunity mistress. She may not have enjoyed sex with men, but it looks like she enjoyed dominating them."

"Men and women," Hollis said. "She really did want to be boss, didn't she? I wonder what would happen if she ran into somebody who wanted to be boss even more than she did?"

"A trigger, maybe," Isabel said in an absentminded tone.

"His trigger?" Rafe asked. "He wanted to be the one on top—so to speak—and it wasn't a position Jamie was willing to allow him to assume?"

"Maybe." Isabel's tone was still abstracted. "Especially if we find out the other two primary victims from the earlier murders were unusually strong women. Dominant women. That could be his trigger, his hot button. Finding himself interested in women literally too strong for him."

"Some men just prefer their women to be sweet and submissive, I guess," Hollis said dryly.

"Jerks," Mallory said, then lifted a brow at Rafe. "Forensics?"

"Yeah, get them out here," Rafe said. "But only T.J. and Dustin with their kits, not the van. I'd still like to keep this quiet as long as we've got a hope in hell of it."

"Right." She pulled out her cell phone.

Rafe walked over to Isabel, still uneasily sensing that something wasn't right with her. She was no longer touching the mattress but was gazing off into space with that distant expression he was beginning to recognize in her eyes. But this time she seemed to be looking so far away that it sent a chill through him.

"Are you okay?" he asked.

"There is," she said slowly, "a lot of pain in this room."

"You don't feel it, do you?"

"No. No, I'm not an empath. I feel during the visions, but not this. I just . . . I just know there's a lot of pain in this room. Physical. Emotional. Psychological." She reached both hands up and rubbed the nape of her neck. Her hair was in its accustomed neat, high ponytail, and Rafe could see how hard she was kneading the tense muscles of her neck. But before he could ask about that, she went on in the same level tone.

"Jamie was strong. Very strong. But she'd spent her life being the good girl. Pretending to be what everybody wanted her to be. Hiding inside that shell. But this part of her life . . . this is where she could be in control. Really in control. Where she could be herself and be respected—demand respect—for who she really was."

Hollis stepped closer, her frown deepening. "Isabel—"

"This is where she called the shots. Her partners, male or female, were never her lovers, never close to her emotionally; they were . . . validation. That she was strong and certain. That she was the one in control. They did anything she told them to do. Everything. No matter what, no matter how wild she got. No matter how much she hurt them."

When Rafe realized that Isabel's nails were literally digging into her own skin despite the gloves she wore, he stripped his own gloves off and reached up and grasped her wrists, ignoring the again visible and audible flash that was a hell of a lot stronger than any static shock he'd ever felt. He pulled her hands away from her neck.

"Wow," Hollis murmured. "Talk about sparks."

Rafe ignored her. "Isabel."

She blinked, those vivid green eyes still distant but seemingly focusing on him. "What?"

127

"You've got to stop. Now."

"I can't."

"You have to. This is hurting you." He wasn't entirely sure she knew who he was. She was looking at him, he thought, as though he were the only Technicolor object in a black-and-white universe. Puzzled and wondering.

"It always hurts," she said matter-of-factly. "What difference does that make?"

"Isabel—"

"Bad things happened here, you know. It's been going on for years. Years. But Jamie was always in control. She had to be. Always. At least until . . ."

She frowned. "They sold insurance here, and before that—no, after that—somebody sold bootleg whiskey out of here for nearly a year. Moonshine, just like you said. How strange. And a preacher spent some time here, a few weeks. Except that he wasn't a preacher anymore, because he'd been caught in bed with a deacon's wife and it hadn't been the first time. He thought God had abandoned him, but it was the other way around . . ."

Hollis said, "Take her outside. There are too many secrets in this place. Too much pain. Too much information for her to sort through all at once."

Rafe didn't wait for a more complete explanation; Isabel was pale, he could feel her shaking, and it didn't require anything more than common sense to know she was very close to some kind of collapse. So he took her outside.

Isabel didn't really protest, although once they were outside she did mutter under her breath, "Shit. I *hate* it when this happens."

He put her in the passenger seat of his Jeep and got the engine and air conditioner running, then dug into his first-aid kit and pulled out a gauze pad.

"What's that for?"

He tore open the wrapping and reached over to place the pad against the nape of her neck, again ignoring a strong shock.

"Ouch," she said.

"You drew blood," Rafe told her. "Even with the gloves on. Jesus, does this happen often?"

Isabel looked down at her hands with a faint frown, then stripped off the gloves. "Oh . . . from time to time. Bishop keeps telling me I should wear my nails short. Maybe I'd better start listening to him. Got any aspirin in that box?"

"Ibuprofen."

"Even better. If I could have a couple? Or . . . a dozen?" She reached up to hold the pad in place herself while he got the pain reliever and then a bottle of water from the cooler he kept in the Jeep.

By the time she had swallowed four capsules, the faint scratches had stopped bleeding, and Rafe used an antiseptic pad to wipe the nape of her neck while she sat with her head bowed and eyes closed.

Every time he touched her, the shock was definite, but she didn't react or comment and Rafe thought he was getting used to it. In fact, it seemed to clear his head.

Which was more than a little unnerving.

Her pale gold hair felt even silkier than it looked and seemed to want to cling to the back of his hand as he worked on her neck. Static, of course. Had to be. He concentrated on treating the scratches she had inflicted on herself, though he admitted silently that it took him longer than was strictly necessary.

"Thanks."

"Don't mention it. Are you going to be okay?"

She nodded slightly, still without opening her eyes. "When the painkillers kick in. And as long as I don't go back in there right away."

"Isabel—"

"Look, I know you have questions. Can we save them for a while, please?" She raised her head and opened her eyes finally, looking at him. The distant expression was gone, but she looked incredibly tired. "For now, your forensics team should be here any minute; why don't you go back inside and get everybody doing their thing? Hollis may be able to help. I felt something weird in there."

Rafe thought there had been a lot of weird in there, but all he said was, "Meaning?"

"That increasing nervousness and fear Emily had been seeing in her sister. I don't think it was just because Jamie was afraid her secret life would be exposed. I think she had another secret, a far worse one. And a much greater fear. I think something went wrong in there. I think she went too far."

"What are you saying?" He asked the question, even though he knew what she would answer.

"Have your team look for signs of blood. A lot of blood."

"No sign of that box," Mallory said after both women had thoroughly searched the back room. "No sign of anything she wanted to keep hidden—outside that closet, I mean."

Hollis nodded. "There's an attic, but it's wide open and empty."

"Um . . . on another subject, I gather from your reaction that it isn't normal for somebody touching Isabel to literally strike sparks?"

"I've never seen it happen before, though I've only known her a few months." Hollis frowned. "I was given a pretty thorough knowledge of the other SCU members, and that definitely wasn't mentioned. Could be something new for her, caused by this particular situation."

"Or it could be Rafe."

"Or it could be Rafe, yeah. Don't quote me on this, because I'm certainly no expert, but I guess if the right two energy signatures came in contact, there could be something like those sparks."

"Don't tell me this is what all the poets wrote about," Mallory begged.

Hollis smiled in response, but said, "Who knows? Maybe it's as much an emotional connection as it is literal energy fields. In any case, those two are reacting to each other, and on a very basic level."

"Is that a good thing or a bad thing?"

"I have no idea. But it might explain why Isabel seems to be having a rougher than usual time with this investigation."

"What might explain it?" Rafe asked, entering in time to hear the statement.

"You."

"Come again?"

"Hey, I'm just guessing," Hollis told him. "And I'm a long way from being an expert on any of this stuff, as I just told Mallory. But I was taught at Quantico that sometimes electromagnetic fields—those of individual people or places—come together in a particular way that tends to change or enhance a psychic's natural abilities. Or at least alter the limitations of those abilities. I have never seen Isabel so wide open, and as far as I can tell it's all been hits. No misses. That is very unusual. I'm thinking that sparking thing between you two has something to do with it."

"We can't be sure everything she's picked up is factual, not yet," Rafe said without commenting on the sparking thing.

"I wouldn't bet against her."

"Well, I sure as hell hope she's wrong about one thing. She thinks one of Jamie's little games got out of hand. We're now looking for evidence of a death here."

"Shit." Mallory stared at him. "You mean separate from our serial killer?"

"God knows. Hollis, are you getting anything?"

"I haven't tried." From the slightly stubborn set of her jaw, it didn't appear she planned to anytime soon.

After seeing what had happened to Isabel, Rafe wasn't about to push either psychic, but he was still curious. "Isabel never seems to try. I mean, it doesn't seem to be an effort for her."

"It isn't. For her."

He waited, brows raised.

After a moment, Hollis said, "You know the bit about me not being able to hear what these victims have tried to tell me? So far, I mean."

Somewhat warily, Rafe said, "Yeah, I think I get that."

"There's a barrier, something virtually every psychic has. We call them shields. Think of it as a bubble of energy our minds create to protect us. Most psychics have to consciously make an opening in that shield in order to use our abilities. We have to reach out, open up, deliberately make ourselves vulnerable."

"You didn't seem to be doing it deliberately," Rafe noted.

"I'm new at this. My control isn't as strong as it should be yet, so sometimes I reach out—or at least open a door or window in my shields—without meaning or wanting to. Usually when I'm tired or distracted, something like that. Eventually, they tell me, I should be able to shut this stuff out unless and until I very specifically want it. Most psychics can do that. Isabel is the very rare one who can't."

"You mean—"

"I mean she lacks the ability to shield her own mind. She's always wide open, always picking up information. Important stuff. Trivia. Everything in between. All that stuff always coming at her, crowding into her mind, like the voices of hundreds of people all talking at once. It's a miracle she can make sense of it at all. Hell, it's a miracle she isn't locked up in a padded room somewhere, screaming her guts out."

Hollis drew a breath. "When she told you she couldn't stop it, she meant it literally. She can't shut it off, ever."

Isabel sat in the cool Jeep and stared down at her hands. Watching them shake.

"Okay," she murmured, "so this one was bad. You've had bad ones before. You've heard all the ugly voices before. You can handle them. You can handle this."

She heard the ghost of a laugh escape her. "But *not* if you keep talking to yourself."

She laced her fingers together in her lap and raised her head, staring through the windshield at the building where Rafe and the others were.

It was where she should be, dammit, and never mind the pain. In there trying to sort through all the impressions, listening to the voices still echoing too loudly in her head. Even the ugly ones. Maybe especially the ugly ones.

Doing her job.

Isabel drew in a deep breath and let it out slowly, trying to focus, to soothe raw nerves and regain control of her senses, all her senses. Control. She had to find control.

Jamie had liked controlling people.

And that preacher . . .

God, my God, why have you abandoned me?

Obey your mistress! Crawl!

Just three quarts more, and—

Bones bend before they break, you know. Bones bend—

Blood . . . so much blood . . .

Her shaking hands lifted to cover her face, fingertips massaging her forehead and temples hard, and Isabel drew another breath, fighting to close out the voices. Not that she could.

Not that she'd ever been able to. Still, she tried.

Concentrate.

Focus.

Don't listen to them.

She tempted me, that's what it was. Tempted me down the road to damnation. I was weak. I was . . .

I can make the rope tighter. I can make the rope much tighter. You want me to, don't you? You want me to hurt you. You want me to hurt you until you scream with the pain.

Bones bend . . .

And Bobby Grange, over to Horton Mill, he wants enough to fill a keg. Must be having a party, I guess. Guys like him keep me in business, that's for sure. And it ain't my business, what else they do. It just ain't any of my affair.

It wasn't my fault! She tempted me!

Do you know what happens when you feel all the pain you can feel? When your nerve endings are hot and raw, and your voice is gone from screaming? Do you know what it feels like to go beyond pain? Let's find out . . .

Bones bend before they—

Isabel.

Iss . . . a . . . belll . . .

Her hands jerked away from her face, and Isabel stared all around her, a bit wildly at first. There it was. A different voice. Male. Powerful. Crouching in the darkness . . .

But . . . there was no one. No one. Her head was pounding, her heart pounding, and the voices were only whispers now. Only whispers, none of them calling her name.

"Okay," she said aloud, shakily, "that was new. That was different."

That was terrifying.

8

T.J. MCCURRY FINISHED spraying an area of the floor about two feet from the bed platform and said, "Kill the lights."

They had already draped the high window, so when T.J.'s partner, Dustin Wall, turned off the lights in the room, they could all see the eerie greenish-white glow.

"Bingo," Dustin muttered, and began photographing the evidence.

T.J. said, "Lotta blood here, Chief. There are some older spatters in other areas of the room, especially there around the bed, but here's the only place where somebody bled like a stuck pig."

"Bled enough to die?"

In the glow of the Luminol, T.J.'s round face looked peculiarly gaunt. She shrugged and looked down at the old vinyl floor covering. "Somebody's done a fair job of cleaning, but you can

136

see how strongly the Luminol is reacting. I'm betting that when we pull up this floor covering, we'll find even more soaked into the concrete underneath. This is the old style of vinyl that was put down in tiles, not in a solid sheet, so the blood would have found all the crevices."

"T.J., did somebody die here?"

"You know I can't be absolutely certain about that, Chief. But if you want an educated guess, I'd say somebody did. Either that or a lot of somebodies bled a little bit here at different times—which, given the obvious purpose of the room, is entirely possible. We'll sort it out, get a blood type or types for you, DNA if you want."

"I want. Especially since I don't have a body."

Dustin said, "The state crime lab has cadaver dogs, if you want to start looking."

"Not yet. Not without more information. As edgy as this town is, the last thing we need is to have people and dogs out looking for another body, unless we're very sure one is actually out there." Rafe didn't say anything about psychic help, and he didn't look at Hollis, who was standing only a couple of feet away from him. "T.J., can you tell me if there's a blood trail out of this place?"

"I'll work on it. Dustin, do you have the shots? Then let's get the lights back on so we can see what we're doing."

Rafe left her to it, admitting silently that he was relieved when the lights came back on. He'd seen Luminol used before, and it always struck him as chilling. Invisible to the eye until the chemicals in the Luminol reacted with it, the blood was a silent, ghostly accusation.

He joined Hollis, saying, "Would I be out of line in suggesting that Isabel go back to the inn and call it a day?"

"Arguable point, I suppose, but she won't go, so it hardly matters."

He sighed. "You people are a very stubborn lot."

Hollis didn't ask whether he meant FBI agents or psychics; she knew the answer to that one. Instead, she said, "There are only a handful of team leaders in the SCU, agents Bishop trusts to head up investigations. Isabel is one of them, and has been from the beginning."

"You said it was a miracle she hadn't gone insane." Rafe kept his voice low.

"Yes. But she didn't go insane, that's the point. She is an exceptionally strong lady. She lives her life and she does her job, whatever the effort or the cost. What you saw happen in here is a rare thing, but similar things have happened before. It hasn't stopped her in the past, and this won't stop her now. If anything, the strong connection will probably make her even more determined to put all the puzzle pieces in place and get this killer."

"He's gotten away from her twice before," Rafe said, more to himself than to Hollis.

But she nodded. "Yeah, it's personal. How could it not be? It was her best friend he killed ten years ago, in case you didn't know that. She and Julie King grew up together, practically sisters. Isabel was only twenty-one when it happened, in college, trying to decide what to do with her life. Taking the most amazing variety of subjects, like classical Latin, and computer science, and botany. Nerdy stuff."

Hollis shrugged. "She was drifting, mostly. Getting by with good grades because of a good mind, not effort. Sort of . . . shut in herself, detached, uninvolved. From all I've been told, Julie's murder changed her completely."

"That isn't what . . . triggered her psychic ability?" It wasn't really a question.

"No. That had already happened." Hollis didn't offer to elaborate.

Rafe wasn't surprised. "But her friend's murder more or less started her life as a cop."

"I'd say so. In the beginning, she just wanted to find out who had killed Julie. That's what motivated her, what began to shape her life and future. By the time he surfaced again in Alabama five years later, she had a degree in criminology under her belt and worked for the Florida State Police. She apparently did routine searches of law-enforcement databases on her own time, waiting for the killer to strike again. Just after he killed the second victim in Alabama, Isabel took a leave of absence and turned up there. That was when she met Bishop."

"And turned in her state badge for a federal one."

"Pretty much, yeah."

Rafe drew a breath and let it out slowly. "So now she uses her knowledge, training, and psychic abilities to try and ferret out killers. Especially this one. Tell me something, Hollis. How many more times can she go through what she did in here before it breaks her?"

"At least one more time." Hollis grimaced at his expression. "I know it sounds harsh. But it's also the truth; we take this stuff one . . . experience . . . at a time, and none of us can be sure when the end will come. Or how."

"Wait a minute. You're telling me you guys *know* this stuff you do is going to kill you one day?"

"I'd call that a radical interpretation of the text," she murmured.

"Hollis."

"We're not the only stubborn ones, I see."

"Answer my question."

"I can't." She shrugged, more than a little impatient now. "Rafe, we don't know. Nobody really knows. We're all checked out medically after assignments, and the doctors have noted some changes in some agents. They don't know what that means, *we* don't know what it means. Maybe nothing."

"Or maybe something. Something fatal."

"Look, all I can tell you is that for some agents, there's a price for using their abilities. Some, like Isabel, live with pain most of the time, usually headaches. Some finish up assignments so exhausted it takes them weeks to fully recover. I know one agent who eats constantly during a case, and I mean constantly; it's like her abilities cause her metabolism to shoot into high gear and she has to fuel her body continually in order to do her job. But there are other agents who never seem affected physically by what they do. It varies. So, no, I can't tell you using our abilities is going to kill us one day. Because we just don't know."

"But it's possible."

"Sure, it's possible, I guess. It's also possible—more than possible, really—that we'll be killed in the line of duty by a regular old bullet or knife or explosion of some kind. The risk comes with the job. We all know the potential hazards, believe me. Bishop is very careful to make certain we understand what we might be risking, even if it's only a theoretical possibility. Anyway, Isabel made the decision that was hers to make, to use her abilities this way. She's been doing it for years, and she knows her limits."

"I don't doubt that. What I doubt is that she'll stop before those limits are reached."

"She's dedicated" was Hollis's only response.

"Yeah, I get that."

"You face risks in your job. Why keep doing it?"

Rafe didn't answer, just shook his head and said, "T.J. and Dustin will be a while, and there's really nothing more you and Isabel can do here. Is there?"

It was Hollis's turn to avoid the direct question. "We can go back to the station, work there while you guys finish up here. Get the information on the two previous series of murders posted on the boards."

"Good idea," Rafe said.

Hollis took the first chance she got to call in, which turned out to be about an hour later, when Isabel left the conference room to make copies of a stack of paperwork.

The number was still a bit unfamiliar, but her cell phone's address book had been carefully programmed, so it was easy to find the number and make the call.

As soon as he answered, Hollis said, "I didn't like doing that. Isabel's business is her own. She wouldn't talk about me behind my back, not that sort of personal stuff."

"He needed to know," Bishop said.

"Then Isabel should have been the one to tell him."

"Yes, but she wouldn't. Or, at least, wouldn't tell him right now. He needs to know now."

"And why is that, O wise Yoda?"

Bishop chuckled. "I'm guessing 'Because I say so' is not going to be a satisfactory answer for you."

"I didn't accept that even from my father; it definitely won't work for you."

"Okay. Then I'll tell you the truth."

"I appreciate that. The truth being?"

"The truth being that certain things have to happen in a certain order if we're to avert a catastrophe."

Hollis blinked. "And we know that catastrophe lies ahead because . . . ?"

"Because some of us occasionally catch a glimpse of the

future." Bishop sighed. "Hollis, we can't fix everything. We can't make the future all bright and shiny just because we know before they happen that there are troubles and tragedies waiting there for us. The best we can do sometimes, the absolute best, is to chart a careful path somewhere between bad and worse."

"And that path requires that I spill part of Isabel's story to Rafe."

"Yes. It does. This time. Next time, you may be asked to do something else. And you'll do it. Not because I say so, but because you can trust in the fact that Miranda and I would never do anything to injure or betray any member of the team—even to save the future."

Hollis sighed. "I wish that sounded melodramatic, but since I know the stories and I've seen a few things myself, I'm afraid it's the literal truth. The saving-the-future business, I mean."

"We have to do what we can. It's seldom enough, but sometimes the right word or the right information at the right moment can change things just a bit. Shift the balance more toward our favor. When we can even do that much. Sometimes we can't interfere at all."

"Going to tell me how you know that this is one of the times you can interfere?"

"Miranda sees the future and takes me along for the ride. Sometimes we see alternate futures; that's when we know we can change things. Sometimes we see only one future. We see what's inevitable."

"That's when you know you can't."

"Yes."

"And the future I just changed by telling Rafe some of Isabel's past?"

"Was a future in which he died."

"So why hasn't her cameraman reported her missing?" Isabel asked Dana Earley.

"I think he's ashamed of himself. Apparently, she told him to wait in the van while she went to check something out. He claims he doesn't know what. Anyway, she hadn't been gone ten minutes before he was asleep. And he didn't wake up until Joey and I banged on the side of the van about half an hour ago."

"That's a long nap."

"He says he's been running short on sleep for days. Probably true; a lot of our technical people get fascinated with their toys and keep the weirdest hours you can imagine."

Isabel frowned. "You've checked with her station, with the other media people across the street?"

Dana nodded. "Oh, yeah. The last anybody saw of Cheryl was just before dark last night. Dammit, I warned her to watch her back, brunette or not."

"Why?"

"Because I think the spotlight on a small town like Hastings can get pretty uncomfortable, and I wouldn't be surprised if this maniac targeted a journalist just to get us to back off."

Isabel rested a hip on the corner of an unoccupied desk, where the conversation was taking placc. "That's not a bad theory, assuming he isn't too far gone to think logically. Off the record."

Dana nodded again, this time somewhat impatiently. "And I'm no profiler, but I'd expect him to target somebody who doesn't fit his clear preferences so far, just to make a statement."

"You're not the one I want, but you're in my way. Nobody's safe," Isabel murmured. "Go away."

"It makes sense, doesn't it?"

"Unfortunately, yes. Thanks for filing the report, Ms. Earley."

"If there's anything I can do to help look for that kid—"

"The best way you can help her and us is not to get yourself added to our missing-persons list. Don't go anywhere alone. I mean anywhere, unless it's into a locked room you know damned well is safe. Pass the word to the other journalists, will you?"

"Will do."

"Male and female journalists," Isabel added.

Dana nodded wryly and left.

Isabel remained where she was for several minutes, frowning at nothing. She was tired. Very tired. And worried.

If this bastard *had* grabbed a brunette journalist, *had* been angry enough to stray so far from his preferences, then why hadn't Isabel felt it?

"What's wrong with me?" she murmured.

There was no answer, except for the feeling she had of something crouching in the darkness. Watching.

Waiting.

When Rafe walked into the conference room just before four that afternoon, he wasn't especially happy to find Alan Moore there with Isabel.

"Hollis and Mallory are out running down a couple of leads," she told him, without going into detail. She seemed none the worse for what had happened in Jamie Brower's secret playroom, though something about her eyes told him she was still suffering a pounding headache.

Rafe nodded without commenting on either her info or his own hunch, and said to Alan, "Please tell me you have a reason other than idle curiosity for being here."

"My curiosity is never idle."

"I should have warned you about him, Isabel. You can only believe about half of what he says. On a good day."

"See, this is what happens when you grow up with a guy who becomes a cop," Alan said. "He turns into a suspicious bastard right before your eyes."

"Not without reason," Rafe retorted. "You've been a pain in my ass since I was appointed."

"I've been doing my job."

Isabel intervened before they could begin rehashing past offenses, saying, "Alan received something a bit unexpected in yesterday's mail."

Rafe stared at Alan. "And you're just now bringing it in?"

"I've been busy."

"Alan, one of these days you're going to go too far. Consider this a warning."

Despite the calm tone, Alan was perfectly aware that his boyhood friend was deadly serious. He nodded, not really having to fake the sheepish expression. "Noted."

Without commenting on the byplay between the men, Isabel handed Rafe a single sheet of paper in a clear plastic evidence bag. "I've already checked it. No prints, except his."

The note, block-printed yet virtually scrawled in a bold, dark hand on the unlined paper, was brief.

MR. MOORE, THE COPS HAVE GOT IT
ALL WRONG. HE ISN'T KILLING THEM BECAUSE
THEY'RE BLONDES.
HE'S KILLING THEM BECAUSE THEY'RE NOT

"Not blondes?" Rafe said, looking at Isabel.

"Yeah, but they were," she said. "At least, Jamie and Tricia were natural blondes; Allison Carroll used hair color."

"But she—" He stopped himself.

Isabel finished the comment for him. "She matched top and bottom. But the lab results are in, and they say she used hair color. It's not all that uncommon for a woman to dye her pubic hair, especially when the change is so drastic and she's at a stage in her life when looking good naked is a major goal. In any case, Allison's natural hair color was very dark."

Rafe met Alan's interested gaze, and said, "This is off the record, you realize that?"

"Yeah, Isabel's already warned me. Giant red federal warning, accompanied by flags, stamps, sealing wax, oaths of secrecy, and appropriate threats of being transported to Area 51 and turned into a lab rat."

Isabel smiled but said nothing.

"Just as a point of interest," Alan commented, "Cheryl Bayne is a brunette."

"Cheryl Bayne," Isabel said, "is missing. As are others on an unfortunately lengthy list. We don't know that anything has happened to any of them."

"Yet."

"Yet," she agreed.

Alan eyed her, then continued, "Anyway, when all is said and done and you've got the guy, I reserve the right to inform the public that I was contacted by the killer."

"Were you?" Isabel murmured.

"Third person," Rafe noted, studying the note. "*He* isn't killing them because they're blondes. This could have been written by someone who knows the killer. Knows what he's doing."

"Or maybe," Alan offered, "he's schizophrenic and believes it's not really him killing these women."

"You just want this to be the killer," Rafe said in an absent tone.

"Well, yes. This story could be my Watergate."

Isabel pursed her lips. "No. Your Ted Bundy or John Wayne Gacy. Not your Watergate."

"It could make my career," Alan insisted.

"Yeah?" Isabel was politely interested. "And do you happen to remember the name of the journalist who was supposedly contacted by Jack the Ripper?"

Alan scowled. "Shatter a man's dreams, why don't you?"

"Do you remember?"

"It was over a hundred years ago."

"And the most famous serial killer of modern times. Countless books have been written about him. Movies made about him. Theories as to his identity endlessly debated. And yet the name of that journalist doesn't exactly spring readily to the tongue, does it?"

"Do you know it?" Alan challenged.

"Of course. But then, I specialize in serial killers. More or less. Everybody in the business has studied the Ripper case. It's practically Murder 101 in Behavioral Science at Quantico. Everybody wants to be the one to solve it."

"Including you?"

"Oh, I don't think it'll ever be definitively solved. And I don't believe it should be. Some things should remain mysteries."

"You don't really believe that."

"Yes, I do. We should never, ever believe life—or history—holds no surprises for us. That way lies arrogance. And arrogance can blind us to the truth."

"Which truth?"

"Any truth. All truth." Her voice was solemn.

Alan sighed and got to his feet. "Okay, before you start calling me Grasshopper, I'm going to leave."

"I'm sure I have a pebble around here somewhere, if you want to stay and test your readiness," Isabel said, still solemn.

"Somehow, I don't think I'm fast enough," Alan said, not without a note of honest regret. He offered them both a casual salute, then left the conference room, closing the door behind him.

"Good job of distracting him," Rafe said.

"Maybe. With any luck he'll spend at least the next few hours on the Internet or in the library reading up on Jack the Ripper— just so he can tell me the name of that journalist the next time I see him. It'll occupy his mind a little while." She leaned back in her chair and rubbed the nape of her neck with one hand, frowning slightly.

"Still got that headache?"

"It comes and goes. So far, there's no sign of Cheryl Bayne; her station has backed up Dana Earley's missing persons report with one of their own. And Hollis and Mallory are checking out the rest of the properties owned by Jamie Brower."

"You still want to find that box of photos."

"I want to find whatever is there. Speaking of which, your forensics team confirmed blood in Jamie's playhouse, I gather. A lot of blood."

He nodded. "Yeah, you were right about that. And a faint blood trail to the door. T.J. figures the body was wrapped in plastic. I'm guessing it was put into a car and hauled somewhere. They're going over Jamie's car now, but we didn't find anything when we checked it bumper to bumper after she was killed."

Isabel shook her head. "She wouldn't have panicked, and she was too smart to transport a body in her own car. It would have been her playmate's car. And I'm betting she got rid of it afterward. Very rid of it. Like maybe sank it to the bottom of one of the lakes in the area. With or without the body inside."

"That," he agreed, "is all too likely." He hesitated, then added, "Did you pick up anything from Alan?"

"No, he's a very closed book. Not uncommon for a journalist;

they keep a lot of secrets, as a rule. Most of us find it difficult to read them, even the telepaths."

"You think his guess about the killer being schizophrenic was right?"

"I think it's at least as likely as any other theory we have. Maybe more than likely." She drew a breath and spoke rapidly. "One school of thought proposes four different types of serial murderers: visionary, mission-oriented, hedonistic, and control-oriented. The mission-oriented is out to eliminate a particular group he feels is unworthy of living. Common victims for this type of killer are those easily categorized: prostitutes, the homeless, the mentally ill. Or—plumbers."

Rafe blinked. "Plumbers?"

"I'm just saying. Mission-oriented serial killers target groups. Unless our guy is out to kill all women, or at least all successful women—a task even a madman would have to find daunting— then I don't believe he's mission-oriented."

"Sounds logical to me. Next?"

"The hedonistic killer is after pleasure or thrills when he kills. He may get his jollies from the kill itself, from the arousal and gratification of what's basically a lust murder; he may enjoy the planning stages, the stalking of his prey. Or he may find pleasure in the consequences of the kill if, for instance, he gains a kind of freedom by killing family or people he perceives as tying him down somehow."

"Control-oriented type?"

"His thing is having power over the victim, especially the power of life and death. If he rapes, it's for control and domination, not thrills. And this type generally doesn't kill his victims immediately. He likes to torture, both physically and psychologically. He wants to draw it out, savor his power over them, watch their helplessness and terror."

"You must have hellacious nightmares," Rafe said.

She looked at him with a little half smile. "Oddly enough, no. My nightmares tend to come while I'm awake."

Rafe waited a moment, giving her an opening, but it was obvious she didn't intend to take it. "So our guy is not likely to be control-oriented, or at least not driven by that, since he doesn't waste any time at all in killing his victims. And the visionary type of serial killer I'm assuming is the nail Alan may have hit on the head?"

"Umm. Alan . . . and the note sent to him." She tapped a red fingernail against the plastic-sleeved note Rafe had placed atop the stack of papers on the conference table in front of her. "This makes me wonder, it really does. If it's not purely a ruse designed to throw us off track—and we have to assume that's at least possible—then this note could tell us a lot about our killer. I'll need to make a copy for us and send the original to Quantico, by the way. The handwriting experts may be able to tell us something. As for what the note says . . ."

"He wants us to stop him?"

"If we accept this as written, and as written by the killer, then some part of him does. The sane part." Isabel paused, frowning. "The least common type of serial killer is the visionary, someone who sees visions or hears voices commanding him to kill."

"As in Son of Sam."

"Yeah. He usually attributes the voices to God or some kind of demon and feels himself helpless to disobey them. He's not in control, the voices are. They tell him to kill, who to kill, when to kill. Maybe why those particular people have to be killed. He may hear the voices from childhood, or it may be a sudden psychosis brought on by stress or trauma. Some people believe a chemical change in the brain is responsible, but, as I said, we don't know a whole hell of a lot about how the brain really works.

"In any case, the visionary killer feels he's controlled by something alien, something that is no part of himself. Sometimes he ignores or fights the voices or visions for years before they finally overpower his will. Bottom line, he's a puppet with someone else—or something else—pulling his strings."

"Okay," Hollis said, studying the notes in her hand and then looking up as Mallory pulled the police Jeep to the curb and parked. "This should be it. Last place on Jamie's list of properties."

"What're we expecting to find here?" Mallory wondered, eyeing the boarded-up front window of what had once, years before, been a gas station. "According to her broker, Jamie planned to sell this place."

"Yeah, but he also said that wasn't the original plan. She bought this property meaning to raze what's here and build a nice little place to fit in with the boutiques popping up at this end of town. It would have vastly increased the value of the property. Then she very suddenly decided to just sell out."

"But she made that decision about several of the properties we've looked at. And the broker didn't say suddenly, he said somewhat unexpectedly."

"Somewhat unexpectedly about three months ago. Isabel says that fits the time frame; it's when Jamie started showing signs of nerves. Deciding to unload so much of her property virtually all at once even if it meant taking a loss was out of character, and when people do things out of character there's usually a good reason behind the actions."

"Like she accidentally killed a lover, maybe. But what was the plan after she sold out? Did she mean to get her hands on all the cash she could so she could leave town?"

"Could be. Isabel thinks there's a possibility."

"Then why are we checking out these places? She wouldn't have hidden the photo box—or any other keepsake—in a place she was going to sell. You don't think we're going to find a body in there?"

"Well, you know as well as I do, the state crime network coughed up a list of at least three women of roughly the right age reported missing in this general area at about the same time Jamie got nervous. The police in each district believe all three women did not leave of their own free will, which makes homicide at least a possibility. And . . . if things did get out of hand in one of Jamie's little games, she had to do something with the body."

"Hide it in a building she owned herself and was planning to sell?"

"I wouldn't call it a smart thing to do. Unless she figured out a way to completely destroy the body or completely hide it even if the building came down. Or unless she planned to be far away and living under an assumed name or something by the time anything was discovered."

"Interesting possibilities," Mallory agreed. "Okay. Grab your flashlight and let's check it out."

Isabel turned her gaze to the bulletin boards across the room, which had, Rafe noted, acquired what looked like canvas drop cloths that could be conveniently lowered to cover the boards whenever unauthorized persons were present.

The cloths were lowered now, presumably because Alan had been in the room.

Absently, she said, "Mallory thought the drop cloths would be a good idea, so she fixed them. We can keep the boards covered most of the time, unless we're in here working. Less chance of too much information leaking out."

"Isabel? Could a visionary killer gain control over his voices for years between killing sprees? Could he live normally during those years?"

"That would be . . . unusual."

"But would it be possible? Could it be? Are we dealing with a killer who really isn't responsible—at least legally—for what he's doing?"

"That might depend on the trigger—and the reason or reasons behind all this."

"What do you mean?"

"I mean the human mind, the human psyche, is a very complicated beast. Generally speaking, it knows how to protect itself, or the most fragile aspects of itself. If he's hearing voices or seeing visions, and they're commanding him to do things utterly alien to his nature, then sure—he could forget about them the moment the voices or visions stop."

"For years on end?"

"Maybe. And then something happens in his life to trigger this psychosis, and his sick and twisted alter ego comes out to play."

"For six weeks. Six women. Six murders."

"The number, the time period, both have to be relevant, either tied to an event somewhere in his past or tied to the psychosis. To his voices."

"Which is your guess?"

Isabel thought for a moment, then said, "Childhood. The majority of the traumas that affect us most deeply occur in childhood. It's when we're most vulnerable."

"What about the idea that he's schizophrenic?"

"There are schizophrenics able to function, with medication and other treatment. No pharmacy within a hundred miles has filled a prescription for the sort of medication that would be needed."

Rafe lifted his brows. "Already checked that out?"

"Well, the profile noted the possibility of schizophrenia, so it seemed prudent. An inquiry from the Bureau tends to carry a bit of weight, and since we weren't asking for specific patient information or identification, all the pharmacies were happy to cooperate."

"Okay. So we can be pretty sure he isn't being treated for schizophrenia."

"Which doesn't rule out him having it. Or that he's getting psychiatric treatment without medication. We haven't checked with doctors."

"Because they wouldn't disclose the information."

"Not willingly. They have a responsibility to report it if they believe a patient has committed or is about to commit a violent crime, but that sort of treatment can take years before the doctor truly begins to understand his or her patient."

"And understand what the voices are making him do."

"Exactly. In any case, my guess is that our guy isn't getting treatment of any kind. Whether he's aware of being sick is an open question; whether he knows what he's done is another one. From the information we've gathered so far, there's just no way to be certain."

"Earlier, you said some schizophrenics were, literally, possessed by another person, another soul trying to take over. Is that possible in this case?"

Isabel shook her head. "So far, we've never encountered a person in that condition who wasn't in a mental institution and under restraints or drugged into a stupor. We don't believe such a person could function normally under any conditions—far less something like this. There's just too much violence going on in the brain itself to allow even the appearance of normalcy."

"And our killer appears normal."

"Yes. No matter how screwed up his childhood may have been, or how many voices he might be listening to, he's able to function normally to all outward appearances."

After a moment, Rafe said, "I think I'd prefer an evil killer who knows exactly what he's doing, sick as it is. At least then it would be . . ."

"Simpler," she agreed wryly. "Black and white, no shades of gray. No agonizing over who or what is really responsible. No reason to hesitate or regret. But you know as well as I do that it's seldom that easy."

"Yeah. As Hollis said, the universe never seems to want to play it that way. Listen . . . we aren't talking about a psychic killer, are we?"

"Christ, I hope not." With a sigh, she returned her gaze to his face. "True visionary killers are delusional, Rafe. They believe they hear the voices of demons or the voice of God. They're being commanded to do things they wouldn't ordinarily do, for reasons the sane among us would find completely nuts. They aren't psychic; what they're experiencing isn't real except inside their own twisted minds."

9

IT HADN'T TAKEN ALAN long to find the information he was looking for on Jack the Ripper, and he was somewhat chagrined to see just how much information was readily available via the Internet on the case.

Just as Isabel had said.

She hadn't exactly thrown a gauntlet at his feet, but Alan nevertheless felt challenged to somehow best the federal agent. And Rafe, of course. It would be nice, he thought, to get the upper hand with Rafe.

Just once, for Christ's sake.

The problem was, Alan hardly had access to the sort of databases of information the police and feds could command. But there was one thing he did have, and that was knowledge of this town and its people.

The question was, could he use that?

He wasn't able to speak to Mallory as he left the station, since she wasn't there, so he didn't know whether to expect a visit from her tonight. After last night, he figured he probably wouldn't see her for days; whenever she showed him any signs of vulnerability—falling asleep in his arms would definitely be listed in that column, he knew—she tended to retreat for a while both literally and figuratively.

In any case, he had learned the hard way not to plan his days or nights around her. He got in his car at the station and checked his watch, debating silently, then started the car.

It was time he tapped *all* his sources.

4:45 PM

Rafe had a hunch Isabel's explanation contained a *but*, so he asked. "But?"

"But . . . we've encountered serial killers before who also happened to be psychic, so the two aren't exactly mutually exclusive. In fact, some researchers believe that serial killers and psychics have something in common: an unusual amount of electromagnetic energy in the brain."

"Which means?"

"Which means we are or could be kindred spirits, scary as that sounds. The *excess* energy in a psychic seems to activate an area of the brain most people don't appear to use, an area we believe controls psychic abilities. The energy in a serial killer tends to sort of go wild, building up in different areas of the brain, especially in the rage center, and since it has no way to be channeled, you end up with synapses misfiring right and left. Burned-out or overloaded areas of the brain could trigger the compulsion to kill."

"So that's one theory."

"One of many. And that theory holds something else to be a possibility. That a serial murderer can also become psychic. Which comes first in that case, the psychic ability or the insanity, is still an open and much debated question."

"Does it matter?"

"Well, yeah, for some of us." Her voice was light. "I hear voices, Rafe, remember?"

"Voices you don't attribute to God or a demon. Voices that don't command you to kill."

"Not even on the worst day yet, I'm happy to say. So far, so good." She shook her head slightly. "But returning to the point—a psychic killer is possible."

"Would you know? I mean, could you tell if that were the case?"

"Not necessarily. Psychics can often recognize each other as psychic, but not always."

"Shields," he said, remembering what Hollis had told him. "Yet another instance of the mind protecting itself."

"Hollis said she mentioned that." Isabel didn't seem disturbed by it. "And it is one reason we don't always recognize each other. Also, nonpsychic people frequently develop shields of their own, for privacy or protection, especially in small towns where everybody tends to know everybody else's business. It's a lot more common than you might think. Hell, I could talk to the killer every day, never knowing he's the murderer and never picking up psychic ability—or psychotic voices in his head."

For the first time since he'd returned, she sounded tired, and it made him say, "How close are Mallory and Hollis to finishing up?" He was about to suggest calling one of them, but Isabel automatically used a more direct line of communication.

"They are . . ." She frowned, concentrating. ". . . at the last property on the list, I think. What used to be a gas—" Her face changed, tightened.

Watching her, Rafe was conscious of the same uneasiness he'd felt in Jamie's "playhouse." She was somewhere else, somewhere distant from here. He wanted to reach over and touch her, anchor her here somehow.

She came abruptly to her feet. "Oh, Christ."

"You know, for a gas station, this is a huge building." Mallory's voice echoed.

They were in the rear area, which was divided into at least three separate rooms, all apparently cavernous; the one they were presently exploring had a concrete floor and high windows so dirty they admitted almost no light. Rusted pieces and parts from old cars still hung on hooks and racks on the cinder-block walls, and piles of junk lay everywhere.

Every time Mallory moved the beam of her flashlight, it seemed to catch something metallic and glare back at her, like something springing out of the shadows.

Unsettling.

"Tell me about it. I'm guessing it didn't start out life as a gas station." Hollis pointed her flashlight into a dark corner and jumped when an unexpectedly shiny chrome bumper glinted brightly. "Jesus."

Mallory jumped in the same instant, but in her case it was because something skittered across her foot. "Shit. I hate rats, but I hope that's what just ran across my foot."

Hollis didn't care for rats herself, but she was standing before what looked like a solid steel door that held her interest at the moment. The door was padlocked. "Never mind the rats. Take a look at this."

Mallory joined her. "I can't never mind rats. I hate rats. And I'm going to throw these shoes away. Yuck." Her flashlight beam joined Hollis's. "Is that a new lock?"

"I'd say so. Hold on a minute." She juggled her flashlight briefly before tucking it under her arm as she dug into the waist pack she was wearing. She put on a pair of latex gloves, then produced a small, zippered leather case.

Mallory watched with interest. "Burglar's tools? You didn't bring those out at Jamie's playhouse."

"I didn't have to, you had the locksmith's tools." Hollis smiled suddenly. "I've been hoping there'd be an opportunity for me to try out my lock-picking skills. They haven't been field-tested yet." She selected a couple of tools and bent to begin working on the lock.

"You learned this at Quantico?"

"From Bishop. It's sort of fascinating which skills he determines to be most important to a new agent. Handling a gun without shooting myself in the foot and with reasonable accuracy—check. Being able to use a form of autohypnosis and biofeedback to focus and concentrate—check. Ability to talk to the dead—a major plus. Being able to pick various and sundry locks—check. Or, at least, so I hope."

Mallory laughed under her breath. "You know, I'd really like to meet this Bishop of yours. He sounds like a very interesting man."

"He certainly is. Damn. Shine your light right here, will you?"

Mallory complied.

"Wait—I think—" There was a soft click, and Hollis opened the padlock with a flourish. "Ta-da. What do you know, I can do this. I wasn't at all sure I could."

"Congratulations."

"Thank you." She put away the tools, then had to put her

shoulder against the door to push it inward. And the moment it was open a few inches Hollis immediately stepped back. "Oh, shit."

The two women looked at each other, and Mallory said, "I haven't had the misfortune to stumble across a decomposing human corpse, but I'm guessing that's what one would smell like. Please tell me I'm wrong."

Breathing through her mouth, Hollis said, "I'm pretty sure that's what it is. Part of the training I got was a visit to the body farm—where students and forensics specialists study decomposition. It's not an odor you easily forget."

Mallory stared at the partially open door. "I'm not looking forward to seeing what's inside there."

"No, me either." Hollis eyed her. "Want to wait and call in reinforcements?"

"No. No, dammit. With a padlocked door and that smell, there's obviously nothing dangerous in there. Nothing alive, I mean. We have to open the door and look, make sure it's not some dead animal in there. Then call it in."

Hollis braced herself mentally and emotionally—and did her best to shore up her psychic shields. Then she and Mallory shouldered the door all the way open and stepped inside.

"Jesus," Mallory whispered.

Hollis might have echoed her, if she could have forced words past the sick lump in her throat.

It was a bare room, for the most part, with only a few shelves along one wall to show it had been used at least once for storage. The high windows admitted just enough illumination, from the southwestern corner of the building and the hot sun low enough in the sky, to provide mote-filled beams of light focused on the center of the room.

On her.

One end of a thick, rusted chain was wrapped around a steel I-beam overhead, while at the other end of the chain a big hook jutted from between her rope-bound wrists. She dangled, literally, from the hook, her feet several inches above the floor. There was nothing beneath her except rusty stains on the concrete.

Thick, dark hair hung down to mostly obscure her face. The clothing she had worn, a once-demure blouse and skirt, had been shredded, but very neatly, methodically, almost artistically. The material provided a fringe that almost hid what had been done to her body.

Almost.

"Jamie didn't do this," Mallory whispered. "She couldn't have done this."

"Nothing human could have done this," Hollis responded, her own voice thin. "It's like he was curious to see what color her insides were."

Mallory backed out of the room, gagging, and Hollis didn't have to follow to know the other cop was throwing up everything she'd eaten today.

Her own stomach churning, Hollis reached for her cell phone, her gaze fixed on the dangling and decomposing body of a woman who'd been gutted like a fish.

6:00 PM

The medical examiner for the county, Dr. David James, was a normally dour man, and a scene like this one didn't make him any more cheerful.

"She's been dead at least a couple of months," he told Rafe. "The fairly cool, dry conditions in here probably slowed decomp a bit, but not much. I can't be positive, of course, but from the

162

bruising on her neck I'm guessing strangulation, probably with a rope of some kind. Whoever cut her did it postmortem, probably days afterward; there was almost no bleeding from those wounds."

"Anything missing?" Rafe kept his own voice as level as the doctor's, but it required a tremendous effort.

"I'll be able to tell you more when I get her on the table, but it does look like one kidney is gone, some of the intestines, part of her stomach."

"Christ."

"Yeah. I may be able to get you prints from her, and it looks like she's had some dental work done, so we have a fair shot at an I.D. if she's one of the missing women on your list. Get this guy, Rafe. What he did to the other women was bad enough, but this . . . He's worse than a butcher."

Rafe didn't comment on the doctor's assumption that the same killer was responsible for this woman's death. "We're doing our best."

"Yeah. Yeah, I know." Dr. James hunched his shoulders a little, weariness in the gesture. "My guys are standing by to bag her as soon as yours are finished."

"Right."

"I'll get the report to you ASAP."

Rafe watched the doctor make his way back toward the front of the former gas station, then returned his gaze to the activities in the back room. T.J. and Dustin were working methodically, their faces grim. Off to one side, Isabel stood with Hollis as they studied the dead woman.

If he'd been asked to guess, Rafe would have said that Hollis was feeling queasy and Isabel was exhausted. He was pretty sure both hunches were on the mark.

Mallory joined him in the doorway and nodded toward the

federal agents, saying, "They still believe she was one of Jamie's playmates, the one accidentally killed."

"But they don't believe Jamie did this," Rafe said, a statement rather than a question.

"No."

"Which begs the question . . ."

"Who did. Yeah. Didn't Doc say she died two months ago at least?"

Rafe nodded. "Before the murders started. Isabel?"

She and Hollis immediately walked over to join them at the doorway.

"The doc says she didn't bleed to death," Rafe said to Isabel without preamble.

She nodded. "Yeah, I missed that one. I'm guessing the lab work from Jamie's playhouse will come back showing several people bled in that spot over a long period of time. Some of her clients, probably, but others as well. There might even have been a murder there a long time ago."

"That blood trail to the door," he noted.

"Possibly. Or one or more of Jamie's clients." Isabel shrugged. "In any case, I missed."

Mallory said dryly, "All will be forgiven if you just help us get this bastard."

"Was this his trigger?" Rafe asked.

"I don't know," Isabel replied.

"An educated guess?"

"If you want that . . . then maybe. Maybe he saw this woman die accidentally at Jamie's hands, and maybe it pissed him off. Or maybe he got his hands on a cold body and wondered what a warm one would feel like. Or maybe she was just a toy he played with because she happened to be handy."

"You're not picking up anything?" He kept his voice low.

She grimaced slightly. "Lot of old, old stories; this building has been here a while. Arguments, mostly, but . . ."

Whispers.

Jesus, George, we have to do it in the backseat?

I told you I can't afford a motel room.

Yeah, but . . .

Hide the stuff inside the hubcap. I'm tellin' you, the cops'll never find it there . . .

That Jones bitch wants her car done by tomorrow or she won't pay . . .

You're fired, Carl! I'm fucking sick and tired of . . .

Bones bend before they break.

She's all colors inside.

Isabel.

Isss . . . a . . . bellll . . .

"Isabel?"

She blinked and looked at Rafe. "What? Oh. Just old stuff, mostly. But he was here. A day or two ago."

"How do you know that?"

There was no way Isabel was going to tell Rafe that their killer had been looking at this poor woman and thinking about what he wanted to do to Isabel.

No way.

So all she said was, "He . . . looked at her. Thought about how she had deserved to die because she was bad."

Rafe frowned. "Bad?"

"I get the sense he saw her with Jamie. Watched them. And what they did together bothered him on a very deep level. Sickened him, believe it or not."

Something in the dark, crouching, waiting.

Watching.

Isabel shivered. "It feels cold here. Really cold."

He was a little surprised. "Cold?"

"Yeah." Her arms were crossed beneath her breasts, the goose-flesh on her skin actually visible. "Chilled, cold. Like a gust of icy air blowing through me. Yet another fun new experience."

"You said you weren't an empath."

"I'm not. I have no idea why I'm beginning to feel things rather than simply know them. Until now, feelings, sensations, only came with visions. Now . . ." She shivered. "No visions. But, man, I'm cold. I'm thinking that's not normal for June, never mind it not being normal for me."

"Maybe you're coming down with something," Rafe suggested prosaically.

"I sort of doubt it."

"It's just in here?" Hollis asked.

"Seems to be. Outside, I was fine."

"Then you should be outside."

"We both should," Isabel said. "You feel the cold too." She gestured slightly, and they all saw the goose bumps on Hollis's bare arms.

Rafe looked at both agents, then said to his detective, "Mal, would you mind staying to supervise until T.J. and Dustin are finished and the body is removed?"

"No problem."

"Thanks. I'll be right back." Rafe gestured slightly, and the two other women walked with him toward the front of the building. "It's after hours for most of the businesses around here, so there's not too much traffic in the area, but I've posted a few of my people on the block to stop the curious from gathering. Or, at least, from gathering close by."

When they stood out on the sidewalk, Isabel could indeed see both uniformed cops and passersby at a perimeter about half a block away.

"Great," she muttered. "Well, at least the icy breeze stopped blowing." She rubbed her upper arms briefly with both hands, relaxing visibly.

To Hollis, Rafe said, "I gather you didn't pick up anything helpful in there either?"

"No."

He couldn't tell whether it was because there'd been nothing for her to pick up or because she hadn't tried. He decided not to ask.

"I was about to suggest we call it a day before Hollis and Mallory found the body. It still sounds like a good idea. First thing tomorrow we'll have a preliminary forensics report, and if I know Doc we'll have the postmortem as well. We'll have a decent shot at making an I.D. of the body, and we can start trying to piece together what happened to this lady. Between now and then there isn't much we can do. Except get some rest for tomorrow."

"I will if you will," Isabel said.

He eyed her, but before he could say anything, Hollis was speaking calmly.

"I, for one, would just as soon start fresh tomorrow. I want to shower about six times, watch something funny on television, and maybe call my mother. If I ever feel like eating again, I'll order a pizza. You two want to be gluttons for punishment, have at it. I'm going back to the inn."

Isabel grimaced slightly. "A shower definitely sounds like a good idea; nobody wants to smell like death. But I'm way too restless to call it a day." She looked at Rafe, brows lifting inquiringly. "Buy you dinner?"

He checked his watch but didn't hesitate. "I'll pick you up at eight."

"See you then." Isabel walked with Hollis back to their rental and got in the driver's seat. Hollis got in beside her and didn't say anything for about half a mile.

Then she spoke slowly. "He's blocking you, isn't he? No—he's shielding you."

Isabel gave her partner a surprised glance, then fixed her gaze on the road again. "Bishop said you picked up on things quickly. Once again, he wasn't wrong."

Absently, Hollis said, "You relax a bit whenever Rafe is nearby, as if some of the strain is lifted. Maybe I see it because I used to be an artist. It started in Jamie's playroom, didn't it? When he put his hands on your wrists."

"Yeah."

"You felt something?"

"The shock first. And then a muffling quality. Didn't shut out the voices, just . . . quieted them a bit, as though I were suddenly insulated. Just enough for me to notice. Out in the Jeep, when he was putting disinfectant on my neck and sitting so close, the voices were barely whispers. When he left to go back inside, they got louder again."

"And just now, back there?"

"If he was within five feet of me, all I heard were whispers. Creepy whispers, but whispers. And felt that goddamned icy breeze; he doesn't seem to have had any effect at all on that."

"So what does it mean?"

"I don't know. I seem to have been saying that a lot today. I don't like saying it, for the record."

Hollis looked at her. "What do you hear now?"

"Usual background hum. Like listening to a party in the next room. That's normal."

"Headache?"

"Dull throb. Also normal."

"Rafe shielding you—is it getting stronger as time goes on?"

Isabel shrugged. "Hard to say, since it just started hours ago. I'll have to wait and see. It could get stronger. Or it could go away entirely. God knows." She smiled suddenly, wryly. "But if it turns out he can silence the voices, if only for a while, I may just have to move in with the man. Or at least take vacations with him."

"It would be nifty to have that quiet place to go to from time to time," Hollis said seriously. "A refuge."

Shaking her head, Isabel said, "Something else you'd better catch on to: the universe never offers something for nothing. There'll be a price tag. There always is."

"Maybe it's a price you can pay."

"And maybe it's a price he'll have to pay instead of me. Or would, if we went in that direction. It's the sort of thing the universe demands. Cosmic irony."

"Doesn't seem fair. And you don't have to remind me that the universe isn't about fairness."

"No, it's about balance."

"Then maybe that's what Rafe is, for you. Balance. Maybe the universe is offering you a refuge because you push yourself so hard."

"Yeah, and what's it offering him? A clairvoyant, career-driven federal agent who reads up on serial killers for fun, travels all over the country on a regular basis to get shot at and *talk* about serial killers, not to mention meeting a few of them in deadly situations, and, oh, by the way, hasn't had a successful romantic relationship in her entire adult life?"

"Great breath control," Hollis murmured. "The meditation exercises must really work."

Ignoring that, Isabel said, "I'm fairly sure Rafe hasn't pissed off the universe enough to be offered that little *balance* for his life."

"Maybe there are qualities in you he needs for his own balancing act."

"And maybe," Isabel said, "it's just a chemical or electromagnetic thing. Energy fields, nothing more. Basic science, emotions and personalities not involved."

She didn't have to be psychic to know she was being warned off, so Hollis didn't say anything else until her partner pulled the car into the parking lot of the inn. And then all she offered was a mild "I hear there's a surprisingly good Mexican place here in Hastings. You like Mexican, don't you?"

"I do."

"And does Rafe?"

Isabel hesitated, then said with clear reluctance, "Yes. He does."

As both agents got out of the car, Hollis said, again mildly, "Handy to already know so much about him. Likes and dislikes, habits, background. Sort of shortens the getting-to-know-each-other dance."

"For me. Not for him."

"Oh, I don't know about that. I have a hunch Rafe Sullivan already knows most of what he needs to about you. Except for one thing, I guess. And sooner or later, you're going to have to tell him."

"I know," Isabel said.

Special Agent Tony Harte scowled at the window as lightning flashed, then said, "Why is it that we always get the lousy weather, you want to tell me that?"

"Just lucky, I guess," Bishop responded absently as he worked at his laptop.

"This is not lucky. This is The Universe Hates Me. Me, personally. Who got a flat tire in the rain last night? Me. Who got grazed by a bullet when a pissed-off guy who wasn't even our suspect got even more pissed off and started shooting? Me. Who had to observe what was without doubt the most gross autopsy on record? Me."

"Who has to put up with your bitching? Me," Bishop said.

"And me," Miranda said as she came into the room. "What's he going on about now?"

"Usual," Bishop replied. "The universe hates him."

"Persecution complex."

"Yeah, that was my diagnosis."

"You two are not nearly as funny as you think you are," Tony informed them.

"Neither are you," Miranda said, then smiled. "Kendra will be fine, Tony."

"I hate it when you do that. Here I am, working up a really good, strong mad to let off steam, and you pat me on the head—metaphorically—and tell me, there, there, sit down and be a good boy."

"I did no such thing. I just said Kendra would be fine. And she will."

"She's in *Tulsa*," Tony said witheringly. "Setting aside the deranged killer she's looking for, they have tornadoes out there. Did you see today's weather?"

"Must have missed it." Miranda sent a glance toward the window, where another flash of lightning showed the heavy rain battering Spokane. "There was so much weather here that I didn't bother."

"There's a storm cell," Tony fretted. "Big, nasty one. Bearing down on Tulsa."

"Tony. Kendra will be fine."

He eyed her cautiously. "Are you just saying that, or do you know?"

"I know."

Looking up from his laptop, Bishop said mildly, "That's breaking the rules."

"You really want to listen to him bitch for the next few hours?"

"No."

"Well, then."

Tony was staring at Bishop in some indignation. "You knew? You knew Kendra would be fine and just sat there without easing my mind?"

"I thought you wanted to let off steam."

"There wouldn't have been any steam to let off if you'd told me Kendra would be all right. Dammit."

"See what you started?" Bishop said to his wife.

"Sorry. I just came in for—"

Whatever she'd come in for, what she got was a vision.

Even though he was relatively accustomed to seeing it happen, Tony nevertheless felt a little chill go through him as both Miranda and Bishop paled and closed their eyes, perfectly in sync. He waited, watching them, his own extra senses telling him this was a strong one, a painful one.

Finally, they opened their eyes, each reaching up to massage one temple. Miranda sat down across from her husband, and they looked at each other, both wearing an expression Tony had never seen before.

It caused another chill to go through him.

"We can't interfere," Bishop said. "We've done all we can do."

"I know. She'd probably ignore a warning anyway."

"Probably. She's stubborn."

"That's one word for it."

Tony cared about all the members of the SCU, not only his absent fiancée, and he was anxious. "What is it?" he demanded. "What did you see?"

Slowly, still gazing at her husband, Miranda said, "If it's literal and not symbolic, then Isabel is about to make a choice that will change her life. And put her on a very, very dangerous path."

"What's at the end of the path?"

Miranda drew a breath and let it out slowly. "The death of someone she cares about."

10

CALEB HEARD THE NEWS about a fourth woman's body being found when he stopped by the coffee shop for a cup to take home. The girl behind the counter—he couldn't figure out how on earth they could be called "sales associates" when they worked in a coffee shop—was only too happy to fill him in on the latest details while she prepared his latte.

Gory details.

"And you know the worst part?" she demanded as she put a lid on the cup.

"Somebody died?" he suggested.

She blinked, then said anxiously, "Well, yeah, but I heard she'd been dead for months."

Caleb resisted the impulse to ask what the hell difference that made. Instead, he said, "And the worst part is?"

"She was brunette," Sally Anne, sales associate for the coffee shop and a brunette herself, whispered.

"Ah."

"So none of us is safe. He's not just going after blondes now, he's—he's going after the rest of us."

Caleb paid for his coffee and said with ruthless sympathy, "If I were you, I'd leave town."

"I might. I just might. Thanks, Mr. Powell. Oh—can I help you, ma'am?"

"One iced mocha latte, please. Medium."

Caleb turned quickly, surprised to find Hollis there. "Hi."

"Hi." She looked tired and also more casual than he'd yet seen her, in jeans and a black T-shirt that demanded to know if the hokey-pokey was *really* what it was all about.

"You're not still working?"

"No, we've pretty much called it a day." She shrugged. "Can't do a lot in the way of investigating the body Sally Anne just told you about until we get forensics and a postmortem."

Something about her wry tone made him say, "You didn't expect the news to *not* get around, did you?"

"No. But this town sets the land speed record for gossip, I've realized that much. The unfortunate thing is that it tends to be so damned accurate."

"I'll say. I didn't grow up here, but when I started my practice fifteen years ago, it took less than a week for everyone in town to know that my parents were dead and my younger brother had gotten his girlfriend pregnant and married her literally at the business end of her daddy's shotgun." He paused, then added, "I told no one, absolutely no one."

Hollis smiled slightly and paid Sally Anne for her coffee. "They do seem to find out what they want to know. Which begs the question . . ."

"How can a killer walk among us, unseen?"

"Oh, not that question. Killers always have walked among us unseen. No, the question I'm asking myself is: how is it possible that a woman's decomposing body hung inside a derelict gas station less than three blocks from the center of town for months without anybody noticing?"

Sally Anne uttered a choked little sound and rushed toward the back of the shop.

Hollis grimaced. "Well, that was definitely indiscreet. To say the least. I must be more tired than I thought. Or, at any rate, that'll be my story."

Caleb shook his head slightly. "Look, I know you've had a hell of a day, but can we sit down here and talk for a while? There's something I want to ask you."

She nodded and joined him at one of the small tables by the front window.

"Have you eaten?" Caleb asked. "The sandwiches here aren't bad, or—"

Hollis shook her head, almost flinching. "No. Thank you. I'm reasonably sure the coffee will stay down, but only because I was practically breast-fed the stuff. I'm not planning to eat anything for the foreseeable future."

It was Caleb's turn to grimace. "So I take it Sally Anne's gory details about the body were on the mark?"

"Oh, yeah."

"I'm sorry. That had to be rough."

"Not destined to be one of my more pleasant memories. But I was warned what to expect when I signed on for this gig." She sipped her latte, adding, "You wanted to ask me something?"

"Why *did* you sign on for this gig?"

Surprised, Hollis said, "I . . . didn't expect a personal question."

"I didn't expect to ask one," he confessed.

She smiled. "I thought lawyers always rehearsed what they said."

"Not this one. Or, at least, not this time. If it's too personal, we can forget I asked. But I'd rather not."

"Why so curious?"

Even experienced as he was at reading juries, Caleb couldn't tell if she was stalling or really wanted to know. "That explanation would undoubtedly involve a lot of me backpedaling and trying to justify my curiosity to myself, let alone you, so I'd just as soon skip the attempt. Let's just say I'm a curious man and leave it at that."

She gazed at him for a long moment, blue eyes unreadable, then said in a queerly serene voice, "I was assaulted. Beaten, raped, stabbed, left for dead."

Not what he had expected. "Jesus. Hollis, I'm sorry, I had no idea."

"Of course not, how could you?"

He literally didn't know what to say, and for one of the very few times in his life. "That's . . . why you became an agent?"

"Well, my old life was pretty much in tatters, so it seemed like a good idea when I was offered a chance at a new one." Her voice retained that odd tranquillity. "I was able to help—in a small way—stop the man who had attacked me and so many other women. That felt good."

"Revenge?"

"No. Justice. Going after revenge is like opening a vein in your arm and waiting for somebody else to bleed to death. I didn't need that. I just needed to . . . see . . . him stopped. And I needed a new direction for my life. The Bureau and the Special Crimes Unit provided that."

Tentatively, because he wasn't sure how far she would be willing to go in talking about this, he said, "But to devote your life

to a career that puts you face-to-face on a regular basis with violence and death—and evil? How healthy can that be, especially
after what you've gone through?"

"I guess it depends on one's reasons. I think mine are pretty
good, beginning with the major one. Somebody has to fight evil.
It might as well be me."

"Judging by what I've seen in my life, it'll take more than an
army to do it. No offense."

Hollis shook her head. "You don't fight evil with an army.
You fight it with will. Yours. Mine. The will of every human soul
who cares about the outcome. I can't say I thought much about it
until what happened to me. But once you've seen evil up close,
once you've had your entire life changed by it, then you see a lot
of things more clearly." Her smile twisted, not without bitterness.
"Even with someone else's eyes."

He frowned, not getting that last reference. "I can understand
feeling like that after what you went through, but to let it change
your whole life—"

"After what I went through, it was the only thing I *could* do
with my life. I not only saw some things more clearly, I also saw
things differently. Too differently to ever go back to being an
artist."

"Hollis, it's only natural to see a lot of things differently after
such a horribly traumatic experience."

A little laugh escaped her. "No, Caleb, you don't understand.
"I *saw* things differently. Literally. Colors aren't the same now.
Textures. Depth perception. I don't see the world the way I used
to, the way you do, because I can't. The connections between my
brain and my sight are . . . man-made. Or at least man-forged.
Not organic. The doctors say my brain may never fully adjust."

"Adjust to what?"

"To these new eyes I'm wearing. They weren't the ones I was

born with, you see. When the rapist left me for dead, he took a couple of souvenirs. He took my eyes."

By the time Mallory got back to the station, it was nearly eight and she was tired. Tired as hell, if the truth be known. Also queasy, depressed, and not a little anxious.

"Mallory—"

"Jesus."

"Oh, I'm sorry," Ginny McBrayer said. "I didn't mean to make you jump."

"These days, everything is making me jump." Mallory sighed. "What is it, Ginny?"

"You asked me to check with the other women in the department and find out if anybody had the sense of being watched lately."

"Yeah. And have any of them?"

Ginny shrugged. "It's sort of hard to say. Everybody's jumpy. Two or three said they'd gotten the feeling of being watched at least a couple of times in the last few weeks, but even they admitted they weren't sure of anything. Of course, now that I've brought up the subject, everybody's talking about it, the guys too."

Mallory sat down at her desk and rubbed her eyes wearily. "Well, hell. Dunno if that helps."

"We'll all be alert, anyway. Have you talked to the FBI agents about it?"

"Not yet. Need to, though, I suppose." She sighed. "The dairy farmer's wife; she turn up yet? And what is her name, anyway? Helton. What Helton?"

"Rose Helton. Not a sign of her. And we still have two other women reported missing in Hastings during the past month, not counting that news reporter who vanished last night. Sharona Jones and Kate Murphy. Plus the dozen or so missing from the general area outside Hastings in the same time period."

"I know Sharona—she doesn't fit the profile, she's black. She's missing?"

"Well, her boyfriend claims she is. But her dog is also missing, as well as her car and a lot of her clothes, and her mother says she's always wanted to see the world, so we're thinking she might have upped and left."

"If Ray Mercer was my boyfriend, I'd up and leave too." Mallory sighed again. "Still, we have to make sure, so keep everybody on it. What about Kate Murphy?"

"More troubling, in that she *does* fit the profile. Late twenties, blond, successful; she owns one of those new little boutiques on Main Street. Was doing pretty well with it too. Didn't show up for work on Monday, so her assistant manager has been running the shop."

"We've checked out her house or apartment?"

"Uh-huh. No sign she's been taken—but no sign she left voluntarily either. Her car is in its slot at her condo, and far as we can tell it's clean. Haven't found her purse or keys, though. She didn't—doesn't—have any pets, and no family in Hastings. We're trying to track down relatives now."

"And still no sign of Cheryl Bayne."

"No. The station in Columbia has sent another reporter, this one male, to cover this new . . . angle."

"How caring of them."

Ginny nodded. "Yeah, even the other reporters are being pretty scathing about that."

"While doing their own reports."

179

"Uh-huh."

Mallory shook her head in disgust. "Okay. Let me or the chief know if anything changes."

"Right."

When she was alone again, Mallory sat for a moment with her elbows on her desk and her hands cupping her face, fingers absently massaging her temples. She should stay, but Rafe had made it plain she was to go home as soon as the body had been taken from that old building and the forensics team finished.

Both of which had been done.

Mallory was tired but also curiously wide awake. She didn't want to go home. Didn't want to be alone. She wanted something to get the image of that poor woman out of her head.

With only a slight hesitation, she picked up her phone and called Alan's cell. "Hey, are you home?" she asked without preamble.

"Headed that way. Pulling into the parking lot now, as a matter of fact."

"Have you eaten?"

"Nothing you could truthfully define as food," he replied. "There was something a charitable person might have called a sandwich hours ago, but it may have been just a figment of my imagination. Are you offering?"

"I'm offering takeout Chinese. I'll even pick it up on my way to your place. Deal?"

"Deal. Stop for wine if you feel like that. My place is dry as a bone. Oh—and I have a splitting headache, so if you could pick up some aspirin as well? I don't think I have any."

"Okay. See you in a few minutes." Mallory hung up, telling herself this wasn't a bad idea at all. So what if she had spent most of the previous night in his bed? It didn't mean anything. It didn't have to mean anything. Alan could be an amusing and entertaining companion, and he was good in bed.

Very good, in fact. And she couldn't deceive herself into believing she wasn't looking forward to a little body-on-body comfort, because she was. Two clean, healthy, sweaty bodies tangled together in the sheets sounded like a dandy way to affirm that both of them were alive.

Alive. Not hanging from a beam like a weeks-old gutted fish. Not lying in a boneless, bloody sprawl in the woods off some highway. Not laced into an impossibly tight leather corset and smothered with a hood while a woman with a whip and chains tortured—

"Christ," she muttered. "I've gotta get out of here."

It took a few minutes, of course, to do what she had to in order to leave for the night, but she took care of things quickly and bolted before anyone could come up with anything that required her continued presence at the station.

She called and ordered the food on her way to the restaurant, so it'd be ready and waiting for her, and did stop for wine even though she wasn't usually much of a drinker. She even remembered Alan's aspirin. Still, it was barely half an hour after she talked to him when Mallory entered his apartment with one bag full of little cardboard cartons and another holding the wine and aspirin.

"You look jumpy as hell," he commented as soon as she walked through the door.

"It's a jumpy time." Mallory knew the way to the kitchen, of course, and lost no time in getting the wine out and hunting through his cupboards for glasses. "Jesus, Alan, not a single wineglass?"

"Housewares aren't a priority with me. Sue me."

"My life has come down to drinking wine from jelly glasses. Could this day get any better?"

Alan had swallowed several aspirin dry, then began setting out the cartons on his breakfast bar, where they normally ate. He paused to look at her intently. "I heard. Couldn't have been much fun, finding that body."

"No."

"Want to talk about it?"

"No." She poured wine into one of the glasses and immediately took a swallow. "I intend to drink at least half this bottle, part of it while I shower away the assorted smells of today, then choke down some shrimp and vegetables. After that, unless you object, the plan is to adjourn to your bedroom and fuck like bunnies. Possibly all night. Unless you still have your headache, of course. Tell me you won't."

"I expect the aspirin to work any minute," Alan replied. "And that plan suits me just fine."

The Mexican restaurant wasn't crowded despite the fact that Saturday night was usually one of the busiest. As the owner had told them mournfully when he escorted them personally to a cozy table back in the corner, people were going out less at night since the murders had started. And after what had been found today, undoubtedly most of his usual patrons were home with their doors locked.

So if Rafe and Isabel didn't have the restaurant to themselves, they did have their own secluded corner of it. With quiet music playing in the background and an attentive but unobtrusive waiter, they were almost in their own world.

Almost.

"You still believe Jamie didn't mutilate Jane Doe?" Rafe

asked as they were finishing up the main course. They had been talking generally about the murders and the investigation, both with too much experience as cops to allow either the clinical details of brutal death or the bloody images they had seen all too recently to affect their appetites. And both shying away from anything more personal.

"I'm positive. My guess is, he was watching Jamie and saw her put the body into the trunk of Jane Doe's car. I don't know if she drove the car to wherever she planned to leave it, or if he did—and when she came back either to the playroom or to the car for some reason and didn't find the body, that was when she really freaked out. In any case, I think he put the body in that old garage. And amused himself with it."

"That's sickening," Rafe said.

"Definitely. He's very twisted, our boy."

"So his reasons for picking Jamie as his first victim in Hastings were probably twisted as well."

"Well, it may have been about Jamie being a dominatrix rather than a lesbian. Her wielding so much power over other women, power he wanted and didn't have. Maybe sheer jealousy was the trigger. Or envy. Maybe he couldn't stand the fact that she could control the women in her life."

"And he couldn't control the women in his."

"Maybe. Or it could have been the fact that her partners came to Jamie, willingly put themselves into her hands, submitted to her. And no matter how hard he tried, he couldn't get that response from women. Ironic, really. He always goes for the smart, successful ones, the ones least likely to allow themselves to be dominated in a relationship, and yet to dominate women is what he desperately wants."

"So for him it really is the unattainable."

"Unless his taste in women changes, yeah." Isabel's voice was wry. "He'll never get what he wants—except by killing them. It's only when they're dying and then lifeless that he's the one in control, stronger than them.

"In killing Jamie, he could have achieved a particular sort of satisfaction, because she was a dominatrix. For the first time, he was able to dominate a woman whose specialty was dominating others. Even if he had to kill her to do it."

"She possessed traits he wants to destroy?"

"That's usually the case with a sexual sadist."

"But not this time? Not our guy?"

Isabel frowned. "Targeting the breasts and genitals is a classic sign of a sexual obsession. But this guy, our guy, the sense I get is that he seems to be . . . punishing them for being women. So maybe he is trying to destroy the feminine traits in his nature. Or maybe he's furious with them because they're too female for him, literally too much woman for him to handle."

"And that isn't a sexually driven motivation?"

"Not really. More a question of identity. His."

"This is fascinating," Rafe said.

Isabel stared at him for a moment, then sat back in her chair with a sigh. "See, this is why my social life sucks. I always end up talking about killers."

"My fault. I did ask."

"Yeah, but the subject sprang to mind. Doesn't say much about my sex appeal."

Rafe eyed her. "It says we're in the middle of a murder investigation. And so."

"That's a handy excuse. Can't you tell when a woman is fishing?"

"You're not serious? Isabel, you have to know you're gorgeous."

"My mirror tells me all the pieces fit together nicely, but that

184

doesn't mean I'm your type. Lots of men prefer petite redheads, or very slender brunettes. Or—women who don't carry guns and know a dozen different ways to *really* hurt a guy if he pisses her off."

He had to laugh. "I admit that last bit is enough to give any man pause, but you don't see me taking to my heels, do you?"

"No, but since we sort of have to work together—"

"We don't have to go out to dinner together. Isabel, I'm here because I want to be, period. Just for the record, I don't prefer petite redheads or slender brunettes. And I never figured you for the insecure type."

"And here I was thinking I was coming on too strong."

Their attentive waiter appeared to clear the plates and take their order for coffee and dessert, and Rafe waited until he'd gone again to respond to her somewhat mocking comment.

"So what happened today?"

Isabel blinked. "You know what happened today."

"What don't I know? What's got you so rattled that you're pushing yourself to . . . make a different kind of connection with me when you're not sure it's what you want?"

"Who says it's not what I want?"

"I do. Hell, you do. Look at your body language, Isabel. As soon as you decided to end the shop talk and get into more personal territory, you leaned back. Away from me. That's not as good as a sign, that *is* a sign. Your words say you're interested, but your body says stay away."

"Dammit," she muttered. "What was that I said earlier about you making a fair profiler? I'm changing my assessment. You'd make a very good one."

"So I'm on target?"

"Well, let's just say you're not far off it. I am just not very good at this sort of thing."

Rafe had to smile at her disgruntled tone. "You're a very confident woman, Isabel—almost always. Very sure of yourself. But right now, at this moment, you're scared. Why?"

She was silent, frowning down at the table.

"Something happened. What was it?"

"Look, this investigation is . . . different, that's all. Odd things are happening. My abilities seem to be changing. And I don't quite know what do to about it."

"Have you reported this to Bishop?"

"No. Not yet."

"Why not?"

"Because . . . I don't know why not. Because I want to figure it out for myself."

"And making a move on me seemed like a good way to do that?"

"Stop rubbing it in."

"What?"

"My failure."

Dryly, he said, "Who says you failed? Isabel, I realized I wanted you sometime yesterday. Early yesterday. Or possibly about ten minutes after we met. I also realized it was going to hellishly complicate the entire situation, so I've been doing my best not to think about it."

"Maybe thinking about it would be good," she said earnestly. "And doing something about it even better."

"You're still leaning back in your chair," he pointed out.

"I can lean forward." But she didn't. She frowned again, honestly baffled.

"See?" Rafe said. "Conflicting signals. Even consciously, you're not sure what you want."

With a sigh, she said, "Trust me to find myself attracted to the one man who isn't willing to take what he's offered, no questions asked. Keep this up, and I'll have to start believing in leprechauns. And unicorns."

"Sorry about that. But I'm not a kid, Isabel. I'm a twenty-year veteran of the sexual wars, and I've learned a few things along the way. One being if you're going to get involved with a complicated woman, you'd better damned well know what the complications are. Ahead of time. Before you trip over them."

"That does sound like bitter experience."

"It was. Not bitter, really, but I learned a hard lesson. And it's more or less my own fault. You said the sort of energy that makes you psychic is something you have in common with our killer; well, I have something in common with him too. I like strong women. With strong, I've discovered, comes complicated, which can cause problems. Unless I know about the complications going in."

"Okay. Well, I hear voices. There's that."

"Uh-huh. And?"

"I need coffee in the morning before I'm human. And cornflakes. I like cornflakes. I take really hot showers, always, so I tend to steam up the room. I hate silence in strange places, so I travel with a sound machine. Ocean waves. I have to have air-conditioning on full blast even in the dead of winter to sleep well. Oh—and I hate moonlight shining in the bedroom."

"Isabel."

"Not those sorts of complications, huh?"

"No."

"Dammit."

"If I *were* a profiler," he said slowly, "making an educated guess, I'd say that your breezy manner and humorous attitude cover up a lot of pain. And I'm not talking about the headaches your voices give you. That evil face you saw—it really did change your life, didn't it?"

Their waiter placed coffee and dessert on the table and went silently away again, and still Isabel said nothing. She picked up a spoon and poked at her dessert, then put it down again.

"Still not ready to tell me?" He fixed his coffee the way he liked it, his gaze remaining on her face, trying to make his own posture and expression as relaxed and unthreatening as possible.

She sipped her coffee, then grimaced and dumped cream and sugar in before trying a second sip.

"Isabel?"

Abruptly, as if against her will, she said, "It was beautiful."

"What was?"

"The face evil wore. It was beautiful."

It was late when Ginny left the police station, much later than usual for her. And after talking to the other women and hearing how jumpy they were, she made a point of walking out to her car in the company of a couple of male officers who were also leaving. Though none of the guys had said anything openly to the female officers, Ginny had noticed that in the last week or so all the women had an escort coming or going.

She doubted any of the women were complaining. She certainly didn't; anytime she was outside alone, she tended to spend a lot of time looking back over her shoulder and jumping at shadows.

By tacit consent, neither of the men left her until her car was unlocked, the door open, and the interior light showing them all an empty, unthreatening little Honda.

"Lock your doors," Dean Emery advised.

"You bet. Thanks, guys." She got in and immediately locked the doors and started the car, absently looking after them until both reached and safely entered their own cars.

Not that the guys had to worry, really.

So far, anyway.

Ginny was hardly a profiler, but she did have a semester of Abnormal Psychology under her belt, and she vividly recalled the section about serial killers, especially since it had given her night-mares for weeks.

Very few serial killers murdered both men and women. There had been killers who targeted both male and female children or young people, but when the targets were adults, they were almost always one sex.

A homosexual serial killer targeted men or young males, and a heterosexual killer targeted women or girls, as a rule. Though some homosexual killers, or men who were insecure sexually and feared they might be homosexual, had been known to target women out of sheer rage. They didn't want to be whatever they were, and they blamed women for it.

The very rare female serial killers went after men, or appar-ently had so far—except in the rather frighteningly common cases of women poisoning children or other family members, when they tended not to differentiate between the sexes.

Have some soup, dear. Oh, it tastes funny? That's just a new spice I'm trying out.

Jesus.

The things people got up to.

Ginny pulled her car out of the lot and headed for home, still pondering, mostly because her mind refused to let go of the subject.

What did he look like? Did she pass him on the street every day? Did she know him? He was strong, very strong; the medical report on Tricia Kane said that he'd driven a large knife into her chest to the hilt.

Ginny shivered.

What kind of rage did it take to do something like that? And how had Tricia aroused it in him? Just by being blond and successful? Just by being female?

Just by being?

When Ginny had colored her bleached hair back to something approximating its natural dark brown a week or so before, not a soul at the station had laughed or even commented, and her friends said it was wise of her. No reason to take stupid chances, after all, not when she was a cop in the thick of things.

Her mother had been visibly relieved.

Her father had said at least it made her look less like a whore.

As she pulled her car into the driveway, Ginny felt all her insides tighten. He was home, and judging by the crooked way his car was parked, he had, as usual on a weekend, spent the afternoon drinking.

Shit.

Still in the car, she removed her holster and locked it securely away in the glove compartment. When she got out, she locked the car up as well.

She never took the gun with her into the house. Never.

It was too tempting.

She went up the steps and used her key to let herself in, silently telling herself for the hundredth time that she had to get her own place, no matter what. And soon.

"Hey, little girl." His voice was slurred, his mouth wet. "Where you been?"

Her own voice deadened, Ginny replied, "At work, Daddy," and pushed the door closed behind her.

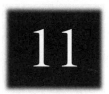

11

ISABEL LOOKED AT RAFE with a faint smile. "You didn't expect that, did you? That evil could be beautiful." She wondered if he understood. If he could even begin to understand.

"No."

"Of course not. It should be ugly, that's what everyone expects. Red eyes, scaly flesh, horns and fangs. It should look like it was born in hell. At least that. At least. It should breathe fire and brimstone. It should burn to the touch."

"But it doesn't."

"No. Evil always wears a deceptive face. It won't be ugly, at least not until it really shows itself. It won't look like something bad. That would be too easy to recognize. Too easy for us to see. Because the important thing, the thing evil does best, is deceive."

"And it deceived you."

She laughed, the low sound holding no amusement. "It wore a handsome face, when it first showed itself to me. A charming smile. It had a persuasive voice, and it knew all the right words to say. And the touch of it was kind and gentle. At least in the beginning."

"A man. Someone you cared about."

Isabel crossed her arms beneath her breasts, unconsciously adding yet another barrier between them, but she continued speaking in a toneless voice.

"I was seventeen. He was a little older, but I'd known him all my life. He was the boy in the neighborhood everybody depended on. If an elderly widow needed her yard mowed, he'd do it—and refuse payment. If anybody needed furniture moved, he'd offer to help. Stuck for a baby-sitter? He was there, always reliable and responsible, and all the kids—all the kids—adored him. The parents trusted him. Their sons considered him a buddy. And their daughters thought he walked on water."

"Deceiving everyone."

She nodded slowly, her gaze fixed on the table now, eyes distant. "The weird thing is, after taking all the time and trouble to deceive everybody around him for such a long, long time, when it came right down to it, it didn't take much at all to start revealing the beast inside."

Rafe was very much afraid he knew where this was going, and it required an effort to hold his voice steady when he asked, "What did it take?"

"*No.* Just that. Just one little word." She looked up, focused on him. "That was the beginning. He asked me to a school dance, and I said no."

"What did he do, Isabel?"

"Nothing then. I told him I didn't feel like that about him, that he was more of a brother to me. He said it was a shame, but he understood. A few days later, I saw him in the bushes outside my house. Outside my bedroom. Watching me."

"You didn't call the cops," Rafe guessed.

"I was seventeen. I trusted him. I thought he was just . . . taking the rejection badly. Maybe I was even a little bit flattered on some level of myself, that it mattered so much to him. So I just closed the curtains. And kept them closed. But then he started . . . turning up wherever I was. Always at a distance. Always watching me. That was when I started to be . . . just a little bit afraid."

"But you still didn't report it."

"No. Everybody loved him, and I think I was half afraid nobody would believe me. I confided in my best friend. She was envious. Said he had a crush on me, and I should be flattered." She laughed, again without humor. "She was seventeen too. What do you know, at seventeen?

"I tried to feel flattered, but it was getting more and more difficult to feel anything but scared. I could take care of myself, I knew self-defense, but . . . there was something in his eyes I'd never seen before. Something angry. And hungry. And I didn't understand why, but it terrified me."

Rafe waited, unable to ask another question. He wished they were somewhere more private yet had a strong hunch that, if they had been, Isabel wouldn't have been willing—or able—to confide in him about this. He thought she needed the insulation of a semi-public place for this. There were people here, even if not close by. Food and music and an occasional quiet laugh from another part of the room.

Normality here.

He thought Isabel was afraid she wouldn't be able to hold it together enough to talk about this if they were alone. Either that or she had chosen, quite deliberately, to tell him this without even a shadow of intimacy. With a table between them in a public place, where the ugliness could be softened or blurred or even discarded at the end with a game shrug and a bland *But it happened years ago, of course.*

Depending on his reaction to what she was telling him.

Depending on how well *he* held it together.

"Of course, it wasn't talked about so much in those days, stalking." Her voice was steady, controlled. "I mean, that was something that happened to celebrities, not ordinary people. Not seventeen-year-old girls. And certainly not involving boys they'd known their whole lives. So when I finally did tell my father, he did the logical thing in his mind. He didn't call the police—he confronted the boy. Very reasonably, no yelling, no threats. Just a friendly warning that I wasn't interested and he should, really, stay away."

"His trigger," Rafe muttered.

"As it turned out, yes. My father couldn't have known. Nobody could have known. He'd hidden his true face all too well. If my father had gone to the police and everyone had taken the threat seriously, maybe the ending would have been different. But after it was all over, they told me . . . it probably wouldn't have. Delayed things, maybe, but he hadn't actually done anything, and he was such a *good* boy, so they couldn't have held him for long. So it probably wouldn't have changed anything if I had acted differently, if my father had. Probably."

"Isabel—"

"It was a Wednesday. I came home from school, just like always. Rode with a friend, because my father didn't believe I was old enough to have a car yet. She let me out, and then she headed home while I went into the house. As soon as I closed the front door behind me, I knew something was wrong. Everything was wrong. Maybe I smelled the blood."

"Oh, Christ," Rafe said softly.

"I went into the living room and . . . they were there. My parents. Sitting on the couch, side by side. They were holding hands. We found out later from the note he'd left that he had forced them in there at gunpoint. Sat them down. And then he shot them. Both of them. They hadn't even had time to get really scared; they just looked . . . surprised."

"Isabel, I'm sorry. I'm so sorry."

She blinked, and for just an instant her mouth seemed to quiver. Then it steadied, and she said calmly, "The story could have ended there. If it had, maybe I wouldn't have come out of it psychic. I don't know. Nobody knows.

"But that was really just the beginning. I turned—to run or call the police, I don't know. And he was there. He said he'd been waiting for me. He had the gun, a silenced automatic; that's why the neighbors hadn't heard. I was too scared to scream at first, too shocked, but then he told me he'd kill me if I made a sound. So I didn't. All during those hours, all night long, I never made a sound."

Rafe wished he could drink. He wished he could stop her from finishing the story. But he couldn't do either.

"Looking back, knowing what I know now, I think if I had made a sound he might not have gotten so crazy. I think that's what maddened him, that no matter what he did to me, he couldn't get me to scream. Or even to cry. Without even understanding how or what it would mean, I was taking away his power.

"He—right there on the living-room rug, in front of my dead parents, he tore my clothes off, and he raped me, holding the gun jammed against my neck. He kept saying I was his, I belonged to him, and he'd make me admit it.

"He did things to me I didn't even know were possible. I was just seventeen. Just a kid, really. I was a virgin. I'd never had a boyfriend serious enough to—to do more than kiss. I wasn't ignorant about sex, but . . . I couldn't understand why I didn't die, why what he was doing didn't kill me. But it didn't. I bled. And I hurt. And as the hours passed, the beautiful face he'd worn for so long got uglier and uglier. He started cursing me. Hitting me. He took the gun and—hurt me with that too."

She drew a breath and let it out slowly. "Cracked ribs, a fractured jaw and wrist, a dislocated shoulder. Too many bruises to count. Raw inside. At the end, he was sitting astride me, both hands holding my head as he slammed it against the floor, over and over again. Screaming that I was his and he'd make me admit it."

Isabel didn't shed a tear, but her eyes were very bright, and her voice was very soft when she finished. "And his touch burned. He had red eyes, and horns, and scaly flesh, and his breath smelled of brimstone."

Travis was more pleased than he wanted to admit—or show her—when he found Ally waiting for him outside the police station after work. Waiting on the hood of his car, actually, and wearing a very short skirt.

"You shouldn't be out alone this time of night," he told her, trying not to stare at long legs that looked great even under garish outside lights.

She lifted an eyebrow at him, amused. "I'm in a brightly lit parking lot. At the police station. Other than being inside the building, I doubt there's a safer place right now."

"Maybe not. Some of our female officers think they've been watched, maybe even followed."

"Really?" She slid off the car's hood and shrugged. "Well, I'm not a blonde. And I can take care of myself."

"It might not be just blondes, you know. Or didn't you hear about the body we found today?"

"I heard. Also heard she'd been dead a couple months or thereabouts. So maybe it was a different killer."

Travis didn't want to admit that he wasn't so close to the inner circles of the investigation that he was up on the latest theories, so he merely shrugged and said, "Still, we've got other women missing in the area, and not all of them are blondes. You really should be careful, Ally."

"It's so sweet that you're worried about me."

He grimaced. "Don't make it sound like that."

"Like what?"

"Like you're amused. I'm not some toy you're playing with, Ally. Or, if I am—"

"If you are, what?" She stepped closer and slipped her arms up around his neck.

"If I am . . . then tell me before I make a goddamned fool of myself," he said, and kissed her.

She laughed. "Believe me, sweetie, you are not a toy. I like my men with plenty of muscle and minds of their own. You fit that bill, right?"

"I'd better."

"Great. And now that we both understand that—how about a drink or two to unwind after a tough day?"

He groaned. "I've gotta be up at the crack of dawn. Why don't we just pick up a pizza on the way to my place?"

"Or we could do that," Ally agreed. She smiled at him and kept smiling as he put her into the passenger seat of his flashy sports car and went around to the driver's side.

She wondered how soon she could find a few minutes alone to call in and report what Travis knew.

Before he figured out what she was up to.

———————

Without a word, Rafe placed his hand on the table between them, palm up.

For the longest time, Isabel didn't move. Then, finally, at last, she leaned forward and put her hand in his. The shock this time was almost a crackle, as if it should have been white-hot and burned them. But it didn't. It just felt warm, Isabel thought.

He said, "I can't even begin to imagine how you survived that. And then to survive, sanity intact—only to find yourself hearing voices. That's what happened, isn't it?"

She nodded. "The worst of it, at first, was that I was in the hospital with my jaw wired shut." A shaky little laugh escaped her. "Left-handed, and it was the left wrist that was fractured. So I couldn't even write to the doctors and tell them what I was hearing. I just had to lie there and listen."

"A combination of the head injury and the other shocks and trauma. That woke up your latent abilities."

"With a vengeance. At first, I just thought I was going nuts. That he had damaged my mind even worse than he had my body. But slowly, while I healed physically, I began to realize that the voices were telling me things. Things I shouldn't have been able to know. A nurse would come in to check on me or whatever, and I'd know she was having trouble in her marriage. Then later, I'd hear her out in the hallway talking to another nurse—about having trouble in her marriage. Things like that. Sometimes voices, as though another person were saying something to me conversationally, sometimes . . . I'd just know."

"And when you could finally speak again? You didn't tell anyone, did you?"

"Not even the trauma expert—shrink—I saw for nearly a year

afterward. I went to live with an aunt while I finished high school. Another school, needless to say. In another neighborhood."

"Where no one knew."

Isabel sighed. "Where no one knew. My aunt was very kind, and I loved her, but I never told her about the voices. At first because I was afraid they'd lock me up. Then, later, when I began reading up on what little information I could find on psychic abilities, because I didn't think anyone would believe me."

"Until you met Bishop."

"Until I met Bishop. By then, the only thing I was sure of was that there had to be a reason I could do what I did, a reason why I heard the voices. A reason why that evil hadn't been able to destroy me, hard as it tried."

"A reason you had survived."

"Yeah. Because there had to be a reason. They call it survivor's guilt. You have to get through that, find some purpose in your life. Figure out how you lived when those around you died. And why. I didn't know those answers.

"I drifted through college until my friend was killed. Julie. She died horribly, suddenly. There one day, gone the next. Before I could even begin to grieve for her, more women were dead and their killer had vanished."

"The second traumatic event in your life," Rafe said. "And the second time you encountered evil."

Isabel nodded. "I hadn't seen it coming then either, that was what hit me hardest. These voices that told me things never told me I was going to lose my best friend. That was when I decided to become a cop. I still didn't know how to channel or use the voices—or how to keep myself from being locked away in a padded cell somewhere if I did. But I knew I had to try. I knew I had to look for that evil face. And destroy it when I found it."

———

Dana had finally grown tired of Joey's whining and sent him back to Columbia—but she had also ordered him to make the drive back to Hastings on Sunday morning. And when he whined about *that,* she reminded him that news was a twenty-four-seven business and if he didn't like it he could go use his supposed camera skills elsewhere.

As for Dana herself, she had elected to keep her room at the inn. There were several women staying there, including the federal agents, and it felt safer there.

If anywhere could feel safe in Hastings.

Dana didn't apologize even to herself for being so jumpy, especially since Cheryl Bayne had disappeared. If this maniac was killing anybody who got in his way, anybody who offered a threat to him . . . then Dana now had two strikes against her. She was blond and she was media.

It was enough to make any woman jumpy, and never mind the additional worry of too many guys prowling around town with guns stuck in their belts, also jumpy as hell—

"Hi."

Dana nearly came out of her skin. "Christ, don't do that!"

"Sorry." Paige Gilbert shrugged apologetically. "Like you, I just came out for ice." She was holding an ice bucket in one hand.

Dana looked at her own bucket and sighed, continuing around the corner of the hallway to the alcove where the ice machine lived on this floor of the inn. "Why're you staying here?" she asked the other woman. "You live in Hastings, don't you?"

"I live alone. So I thought I'd stay here at the inn for the duration."

Dana scooped ice, then eyed Paige. "But you aren't a blonde."

"Neither was—is—Cheryl Bayne. And then there's the body they found today."

Wary, Dana said, "I know they found one. Been dead a while, I heard."

"Yeah." Paige scooped ice into her bucket and straightened, adding, "My sources claim she was brunette."

"Brunette."

"Yeah."

"Did your source also say she was . . . tortured?"

"Mangled."

"The difference being?"

Paige hesitated, then said, "Tortured means she was alive when it happened. Mangled means she was dead."

"Oh, shit."

"I've got a bottle of scotch in my room. Want some?"

Dana didn't hesitate. "Bet your ass I do."

Rafe didn't push his luck by asking too many questions. He knew Isabel had been exhausted even before the evening began, and by the time she'd confided the unspeakable tragedies in her life, it was obvious what she needed more than anything was sleep and plenty of it.

So he took her back to the inn, some instinct urging him to maintain the physical contact between them as much as possible. He was still holding her hand when they walked up the steps to the wide, old-fashioned porch.

Absently, she said, "This place couldn't decide what it wanted to be when it grew up—a bed and breakfast or a hotel. I've never seen a hybrid quite like it."

"Rocking chairs on the front porch, but no central dining

201

room," he agreed. "Strange. But nobody has to share a bathroom, and there's cable."

Isabel smiled faintly, looking at him in the yellow glow of the front porch lights. "I think Hollis and I, and a few of the news-people, are the only guests."

"Hastings was never a favored tourist destination, just a little town on the way to Columbia. Nothing much to see. But if we manage to stop this guy here, before he slips away again, I have a feeling it'll put us on the map. For all the wrong reasons, unfortunately." His fingers tightened around hers. "Isabel . . . that first evil face you saw. He killed himself, didn't he? After he thought he'd killed you."

She nodded. "Left that note I mentioned earlier, explaining what he'd done and why. Then blew his brains out. They found his body draped across my bed. How did you know?"

"Because you never went after him. Once you healed and before your friend was killed, if he hadn't already been dead, you would have gone looking for him."

"Maybe."

"No maybe about it. You would have."

Her smile went a little crooked. "You're probably right. And I probably would have gotten myself killed doing it. Anger and vengeance as motives never offer a happy ending. So it's all for the best that he did the job for me, that evil is as *self*-destructive as it is destructive. Tips the scale a bit toward the good guys on those rare occasions when evil consumes itself with little or no help from us."

"That balance thing."

"Yeah. That balance thing." She looked down at their clasped hands. "Rafe . . . what happened to me is something I recovered from, eventually. Physically, even psychologically. I've had a few relationships in recent years. Not very successful ones, but that's probably due as much to my dedication to my job as to any lingering ... emotional scars. Or maybe it's the voices that men along the way haven't been able to deal with. I do come with lots of baggage."

"You don't want me to be afraid to touch you."

"Stop being so perceptive. It's unnerving."

Rafe smiled. "The only thing I'm afraid of, Isabel, is that you still don't know what it is you want. From me. For yourself. And until you do, taking the wrong step could be the worst possible choice. For the record, I don't think either of us is the type to consider a quick roll in the hay as a great way to de-stress."

"No."

"And neither one of us is a kid. At our age, we should know what we want—or, at least, know what we're risking by getting involved with each other."

Isabel eyed him, not without a certain humor. "I've always been impulsive as hell. Jump, then look for a place to land. Obviously, you look before you jump."

"They do say opposites attract."

"They certainly do." She sighed. "You're right, I don't know what I want. And I have been feeling rattled all day because of the changes in my abilities. Not the best time to make this sort of decision, I guess."

"No. But for what it's worth ..." He leaned over and kissed her, his free hand lifting to the side of her neck, his thumb stroking her cheek. There was nothing especially gentle in the action, nothing in the least tentative; he wanted her, and left her in no doubt of that fact.

When she could, Isabel said, "Okay, that wasn't fair."

Rafe grinned at her and stepped back, finally releasing her hand. "See you tomorrow at the office, Isabel."

"Bastard."

"Night-night. Sleep tight."

"If you say don't let the bedbugs bite, I'll shoot you."

Rafe chuckled and turned away.

She stood there on the porch and gazed after him until he returned to his Jeep, then shook her head and went into the inn's lobby, still smiling.

"Good evening, Agent Adams," the desk clerk said cheerily.

Isabel glanced back over her shoulder at the mostly glass front door and very well-lighted front porch, then at the clerk's face. She looked like the soul of discretion.

Which undoubtedly meant she was already making a mental list of people to call with the latest tidbit of gossip.

Sighing, Isabel said, "Good evening, Patty."

"We provide a continental breakfast on Sunday morning, Agent Adams. From eight to eleven. In case you and your partner didn't know that."

"I'll be sure to tell her. Have a nice night, Patty."

"You, too, Agent Adams." She sounded consoling, sympathetic, obviously since Isabel was going to bed alone.

Isabel escaped up the stairs, hoping that glass front door was, at the very least, soundproofed. She stopped by Hollis's room and knocked softly, reasonably sure her partner was still up but not sure she wanted company.

But Hollis opened the door immediately, saying, "I actually ordered a pizza a couple of hours ago. And ate some of it. Does that mean I'm taking a step closer to becoming accustomed to dead bodies?"

"It means your own body is healthy and needs sustenance, mostly," Isabel replied, stepping into the room. "But, yeah, it's a good sign you can handle the more gross aspects of the job. I'd put it in the plus column."

"Good. I need more checks in the plus column. I was beginning to feel horribly inadequate." Hollis invited her in with a gesture, adding, "I have an extra Pepsi here. Or did you get enough caffeine with dinner?"

"Enough. Plus, I really need a good night's sleep." Isabel frowned slightly, but said, "The plan is to meet up at the station by nine-thirty. Patty, downstairs, says the inn offers a continental breakfast on Sunday morning. We can go down between eight and eight-thirty, if that's okay with you."

"Sure." Hollis studied her thoughtfully as she went to sit on her bed beside a closed pizza box. "You look sort of . . . disconcerted. Rafe?"

"He's a little more complicated than I bargained for," Isabel admitted, wandering around the small bedroom somewhat restlessly. "Even the clairvoyant stuff I picked up didn't warn me about that. Dammit."

"You told him?"

"My horror story? Yeah."

"And?"

"He . . . handled it really well. Didn't freak out, didn't act like I was suddenly a leper. Compassionate and understanding and very discerning." She frowned again and added in a dissatisfied tone, "Also a cautious man."

Hollis grinned. "Wasn't ready to just jump into bed, huh?"

"Now, what makes you think—"

"Oh, come on, Isabel. As soon as we talked earlier, I could see the wheels turning. You saw a potential emotional complication looming and, characteristically, your response was to charge toward it head-on. If he was going to be a problem in any way whatsoever, you intended to deal with it *now*. Whether he was ready or not."

"Why is everybody else suddenly so perceptive as to my motives?" Isabel demanded. "I'm supposed to be the clairvoyant one. Look, I wasn't after a one-night stand. Necessarily. It's just . . . things are simpler when the physical stuff is out of the way, that's all."

Shaking her head, Hollis said, "Well, now I can understand why your past relationships weren't entirely successful, if that's your attitude about sex. Just something to get over and done with?"

"I didn't say that."

"Yes, you did. You're a lot of things, Isabel, but subtle isn't one of them. You probably as good as told the man you wanted to sleep with him so you wouldn't be distracted having to think about it anymore."

"I was not that blunt."

"Maybe not, but I'm sure he got the gist of it."

Isabel sat down in the chair in the corner of the bedroom and scowled at Hollis. "The SCU therapist says I have a few emotional issues about giving up control."

"No, really?"

"It's not a big thing. I just . . . prefer to make the first move whenever possible."

"Because the last guy you allowed to make the first move turned out to be a twisted, evil bastard. Yeah, I get that. I imagine Rafe gets it as well."

"I don't like having transparent motives," Isabel announced. "It makes me feel naked."

Hollis smiled. "Don't snap at the messenger. I'm not telling you anything you don't already know."

Isabel sighed. "It's about control. I know it's about control. Even after all these years, I can't help feeling . . . wary. Not of men in general, just of men who might—possibly—mean something to me. Especially if they're obviously very strong men. Don't you? We both went through similar experiences, after all, and yours was just a few months ago."

"I had Maggie Barnes," Hollis reminded her. "That empathy thing of hers did a dandy job of taking away a lot of the pain and healing the trauma. Even though what happened to me was just months ago, it feels more like years. Decades. Distant, unimportant, almost as if it happened to someone else. Almost. Do I know if I can feel a normal, healthy desire for a man? No idea. Not yet anyway. Haven't met a man I felt that sort of interest in so far."

Isabel lifted an eyebrow. "You seemed a bit drawn to Caleb Powell, I thought."

"A bit," Hollis admitted with a shrug. "But . . . a big-city-caliber attorney lives and works in a small town for a reason. He wants a simple life. Had one, too, until a lethal killer began stalking his nice little town, and his employee and friend was horribly murdered. Now, like it or not, I'm part of that gruesome series of events that's turning his simple, peaceful existence upside down."

"You're one of the good guys."

"Yeah, points in the positive column for that. But not enough to balance it, I'm afraid. Especially since I have my own horror story."

"Did you . . ."

"Tell him? Yeah. I met him in the coffee shop earlier, by chance, and we talked for a while. He asked questions, so I answered them. He didn't take it all that well. Sort of freaked, actually. In a very quiet, controlled, lawyerish kind of way. But I saw his face. And he certainly didn't offer to drive me home." Her smile was wry. "It was the eye thing that finally got to him. Up until then, he was more or less okay, but that was a bit too much to take."

"Hollis, I'm sorry."

"Oh, don't worry about it. Some things aren't meant to be, you know? I mean, if he couldn't accept a little thing like an eye transplant, then it's a cinch he'd never be comfortable with me talking to dead people."

"No, probably not."

"Some people just . . . can't think outside the box. You're lucky Rafe can."

Isabel was frowning again. Her head tilted a bit, the frown deepening. Absently, she said, "Yes. Yes, I guess I am. The psychic stuff doesn't throw him at all, and he was more than okay with the rest."

"So if you can just deal with these control issues of yours, and always assuming we get this killer before he decides to add you to his blonde collection, maybe the universe really is offering you something special. A man who knows what you've been through, what you are, and doesn't mind all the baggage you have to drag around with you."

"Maybe."

"At least accept the possibility, Isabel."

Isabel blinked at her. "Sure. Yes. I can always accept possibilities."

It was Hollis's turn to frown. "Are you thinking about the long-term complications of him being settled here and you at Quantico?"

"No. I haven't gotten that far. I mean, I haven't really looked past now."

Hollis studied her. "So what's bothering you?"

"It's just . . . I'm tired. Really tired."

"I'm not surprised. You need a good night's sleep."

Still frowning, Isabel said, "I know I do. I can't remember ever being this tired. So that's probably why, right?"

"Why what?"

Softly, Isabel said, "Why I don't hear the voices. At all."

12

GINNY HUNG UP the phone and frowned at the clock on the wall. Three times. Three times she'd tried to call Tim Helton, hoping his wife might have come home and he just hadn't thought to report in.

It was after ten-thirty; dairy farmers got up at dawn, she knew that much. Even on Sundays. And Tim Helton wasn't a churchgoer. Maybe he was out with his cattle. Except he'd given her his cell-phone number and said he always kept it with him. And a body would think he'd be eager to hear whatever the police might have to say about his missing wife. Unless she'd come home.

Or unless he knew she wasn't going to.

Travis wasn't at his desk, so Ginny couldn't ask him, as she usually did, what she should do. This would have to be her call, her decision.

Surprising herself somewhat, Ginny didn't hesitate. She got to her feet and headed for the closed door of the conference room.

Rafe shut the folder and shoved it toward the center of the conference table. "Okay, so neither the post nor any forensic evidence gathered at the scene has told us much more than we knew yesterday."

Mallory said, "Well, the doc's sure she wasn't bound in any way when she died, and there are absolutely no defensive wounds, so we can reasonably infer she didn't put up a fight."

"Yeah," Rafe said, "but if she *was* one of Jamie's partners, submissive might have been her natural state."

"So she wouldn't necessarily have fought an attacker," Isabel agreed. "Still, strangling is up close and personal; if somebody was very obviously trying to kill her, the reflexive survival instinct would have kicked in. At the very least, we should have found some skin cells underneath her fingernails. The fact that we didn't lends weight to the idea that she didn't realize what was happening to her until too late."

Hollis said, "And our killer uses a knife, he doesn't strangle. So that's another argument for an accidental death at someone's hands, probably Jamie's."

Mallory added, "Especially since forensics found bits of that old linoleum floor covering embedded in the vic's knees, which places her *in* Jamie's playhouse and in a kneeling, possibly submissive position. Which is, at least, more tangible evidence to confirm what we were pretty sure of but couldn't have proven in court—that this woman was one of Jamie's partners."

"An unlucky one," Rafe noted. "According to the info we have on the S&M scene, strangulation to the point of unconsciousness is fairly common. Supposedly intensifies orgasm."

"Another thing I don't want *that* much," Mallory murmured.

Rafe nodded a wry agreement, but said, "We'll probably never know why Jamie went too far, if it was anger or just a . . . miscalculation. But we need to I.D. this woman. Notify her family."

Isabel said, "A forensic dentist at Quantico is comparing her chart to those we have from women reported missing in the area; we should know in the next hour or so if there's a match."

"But we didn't have charts for every woman," Mallory reminded her. "Either they used dentists we haven't been able to track down, or no dentists. Lots of people are still scared of sitting in that chair."

"And none of the missing women had ever been fingerprinted," Rafe added.

"Is getting an I.D. even going to help us?" Hollis wondered. "I mean, it's closure for her family, which is great, but what's it going to tell us?"

"Maybe if she was a regular client of Jamie's," Isabel said. "We can talk to her relatives and friends, check her bank accounts, hopefully find a diary or journal if we're very lucky. But, yeah, I know what you mean. It's not really likely to put us any closer to the serial killer. Or help us identify and protect the woman he's undoubtedly stalking even as we speak."

"And we're running out of time," Mallory said.

There was a moment of silence, and then a somewhat timid knock at the door preceded Ginny's entry into the room.

"Chief, excuse me for interrupting—"

"You didn't," Rafe told her. "What's up?"

"I've been trying to call Tim Helton, just to check if his wife came home, and I can't get an answer. He doesn't go to church and by all accounts almost never leaves the farm. He should be there."

"If he's out in his barns—"

"He gave me his cell number, Chief, and he said he always wears it clipped to his belt. I tried the house number, too, but there was no answer. And just the machine at the dairy number. It's like the place is deserted out there."

Isabel said, "I don't much like the sound of that. If this killer is escalating, there's nothing to say he might not have decided to change his M.O. and kill somebody in or near her own home. Or just come back later and take out the husband as well."

"What worries me," Rafe said, "is that Tim Helton is the type to get his gun and go looking himself if he feels the police aren't doing enough to find his wife. The detective I sent out there to talk to him said he was angry and just this side of insulting about our efforts so far."

"He has a gun?"

"He has several, including a couple of shotguns and rifles, and his service pistol. He was in the army."

"That's all we need," Isabel murmured. "A scared and pissed-off guy with a gun—and the training to use it."

"No sign of his wife?" Rafe asked Ginny.

"Not so far. Or any hint from anyone who knew her that she might have gone somewhere on her own. In fact, everybody says the opposite, that she was a homebody and quite happy at the farm."

"Solid marriage?" Hollis asked.

"By all accounts."

"No children?"

"No."

Isabel drummed her fingers briefly on the table. "I say we go check it out. There isn't much we can do here for the present, with no new information to go over. And we need to find Tim Helton, make sure he's all right—and not conducting his own manhunt."

Rafe nodded and looked at Ginny. "Anything new on any of the other missing women?"

"Not so far. Still nearly a dozen unaccounted for, if we go back a couple of months and take in the thirty miles or so surrounding Hastings, but only a handful even come close to fitting the profile. The reporter, Cheryl Bayne, is still missing; we tried the dogs, and they lost the trail a block or so from the van."

"Where, specifically?" Rafe asked.

"Near Kate Murphy's store. She's the other woman missing from Hastings. We're drawing blanks everywhere we check in looking for both of them."

"Okay, keep at it."

As the young officer turned to go, Isabel said, "Ginny? Are you okay?"

"Sure." She smiled. "Tired, like everybody else, but otherwise okay. Thanks for asking."

Isabel held her gaze for a moment, then nodded and smiled, and Ginny left the conference room rather quickly.

Absently, Rafe said, "You know, Rose Helton doesn't fit the profile in one very obvious and possibly important way."

"She's married," Isabel said. "So far, in all three series of murders, he's only gone after single white females."

Slowly, Hollis said, "I wonder what would happen if he found himself interested in a married woman? Would he see the husband as a rival? Would that make the chase—the stalking—even more exciting for him?"

"Could be." Isabel rose to her feet.

Mallory got up with the rest, but said, "Since Kate Murphy and Cheryl Bayne are also still missing, I think they should be up there on the priority list too. If you guys don't mind, I think I'll run through the info we have on them and see if I have some luck in either finding them or at least ruling out a voluntary absence."

"Good idea," Isabel said. "The reporter especially worries me; if he's killing to scare off the media or to make a point, then all bets are off. It would mean he's changed in some fundamental way, and we have no way of knowing how or why."

"Or who he could decide to target next," Hollis added.

He wished he could stop the voices. The other things, the other changes, he could deal with. So far, at least. But the voices really were driving him mad. It had become harder and harder to shut them out, turn them off. They told him to do things. Bad things.

Things he'd done before.

Not that he minded doing the bad things. That was the only time he felt real, felt strong and alive. Felt free. It was just that his head hurt all the time now because of the voices, and he hadn't slept through the night since . . . he couldn't remember when.

The whole world looked surreal when you couldn't sleep, he'd discovered.

And blondes were everywhere.

Tempting, aren't they?

He ignored the question. The voice.

They're just asking for it. You know they are.

"Go away," he muttered. "I took care of the other one. The one you said nearly found us. Leave me alone now. I'm tired."

Look at that one on the corner. If she swung her ass any harder she'd dislocate it.

"Shut up."

Don't forget what they did to you. What they're doing to you. Even now, they're corrupting you.

"You're lying to me. I know you are."

I'm the only one who's telling you the truth.

214

"I don't believe you."

That's because they've twisted your thinking, those women. Those blondes. They're making you weak.

"No. I'm strong. I'm stronger than they are."

You're a wimp. A useless wimp. You let yourself get distracted.

"I'm not distracted. She has to be next."

The other one's more dangerous. That agent. Isabel. She's different. She sees things. We need her out of the way.

"I can do her later. This is the one I have to do next."

This one can't hurt us.

"That's what you think." He watched as she came out of the coffee shop and continued along the sidewalk, an iced mocha in one hand and her list in the other. She always had a list. Always had things to do.

He wondered idly if she had any idea the last item on today's list was to die.

11:00 AM

On their way to the dairy farm, Hollis said, "If Rafe hadn't had to stay at the station a few more minutes to deal with a call, would you still have suggested separate vehicles?"

"Probably."

"Still no voices, huh?"

"No. I thought getting away from everybody might help, but it didn't."

"Was anything different when Rafe was close by?"

"No. Just silence, same as when he isn't close by. Exactly the way it's been since last night." Isabel glanced at her partner, mouth twisting slightly. "I'd thought the peace and quiet would be nice. I was wrong. This just feels . . . bad. Not natural. I even miss the damned headache. A part of me has suddenly gone deaf, and I don't know why."

"It must have something to do with the sparking thing between you and Rafe, right?"

"I don't know. As far as I can remember, nothing like this has happened to any psychic. I mean, our abilities can change, but this drastically and suddenly to a reasonably stable and well-established psychic? Not without some . . . trigger. Some cause. It just doesn't make sense."

"You still haven't called Bishop?"

Isabel shook her head. "They're wrapped up in their own investigation out there and don't need a distraction."

"You just don't want him to pull you."

"Well, yeah, there's that. I don't really think he would, not at this stage, but he worries whenever any of us have problems with our abilities. Unforeseen problems, I mean."

Hollis hesitated, then said, "How can you be sure this is an unforeseen problem? I mean, Bishop and Miranda see the future on a fairly regular basis. What if they saw this?"

Isabel considered it, then shrugged and said wryly, "That is more than possible. It wouldn't be the first time they'd seen something ahead in the road for one of us—and just let us stumble forward blindly. Some things have to happen just the way they happen."

"Our mantra."

"More or less. You know, I half expected Bishop to call last night, since he always does seem to know whenever something's gone wrong. So maybe this isn't as wrong as I feel like it is. Or maybe he knows and also knows I have to figure out my own way through it."

"Are you going to tell Rafe?"

"Sooner or later I'll have to. Unless he picks up on it himself. Which is also possible."

"Yeah, he's very . . . tuned in where you're concerned. I mean, it's obvious. I think he knew before I did in Jamie's playhouse that it was going to be too much for you. He kept watching you."

"I know."

"You felt that even with all the voices coming at you?"

"I felt it. Him. He wanted to protect me. To keep me from being hurt."

Hollis lifted both eyebrows. "And now you don't hear the voices. You're protected from them. Coincidence? I sort of doubt it."

"Rafe isn't psychic. He couldn't have done this."

Hollis thought about it, then shook her head. "Maybe not consciously, even if he's a latent. But what if it's a combination of factors?"

"Such as?"

"Such as his desire to shield you and the way his and your electromagnetic fields react to each other. It really could be pure basic chemistry and physics, at least the beginning of it."

Isabel frowned. "Even without a shield of my own, I had the training in how to use one. I know how to reach out, break through a barrier. I know what a shield should be, even if I've never had one. This . . . doesn't feel like a barrier. It's not something I can control."

"It's new. Maybe you have to get used to it before you can. Or maybe . . ."

" . . . it's not mine *to* control," Isabel finished.

"If Rafe is a latent, or was, it could be his to control. You didn't pick up any sense that he might be when you first read him?"

"No."

"Nothing unusual at all?"

"No. At least . . . He's very strong. And not very easy to read except for surface, trivial things. I didn't get the sense he was blocking me, but at the same time I felt there was a lot of him I just couldn't get at."

"Didn't you tell me his grandmother was psychic?"

"Yeah."

"Then if I remember what I was taught in the training sessions, there's a better than average chance he could be a latent."

"In our experience, yes. It often runs in families."

"Isn't that the most likely explanation for all this? That he is, or was, a latent and that the way you two reacted to each other somehow activated it and made him a functional psychic, even if only on an unconscious level?"

"So far, everything we've seen and experienced tells us that activating a latent ability requires a traumatic event."

"Maybe Rafe will add something different to that experience."

"Maybe."

"You could ask him."

"Ask him if he's psychic? Oh, he'll love that."

"If he is, and functional, he needs to know. He needs to begin learning how to control what he can do. Especially since he may be shielding you. That urge to protect you may have him wrapping you in psychic cotton wool. A nice respite for you, at least in theory, but we do need your abilities to help us find and catch this killer."

"Tell me something I don't know."

Hollis pushed her sunglasses to the top of her head and studied her partner thoughtfully. "Maybe when you and Rafe connected, you did it in an unusual way, something every bit as direct and potent as actual physical contact—and magnified by sheer power. That sparking thing we all find so fascinating. Maybe it created a link between you."

"It didn't create a shield. I've told you, at first it was just a slight and gradual muffling of the voices. It wasn't until last night that the voices suddenly went silent."

"It *was* sudden? You didn't tell me that. Can you remember exactly what was happening when you lost them?"

Isabel had to think about it, but only for a moment. Slowly, she said, "Actually, it's so clear I don't know why I didn't notice it at the time. Because I was so tired, I suppose. I thought it was that. And the relief."

"Relief?"

"That he didn't draw away. I told him all about my chamber of horrors, and he didn't draw away. In fact, he reached out to me. Physically. And that's when the voices went silent."

"Travis, any luck reaching Kate Murphy's sister in California?" Mallory asked.

Without needing to check the notes on his legal pad, Travis shook his head. "Nada. It's awfully early on a Sunday out there, so you'd think she'd be home, but if so she isn't answering her phone."

"Machine or voice mail picking up?"

"No, it just rings."

"Shit. I thought everybody had voice mail."

"Guess not."

"Well, keep trying." Mallory headed back toward her own desk, pausing as she passed Ginny to ask, "Still nothing new on Rose Helton?"

"I finally got hold of her brother in Columbia, and he says last he heard, Rose was happy on the farm with Tim. No family occasions or visits to other relatives that he knows of. He didn't even know Rose wasn't home. Until he talked to me."

Mallory grimaced. "I hate it when that happens. When we're following up leads or looking for them—and shatter somebody's day, possibly their life, with news they really don't want to hear. That is never fun."

"I'll say. Oh—and for what it's worth, it doesn't seem to have even occurred to Rose's brother that her husband might have had something to do with her disappearance."

"That might be worth a lot. Relatives often know, even if only subconsciously, if there's trouble in a marriage."

"He obviously thinks not. In fact, he asked immediately if we thought it was this serial killer, even though Rose isn't really a blonde."

"Come again?"

"Apparently, the last time he saw Rose at Christmas, she was blond. Trying it out, he said."

Mallory was frowning. "That isn't in the report."

"I know. When Tim Helton gave us a description of his wife, he said brown hair. Just that. The photo he gave us shows a brunette. And none of the people we've talked to in the area described her as blond."

"But she was blond last Christmas."

"According to her brother."

"Shit. Does the chief know?"

"I was just about to call him. He should be getting to the Helton farm any minute now."

"Call him. He needs to know Rose Helton just moved a step closer to the victim profile."

The Helton dairy farm seemed as deserted as the main house when Isabel and Hollis parked their car near the gates to the barn area and got out. Standing at the front bumper of the car, Isabel

220

absently checked her service weapon and then returned it to the holster at the small of her back.

Automatically, Hollis followed suit.

"Storm's coming," Isabel said, pushing her sunglasses up to rest atop her head as she looked briefly at the heavy clouds rolling in. The day had started out hot and sunny; now it was just hot and humid.

"I know." Hollis shifted uneasily. Storms always made her feel especially edgy. Now, at least. It made her wonder if Bishop had been entirely joking when he'd once told her that some people believed storms were nature's way of opening up the door between this world and the next—like a steam valve relieving pressure.

"And this place feels very deserted to me," Isabel added, looking around restlessly.

"You're not picking up anything at all out here? I mean, it's not just no voices, is it? It's nothing the usual five senses can't get?"

"Just the usual five. I'm getting nothing, no sense of anything that isn't visible to me. Dammit. I can't even tell if Helton is anywhere near. He could walk up behind me and I wouldn't feel it. And I've been able to feel that since I was seventeen years old."

"Don't worry, I'm sure it's temporary."

"Are you? Because I'm not."

"Isabel, even without the psychic edge, you're a trained investigator. You'll just have to . . . use the usual five senses until the sixth one comes back."

Eyeing her partner, Isabel said, "Do I detect a certain satisfaction in your voice?"

Hollis cleared her throat. "Well, let's just say I don't feel quite so useless as I did before."

"Fine pair we are. Two psychics who can't use their abilities. Bishop couldn't have seen this one coming."

"Look, we're cops. Federal agents. We'll just *be* federal agents and use our training to look for Helton," Hollis said practically. "When Rafe gets here."

Isabel looked around her, frowning. "Where *is* he? Rafe, I mean. And is it just my internal silence, or is this place way too quiet?"

It really was peculiarly still, the hot, humid air surrounding everything in a heavy, smothering closeness.

"Pretty quiet for a working dairy farm, I'd say. But it's just a guess on my part." Hollis studied the cluster of outbuildings and surrounding pastures. "Maybe all the cows are out in the fields. That's the deal, isn't it? They're milked in the morning, then go out and eat grass all day?"

"You're asking me?"

"Somebody told me you rode horses, so I just figured—"

"What, that I'd know cows? Sorry. You get milk from them; that's all I know." Isabel drummed restless fingers on the hood of the car. "Time to be a federal agent. Okay. We checked the house first and got no answer at the door. At either door. Both doors are locked, and we have no probable cause to enter."

"Can we enter the barns without cause?"

"Being federal agents, we have to walk carefully, at least until Rafe gets here; under the mantle of his local jurisdiction, we can do more." Isabel eyed the cluster of buildings. "The barns that are open are fair game, I'd say. That big central barn looks closed up, though, at least on this end."

Before Hollis could comment on that, they both saw Rafe's Jeep turn in at the end of the long driveway.

"No luck at the house?" he asked as soon as he got out of the vehicle.

"No," Isabel replied. "And haven't heard a sound out here. Is this normal?"

"Well, I wouldn't call it abnormal. The cows will be out in the pastures, so the barns would be quiet. Helton runs this place on his own except for the crew that comes to pick up the milk, and part-time afternoon help, so he has plenty to do around here most of the day. Have you tried yelling for him?"

Without a blink, Isabel said, "We thought your bellow would carry farther."

Rafe eyed her for a moment, then cupped his hands around his mouth and yelled out Helton's name.

Silence greeted the summons.

"Okay," Rafe said, "let's start looking around, before it gets even hotter out here."

"Private property, even if it is a business," Isabel reminded him.

"Yeah, but we've got cause with the wife missing and Helton out of touch. Judge'll back me up on that." He led the way, opening the gate at the end of the drive and allowing it to swing back as they passed through and headed for the cluster of barns and other buildings just a few yards away.

A slight breeze disturbed the heavy closeness of the humid air, giving them all a sense of relief from the heat—and offering a rather ripe olfactory experience.

"I love the smell of manure in the morning," Isabel said. "Smells like . . . shit."

Rafe had to laugh, but said, "Looks like he stopped in the middle of unloading a hay shipment." There was a half-ton truck parked alongside the largest, closed barn and facing in the opposite direction, with its tailgate down and a great deal of loose hay piled all around it. A number of bales of hay remained stacked in the bed of the truck.

"I'll check out the cab," Isabel said, and crunched her way through the hay toward the front of the truck.

Hollis was about to say she'd head in the opposite direction and see if the other side of the barn was open, but something about the way Rafe was looking after Isabel made her pause. Just for something to say, she asked, "Why would he have stopped in the middle of unloading?"

"Maybe that's when he realized his wife was missing. He might have been too distracted since then to worry about unloading hay." Rafe frowned as he looked at her, and lowered his voice when he added, "What's wrong with Isabel?"

"What makes you think something's wrong?" Hollis countered, stalling.

Rafe's frown deepened. "I don't know, just something . . . off. What is it?"

Something off. Something turned off. Did you do it?

But she didn't say any of that, of course. Already regretting that she had allowed this, Hollis said as casually as possible, "You'll have to ask her. I should check out the other side of the barn, I guess, and see if there's a door open."

After a moment, Rafe said, "Okay, fine."

Hollis took a step away, then turned back with a genuine question. "Is it just me, or is there a weird smell around this building? Doesn't smell like manure now that the breeze has shifted. Sort of a sweet-and-sour odor."

Rafe sniffed the air, and his rugged face instantly changed. "Oh, no," he said.

"What?"

Before either of them could move, the barn doors burst outward, and a thin, dark man in his thirties stood there between them, one shaking hand pointing a big automatic squarely at Rafe.

"Goddamn you, Sullivan! Bringing feds out here!"

13

A LYSSA TAYLOR KNEW damned well there was no good reason for her to hang around near the police station on a Sunday morning. No casual or innocent reason, that is. She couldn't even pretend to sit nonchalantly in the coffee shop near the station, since it wouldn't open until church let out.

She had toyed with the idea of going to church, but Ally found she couldn't be quite that hypocritical.

She also half-seriously feared being struck by lightning if she crossed the threshold.

"You're lurking, too, huh?" Paige Gilbert, who Ally knew was a local reporter for the town's most popular radio station, leaned against the other side of the old-fashioned, wrought-iron light post, as seemingly casual as Ally.

"I bet we look like a couple of hookers," Ally said.

Paige eyed Ally's very short skirt and filmy top, then glanced down at her own jeans and T-shirt, and said, "Well . . ."

"Catch more flies with honey," Ally said.

"I'll just watch them flit past, thanks."

Ally chuckled. "Travis likes my legs. And it's such a little thing to make him happy."

"A very little thing," Paige murmured. "How's the pillow talk?"

"I don't kiss and tell."

"Except on the air?"

"Well, we all have our boundaries, don't we?"

Paige half laughed and inclined her head slightly in a sort of salute. "You're good, I'll give you that much."

"I usually get what I go after."

"Didn't Cheryl Bayne say something like that?"

"She wasn't careful. Obviously. I am."

"Speculation seems to be she stuck her nose in where it didn't belong."

"Occupational hazard."

"For us too."

Ally shrugged. "My philosophy is, no sense being in the game unless you're willing to play all-out. I am. Like I said, I usually get what I go after."

"You get any news on the body they found yesterday?"

Ally's internal debate was swift and silent. "Not a blonde and not a victim of our serial killer. The theory is, she died by accident."

"And hung her own body in that old gas station?"

"No, our resident ghoul probably did that. A nice toy for him, already dead and everything."

"Yuck."

"Well, we knew he was sick and twisted. Now we know he's an opportunist too."

Paige frowned. "If she wasn't one of his victims, how did he get his hands on her?"

"The mystery of the thing. I'm going to go out on a limb and say she had a connection to either him or one of the victims."

"What kind of connection?"

"Dunno. Friend, family, a lover in common—something. She died by accident, he saw or knew and took advantage of the situation."

Paige was still frowning. "There's got to be more to it. How, exactly, did she die?"

"That I don't know. Yet."

"Is it true she'd been dead a couple of months?"

"About that."

"Then she died before the first victim did. Maybe he liked playing with a dead body so much he decided to make a few of his very own?"

"Maybe."

They stood on either side of the lamppost, leaning against it, and gazed across the street at the town hall. The downtown area was practically deserted. It was very quiet.

"I sort of wish I'd gone to church," Paige said finally.

"Yeah," Ally said. "Me too."

Rafe wore his weapon in a hip holster, with the flap fastened; there was no way he could get to it; Hollis, like Isabel, wore her holster at the small of her back, also out of reach. Both she and Rafe stood frozen, their hands a little above waist height with the palms out, by training and instinct showing this dangerously unstable opponent the least threatening posture possible as his gun wavered between them.

"Tim, settle down," Rafe advised calmly.

"Rose said she'd had enough," Helton said, his voice as shaky as his gun hand. "That's it, that's why you're here. She told you. She come and told you, and now you've brought the feds out here."

From her angle, Hollis caught only a glimpse of what she knew Rafe could see more clearly: Isabel, at the rear bumper of the hay truck. Like the other two, she had frozen the moment the doors had burst open, but unlike them, she wasn't visible to Tim Helton.

Unfortunately, he wasn't visible to her either, since the heavy barn door shielded him from her view.

Worse, she was standing knee-deep in brittle, noisy hay; any movement at all would draw his attention and take away whatever hope she had of surprising him.

Standing still, Isabel silently drew her weapon and held it in a practiced, two-handed grip, thumbing off the safety.

Then she looked toward Rafe and Hollis, brows lifting in a silent question.

"Tim, we haven't heard from Rose," Rafe was saying, still calm. He kept his gaze fixed on Helton, though he could see Isabel from the corner of his eye. "That's why we're here, to look for her."

"Liar. I heard them talking out here a while ago—they're feds. Both of 'em. You bring feds out here and think I don't know why? What am I, stupid? Where's the other one? You tell her to come out, Sullivan, and I mean quick. You know I ain't afraid to use this gun."

"Tim, listen," Rafe said. *"Aspice super caput suum."*

Helton blinked in confusion. "Huh? What'd you—"

The crack of Isabel's pistol was loud, but before Helton could do more than twitch in surprise, the hay bale that had been hanging several feet above his head crashed down, knocking him to the ground—and out cold.

Rafe immediately moved forward to get the unconscious man's pistol, calling out, "Got him, Isabel. Nice shot."

She came around the barn door even as he finished speaking, crunching through the hay, pistol lowered but ready, and said, "Dead-eye Jane, that's me."

Hollis was staring up at the loft door and the winch designed to lift heavy bales of hay inside the building. "I'll be damned. With the barn painted that wheat color, I didn't even notice that up there."

"Neither did I," Isabel said. "Good thing Rafe did. I gather all this was about moonshine, of all the ridiculous things?"

Rafe nodded. "He's got a still in there. You can smell the stuff. Or, at least, Hollis could. I didn't notice when we got here, unfortunately."

"Easy to smell now. On him. He reeks."

"Yeah, he's drunk. Probably since he noticed his wife was missing, and possibly what drove her to leave him. I don't know how long he's been selling bootleg whiskey, but it's obvious he's been drinking and otherwise using it for years."

"Mallory's tractor story," Isabel said, realizing. "He blew up his own tractor using moonshine instead of fuel."

"Right. I really should have remembered that before bringing two *feds* out here. With that level of paranoia and the amount of raw alcohol in him, he could have shot all three of us and not felt a twinge of regret about it until he sobered up."

"I'm confused," Hollis said. "What did you say to him?"

"Not to him. I told Isabel to look above his head. I knew the only clear shot she had was the winch or rope."

"Nice you trusted me to hit either one," Isabel said, then frowned at him. "But how in hell did you know I'd understand classical Latin? I didn't tell you that."

"No, Hollis did, sort of in passing. I remembered because it so happens that I took it in college as well." He sent a sidelong glance at Hollis. "A fairly nerdy thing to do, I admit, but it has been useful here and there."

"Especially here," Isabel said. "Another few seconds, and this lunatic would have shot one of you. Probably killed you."

Hollis uttered a shaken laugh and, when the other two looked at her inquiringly, said, "Okay, now I'm a believer."

It was nearly five that afternoon when Rafe came into the conference room and found Isabel, for the first time that day, alone. He closed the door behind him.

Sitting on the table studying autopsy photos of the woman found hanging in the old gas station, she said, "Please tell me we finally have an I.D. on her."

"Word just came in from Quantico. They think her name is Hope Tessneer. Age thirty-five, divorced, no children. The dental records are a close, but not exact, match. The record we gave them for comparison is at least ten years old."

"So there's a good chance it's her."

"A very good chance. Mallory's talking to the sheriff's department in Pearson now. That's another small town about thirty miles from here. We'll know more when they give us all the information they have, and when they talk to her family and friends. We do know that Hope Tessneer worked as a real-estate agent."

Isabel looked at him, frowning. "A possible connection with Jamie. How they met, maybe."

"Could be. She's been missing almost exactly eight weeks,

according to her boss. He wasn't all that worried, because she had taken off without warning or explanation at least twice in recent years. Said she wouldn't have come home to a job either time except that she was the best sales associate he had."

"Then she knew how to please people, how to give them what they wanted. That fits."

"For a submissive, you mean."

"Yeah. And a good fit for Jamie. Somebody like that might have been a longtime partner. Someone who wasn't just submissive but really trusted Jamie. It could help explain the lack of defensive wounds."

"That's what I thought."

Still frowning, Isabel said, "I wish we could find that damned box of photos."

"We can't even check for more safe-deposit boxes in the other banks in the area until tomorrow morning."

"I know, I know. I just think it's important. We need to see what's in that box."

"Agreed." Very deliberately, Rafe took a chair on the side of the table where she was sitting. "On another subject . . ."

Her frown vanished, and she smiled. "Where the hell am I, and how do I get to Detroit?"

He smiled slightly in response. "Are you a Richard Pryor fan, or do you just know that I am?"

"Both."

"Any more one-liners you want to throw at me?"

"No. I'll be good."

"Just tell me what's going on, Isabel."

She closed the autopsy file and set it aside, then drew a breath and let it out slowly. "The short, perfectly truthful version is, I don't know what's going on."

"And the long version?"

"I'm not picking up anything from anyone. I don't hear any voices. All my extra senses closed up shop last night, and I think it has something to do with you. And I don't know what the *hell* is going on."

5:10 PM

Mallory hung up the phone and rubbed the back of her neck as she looked at Hollis, who was perched on the corner of her desk. "They'll get back to us once they've interviewed Hope Tessneer's family and friends. But just from the information they already had on her bank accounts, it looks like she'd been paying for *something* about twice a month for the last year or so. Checks made out to cash, and cashed by her."

"For how much?"

"Always the same amount. Fifteen hundred."

Hollis raised her eyebrows. "I guess Jamie's services didn't come cheap."

"I guess not. If we're right about all this, that's an extra three grand in undeclared cash Jamie was pulling in per month—and from just one client. Who knows how many regulars she had?"

"Where the hell did she hide all that money?"

"There has to be another bank. No unexplained deposits show up in any of the accounts she kept at two banks here in Hastings. Her salary, declared income from real estate and other investments—all documented, everything on the up-and-up. The public part of her life was squeaky clean."

"And the secret part was buried deep."

"I'll say. Buried deep and probably under an alias, at least financially; it's obvious she's been hiding at least some of her financial dealings for a long time, maybe years. Hell, her other bank or banks could be out of state. Or out of the country."

"If so, we may never find them. We've got people set to start checking out all the other area banks tomorrow, right?"

"Yeah. With pictures of Jamie and the information that she could have been disguised and using an alias."

"And it seemed like such a nice little town," Hollis said.

Mallory leaned back in her chair with a sigh. "I always thought so."

"You grew up here, I think you said."

"Yeah. Well, from the time I was about thirteen. Both my parents and a brother still live in the area. I thought about leaving when I was in college, but . . . I like it here. Or did. Never knew how many people kept nasty secrets until I became a cop."

"It's been an eye-opener for me too," Hollis confessed. "Still, this sort of thing has got to be unusual for small towns. I mean, a dominatrix practicing her . . . art . . . for paying clients, while also working as a top real-estate agent?"

"If it's not unusual, I'm moving."

"I don't blame you a bit for that."

"You know, she picked a good public job to hide a private second one," Mallory mused. "Real-estate agents often keep erratic hours, so nobody would question if she wasn't in the office at any given time. She could probably meet clients day or night, accommodate their schedules easily."

"And since she was the dominant," Hollis said, "she could probably take on as many clients as her energy allowed. No need to take a day or week off now and again to allow those ugly bruises and burns to heal. Or whatever else there might be. She'd be the one dealing out the punishment. Jesus."

Hearing the distaste in the other woman's voice, Mallory

grimaced in agreement. "A very twisted way to find pleasure, if you ask me."

Ginny joined them in time to get the gist of the conversation, saying, "The things people get up to behind closed doors. We've found Rose Helton."

"Alive and well, I gather?" Mallory said.

"Definitely alive. I'd say pissed rather than well. When I told her that her husband was sleeping it off in a cell after having waved his gun around at the chief and two federal agents, she said she hoped the judge would throw away the key."

"Where is she?" Hollis asked.

"In Charleston, with a college friend."

"She went to college?" Mallory asked in surprise. "And still married Tim Helton?"

Pronouncing the words carefully, Ginny said, "She said it had been a cosmic karmic mistake. And that she'd already filed for divorce and wasn't coming back here. And, oh, by the way, in case we hadn't found it, there was also a still in an old shed in the back pasture."

"We found it," Hollis murmured.

"Everybody said they were so happy." Mallory shook her head. "Christ, you really don't know about people."

Hollis said, "Well, anyway, we can cross her off the missing list."

"One less to worry about," Ginny agreed.

"How's the rest of the list coming?" Mallory asked her.

"No change. No sign of Cheryl Bayne. Plus, we still have several women missing in the general area, and nothing new on Kate Murphy." Ginny sighed, clearly weary. "It's like she disappeared into thin air. She fits right in with the other victims too."

"But not Cheryl Bayne."

Hollis said, "I think Isabel's probably right about Cheryl. If the killer got her, it wasn't specifically because she was—is—a reporter, but because she somehow got too close. Or he was afraid she had. And if so, it's only going to get more difficult to even try to predict what he might do next."

"Except kill," Mallory offered wryly.

It was Hollis's turn to rub the back of her neck. "And there's something else. Isabel's the profiler, but I've got to say, if Kate Murphy is a victim, why haven't we found her? So far, the rule's been that if he kills them, he does it quick and leaves them out in the open where they're easily found. Assuming he has killed again, or that he has Kate Murphy, why would he change his M.O. now?"

"Our patrols are checking out every highway rest stop," Ginny said. "Most of them two or three times a day."

"Maybe we've spooked him," Mallory suggested. "He could be killing and leaving the bodies in places we aren't keeping under observation."

Hollis glanced toward the closed door of the conference room. "Maybe it's time we discussed that possibility."

Mallory didn't move. "Rafe had a sort of determined look on his face when he closed the door. I'm not so sure I want to be the one to disturb them."

Hollis continued to look at the door intently, focusing, tentatively trying out the spider sense. After a long moment, she said, "Um . . . let's give them a few more minutes."

"You're serious?" Rafe leaned forward and touched her hand, not even reacting now to the spark.

Isabel looked down at their hands for a moment, then back at his face. "Entirely serious. For the first time in more than fourteen years, there's silence in my head."

"That's what's been wrong all day."

"That's it," she said, unsurprised that he had noticed. "The question is: why?"

They both looked down at their touching hands, and Rafe said, "Frontier territory, huh?"

"Yeah. Scary, isn't it?"

"Today, looking at the wrong end of a gun being waved around by a paranoid drunk, was scary. This? This is just a very interesting turn my life has taken."

"You're a very unusual man," she said.

"Which is probably a good thing," he said, "considering that you're a very unusual woman."

There was a part of Isabel that wanted to shy away, to pretend he hadn't said that or that she hadn't understood what he meant. But Isabel didn't let herself shy away, or draw away, or back away. Whatever this was, it was something she had to deal with.

"Rafe, do you realize what this could mean?"

"Static electricity is more important than I thought it was?"

"Electromagnetic energy. And, no, not that."

"Then I don't have a clue what this could mean. Or even what this is."

"Hollis and I have a theory."

"Which is?"

"The theory is, my abilities are still with me, it's just that now there's something standing between me and the great wide world out there."

"You're not saying—"

"We think it might be you."

"You are saying." He frowned at her. "Isabel, how could it be me? I'm not psychic. I wouldn't even know how to *be* psychic."

"We think that might be the problem."

Rafe waited, brows raised.

"When a latent first becomes a functional psychic, there's an adjustment period. The psychic isn't in control of his or her abilities from the get-go. I mean—look at Hollis. She's been a medium for months and still can't open and close that door at will. It takes concentration, and focus, and practice. A lot of practice."

"I'm not psychic." He said it with more wariness than uncertainty.

"Your grandmother was."

"So?"

"So sometimes it runs in families. Your chances of being a latent psychic are much higher than average."

"I still don't—"

"Look. There was a connection between us from the beginning. Call it an attraction, a sense of understanding, simpatico, whatever. It was there. We both felt it."

"I felt that, yes."

"We feel it now," she said, admitting it.

Rafe nodded immediately. "We feel it now."

"And there's the sparking thing. I told you that was something new for me."

"Electromagnetic energy fields. Basic science."

"Yeah, but the way those fields were reacting to each other and the strength of that reaction was something different. Something that might have affected my abilities."

"Okay. But—"

"Rafe. There was this connection, this . . . conduit between you and me. Maybe the energy opened it, or maybe . . . Maybe the energy opened it. And then when I told you about what had happened to me, you reached out. Through the conduit. You wanted the pain to go away. And it did."

Rafe spoke very carefully. "How could I have done anything to . . . put your abilities in a box?"

"Actually, that's a very good description," she noted.

"Isabel."

"Okay. One of the things we've discovered is that the subconscious is often more in control of our abilities than the conscious mind is, especially in a newly functional psychic. One theory is that it's because these are very old abilities—not new ones. They were born out of instinct, when primitive humans needed every possible edge just to survive."

"Makes sense," Rafe said.

"Yes, it does. And if you subscribe to that theory, it also makes sense that our subconscious minds—the deeply buried, primitive id—would not only be able to master psychic abilities but would do so immediately and skillfully. To that part of us, being psychic would be perfectly natural."

"My id put your abilities in a box?"

Thoughtfully, Isabel said, "Has it occurred to you that we have very strange conversations?"

"Constantly. Answer my question."

"Yes. More or less. Rafe, your nature is very protective, and even though you like and respect strong women and are perfectly able to work alongside us on equal terms, deep down inside, you will always want to protect anyone you . . . care about. That is your instinctive response."

"Anyone I care about."

"Yes. And, obviously, the more you care, the more . . . passionate . . . your feelings are, the stronger your protective instincts will be."

His mouth twisted slightly. "Want to stop tiptoeing around that part of it and just say it?"

"Do I have to?"

"We might as well get it out into the open. This is happening because I'm falling in love with you."

Isabel had to clear her throat before she could say, "With or without my extra senses, you keep surprising me. That is very disconcerting."

"What would you have said? That I had a crush on you?"

"Well . . ."

Dryly, he said, "We're talking about my feelings here, Isabel, not yours. I am not trying to corner you, not even asking how you feel about me. So you can stop backpedaling."

"I was not—"

"But I'm guessing honesty on my part is important right now, since I may be—unconsciously—affecting your abilities. Yes or no?"

She cleared her throat again. "Yes. We think so."

"Okay. So despite the reasonable and logical certainty of my conscious mind that you can take care of yourself, and today's ample demonstration that you can also take care of me if the occasion demands, my subconscious thinks you need a shield."

"Apparently."

"And gave you one."

"That's the theory."

"How?"

"That part's a little fuzzy."

"Meaning?"

"We haven't got a clue."

"Shit."

Isabel had to laugh at his expression, even if the sound held virtually no humor. "Frontier territory, remember? We don't know how it happened, *I* don't know how it happened, but it's

the only thing that makes sense. I'll tell you now, if we both survive this, Bishop is going to want to study us. Because as far as I
know, this has never happened before."

"Never mind Bishop. What do we do about this? You need
your abilities, Isabel. Hell, *I* need your abilities. If we don't stop
this bastard, he'll murder at least three more women. And you're
on his list."

"A fact that makes me far more uneasy today than it did yesterday."

"Because yesterday you had an edge none of the other women
did. You believed you'd see him coming," Rafe said.

It's time.

He tried to ignore the voice this time, because there were people around. People who'd hear.

*Wimp. You really aren't a man, are you? You're worse than a
neutered dog, following them around, sniffing at them, unable to
do anything else. That's it, isn't it? No balls.*

His head hurt. The voice echoed inside, bouncing off his skull
until he wanted to pound it against a wall.

*You know who they are now. The three that matter. You know
them.*

Yes, he knew them. He knew all of them.

And you know they'll tell.

"But not yet," he whispered, fearful of being overheard.
"They won't tell yet."

*That agent will. That reporter will. And the other one, she'll
tell too.*

He didn't say it out loud, because he knew people would hear,
but it was the other one that worried him most. The other one
wouldn't just tell.

She'd show.

She'd show it all.

Isabel nodded slowly. "Even though twice before in my life I've been blindsided by evil, I believed I'd see it this time. I believed that this time . . . I'd fight it face-to-face. For some reason, I was sure even before I got here that that's how it would end." She hesitated, then said, "I need to do that, you know."

"Yes. I know."

Isabel was very much afraid he did know. Almost unconsciously, she drew her hand away from his and leaned back a bit, crossing her arms beneath her breasts. "So we need to figure out how to undo this," she said. "How to take away the box, or at least punch a hole or two in it so I can reach out and use my abilities."

After a moment, Rafe leaned back in his chair and laced his fingers together over his middle. "Whether you're right about it or not, the only thing I know about psychic abilities is what you and Hollis have told me. So all I can contribute is willingness to try . . . whatever you think I should try."

She nodded, but said, "Before we try anything, we need to be sure. Sure that psychic ability has been triggered in you and you're a functional psychic."

"I'm beginning to have fewer doubts about that."

"Oh? Why?"

"Because as soon as we stopped touching, your voice became a little muffled."

"As if there's . . . something between us."

Rafe nodded.

"Psychic cotton wool," Isabel said. "That's what Hollis called it."

He looked at her in silence for a moment, then shook his head slightly. "Brave new world. Not something I expected to be part of."

"No. Me either." Before he could say anything to that, she added, "Anyway, we need to know for sure."

"How can we find out?"

Very casually, Isabel said, "It just so happens that there's a telepath in town. A telepath with the ability to recognize another psychic at least eighty percent of the time. That's the highest percentage we've ever found."

"A telepath," Rafe said. "SCU?"

"Yes."

"Undercover, I gather."

"Bishop often sends in a secondary agent or team to work behind the scenes whenever possible. We've found it a very effective method of operation." Her tone was a little wary now, and she watched him uncertainly.

"Waiting for me to blow my stack?" he asked.

"Well, law-enforcement officials we work with tend to get a little upset when they find out they've been left out of the loop. Even for a very good reason. So, let's just say it wouldn't surprise me if you did."

"Then," Rafe said, "your senses really are in a box. And I'm not just talking about the extra ones." His voice was very calm, almost offhand. He got to his feet. "When do I meet this telepath?"

Isabel checked her watch. "Forty-five minutes. We'll have to leave in thirty to make the meeting."

"Okay. I'll be in my office until then."

She watched him leave the room and continued to gaze at the open doorway until Hollis appeared just a minute or two later.

"Isabel?"

"The thing that actually scares me," Isabel said as though they were continuing a conversation begun sometime before, "is that I have this uneasy feeling he's at least three steps ahead of me. And I don't understand how he's doing that."

"The killer?"

"No. Rafe."

Hollis closed the door behind her, then came in and sat down at the conference table. "He's still surprising you, huh?"

"In spades. He just never reacts to things the way I think he's going to."

Mildly, Hollis said, "Then maybe you're thinking too much."

"What do you mean?"

"Stop trying to anticipate, Isabel. Instead of thinking about everything, why not try listening to your instincts and feelings?"

"You sound like Bishop."

Hollis was a little surprised. "I do?"

"Yes. He says I only get blindsided when I forget what my senses are *for.* That I have to accept and understand that what I feel is at least as important as what I think."

"More important," Hollis said. "For you. Especially now, I imagine."

"Why now?"

"Rafe."

Isabel frowned and looked away.

"He reached out to you, Isabel. You wanted him to. You let him. But you couldn't reach back. You weren't quite ready to take that chance."

"I've known the man a grand total of about four days."

"So? We both know time has nothing to do with it. You and Rafe connected in those first few hours. You were wide open because you always are—or were. He was definitely attracted and unusually willing to open himself emotionally, or so it seemed to me. Jesus Christ, Isabel, you two strike sparks when you touch. Literally. Are you telling me you can't see a sign from the universe *that* clear?"

"We're going over old ground here," Isabel said tightly.

"Yes, but you keep missing the point."

"And what is that?"

"Those control issues of yours. You can be flip about them if you want, but we both know they're at the heart of this entire situation."

"Yeah?"

"Yeah. You came into this as confident as always, sure of yourself and your abilities. In control. I don't know, maybe you were a little more vulnerable than usual because it's this particular killer, this old enemy, that you were after. Or maybe that had nothing to do with it. Maybe it was just a case of right place, right person—and really lousy timing."

"I'll agree with that much, anyway," Isabel muttered.

"Doesn't really matter. The fact is, you found yourself losing control, and not just of your own emotions. Your abilities were suddenly different. You were so wide open you didn't have a hope in hell of being able to even filter all the stuff coming at you. You could do that before, I'm told. Filter what came through, exert a kind of control over it even if you couldn't block it out. But once you got to Hastings, once you connected with Rafe, you didn't even have that."

"What happened here was nothing that hadn't happened before, as far as my abilities go."

"No, but the scale of it was different. You've already admitted that much yourself."

Reluctantly, Isabel nodded.

"And there he was, so close. Too close. All of a sudden, you got very spooked. So you opened the door to your chamber of horrors, thinking that would drive him away and things could get back to normal. But it did just the opposite. It brought him even closer, and it strengthened the connection between you two. So much so that he was somehow able to use it himself, even if only unconsciously."

Hollis shook her head slowly. "I guess it was easier for you to just let him be the one in control for a while. Let him do what he wanted to do, needed to do. Protect you, shut out all the pain. Even if it meant shutting off your abilities and blinding you to the evil you know is almost close enough to touch."

14

THE POUNDING IN HIS HEAD was almost as rhythmic as his heartbeat, as though his very brain pulsed inside his skull.

The imagery pleased him briefly.

The pain made him reach for yet another handful of painkillers. He'd considered going to a doctor and getting the stronger prescription stuff but was wary of doing anything that might call attention to himself.

That bitch agent, it might occur to her that the change kept him in pain most of the time, and she might start calling doctors, checking for just that.

No, he couldn't take the chance.

But he had a hunch that all the painkillers on top of not being able to eat much these days might be causing other problems. There was a new pain, deep in his gut, a burning. It got better when he was able to eat something, and he knew what that meant. An ulcer, probably.

Was that part of the change? Was it intended that his own digestive acids—helped along by handfuls of painkillers—would eat through the lining of his stomach?

He didn't see how that would help him become what he had to be, but—

It's punishment, wimp.

"I haven't done anything wrong." He kept his voice low, so nobody else would hear.

You're dragging your feet. You haven't done that agent. You haven't done the reporter. Or the other one. What're you waiting for?

"The right time. I have to be careful. They're watching me."

I knew I wouldn't be able to count on you to keep it together. You're paranoid now.

"No—"

You are. All you should be thinking about is what those women have done to you. Those bitches. You know what they've done. You know.

"Yes. I know."

Then there's nothing else to think about, is there? Nothing else to worry about.

"I just have to kill them. All six of them. Just like I did before."

Yes. You just have to kill them.

"I'm not that self-destructive," Isabel said.

"You're that scared."

"And you know that because of your degree in psychology?"

"I know it because I was brutalized too."

After a long moment, much of the tension drained visibly from Isabel and she said, "Yeah. We belong to a very select club, you and I. Survivors of evil."

"It doesn't have to be a lifetime membership, Isabel."

"Doesn't it?"

"No. And if you let it be, then you let him win. You let evil win."

Isabel managed a faint smile. "If this is what Maggie Barnes did for you, then I wish I'd had her around fourteen years ago."

"What Maggie did for me," Hollis said, "was put me in the same place you're in now. As if years have gone by. The memories are still there, the pain is only an echo—and the scars are fear. I can be more objective than you because I'm not the one falling in love."

"And if you were?" It was a tacit admission.

"I'd be scared to death."

"I'll remind you that you said that."

It was Hollis's turn to smile faintly. "Believe me, I'm counting on you to help me through, if it ever happens."

"The blind leading the blind."

"You'll have figured things out by then. You'll have to. As our esteemed leader says, the universe puts us where we need to be. You obviously need to be here, now. With Rafe."

"And a killer."

Hollis nodded. "And a killer. Which is why I think you can't try to ignore or deny your own feelings. Not now, not this time. You don't have that luxury, not with a killer in the equation. You need your abilities at full strength, *plus* whatever Rafe brings to the relationship."

In a slightly suspicious tone, Isabel asked, "Did Bishop tell you anything else about what's happening here? I mean, aside from having you give Rafe just the information he needed to keep that little confrontation at the dairy farm from having a tragic ending?"

"No, but I've been thinking about that."

"I'm almost afraid to ask."

"Oh, it's nothing definitive. You know how Bishop and Miranda are when it comes to seeing the future. Maybe they did see this and knew that Rafe needed to be part of it; maybe that's why they made sure he'd survive Helton's drunken paranoia. But even if they did, they'd hardly tell me anything about it."

"Probably not," Isabel agreed wryly. "They feel very responsible for what they see and the actions they take or don't take, so they don't say a whole lot about it to the rest of us."

"One of these days," Hollis said, "I'd love to talk to them about the whole philosophical question of playing God."

"Good luck."

Hollis smiled faintly, but said, "Getting back to the point I wanted to make, I think there's a very simple reason why you and Rafe reacted to each other so instantly and on a basic chemical and electromagnetic level."

"I guess you're going to tell me even if I don't ask."

"Yes. It's that balance thing the universe tries to keep going. In your case, you needed something outside yourself to be whole, balanced. And so does he. I think you two were meant to be a team, Isabel. Just like Bishop and Miranda. The two of you together are potentially . . . greater than the sum of your parts. A perfect balance, something the universe keeps aiming for and so often misses."

"Hollis—"

"I don't know why I believe that, but I do. Maybe it's the sparking thing. Or just the way you talk to each other, as though you've been close for years. All I know is that I believe what I believe. And I think the only difference between you two and

Bishop and Miranda is that it took them years and a lot of tragedy to figure things out."

"What makes you think I—Rafe and I—can get there any faster or easier?"

"You do. You charge at things head-on, Isabel. It's your instinct as sure as Rafe's instinct is to protect. So stop holding back. Stop being afraid. Trust yourself."

"Easy for you to say."

"Yeah, it is. Like I said, I'm not the one falling in love and trying to cope with all this. But the universe put me here for a reason, too, and maybe it wasn't to talk to dead victims. Maybe it was to talk to you. Maybe it's not time for me to learn to control my abilities."

"That's a handy excuse," Isabel said, not unkindly.

"You don't have to worry that I'll stop trying." Hollis grimaced slightly. "Okay, you don't have to worry that I'll keep on not trying."

"I was beginning to wonder."

"I know I need to learn to control this. And I know I won't be able to if I don't start trying. So I will. You have my word on that. My abilities might be the only edge we've got in this. Especially if it's going to take time for you and Rafe to get this shield thing figured out."

"The thought had occurred."

"So we both have a lot of work to do. And Rafe'll have to get a crash course in being psychic."

Isabel sighed. "Well, after my last little discussion with him, Rafe may not be all that willing, no matter what he said. I don't need any extra senses to know he was not happy with me."

"If I have to say it again, I will. Subtle is not your strong suit, pal."

"It comes of being a platinum blonde almost six feet tall," Isabel said wryly. "Like being a neon sign in human terms, at least according to what the therapists say."

"Since you've never been able to melt into the background physically . . ."

"Exactly. Another reason I—to use your phrase—charge at things head-on. Usually. Everybody tends to be watching me, might as well give them something to see. Never really got much of a chance to practice subtle."

"It shows."

"Yeah, I'm getting that."

"Mmm. In any case, I've got a strong hunch that Rafe will meet you halfway even if he is pissed at the moment. But only halfway. You're the profiler, so consider this: what is it you have that Rafe needs to balance himself—and vice versa? And I'm not talking about the shield thing. Emotionally. Psychologically."

"You obviously think you know the answer."

"Yeah, I think I do. I also think it's something both of you will have to figure out for yourselves."

"Jesus. You really are beginning to sound like Bishop."

Hollis considered a moment, then said, "Thank you."

Shaking her head, Isabel checked her watch, then got herself off the conference table. "I'm taking Rafe for his . . . psychic litmus test."

"Say hello for me."

"I will. In the meantime, the focus of the investigation needs to be on locating that box of photographs and the missing women, *and* trying to figure this bastard out before he kills another one. In other words, same old, same old."

Hollis nodded, then said, "This morning, you asked Ginny McBrayer if she was feeling okay."

"Yeah."

"You saw the shiner, didn't you? It got more obvious as the day wore on, despite her attempts to cover it up."

Isabel sighed. "She did a good job with the makeup, which makes me think it's not the first black eye she's had to hide. What do you know about her home life?"

"I asked Mallory, casually. Ginny still lives at home, with her parents. She's trying to pay off college loans and save for a place of her own."

"Boyfriend?"

"Mallory didn't know. But I can ask Ginny outright. I'm not especially shy."

"I noticed that." Isabel thought about it, then nodded. "If you get the chance, do. She may think we're butting in to something that's none of our business, but there's a lot of tension in this town, and borderline situations can get pushed over the edge really fast."

"An abusive boyfriend or parent could get worse."

"Much worse. Besides, she's got a lot on her plate as a young officer, especially right now, and stress can cause different reactions in people. Like the rest of us, she takes her gun home with her."

"Oh, hell. I hadn't even thought of that."

"Let's hope she hasn't either."

"So, are you still mad at me?" Isabel asked Rafe as they got into her and Hollis's rental car.

"I wasn't mad at you."

"No? Then I guess an arctic cold front swept through the conference room despite all those walls. I nearly got frostbite. Amazing."

"You know," he said as she started the engine, "you don't talk like any other person I've ever met."

"One of a kind, accept no substitutes."

He looked at her, one brow rising. "Where are we going?"

"West. That little motel on the edge of town."

"Great. The only motel in Hastings that charges hourly rates."

"Oh, I doubt anybody will pay attention to us going in, if that's what you're worried about. I took Stealthy 101 at the Bureau."

Rafe's mouth twitched. "You don't play fair either."

"Well, at least we both have our little tricks. You can kiss me until my knees get dizzy, and I can make you laugh even when you're pissed."

He laughed, but said, "I was not pissed. Just . . . annoyed. You are a very difficult woman, in case no one has ever told you that."

"I have been told, as a matter of fact. It doesn't seem to help, knowing about it. Sorry."

He turned slightly in his seat to watch her as she drove, but let a few minutes pass before saying, "Dizzy knees, huh?"

"Oh, don't say you didn't know."

"I knew there was some effect. That was the only reason I didn't get pissed in the conference room when you were so busy backpedaling."

"You weren't supposed to see me backpedaling. Hollis says I don't do subtle real well."

"You don't do subtle at all."

"Then I'll stop trying, shall I?"

He grinned. "So you do have a few buttons."

Isabel got hold of herself. Or tried to. "Apparently. Look, it's not all that much fun to keep hearing how blatant you are. I'm an almost-six-foot blonde, which makes me real visible; I'm a clairvoyant without a shield—usually—which makes me a high-wattage receiver for an amazing range of trivia that tends to come at me like painful bullets, and now I find out I might as well be wearing my heart on my sleeve. Just look for my picture beside the word *obvious* in the dictionary."

"You do defensive very well."

"Oh, shut up."

Rafe chuckled. "You'll feel much better when you just admit it, you know you will."

"I don't know how I'll feel. And neither do you."

"You're wasting a lot of energy, I know that. Want to talk about our primitive instincts? You're a fighter, Isabel; backing away from this isn't doing anything except keeping you rattled and off balance."

"All of a sudden everybody has a degree in psychology," she muttered.

"Just tell me this much. Is it going to make a difference, finding out whether I'm psychic?"

Isabel knew that was a serious question and answered it seriously. "You mean will I love you more if you can provide a shield for me? No. Being shielded for nearly twenty-four hours has taught me I'd rather be without one. I mean, nice place to visit now and then, but I really do feel like I've suddenly gone deaf, and I don't like it."

"So if I am psychic and have somehow put a shield around your abilities, you're going to run to the ends of the earth to escape it?"

"I didn't say that. And no. We'll just figure out a way for one or both of us to control the damned thing, that's all. Having psychic abilities never makes life easier, but the whole point is learning to live with them."

"So you'll love me either way?"

Isabel opened her mouth, then closed it. She allowed the silence to lengthen for a moment before saying, "You're very tricky."

"Not tricky enough. Apparently."

"Here's the place."

Rafe smiled slightly but didn't say anything else as she pulled the car into the motel's secondary drive and around to the back of the building.

It was a somewhat seedy motel, an L-shaped single floor, and the neon VACANCY sign was flickering on the point of going dark. Only two cars were parked at the front; around the back there were half a dozen more scattered vehicles.

Isabel parked the unobtrusive rental beside a small Ford with a dented rear bumper, and they both got out. She went immediately to the room in front of the Ford and knocked quietly.

The door opened. "What, no pizza?"

"I forgot," Isabel said apologetically, stepping into the room.

"You owe me one. Hey, Chief," Paige Gilbert said. "Come on in."

"We're just concerned," Hollis told Ginny quietly.

The younger woman shifted a bit in her chair at the conference table, then said, "I appreciate that. I really do. But I'm fine. In a few more months, I'll have enough saved to move out on my own."

"And until then?"

"Until then I'll just stay out of his way."

"Like you did last night?" Hollis shook her head. "You've had enough training to know better, Ginny. He's mad at the world and you're his punching bag. He won't stop until somebody makes him."

"When I move out—"

"He'll go back to beating your mother."

"I didn't tell you that."

"You didn't have to."

Ginny slumped in her chair. "No. It's textbook, isn't it? He's a bully who beat her up until I got old enough to intervene, and now he hits me. When I'm not fast enough to stay out of his reach, that is. Usually, he's so drunk he passes out or knocks himself out trashing the house, at least now that he's older."

"Your mother?"

"I haven't been able to talk her into leaving him. But once I'm out, I think she'll go live with her sister in Columbia."

"And what will he do?"

"Go down the drain, probably. He hasn't had a regular job in years because of his temper. He's stupid and sullen and—like you said—mad at the world. Because, of course, it's not his fault that his life sucks. It's never his fault."

"It isn't your fault," Hollis said. "But when he goes too far and assaults someone else, or drives drunk and causes an accident, or does something else stupid and destructive, you'll blame yourself. Won't you?"

Ginny was silent.

"You're a cop, Ginny. You know what you have to do. Press charges, see that he's locked up or forced into some kind of treatment program, or whatever it takes to defuse the situation."

"I know. I know that. But it's hard to . . ."

"To take it all public. Yes, it is. Maybe one of the hardest things you'll ever do. But doing it will take away his power. It's his shame you'll be showing the world, not yours. Not your mother's. His."

Biting her bottom lip, Ginny said, "It's mostly the guys here that I think about. I mean, I took the training, I know self-defense, and still he hits me. So what're they going to think? That I'm some weak little girly-girl who needs them to protect me all the time? I wouldn't be able to take that."

"You might get that reaction at first," Hollis admitted. "Not because they think you aren't capable, but because they wouldn't have become cops if they didn't want to help people. Protect people. Especially one of their own. But you'll show them, in time. Earn another marksman's medal or another belt in your karate classes, and they'll notice."

"How did you know—"

"A little birdie told me." Hollis smiled. "Look, the point is that you have friends. And they'll be supportive. But this is not the time to back off, to avoid taking action against your father. With this killer on the loose, everybody's on edge and in full defensive mode. If your father pushes *anybody* the wrong way, he's likely to provoke a situation with a tragic outcome."

"You're right." Ginny got to her feet and managed a smile. "Thank you, Hollis. And thank Isabel for me, will you? If you hadn't said something, I probably would have let this go on, and God knows what might have happened."

"You have friends," Hollis repeated. "Including us. Don't forget that."

"No. No, I won't. Thanks." She went quietly from the conference room.

Hollis sat there frowning in silence for a moment, her gaze fixed on the bulletin boards covered with photographs and reports, then reached for her cell phone and punched in a number.

"Yeah."

"I know this isn't a good time," Hollis said, "but when you've finished up there, ask Rafe about the McBrayer household, will you? He might know just how volatile Hank McBrayer is, how dangerous."

"She's going to press charges?"

"I think so. And I have a very bad feeling about how he might react."

"Okay. Keep her busy there, if you can; she might feel the need to go confront him before she takes official action."

"Shit. Okay, I will. Oh—and we've got a small lead on Kate Murphy; after the latest round of radio announcements asking for help, a witness came forward to report he thinks he might have seen her getting on a bus the day she disappeared. We're checking it out."

"Good. It'd be nice to know we aren't looking for another body. Yet."

"I'll say. How's it going there?"

"I'll fill you in when I get back."

"That bad, huh?"

"*Tense* is the word I'd use. Talk to you later."

"Is who going to press charges?" Rafe asked as Isabel ended the call.

"Tell you later."

He frowned at her. "I am not tense."

Isabel lifted both brows at Paige.

"He's tense," Paige said.

Rafe, sitting on one of the two rather unsteady chairs near the front window, rubbed the back of his neck and stared at the two women warily. "I'm still trying to deal with you being a fed," he told Paige. "And the fact that you've been here longer than Isabel."

Isabel shook her head. She was sitting in the other rickety chair, both of which faced Paige, who sat on the bed. "I'm still pissed at Bishop for that part of it. All the time I was arguing with him about sending me down here, and he already had an agent in place—and had sent her here right after the first murder, even before you asked for a profile."

"Not much gets past him," Paige reminded Isabel. "Neither of them has said, but I get the feeling he and Miranda keep an eye on any investigations that might even possibly involve any of the killers in our cold-case files. Hell, Kendra probably wrote a program for them purely to do that—scan all the police and law-enforcement databases looking for specific details or keywords."

"He might have told me," Isabel said.

"And he might have told Hollis why she was supposed to make sure Rafe knew you understood Latin. Of course, if he had, then she might have been self-conscious about what she was doing, and Rafe might have picked up on the wrong part of the conversation, and you might never have had to bring him to me to find out if he's psychic because he'd be dead."

"If my vote counts," Rafe said, "I vote we let Bishop continue to do things his own way."

"Okay, point taken. But Hollis is right: one of these days, one of us is going to have to sit down and have a long talk with Bishop and Miranda about the philosophical and actual consequences of playing God."

"Later," Rafe said. "Can we please do what we came here to do and find out what's going on inside my head? How *do* we find out, by the way? And does it involve something unspeakable like . . . chicken entrails?"

"What *have* you been reading?" Paige demanded.

"Well, since nobody offered me a copy of the psychic newsletter . . ."

Isabel frowned and looked at Paige. "Isn't that a joke Maggie uses sometimes?"

Paige nodded, her gaze thoughtfully fixed on Rafe. "Yeah.

He's very plugged-in. Aside from Beau, I've never met anybody else who could do that. He's sort of picked up the rhythm of the way you talk too."

"Yeah, I noticed that."

"Ladies, please." Rafe was beginning to look profoundly uneasy.

"Oh, you're psychic," Paige said matter-of-factly.

Rafe had braced himself to be told that, but the abruptness and utter calm of the disclosure threw him more than a little. "You don't have to touch me to make sure?"

"No. I'm not a touch telepath, I'm an open telepath. All I have to do is focus on someone and concentrate. If I can read them at all, I know right away. I can read you, and you're psychic."

"I am?"

"You are." Paige looked at Isabel. "I was pretty sure he was, at that news conference before you showed up on Thursday. When you walked into the room, I was positive."

"That's when everything changed," Rafe murmured. "I felt it."

"I'm not surprised," Paige said frankly. "The hair on the back of my neck stood straight up. It was like an electrical current was let loose in the room."

"Why didn't you tell me?" Isabel demanded. "Then would have been nice, but when I called you today—"

"I reported in to Bishop on Thursday, and he told me to wait. That you and I shouldn't have any contact at all until you called me. On Sunday."

"He knew I'd call today."

"Apparently, yes."

"At least tell me he didn't give you a whole list of things to say to one or both of us."

Paige grinned. "No. He just said you'd call, and it would be safe for us to meet, that I should follow my training and instincts. So that's what I'm doing."

Isabel was looking thoughtful, her irritation with Bishop a fleeting thing. "Wait a minute. Rafe was already a functional psychic before I came into the room?"

"Yeah, but not consciously."

"Then the original trigger was—"

"Dunno. It had to be recent, and probably some kind of emotional or psychological shock."

Slowly, Rafe said, "I don't recall anything like that happening. My life was very ordinary until all this started. Having a serial killer loose in my town was a shock, I admit, but nothing I'm not trained to deal with."

"Could have been some kind of subconscious shock, I suppose, though that's really rare. We're usually completely aware of the jolts we get through life. Whatever it was, I can't get at it; it's behind his shield."

Isabel rubbed her forehead briefly. "Okay, let's try something a little easier. What happened when I came into the room that day?"

Readily, Paige said, "As near as I can tell, you were the catalyst. Or it was a combination of the two of you in close proximity for the first time. On a purely electromagnetic level, it was like energy going to energy. I felt it come through the room between you. Jeez, I could almost see it."

"And what did that do to Rafe's abilities?"

"Same thing it did to yours. Started to change them."

"Wait a minute," Rafe said. "Change them from what? And into what?"

"Here's where we get into educated guesswork," Paige told them. "From what I was getting before Isabel walked into the room, I think your natural ability would have been precognition."

"Seeing the future?"

"Like your grandmother," Isabel said. "She had the sight."

Rafe leaned forward, elbows on knees, and frowned at Paige. "But I'm not precognitive now?"

"No, not actively. When Isabel walked in, everything changed. Her energy added to yours closed that door and opened another one."

"I'm afraid to ask," Rafe said.

"I'm not," Isabel said. "What's behind door number two?"

"Clairvoyance."

Startled, Rafe said, "Like Isabel?"

"Yeah, except that as we all know you have a shield. Dandy one, as a matter of fact. So dandy you've got it wrapped around both of you."

"How is that possible?" Isabel demanded. "He's not consciously controlling any of this."

"That's how it's possible." Paige eyed Rafe thoughtfully. "In case you don't know this, your conscious mind is always second-guessing your hunches and instincts. For most of your life, I gather."

He nodded without comment.

"Well, your instincts are fighting back. Once your abilities became functional, your subconscious took them over. With a vengeance."

Isabel frowned. "Wait a minute. If this shield of his is so powerful it can even enclose my mind—"

"Then how am I able to read him? It's *because* he's doing all this at a subconscious level. Just beneath his conscious mind is a solid wall." Paige lifted her brows at Isabel. "Same one that's just beneath your conscious mind. It's really no wonder you can't hear the voices anymore."

With a sigh, Isabel said, "You know, Bishop was right—as

usual, damn him—to send Hollis with me. She's been pretty much on the mark about all of this."

"Yeah, the rookies often are. Sometimes knowing just the basics can offer you more room to speculate and the imagination to do it," Paige said. "The rest of us tend to get tripped up by our own assumptions."

"I'm still trying to figure out the basics," Rafe told them. To Paige, he said, "So I'm not stripped naked to you, just down to my underwear."

"Pretty good analogy." She smiled. "And accurate, as far as it goes. I'm not picking up thoughts from you—I mean clear thoughts like sentences. It doesn't work that way for me. You could be calling me rude names in your head or worrying about some deep dark secret you don't want anybody to know, and I wouldn't necessarily read either."

"Because you specialize in reading psychic ability in other minds?" he guessed.

Paige nodded. "Exactly. My own energy seems to be tuned for that, picking up on that particular frequency. So I usually know if somebody else is psychic, how they're psychic, and what's going on in that area of their minds. But the human brain is vast, mostly unmapped terrain, and the larger part of it is as alien to me as it is to most everybody else."

Rafe shook his head as he sat back in his chair, but said, "Okay, how do I control this?"

"Simple. Get your conscious mind in control."

"And you're going to tell me how to do that?"

"Wish I could. Sorry. This is the sort of thing almost every psychic has to figure out more or less alone. The only advice I have to offer is that you two work together on it. Clearly, you're meant to."

It was Isabel who said, "So tell us why."

Paige didn't hesitate. "Do me a favor and hold hands for a minute."

Rafe looked at Isabel, then held out his hand. With only a slight hesitation, she put hers in it.

At the spark, Paige's eyes widened. "I'd heard about it but not seen it. Interesting, to say the least." She frowned, obviously concentrating.

But then something really weird happened.

While Isabel and Rafe watched in fascination, Paige's shoulder-length dark hair began to lift and stir as though a breeze had wafted through the room. There was a soft popping and crackling, and a low hum began to fill the silence.

15

HOLLIS LOOKED UP as Ginny stuck her head in the conference room to say, "Caleb Powell is here to see you. Should I show him in here, or to one of the offices?"

"In here, I guess. Thanks, Ginny." Hollis went to cover the bulletin boards, then returned to a chair on the far side of the table. She was more than a little surprised that he wanted to see her at all; to seek her out here at the police station, and on a Sunday, definitely made her wonder.

Especially after their last meeting.

"Hi," Caleb said as he came in. He didn't shut the door behind him, and Hollis didn't suggest that he do so.

"Hi yourself. What's up?" With a gesture, she invited him to sit down on the opposite side of the table.

He hesitated, then sat down. "I wanted to apologize."

"For what?"

"You know. I acted like a jerk when you told me about your eyes."

She couldn't help but smile. "You didn't act like a jerk, you were just a little unnerved. I can hardly blame you for that, since I am too. And I've had months to get used to them."

"Still, it was a lousy way for me to act. I'm sorry."

"Apology accepted."

Caleb moved half-consciously in his chair. "Then why do I get the feeling I've damaged . . . something . . . beyond repair?"

Having watched Isabel and Rafe circling each other like a couple of wary cats, Hollis was in no mood to play games. "Caleb, you seem like a nice guy, with a nice, satisfying life here in Hastings. And I hope that after we've done our job and gone away, you get your nice little town back again. I hope we can offer you some sense of closure in Tricia's death by finding the animal who killed her."

"But?"

"But nothing. There isn't anything else. There never was, really."

"There might have been."

Still being honest, she said, "I sort of doubt it. Not because of anything you said or did, but just the timing."

"And there's no use even trying?"

"I think . . . that right now my life and your life are so different we could never even find a bit of common ground to stand on. Honestly. You don't know me, Caleb. The little bit you do know is just the tip of a pretty dark and unsettling iceberg."

He leaned back in his chair with a sigh. "Yeah, I was afraid you'd say something like that."

"Admit it. You're relieved."

"No. No, not relieved. In fact, I have the distinct feeling I'm missing out on something I'll regret one day."

"Nice of you to say so."

He smiled a bit ruefully. "Look, there's something else I came here to tell you. Show you. Something that could possibly be related to Tricia's murder."

Hollis had no problem in shifting from the personal to the professional—which told her a lot. "What is it?"

"I found something in the desk. My desk, not hers. It was in a drawer I never use because it's in an awkward position in the desk layout, and apparently she'd been using it to store work-related things she no longer used. Mostly old notebooks. I went through all of them, and they were all the shorthand notes she'd taken. Dictation, notes about schedules and appointments, that sort of thing."

"What was unusual about that?"

"Nothing. But when I was going through the last notebook—which was actually the one that had been on top, by the way—a slip of paper fell out. I'm guessing it was something she wrote down during a phone call, and the date puts it just before the murders began." He reached into the inner pocket of his jacket, adding, "My prints are all over it, but I figured it didn't really matter. It's clearly a private note, since it doesn't match anything in my schedule, and I doubt it has any value as evidence—except to maybe point the investigation in a different direction." He placed the small piece of paper on the conference table and pushed it across to her.

Out of habit, Hollis nevertheless used the eraser of the pencil she was holding to draw the paper closer so she could study it. "Looks like her handwriting," she said.

"I'm no expert, but I've seen a lot of her handwriting over the years. She wrote that. Plus, that's the sort of doodling she tended to do when her mind was on something else."

The "doodles" were clear enough. A little cat face; a couple of hearts with arrows through them; stairs leading to nowhere; a sun setting off the edge of the paper with its rays beaming; a female eye, with long lashes and carefully detailed iris; and two circles connected by a series of smaller circles.

The paper was clearly from a notepad; it was a neon green, and across the top was printed: *It works in practice, but not in theory.*

"There were other notepads like this one in her desk," Hollis remembered. "The kind with preprinted cartoons or funny sayings on them."

"Yeah. She said they lightened up the serious tone of a lawyer's office, but she only used them for personal or throwaway notes."

Hollis nodded, and studied what Tricia had written in the center of the notepad.

J.B.

Old Hwy

7:00 5/16

It was followed by two large question marks.

"Did Tricia know Jamie Brower?" Hollis asked.

"She never mentioned it, if she did."

"How did she react when Jamie was murdered?"

"Shocked and horrified, just like the rest of us." Caleb frowned. "She did take a few vacation days unexpectedly, now that I think about it."

"Did she leave town?"

"She said she was going to. The time off was because her sister had had surgery, and Tricia needed to go to Augusta and help take care of the kids."

Hollis pushed the note to one side and hunted through the folders stacked on the table until she found the one she wanted.

She looked through several pages, frowning, then paused. "Okay. According to her sister's statement, at the time of Tricia's death she hadn't seen her in more than three months. I thought I remembered reading that."

"Tricia lied to me?" Caleb was baffled. "Why? I mean, it's not like I even asked her why she needed the time off. She had so much vacation and sick time accumulated, I remember telling her to take a week or two if that's what she needed. But she came back to work about . . . four days later."

Hollis looked through the folder for several more minutes, pausing here and there, and finally closed it. "We've backtracked every victim's life for about two weeks prior to their murders, which means we have information that starts tracking Tricia just a few days *after* Jamie was killed."

"So you don't know if she was here in town or went somewhere else."

"No. Shouldn't be too difficult to find out, though. Her apartment manager has been very cooperative, and Tricia was a friendly neighbor, so *her* neighbors noticed her."

"A lesson to all of us not to become too isolated, I guess."

"One way to look at it." Hollis hesitated, then said, "Did Tricia ever show up to work with unexplained bruises or burns, anything like that?"

"No. I told you her former boyfriend showed no signs of abusing her. I never saw a bruise, and since she seldom wore makeup I think I would have noticed."

"True enough." Hollis smiled. "Thanks for bringing this in, Caleb."

He took the hint and rose to his feet. "I only hope it turns out to be helpful."

"I'll let you know," she promised. "That closure we were talking about."

"Thanks, I appreciate it." He hesitated just an instant, then turned and left the conference room.

Hollis was just about to call Ginny in and find out if the younger officer wanted to share a pizza and do some brainstorming when she felt a sudden chill, as if someone had opened a window into winter.

She watched gooseflesh rise on her arms and had to force herself to look up, toward the doorway.

Jamie Brower stood there.

"Oh, shit," Hollis murmured.

She wasn't solid flesh, but neither was she a ghostly, wispy thing; she was definitely clearer and more distinct than Hollis had yet seen her. In this form, anyway.

Her expression was anxious, worried; Jamie said something—or tried to. All Hollis heard was that peculiar hollow silence.

"I'm sorry," she said, trying to hold her own voice steady. Trying not to feel terrified. "I can't hear you."

Jamie moved a step closer to the table and Hollis. Or rather—and very eerily—floated closer, since she didn't seem to actually take a physical step.

Again, she tried to say something.

This time, Hollis could—almost—hear something. Like a quiet voice speaking from the far end of a huge room.

She focused, concentrated. "I can just barely hear . . . Try again, please. What do you need to tell me?"

Jamie's mouth moved as she tried to communicate, the intensity of her need so obvious that Hollis could literally feel it, like something pushing at her.

Unnerved, Hollis lost both concentration and the desire to keep trying. "I'm sorry. I'm really sorry, but I just can't hear you," she said, her own voice unsteady now.

An expression of pure frustration crossed Jamie's lovely face, twisting it, and she threw up her arms in the gesture of someone reaching the end of her limits.

Half the folders on the conference table spewed their contents into the air.

When the rain of paper and photographs had ended, Hollis found herself sitting in the middle of a mess.

Alone.

Ginny came into the room a moment later, looking around in surprise. "Hey, it looks like somebody lost her temper."

"Yes," Hollis said. "Somebody did."

"Okay," Paige said, "getting creeped out here."

Isabel and Rafe looked at each other, then stopped holding hands.

Paige reached up to smooth down her hair, and they could all hear the crackle. "Jesus," she muttered. "I'm going to have to write a detailed report on this one. It's the first time that my ability to tap into other psychics' abilities actually manifested itself physically."

"Some psychic abilities do manifest themselves physically," Isabel reminded her.

"Yeah, but not many. I know your visions do that. Have you had one of those, by the way?"

"Not since I've been in Hastings."

"I wonder if you could now."

"I don't know. I assume not, since the visions are just another aspect of the clairvoyance."

"And both are boxed up inside a shield that might as well be Fort Knox."

"You're serious? It's that tough?"

"And then some. Bishop had me test his and Miranda's shield once, and it hit about eight or nine on our scale. Of course, we don't know how consistent that sort of ability is; it may vary widely according to the circumstances—i.e., why the shield is being used by the psychic at that particular moment. When we did the test, they weren't especially motivated or feeling driven to protect themselves. If they had been . . . who knows?"

It was Rafe who said, "So if the reasons were powerful enough, or the—the psychic desperate enough to protect himself or herself from some perceived attack, then the shield would be even stronger than . . . normal." He felt odd just using the word— hell, any of these words. But Paige was nodding, again matter-of-factly.

"The human mind has a hundred ways to protect itself, and it'll use whatever it can whenever it has to. Fear creates energy, just like any other strong emotion does, just like psychic ability itself does. A psychic's mind virtually always uses that extra energy for some kind of wall or shield."

"Except for Isabel."

Isabel shrugged. "We've never been able to figure out why my abilities won't shield themselves."

Rafe looked at her oddly. "No?"

"No." She frowned at him. "Why are you looking at me like that?"

"No reason." But when he looked back at Paige, he lifted his brows slightly.

"Even those of us with extra senses can be incredibly blind to some things," she said. "Keep doing that, by the way. It's working."

Isabel looked from one to the other of them, baffled. "What's he doing?"

"Reaching through his shield."

"He is?"

"I am?"

Paige nodded. "I'm sure you'll both figure it out. Problem is, there's this killer, which doesn't give you a whole hell of a lot of time in which to do it."

"Any advice?" Isabel asked wryly.

"Yeah. Hurry."

Hollis propped her elbows on the table and pressed her fingers against her eyes. "God, I'm tired. What time is it, anyway?"

"Nearly nine," Isabel told her. "I was ready to call it a day hours ago."

Rafe looked at her but didn't say anything, just as he hadn't said much since they'd left Paige at the motel. Isabel had filled the silence—and possibly tried to distract him—by briefly discussing Ginny's situation, a matter Rafe was kicking himself for having completely missed and one he wasn't at all sure how to handle.

Oh, yeah, he was psychic. Sure he was.

In any case, Isabel had offered a few suggestions, and Rafe was more than ready to accept her counsel and approve her plan. He just wished she was as forthcoming with advice regarding this peculiar new ability he supposedly had.

Hell, she hadn't even mentioned it since they'd left the motel, and that bothered him more than he wanted to admit. He knew Isabel was dealing with issues of her own at the moment, and he knew he was a complication in her life. He was even reasonably sure that the simplest thing he could do would be to leave her alone to sort out what she had to.

But as Isabel herself had said, the simplest thing wasn't always the smartest thing.

So what was the smartest thing?

Studiously not looking at him, Isabel said, "Okay, we're agreed that the note doodled by Tricia Kane suggests she was one of Jamie's clients."

"More than suggests," Hollis said. "The only thing on that old highway of any interest is Jamie's playroom."

"Agreed, but that doesn't mean Tricia was a client. We don't know why she was meeting Jamie. Hell, maybe she was painting her."

"There were no sketches of Jamie or anybody who looked like her among Tricia's work. Besides, do you really think Jamie would commission a painting of herself in full S&M ensemble?"

"No."

"Then what other reason could they have for meeting there?"

"Maybe Tricia was interested in buying the building. It was one of those Jamie planned to sell after what happened with Hope Tessneer."

"We checked that out," Mallory said. "At least as far as we could. Jamie kept her official appointments in her date book, and that included appointments to show her own properties during the last couple of months. No appointment listed for May sixteenth."

Rafe spoke finally, saying, "Odds are, Tricia was a client. Or a potential client. You did say at least one of Jamie's partners could have been from Hastings."

Isabel nodded. "I did say that, yes."

Hollis looked from Isabel to Rafe curiously. There had been no opportunity to discuss what they had found out from Paige, since both Mallory and Ginny had been in the room and other officers had come and gone fairly steadily, but it didn't take a sixth sense to feel the tension between them.

Hollis had been debating whether to tell them about the visitation from Jamie, though she had pretty much decided just to tell Isabel later, when they were alone. After all, it wasn't as though she could provide anything new in the way of information or evidence.

Rafe said, "Then Tricia might have been a regular."

"Another Hastings blonde with a secret sexual life?" Isabel leaned back in her chair with a sigh. "And it seemed like such a nice little town."

"I said the same thing," Hollis murmured.

"It was a nice little town," Rafe said. "And will be again. Just as soon as we catch this bastard."

"And all we've got to help us catch him," Isabel reminded the group at large, "is a fairly useless profile and what we know about the victims."

"You haven't revised the profile as you've gotten deeper into the investigation?" Rafe asked Isabel almost idly.

"Not really. This guy leaves so little behind that the only real thing we have to study are the victims he kills. All single white females, all smart and savvy, all successful. Beyond that, and until now, all we really had connecting them was the color of their hair. Cheryl Bayne's disappearance puts the importance of that into question—definitely."

"But even before then," Mallory said, "we found Jamie's secret. And her secret playroom."

Isabel nodded.

"Which could have been an aberration as far as the victims go, having absolutely nothing to do with the killer or his motivations. But then Hope Tessneer's body turned up, having very likely been a . . . toy . . . for our killer after she died, probably accidentally, and probably at Jamie's hands. Connection. And now this note, which is a pretty fair indication that Tricia Kane was or planned to become involved in Jamie's S&M games."

"Another connection," Rafe said.

"But there is absolutely no sign that Allison Carroll led anything but a perfectly traditional sex life. Also no sign that she even knew either of the other victims."

Rafe shook his head. "Maybe we missed something. Or maybe there was nothing there to miss. Maybe she was as good at keeping secrets as Jamie was. As Tricia was."

"Regarding Tricia, there were no regular withdrawals from her bank account in the last few months," Mallory noted. "But that isn't to say she might not have sold some of her sketches or paintings for cash. A couple of her friends mentioned that she'd sold things to them. She could have paid Jamie without leaving any trace of the money."

"Yeah," Isabel said, "but how did she *find* Jamie? I mean, how did she know the services were available? I doubt Jamie advertised in some bondage magazine."

"Word of mouth?" Rafe suggested. "A referral from another client? All these women had something to lose in the sense of not wanting their . . . extracurricular activities to be made public. Jamie could have been pretty sure of their silence."

"Still, she would have wanted to have control—" Isabel broke off with a frown, then continued. "Wait a minute. The photos we have show Jamie unmasked. What if that's the reason Emily took those particular photos? Because they were the only ones that showed Jamie's face?"

Finishing her supposition, Rafe said, "What if Jamie was always masked when she met clients? Except for the client she trusted, the one in the photographs?"

Mallory said, "According to all that info you guys got from Quantico on the S&M scene, that actually makes sense. For the submissive to not know who was dominating her—or him, I guess—could be an important part of the experience. For some of them, it might even be necessary that they not know the identity of their . . . mistress."

"We have got to find that box," Isabel said. "And I want to talk to Emily again first thing tomorrow. The patrol's still watching her, right?"

Rafe nodded. "When she's out of the house, they follow; when she's home, as she was last time I checked, I have a squad car parked across the street from her house. If anybody asks, they're under orders to say they're making sure none of the media bothers the family."

"Good cover story," Isabel said.

"And plausible. Since Jamie was the first victim, the family really has had to put up with a lot of media attention. Allison and Tricia didn't have family in Hastings, so nobody can really know if those families are being watched as well."

"Hey," Ginny said suddenly, "did you guys take a good look at these doodles?"

"I was just looking at the time and place of the appointment," Hollis admitted, unwilling to explain that images often blurred or faded oddly when she looked at them, particularly those drawn two-dimensionally on paper.

"What'd we miss?" Rafe asked his young officer.

Ginny hesitated, then pushed the note across the table to him. "Look at that doodle on the right. The two circles connected with a sort of chain."

Rafe had to look for a moment before he realized what he was seeing. "Jesus. Handcuffs."

"It's about time you got off," Ally told Travis. "I didn't have to hang around the police station waiting for you, you know. I do have other offers."

He grinned at her. "Then why didn't you accept any of them?"

"You're getting too goddamned cocky, I'll tell you that much. Here I am, wandering around downtown on a Sunday evening when the only other women out are brave, and needless to say brunette, hookers—"

"I think those are other reporters, Ally. Hastings doesn't have hookers."

"You sure about that?"

Recalling a certain trip to a certain house when he was about sixteen, Travis felt his face heat up. "Well, not streetwalkers, anyway."

"Don't tell me, let me guess. Your old man took you to a cathouse for your first sexual experience."

"He did not." Travis sighed. "My brother did."

Ally slid off the hood of his car, laughing. "You should send her flowers on every anniversary, pal. She done you proud."

"Thank you. I think." He pulled her close for a long kiss, then said, "Dammit, Ally, it really bothers me that you're wandering around town alone, never mind after dark, especially since Cheryl Bayne disappeared. It's been nearly a week since the last murder; we know we're running out of time. Every other woman in town is jumpy as hell, and you're breezing around like nothing can touch you."

"I'm not blond."

"We don't *know* he's just after blondes. Cheryl Bayne wasn't—isn't—blond. Besides, the other times, he went after brunettes and redheads."

"Other times?"

He grimaced. "You didn't hear me say that."

"Look, I promise I won't report a word until you say it's okay. Scout's honor."

He stared at the fingers she held up. "That's a peace sign, Ally."

"Well, I was never a scout. But that doesn't mean you can't trust me to keep quiet—until I get the word it's okay to report."

He took her arm and escorted her around to the passenger side of his car. "I say we pick up a bag of tacos and head for my place."

"Tacos at this hour? God, you have a cast-iron stomach, don't you? Besides, didn't I see a pizza delivery to the station a couple of hours ago? The poor guy was staggering under the weight of those pizza boxes."

"One of the feds offered to buy," Travis said. "Naturally, we took her up on the offer."

"And you're still hungry?"

"Well, that was a couple of hours ago."

"But tacos? On top of pizza?"

"It's Sunday night in Hastings, Ally; we don't have a lot of choices here."

She sighed and got into his car, waiting until he was behind the wheel to say, "Okay, but only on the condition that you fill me in on the investigation so far."

"Ally—"

"Look, either you trust me by now or you don't. If you don't, please be kind enough to drop me off at the inn."

"So that's it? I talk or it's over?"

"Come on, Travis, give me a break. We're not lovers, we just roll around in the sheets together and have a good time. It's fun and we both enjoy it, but I haven't heard a suggestion that we start picking out china patterns. You're not going to take me home to Mama, and we both know as soon as this maniac is captured or killed, I'm outta here. Right?"

"Right," he said grudgingly.

"So don't get all indignant with me now. I'm having a good time with you, and that's cool, but I also have a job to do. Either I get what I need from you, or I start looking someplace else."

"At least you're up front about it," he muttered.

"I am nothing if not totally honest," she said, lying without a blink.

He eyed her for a moment and then started the car. "Ally, I swear, if you air one single word—or even tell your producer—before I give the okay, I'll figure out a way to throw your ass in jail. Got it?"

"Got it. No problem. So who's Jane Doe, and how did she die?"

"Hope Tessneer, and she was strangled. She lived in another town about thirty miles away."

"And turned up dead here because . . . ?"

"Beats me. I think the chief and the feds know more than they're saying, but they ain't sharing. At least, not with me."

Accurately reading the tone of his voice, she said, "They've brought somebody else into the investigation?"

"Into the inner circle, anyway." He shrugged, trying hard for indifference. "Ginny McBrayer seems to be in their confidence, or at least of the two agents. Figures. You females always stick together."

"Please don't make me call you a sexist pig," Ally requested dryly.

"I'm not. And that's not what I mean. Women talk to each other in ways men just don't. That's all."

Ally looked at him with faint respect. "We do, actually. I'm surprised you noticed."

"I keep telling you I'm not an idiot." He sent her a glance, smiling oddly. "You really should pay attention, Ally."

"Yeah," she said. "Yeah, I guess I really should at that. Where're we going, Travis?"

"The taco place. If I'm going to spill my guts, I'm going to need sustenance first."

"I really wish you'd used a different phrase," Ally said. "Really."

16

ISABEL STUDIED THE NOTE and then nodded, passing it on to Hollis and Mallory. "It looks like a sketch of handcuffs to me. Sort of stylized, the way an artist would maybe do it, which could be one reason we missed it. Nice catch, Ginny."

"I should have caught that," Hollis said, more to herself than to the others, and in a tone that struck her own ears as wistful.

"You're just all a little preoccupied," Ginny murmured.

"Good thing you aren't," Isabel told her. "Okay, a paralegal might have doodled handcuffs, I suppose, but having them on this particular note has got to mean something more than absentmindedness. It's one more indication Tricia Kane was involved, or looking to get involved, with Jamie Brower."

Hollis said, "Any chance Jamie might have trusted Tricia with that box we so badly want to see?"

Isabel started to reply, then looked at Rafe. "What do you think?"

"I'm not the profiler."

"Off the top of your head. What do you think?"

"No," he heard himself reply, and frowned as he went on slowly. "Jamie wouldn't have trusted that box with anyone else—unless it was the partner who saw her unmasked."

"Very good," Isabel said. "And my feeling as well. That box is either stored somewhere Jamie considered safe, or kept by someone she really, really trusted. And we know by now that she didn't trust many people."

Hollis produced the Eyes Only file and opened it to study the photographs. It didn't take long for her to reach a conclusion and close the folder. "This isn't Tricia Kane. For one thing, she had a couple of moles on one arm that would have shown up in the photos. For another, unless the photos were taken months ago, there wouldn't have been time for her hair to grow out."

"But you can't see her hair in the photos because of that hood," Ginny objected. Then she blinked. And blushed. "Oh. That hair."

Isabel smiled at her. "Why don't you go make a few copies of Tricia's note so we can bag the original. And then I really do think we all need to call it a day. Start fresh in the morning."

As soon as Ginny was out of the room, Isabel said to Rafe, "I'm going to go talk to her. Be right back."

"Okay."

"Did I miss something?" Mallory wondered when Isabel had gone.

"We'll be arresting Hank McBrayer," Rafe told her. "Assault charges filed by his daughter."

Mallory looked blank for a moment, then scowled. "Son of a bitch. I'd heard talk, but Ginny never said anything."

"Most victims of abuse don't," Hollis said. To Rafe, she asked, "Is Isabel going to try to convince her to stay in a hotel tonight?"

"She's going to try to convince her to let you two and a couple of officers go back to her house with a warrant for her father's arrest and get him out of there tonight."

"Can we do that?" Mallory asked.

"Yes. I called the judge from the car. The paperwork's almost ready."

Mallory was still frowning. "Why Isabel and Hollis? I mean, why not just send a couple of our officers? I'll volunteer. Since I hate bullies just on principle, I'd love to accidentally break McBrayer's arm while he's resisting arrest."

"So would I," Rafe said. "But it was Isabel and Hollis who realized what was going on and talked to Ginny about it, and Isabel and I both feel Ginny will be more comfortable if they're along for the arrest." He hesitated, then said, "Plus, I think Isabel has something else in mind."

Hollis looked at him. "Do you, now? Like what?"

"Assuming he's sober enough to listen, I think she intends to take him down a peg or two. Without laying a finger on him."

"If anybody can," Hollis said, "it's Isabel. Guys look at that beautiful face and centerfold body, all that blond hair, big green eyes all wide and innocent, and think they know exactly what she is. Boy, do they get a surprise."

"I certainly did," Rafe murmured.

"Speaking of which," Hollis said. "Are you?"

He didn't have to ask what she meant. "Apparently."

Hollis whistled. "Dunno whether to say congratulations or sorry about that."

"I'll let you know when I figure out how I feel about it."

Mallory said, "Hello? What's going on? Are you what?"

"Psychic."

284

She blinked. "You're psychic?"

"So I'm told."

"How could you be and not know?"

"The short answer," Hollis said, "is that he always was, but it was an inactive ability, so he wasn't aware of it. I think we talked about latents when we first got here. Rafe, as it turns out, was a latent. Something happened to activate his abilities."

"What?"

Hollis lifted her brows at Rafe.

"Damned if I know. She—I was told it could have been some kind of subconscious shock, which I suppose it had to be since I don't recall any consciously shocking or traumatic events in my life recently. Other than this killer."

"No bump on the head?" Hollis asked. "Concussion?"

"No," he said. "Never, in fact."

Mallory eyed him somewhat warily. "So what can you do?"

"Not a whole hell of a lot. Yet, anyway. The consensus seems to be I am—or will be—clairvoyant."

"Like Isabel? Just knowing stuff?"

"More or less."

"And that doesn't scare the shit out of you?"

"Did you hear me say it didn't?"

"No."

"Well, then."

Mallory leaned back in her chair, tipped her head back, and addressed the ceiling—and whatever lay beyond. "A few weeks ago, I led a perfectly ordinary existence. No killers. No spooky psychic abilities. Nothing on my mind more weighty than which kind of takeout I wanted for my supper. Those were the days. I'm sorry now I didn't appreciate them." She sighed and looked at the others. "I must be paying off karma for a really, really bad decision in a former life."

"*You* must be?" Rafe shook his head.

Isabel returned to the room before the discussion could continue, saying, "We have a slight change of plan. Hollis, we're going to swing by Ginny's on the way back to the inn and pick up her mother; both of them will be staying there tonight."

"Hank's out on the town?" Rafe guessed.

"Yeah. Seems he often spends Sunday afternoons and evenings drinking in an undisclosed location with others of . . . like temperament."

Rafe sighed. "Yeah, we have a few basement bars in the county. Unlicensed, unregulated, and highly mobile. They tend to change location more often than they wash the glasses."

"Well, apparently Mr. McBrayer has a semiregular habit of drinking all evening and passing out somewhere between the bar and home. Or at the bar, sometimes. In any case, he seldom makes it home on Sunday nights. But on the off chance that tonight would be one of those nights, I've persuaded Ginny to get her mother and come stay at the inn."

"I'll have all the patrols keep an eye out for him tonight," Rafe said. "If they don't spot him, we'll catch up with him tomorrow."

"Good, thanks." Isabel frowned slightly.

"I've also arranged to have all single female officers escorted home and their places checked out before they lock up for the night," Rafe said. "And each is under orders to wait for two male officers to meet them tomorrow morning, if they're on duty, to be escorted back here."

"You're reaching through again," Isabel said.

"I am?"

"I was just thinking about Mallory's report that some of the female officers feel they've been watched or followed and wondering what we should do to help protect those most likely to be at risk if it's our killer—the single ones in the right age range. Don't tell me you read that on my face. I may not be subtle, but I'm not a damned billboard."

Mallory looked at Hollis, who shrugged.

"They've got me, too, this time."

Rafe hesitated, then shrugged. "You looked worried; I wondered why; I knew."

Isabel frowned again. "Okay. Now I'm worried about something else."

Peculiarly enough, Rafe found this answer coming as easily as the one before had, just knowledge in his mind. "Sorry. Since neither one of us knows who the killer is, I don't have a solution for your worry."

"It was," Isabel said, "more fun being the clairvoyant one."

"Yeah, I can see how it would have been."

"You're enjoying this."

"Not all of it. Just . . . some of it."

"I know gloating when I see it. I don't need extra senses for that."

"Good thing too. Since yours are all boxed up, I mean."

Straightening her shoulders, Isabel said, "I'm leaving now. We're going to borrow a patrol to go with us just in case Hank McBrayer shows up unexpectedly while Ginny and her mother are packing overnight bags. If that's okay with you, of course."

"Fine," Rafe said, his tone as polite as hers.

"Great. We'll see you guys bright and early in the morning. Hollis?"

Her partner rose obediently and followed her from the room. As she passed Rafe, Hollis murmured, "You're a lot smarter than you look."

"Christ, I hope so," he responded, equally low.

When the two agents had gone, Mallory looked at Rafe. "Do you know what I'm worried about?"

He frowned at her. "No. Not a clue."

"So it only works with Isabel?"

"Apparently. So far, anyway."

"Um, then I'm worried about two things."

"What's the other thing?"

"We've now got an awful lot of people watching an awful lot of women while we try to anticipate this killer's next move; what worries me is that he may have changed the rules."

It was nearly midnight when Emily Brower's bedside phone rang, and she was more than half asleep when she fumbled hastily to answer it before it could wake her parents.

"Yeah. Hello?" She listened for several minutes, then said sleepily, "Okay, but—now? Why now? Yeah, I understand that, but— Right. Right, okay. Give me ten minutes."

She cradled the receiver, then pushed back her covers and sat up, muttering, "Shit, shit, shit."

It didn't take her more than a couple of minutes to exchange her sleep shirt for jeans and a T-shirt and slide her feet into a worn and comfortable pair of clogs.

Her parents slept like the dead, especially these days with the aid of various sedatives, so she didn't hesitate to leave her bedroom and walk down the lamplit hall, down the stairs, and out the front door, snagging her car keys from the foyer table.

She wasn't surprised not to see the customary patrol car parked across the street, since she'd heard it fire up its sirens and speed away sometime before her phone had rung. An accident somewhere, she assumed.

And, anyway, the reporters always left by dark or shortly after, so there was no good reason for the patrol car to stay out there all night. She'd meant to call the police station and ask the chief or one of the agents about it but kept forgetting.

Shrugging off the question, Emily got in her car and backed it out of the driveway. She knew the way, of course, and hadn't thought much about it until she was almost there. But by the time she parked her car off the side of the road and got out, she was beginning to feel more than a little uneasy.

She got a flashlight from the glove box and carried it to light her way, feeling a surge of relief when she reached the clearing and the light turned the shadowy outline of a person into someone she knew.

"I don't understand what I can show you out here," she said immediately. "And this is creepy, in case you hadn't realized it. We might not have been close, but still—this is where my sister was murdered."

"I know, Emily. She was quite a woman. Very intelligent. It's a pity you aren't."

"What?" Emily moved her hand, the flashlight's beam cutting through the hot, humid night. And that was when she saw the knife.

She tried to scream, but only her killer heard the bloody gurgle that emerged as she was nearly decapitated.

Monday, June 16, 7:00 AM

When the phone rang, he rolled over in bed and had the cordless receiver in his hand even before his eyes opened.

And even before his eyes opened, he smelled it.

"Yeah?"

"We've got another one, Chief." It was Mallory, her voice bleak.

Still holding the receiver to his ear with his left hand, he held out the right one and stared at it in the early-morning light streaming into his bedroom.

His hand was stained with blood.

"Where?" he asked.

"Isabel was right when she said he'd probably start taunting us. He used the same place. As far as I can tell from the report that came in, the victim is exactly where Jamie Brower died. I'm on my way there now."

"Who is it? Who's the victim?"

"It's Emily. Jamie's sister."

"Goddammit, where was the patrol watching her?" Rafe demanded, sitting up in bed.

"They were pulled away from her house last night at about eleven-thirty and were only away a couple of hours. A traffic accident with fatalities."

Rafe drew a breath and let it out slowly. "Which takes precedence over watchdog duty."

"Yeah. As per standing orders."

He shoved the covers away and got out of bed, heading for the bathroom. "Have you called Isabel?"

"Not yet. I only took the report instead of you because I went into the office a bit earlier than usual. I couldn't sleep past six, so I just came in."

"I thought I ordered you to accept an escort."

"You suggested, just like you suggested it for Stacy, the only other female detective in the department. We both passed. She's a black belt, and I can take care of myself. And neither one of us is a blonde. You want me to call Isabel?"

"Yeah. Have them meet us at the scene. I'm on my way."

"Right."

He turned off the phone and literally dropped it on the bathroom rug, immediately turning on the water and washing his hands in the hottest water he could stand.

Again.

Jesus Christ, again.

The gnawing fear that had been with him for so long was less acute this time, and he understood why. Because this morning he knew something he hadn't known all the other mornings.

This morning, he knew there was something new and unfamiliar going on in his brain, and it wasn't homicidal madness.

It was psychic ability.

You could be calling me rude names in your head or worrying about some deep dark secret you don't want anybody to know, and I wouldn't necessarily read that either.

Deep, dark secret. That's what it had been all this time, a secret fear buried so deep he had almost been able to forget about it during the bright, sane light of day. Almost.

He was no killer. He knew that. He *had* known that all along, even with the fear that something inside him might have been capable of such acts.

But if he was no killer, then why had he been waking up with blood on his hands for nearly three weeks?

Yesterday morning, he hadn't had a clue. This morning . . .

Rafe thought he was beginning to understand what was going on—though he only had a hunch as to why. And he thought he understood why his shield was so strong that it not only enclosed Isabel but also blocked her.

Gripping the sides of the sink, he stared into the mirror at his unshaven face and haunted eyes. "I have to be able to control this," he murmured.

Because he couldn't keep blocking Isabel, not even to keep her from knowing his secret fears, his self-doubts and uncertainties, all the demons a man carried inside him if he lived long enough and saw too much. In shutting that away from her, he had both shut her out and imprisoned her.

Imprisoned her abilities, the extra senses that could be all that was standing between her and a killer.

Isabel stood just inside the area blocked off with yellow crime-scene tape, her hands on her hips, grimly studying the clearing.

"Jesus, I don't know where to start," T.J. said as she and Dustin arrived with their crime-scene kits.

"Follow procedure," Isabel advised.

Eyeing the ME, who was examining the body, Dustin said, "Even Doc looks queasy. And he was a state medical examiner, until he got tired of the parade of bodies."

T.J. murmured, "Bet he's sorry he chose Hastings to finish out his professional life."

"I'm having second thoughts myself," Dustin told her.

"I know what you mean. Come on, let's get to work."

Hollis joined Isabel as the two technicians moved away, saying, "Sorry about that."

"Don't be. I lost my breakfast the first three times I was called to an early murder scene."

"I'll remember that. Next time. I thought I could handle something like this, especially after a couple of weeks of classes at the body farm. But, Christ . . ."

"Yeah, he made a real mess this time." Isabel half turned as Mallory joined them. "I'm betting her car's clean, though."

Mallory nodded. "Looks like it. It'll be towed back to the

station so T.J. and Dustin can go over it thoroughly, but the only difference I noticed is that she didn't leave her purse in it."

Isabel said, "If the doctor confirms that she died around midnight, then she'd have had to leave her house just after the patrol was called away for that accident. Maybe she left in a hurry and didn't even bring a purse."

"Had to be to meet someone," Hollis said. "You're a twenty-something blonde in a town where twenty-something blondes are being killed, including your own sister, and you go out alone near midnight? She was either very stupid or really trusted whoever she went to meet. Or both, if you ask me."

Isabel looked at Mallory. "When we were in her home, I didn't get any sense of a steady boyfriend."

"Far as I know, she didn't have one. Dated, but never anybody serious."

Hollis shook her head. "Who could she possibly trust enough to meet, around midnight, at the scene of her sister's murder?"

"And why?" Isabel mused, frowning. "The only reason I can think of is that someone must have told her she could help by coming out here so late. That there was something out here she needed to see, and after dark. If that's true, I can't see any possible answer as to who called her out here except—"

"—a cop," Mallory said. "Has to be."

Hollis looked around at the police technicians and the dozen or so uniformed officers searching the area surrounding the crime scene and in various positions between this clearing and the rest stop at the highway, which had also been roped off, and sighed. "Great. That's just great."

"We still can't rule out some other authority figure," Isabel reminded them. "For that matter, we can't rule out a member of the media. Who's to say some reporter didn't offer Emily a nice big chunk of cash to meet out here where her sister was killed? And being here well after dark was the only real guarantee a passing patrol wouldn't see them, since we've had all these areas under watch. Her car was well off the road and behind that thicket, so either the killer moved it there afterward or told Emily to park there to avoid being seen by a passing patrol."

"But a reporter? For a story?" Hollis said. "That's sick. Would Emily have gone for something like that?"

"To step out of Jamie's shadow? I'm thinking yes."

"That might explain this," Mallory said, "but what about the other victims? Could a reporter have lured them out of their cars and into the woods?"

Hollis said, "You know, maybe we're making a giant assumption that he does it the same way every time. He could be gearing his approach to each woman individually. Isabel, you and Bishop both believe he has to get to know his victims. Maybe this is why. To find the right bait for each catch."

Isabel looked at her for a moment, then said, "If you ever feel useless in an investigation, remember this moment. Damn. Why didn't I see that?"

Hollis was pleased, but nevertheless said, "You've had a lot on your plate."

"Still." Isabel took a step toward the body, then stopped and turned back. The other two women also turned to watch as Rafe approached them from the highway. He looked grim, and on a face as rugged as his, grim was an expression to make even the bravest soul take a step back.

Isabel met him halfway.

"Sorry I'm late," he said. "I got held up at the station."

"What else has happened?" she demanded, reaching out without thinking to touch his hand.

His fingers immediately twined with hers. "The accident that pulled the patrol away from the Brower house," he said. "There were two fatalities."

"I'd heard that much." She waited, knowing there was more.

"Hank McBrayer was one of them," Rafe said flatly. "He was driving too fast, drunk, and apparently crossed over the center line. Hit the oncoming car head-on. The other victim was a sixty-five-year-old grandmother."

"Jesus," Isabel said. "Poor Ginny. This is going to eat her alive."

"I know. I've got the department counselor with her and her mother now." He glanced past her at the taped-off crime-scene area.

"He was incredibly vicious this time," Isabel warned. "He cut her throat, probably first, and with enough force to nearly sever her head. And then he started to enjoy himself."

Without releasing her hand, Rafe continued toward the crime scene. "Has the doc offered his preliminary report yet?"

"No, but I think he's about to."

They ducked under the tape that Mallory and Hollis automatically held up for them.

"If nobody minds," Hollis said, "I think I'll stand right here. I've seen all I want to."

Nobody objected, and as they walked toward the body, Isabel murmured, "Hollis is dealing with her own guilt. She saw Jamie again, last night in the conference room, obviously desperately trying to say something."

"And Hollis couldn't hear her."

"No. At the end, Jamie was so frustrated she apparently focused enough energy to scare the hell out of Hollis by scattering half the paperwork on the table across the room."

Rafe looked at her, frowning. "I seem to remember you telling me something like that would be unusual."

"Oh, yeah. Jamie was a very strong lady. And she was trying very, very hard to communicate. She must have known her sister would be the next victim. Which is another indication to me that Emily knew something dangerous to the killer."

"You don't believe she was killed just because she fit the victim profile?"

"No. She was too young, I think. Not successful enough for his tastes. I also think she would have died no matter what color her hair was. Emily snooped in her sister's life, and it got her killed."

"And we still have a reporter missing."

"Who may also have found out something dangerous to the killer," Isabel said.

They stopped several feet from where Dr. James was still examining the body, and Rafe muttered an oath as he saw her up close for the first time.

Isabel didn't respond to that. Neither did Mallory. There wasn't much they could say.

Emily Brower lay sprawled out almost exactly as her sister had lain and almost exactly three weeks afterward. The slash across her throat was so deep the white vertebra of her neck was visible, and the gaping wound had literally drenched her in blood. Her once-pale T-shirt was soaked with it, and her blond hair lay in a pool of congealing blood and dirt.

"You were right about the escalation," Rafe said, his deep voice raspier than normal. "That son of a bitch. Sick, evil, twisted animal . . ."

The killer hadn't just murdered Emily, hadn't just repeatedly stabbed her breasts and genitals as he had the previous three victims. It looked as if he had stabbed her once in each breast—but had twisted and turned the knife as though trying to bore holes through her body.

And rather than stabbing her genitals through her clothing, he had pulled her jeans and panties down around her ankles, pulled her knees up and pushed them apart, and used the knife to rape her.

"If it helps," Isabel said, holding her voice steady, "she never felt that. Never knew about it."

"For her sake I'm glad," Rafe said. "But it doesn't help."

Dr. James straightened and came to join them, his face very, very tired. "Anything you need me to tell you that you can't see for yourself?" he asked wearily.

"Time of death?" Rafe asked.

"Midnight, give or take a few minutes. She died almost instantly with both the jugular and the windpipe slashed. Blood gushed like a fountain, the last few beats of her heart pumping it out as she fell. He didn't touch her face, but he used something heavy to crush her skull in two places once she was on the ground."

"Why?" Mallory wondered, baffled. "She was already dead, and he had to know it."

"Rage," Isabel and Rafe said in almost the same breath.

She added, "He had to make certain she couldn't see him. Couldn't see his sexual failure."

"He knew before he tried that he'd fail," Rafe said.

Isabel nodded. "He knew. Maybe he's always known."

The doctor looked at them rather curiously but continued with his report in a monotone. "She fell backward, and he didn't move her much. Spread her arms out to the sides, judging by the abrasions I found on the backs of her arms. Fanned her hair out and then pressed it into the pool of blood around her head. God knows why. I don't."

"What else?" Rafe asked.

"What you see. Did his best to gouge out her breasts, then

297

brutalized her with the knife. It was a big knife, and it did a lot of damage. If I had to guess, I'd say he drove it between her legs at least a dozen times."

"Excuse me," Mallory said in a very polite tone. She walked to the edge of the clearing, lifted the crime-scene tape and ducked underneath it, and took several steps beyond, then bent over and vomited.

"I plan to get drunk," Dr. James announced.

"I wish I could," Rafe said.

The doctor sighed. "I'll write up the preliminary report when I get back to the office, Rafe. You'll have the rest when I get her on the table. It's going to be a long day."

"Yeah. Thanks, Doc."

When the doctor walked away, Rafe said to Isabel, "I'm not getting anything but rage here, and just the vaguest sense of that, not even enough to be sure it isn't my imagination—or the training telling me to draw logical conclusions from what I'm seeing here. I don't know how to reach for anything more. You have to do it."

"I can't. I'm not getting anything either. Silence. Like you, I know he was furious from what I'm looking at, not from anything I hear or feel."

"We need more, Isabel."

"I know that."

"We have to stop him here and now. Before he goes after anybody else. Before he comes after you."

"I know that too."

You have to do her. The first chance you get, you have to do her.

He tried to ignore the voice, because it wasn't telling him anything he didn't already know. All it was doing was making his head hurt even more.

She knows. Or she will soon. And he's helping her know. Look at them. You understand what's happening, don't you?

"No," he whispered, because he didn't, he really didn't. All he knew was that his head hurt and his gut, and it had been so long since he'd slept that he'd forgotten what it felt like.

They're changing.

An icy jolt went through him. "No. I'm changing. You said. You promised. If I did it. If I killed them before they told. You promised."

Then you'd better do her. Kill her. Before they finish changing. Or it'll be too late. Too late for you. Too late for both of you.

17

IT WAS NEARLY NOON by the time T.J. and Dustin had done their work and the ME's people had removed Emily's body from the scene. The search of the area had produced nothing, not a scrap of anything that looked even remotely like evidence. There were still officers at the highway keeping the media and the curious away from the scene, but most of the other cops had returned to regular duties.

Isabel had spent the morning prowling the area, restless, watchful, making what she knew was a futile effort to reach through the barrier Rafe had created. To protect her.

She didn't think the irony was lost on either one of them.

"Anything?" Hollis asked as they studied the now empty crime scene.

"Nada. You?"

"No. And I am trying." Hollis shrugged. "But from what

you've said about her, I doubt Emily's is the sort of spirit we could expect to gather enough energy to come back. As for Jamie . . . I didn't hear her when it mattered."

"Don't beat yourself up about it. I'm not exactly firing on all cylinders myself."

"Is that why the watchdogs?" Hollis asked with a slight sideways movement of her head toward an area between them and the highway.

Isabel sighed. "The taller one is Pablo. The other one is Bobby."

"Pablo? In Hastings?"

"Struck me too. But, hey, melting pot."

"I guess." Hollis studied her partner. "So when Rafe went to break the news to Emily's parents, he left two of his uniforms watching you."

"They're not to let me out of their sight. I heard Rafe tell them so. He made damned sure I heard him tell them so."

"Well . . . you could be next, Isabel."

"I can't work hobbled," she said irritably.

"Then take the hobbles off," Hollis suggested mildly. "And I don't mean the watchdogs."

"Don't start spouting Bishop stuff at me, all right? I'm not in the mood. It's hot, it's humid, there's a storm building, and all I can smell is blood."

Hollis grimaced. "Yeah, I was going to ask—how do we turn the spider senses *off*?"

"We don't. Once you learn to enhance, the increased sensitivity is pretty much always with you. There are a few team members who have to focus and concentrate, but for most of us it's just there. Like raw nerves."

"That might have been mentioned *before* I was taught how to enhance."

"Talk to the boss, not me."

"You really are in a rotten mood, aren't you?"

Isabel pointed to the blood-soaked ground several yards away. "This should not have happened," she said. "I should have seen it coming."

"You did. You warned us Emily was a possible victim, and Rafe did everything he could to protect her. It's not your fault or his that a drunk caused a fatal traffic accident."

"That's not what I mean. I should have been . . . tuned in. I should have been listening. Instead, I did just what you said I did—I let Rafe take control. I let him build this shield around my abilities. I went from needing to have absolute control over everything in my life to just . . . handing it over to him. Why in God's name did I do that?"

"You didn't hand over all control. You just let him shut off your abilities."

"Why?"

"Maybe to find out if he could."

Isabel stared at her, baffled. "Okay, if that's Bishop stuff, it doesn't make sense. I mean even more than his stuff sometimes doesn't make sense."

"You're a strong woman, Isabel. You don't want to be dominated, but you *do* want to be matched, if only subconsciously. I think you felt Rafe reaching through this link you guys have, and I think you needed to know, before you decided whether to commit yourself, before you could take that leap of faith, just how strong he was."

"And now that I do know, O wise one?"

Hollis smiled faintly at what was only a token stab at mockery. "Now you know he matches you. He has as much strength of will as you, possibly as much psychic ability as you, and is certainly as stubborn as you."

"So?"

"So stop fighting him. You haven't said, but I'm willing to bet Paige told you that the two of you would have to work together to control his shield."

"Rookies," Isabel muttered.

"I'm right."

"Yeah."

"Then I'd say there's one last little bit of control you'll have to give up. You'll have to stop trying to control the relationship. To guide, or aim, or shape it—whatever it is you've been trying to do since the moment you met Rafe. If you'll forgive the cliché, we don't master love, it masters us. The more you struggle against it, the tighter those hobbles are going to be."

"This should not be about my relationship with him," Isabel said in a last-ditch effort. "Four women are dead in Hastings, five if you count Hope Tessneer, and more are missing. It can't all hinge on my love life, it just *can't*."

"Human relationships are at the heart of everything, you know that. You said yourself they were at the heart of this case. It's about relationships, you said."

"Maybe I didn't know what I was talking about."

"You knew. You know. Relationships matter, Isabel. History's been changed by them, armies toppled, societies rebuilt."

Isabel was silent, frowning toward the bloody ground.

"They have power. Human relationships have power. Family. Friends. Lovers. The closer and more intimate the relationship, the more power it can and does generate. Use that energy. And use it wisely."

"To break through Rafe's shield?"

"No. To make it your own."

———

"Got it?" Rafe asked, meeting up with Mallory in the bullpen at the station.

"Yeah, not that it's helpful. The call Emily received was from a pay phone in town. One of the few remaining pay phones in use."

"Doesn't miss a trick, our guy."

"No. I've got T.J. checking out the phone, but I'm betting she'll either find a million prints or none at all."

"I'll cover that bet. Come on, let's get back out to the scene."

"Isabel and Hollis still out there?"

He nodded, leading the way from the station. "Pablo and Bobby are keeping an eye on them."

"I'll bet Isabel loves that."

"Frankly, I don't give a shit how she feels about it at this point. She's a target, and I have a strong hunch she's next on his hit list."

Mallory looked at him curiously as they got into his Jeep. "Why?"

"Word's getting out. I've had at least two calls from media and one from the town council today asking if it's true we've got a psychic investigator working the case."

"Lovely."

"And the reporter who replaced Cheryl Bayne was one of those calls; he's looking to make a reputation for himself, and it's obvious. His predecessor missing and a psychic working the case? Sounds like a dandy story to him."

"He's going to broadcast that?"

"On today's six o'clock news, he says."

"Shit."

Rafe shrugged. "At this point, I don't think he'll report anything the killer doesn't already know. That's what worries me. If I were him, the killer, I'd go after Isabel, and I wouldn't wait a week to do it. I'm assuming he's thinking the same way."

Mallory sighed and said, "Safe assumption, probably. Plus, if Isabel's right and he really did kill Emily because she knew something rather than because she was one of *his* blondes, then he could have been—for want of a better word—unsatisfied by the murder."

Rafe muttered a curse under his breath and increased the Jeep's speed. He didn't say anything else until they reached the informal rest area and pulled off the highway. Ignoring the questions called out to him by several members of the media still braving the hot day hoping for a photo or a news bite, he headed toward the clearing, relaxing visibly when he saw Isabel and Hollis.

"The phone call?" Isabel asked as the two cops reached the agents.

"No joy," Mallory reported. "Pay phone."

"And there won't be prints," Isabel said with a sigh. "He's using gloves. Not latex, I think, which is odd."

"What do you mean?" Rafe asked.

"Well, latex gloves leave you with a much more tactile sense of what you're touching, you know that. And since they're form-fitting, they don't get in the way."

"No, I mean how do you know he isn't using latex gloves? We haven't found a sign either way at any of the crime scenes."

"I touched them," Isabel said slowly, surprised that she only now remembered that.

"Excuse me?" Mallory's voice was very polite.

Isabel realized she was being stared at, and shook her head. "Sorry. I forgot none of you had seen it here. Or even knew, I guess. I wonder why I forgot that part?"

"What part?" Rafe asked with visible patience.

"I told you that sometimes, rarely, my abilities manifest themselves physically in a vision. During one of those, I *am* the victim. I feel what he or she feels, and I usually come out of it covered in blood. Blood that fades away completely after a few minutes."

"I'd call that creepy," Mallory said.

"Yeah, it's not much fun." Isabel shrugged. "Anyway, what really brought me to Hastings is that I had a vision while Tricia Kane was being killed. I felt what she felt. And when he drove that knife into her chest for the last time before she died, her hands reached up to touch the knife—and touched his hands. He was wearing gloves. Not latex gloves, but thick leather gloves, like working gloves. His hands were big, or at least that was the sense I got."

"And you're just now telling us this?"

"I'm just now remembering." Isabel frowned. "I guess the voices crowded it out. Maybe that's one in the plus column for your shield."

Thunder rumbled just then, and they all glanced upward at the threatening sky.

Half under her breath, Hollis muttered, "Oh, God, I hate storms."

"We're about to have our crime scene washed away," Rafe noted. "Weather's calling for heavy rain today and tonight, with and without thunderstorms."

Isabel hesitated, looking at him. "I've tried," she said. "I've tried all morning to pick up something, and I can't. I can't break through the shield."

"Stop trying to break through it." He held out a hand to her. "Work with me, not against me."

"Rafe—"

"We don't have the luxury of time, not that we ever did. We can't afford to wait any longer. Like it or not, this is it."

"Should we leave?" Hollis asked, indicating herself and Mallory.

"No," Isabel said, then hesitated, recalling what had happened with Paige, and added, "But you might want to step back a little bit."

Both women did, watching the other two warily.

Slowly, Isabel reached out her own hand and felt the spark, felt his fingers closing around hers.

"I wish we had more time," Rafe told her. "I wish we had the luxury of dinners and movies, and hours of talking to each other about what matters to us. But the truth is, we don't have that time. We need every possible tool we can get our hands on—or our minds wrapped around—and we need it now."

"Yes. I know."

"You're next on his list. You know that too."

Isabel hesitated again, then nodded.

"Paige said we'd have to work together. That it would take both of us to figure out how to use this shield."

"Yes." Isabel looked at their hands for a moment, suddenly realizing something. "You're right-handed; I'm left-handed." Those were the hands clasping.

"Like closing a circuit," Rafe said slowly. "Or maybe . . . opening one. All this started when I held your wrists. Both of them."

"Alan, why on earth would I trust you?" Dana Earley demanded.

"Because you want a good story, you want to find out what happened to Cheryl Bayne, and you don't want to be the next blonde on the menu." He paused. "Probably in that order."

Dana didn't bother to be indignant. "So you found out that I have police sources in Alabama you want me to tap, and in

307

exchange you'll share information you got from your own sources in Florida."

"Yes. Look, you're TV and I'm newspaper; if we work this right we can both be heroes."

"Or one of us could be dead. Like me. Alan, if Cheryl is dead it has to be because she got too close. I'm not so sure I want to get too close to this guy, story or no story."

"Which," Alan said, "is why we have to move fast."

"Jesus. I know I'm going to regret this."

Isabel turned slightly so that they were facing each other, glanced down at the bloody ground where the horribly mutilated body of a young woman she had both liked and felt sorry for had so recently lain, and her mouth firmed. "We should be somewhere else," she said.

"No."

She looked at Rafe.

"We should be here. We need to be here, Isabel."

"Why?"

"Because two women died here. Because evil did what it wanted to do, needed to do, here."

The sound of thunder grew louder, more ominous.

"It's disrespectful. Let the rain wash away her blood."

"That isn't the investigator talking," he said.

Isabel smiled wryly. "No. It isn't. I liked her, you know. She felt isolated and misunderstood—and I could relate. I'm sorry she's dead."

"I know. So am I. But the only thing we can do for her now is stop her killer before he does that to someone else."

Before he does it to you.

Isabel could almost hear his words in her head. Or maybe she did hear them. Whichever it was, she knew he was right. "Yes," she said.

"The universe put us *here*. And it put us here, and now, for a reason. Remember what you told me? We leave footprints when we pass. Skin cells, stray hairs. And energy. He left his energy here, and recently. He left his hate, and his anger, and the stamp of his evil."

There was a flash in the distance, and Isabel said, almost to herself and with a touch of fear in her voice, "I can smell it. But it's lightning, not brimstone."

His fingers tightened around hers. "Is it? You said you had to face it this time. Confront it this time. That ugly face evil always hides behind something else. You have to face it. But, Isabel, you won't do it alone. Not this time. Not ever again."

She drew a breath and let it out slowly. "I didn't expect that. I'm not quite sure how to deal with that."

"The same way you deal with everything else," he said, smiling faintly. "Head-on."

"Before the storm gets here."

He nodded. "Before the storm. Before the rain washes away the blood, and the lightning changes the energy here. The energy in this place—his and ours, even anything left of hers—is what we need to help us take the next step. There's nothing disrespectful about that. It's doing our job. It's fighting evil the only way we can."

"How do you know so much?"

"I've been paying attention."

Isabel hesitated only another instant, then held out her right hand. "Okay. Let's see where the next step takes us."

He put his left hand into her right one.

Hollis said, at the time and long afterward, that there should have been something, some outward sign, to indicate what turned out to be a most astonishing event. But, outwardly at least, there was nothing. Just two people facing each other, holding hands, their faces calm but eyes curiously intent.

Mallory took a step closer to Hollis, murmuring, "I get the feeling I've missed something important."

"Beats the hell out of me," Hollis told her. "I mean, I know it has to do with this shield of Rafe's, but I have no idea what they're trying to do about it."

"Get rid of it, maybe?"

"No, from what Isabel told me, that would probably not be such a good idea."

"Why not? I mean, if it's blocking her voices?"

"I don't know. She said something about their combined energy being too strong, especially now when it's new and not under their control. That bad things could happen if they just . . . let go of it."

Mallory sighed. "I long for the days when all we had to deal with was trace evidence, footprints, the occasional half-blind or very stoned eyewitness . . ."

"Yeah, I imagine that was easier. Or simpler, at least."

"I'll say."

After several minutes of silence except for the growing intensity of the thunder rumbling overhead, Hollis ventured a step closer to Isabel and Rafe. "Well?"

"Well, what?" Isabel asked in perfect calm without turning her head.

"What's happening?"

"Good question."

Hollis looked at Mallory, then back at the other two. "Guys, come on. People are beginning to stare. Pablo and Bobby look real nervous. Or real embarrassed, I'm not sure which. What's happening?"

310

After a moment, Isabel turned her head to look at Hollis. "I don't want to sound like a country song, but I can feel his heart beating."

"I know she didn't eat breakfast," Rafe said, also looking at Hollis.

"And he's uneasy because—" Isabel turned her head abruptly to stare at Rafe. "Jesus, why didn't you tell me?"

"You know damned well why I didn't tell you," he replied, meeting her gaze.

"It was your abilities manifesting themselves physically. Which, remember, is a rare thing but not unheard of. In your case, probably caused by guilt because you believed you should have stopped him after the first murder. The blood of the innocent, literally on your hands."

"I realize that. Now. Before we talked yesterday, the possibilities were a lot more creepy."

"So that's why you were blocking me. That was the part of you I couldn't get at?"

"I'm guessing yes. Isabel, I was waking up with blood on my hands every morning and had no idea where it had come from. Women were dead. Other women were missing. You were offering me theories of a serial killer who could be walking around most of the time not knowing he was a murderer. So I was afraid I was blacking out."

"And killing blondes? I could have told you there wasn't a chance in hell of you doing that."

"Well, I was . . . afraid to ask."

"*Guys,*" Hollis's voice was just this side of strident.

Isabel looked at her partner, frowned slightly, and then let go of Rafe's hands. "Oh. Sorry. We were . . . somewhere else."

"I noticed. Where were you?"

"In a galaxy far, far away," Rafe murmured.

"You really are beginning to talk like me," Isabel told him.

"I know. Spooky, isn't it?" He took her arm and guided her toward the yellow crime-scene tape on the highway side of the clearing. "I say we head back to the station before the heavens open up."

Hollis and Mallory went with them, wearing almost identical expressions of baffled interest.

"Blood on your hands?" Mallory said to Rafe. "You were waking up with blood on your hands?"

"Yeah, for the past few weeks."

Hollis muttered, "Man, have you got a great poker face." And waited until they were outside the crime scene to add, "If somebody doesn't tell me, right now, what's going on—"

"I'm not so sure I can." Isabel shook her head. "All I really know is that everything's different."

"Different how?"

"The voices are back. But . . . very, very quiet. Distant."

"What about Rafe's shield?"

"It's still there. Here. I think we punched a couple of holes in it, though. I told you I wasn't sure I could explain."

"And I should have listened," Hollis said.

Addressing his patrolmen, Rafe said, "You two can take your lunch break and then head back to the station; unless you hear otherwise, follow your assignments on the board for the rest of the day."

"Right, Chief."

"Yes, sir."

"No watchdogs?" Isabel asked.

"I'm your watchdog," he replied. "Mallory, if you'll ride back with Hollis?"

"Sure."

By the time they reached the parked vehicles, they saw that the media had vanished, along with any curious passersby.

Isabel said, "Did the weather happen to mention that the storms today and tonight could be mean ones? The sort to keep golfers off courses and reporters with electronic equipment indoors?"

Rafe nodded. "We're not in the Southeast's tornado alley, but close enough."

Isabel didn't say anything else until they were in the Jeep heading back to town, and then her voice was tentative. "Back there at the scene when we . . . did whatever it is we did, I got a flash of something. That box. The box of photographs. We have to find it. The answer is in there, I know it."

"If it's in a bank under an assumed name—"

"I don't think it is. I think we've missed something."

Rafe frowned as thunder boomed again. "We've checked all the properties she owned."

"Have we?" Isabel turned in her seat to look at him. "Jamie had a secret life. A secret self. And she hid her secrets very, very well. What if, once Hope Tessneer died, Jamie decided to bury all the secrets for good?"

"We found her playhouse," Rafe reminded her.

"Yeah, but Jamie didn't count on dying herself. I think if she'd been granted just a little more time, we wouldn't have found anything but an empty storage building there. And nothing at all of her secret life."

"Wouldn't she just have burned everything? I mean, if she had wanted to destroy the evidence of that other life."

"She didn't want to destroy it. Destroy the strongest part of herself? No way. It would have been like cutting off her arm, or worse. She wanted to bury it. To put it where nobody but she would ever find it. Look, when Hope's body turned up missing—and I'm still convinced the killer took it from wherever Jamie had put it—she had to know someone else knew about the death. She had to be afraid that at best the body would turn up and it would be traced back to her, or—possibly worse from her point of view—that someone could be planning blackmail."

"So," Rafe said, "she would have wanted to remove any possible evidence of their relationship."

"Of all her secret relationships. If we found one, we'd find them all; that's what she would have thought. So she started to move, and fast. Listed her properties for sale, maybe started shifting money she wasn't supposed to have, between accounts we weren't supposed to know about."

"We've got people checking area banks today."

"Maybe they'll at least find evidence of those secret accounts. But I don't think they'll find the box. I think Jamie was planning to leave this place, or at least go on a long vacation somewhere until Hope's body turned up and she could determine whether she was going to be suspected of murder."

"And spent the final days of her life trying to erase or hide all the secrets," Rafe said.

"Exactly. I think she found or created a place to bury the Mistress for Hire. The box of photos went there right away, especially since she must have suspected Emily of snooping. The stuff in her playhouse would have followed, but the killer got to her first."

"Okay," Rafe said. "I'll buy the theory. But how do we find out where this hiding place is? We've tapped every source we have, short of going door to door and asking every soul in Hastings. What else can we do?"

Isabel drew a deep breath. "We ask the one soul who knows."

The heavens took their own time in opening up. By three that afternoon, it was twilight, with a hot wind blowing gustily and thunder rolling as though it had miles and miles to go. Flashes of lightning provided eerie strobelike images of very little traffic on Main Street, and clusters of media camped all around the town hall across from the police station. Print media, at any rate; most of those with electronics to consider had, as Isabel predicted, wisely chosen to remain indoors.

"You can feel the nerves," Mallory said, gazing out the window of the conference room. "Even the reporters. I don't have any extra senses, and I can feel it."

"Extra senses make it worse," Hollis told her. She was sitting at the conference table, both elbows propped on it and her hands cupping her face. "My head is throbbing in the weirdest way." She yawned as if to clear her ears. "And I feel like I'm going up in a plane."

"Not the best time to try a séance, I guess."

"God, don't call it that."

"Isn't that what it is? Technically, I mean."

"I don't know, but I can't help feeling a stormy afternoon spent summoning the dead just can't be a good plan."

"We're not doing it in a haunted house."

"Oh, goodie, one for the plus column." Hollis sighed.

Mallory turned her back on the window and half sat on the sill, smiling faintly. "You two are unconventional investigators, I'll give you that much. But, then, this hasn't exactly been a conventional series of murders. If there is such a thing."

Before Hollis could respond, Travis rapped on the open door and said, "Hey, Mallory, Alan Moore is here. He says it's important, and since the chief and Agent Adams are out in the garage with T.J.—"

"Send him in. Thanks, Travis."

Since the bulletin boards were already covered, neither woman had to move, and Mallory remained at the window as Alan came in. She said, "The chief of police has no comment for the media. Didn't you hear him on the front steps a couple of hours ago, Alan?"

"I did," he replied imperturbably. "Which is why I went back to my office. Where I received two bits of news I thought I'd be gracious enough to share with the police."

"I think he rehearsed that," Hollis said to Mallory.

"Probably." Mallory frowned at him. "The news?"

"First, Kate Murphy called a friend who happens to work at the paper. Seems she left town in a hurry—and on a bus—because she got a threatening call from an ex-lover and panicked. Especially with blondes getting killed in Hastings."

Mallory said, "We haven't found a sign of a lover in her past, and we've looked."

"Yeah, but this is about ten years ex. Even she admits the panic was somewhat extreme."

"Sounds like it," Hollis murmured. "Not that I can really blame her."

"Anyway, she's safe," Alan said. "She claims she left a note for her store's assistant manager but hadn't had a chance to call until today. I think she's about four states away, but she refused to say where."

Mallory shook her head. "One less on the list, thank God. And thank you for sharing. What's your other bit of news?"

"This." He produced a folded paper from his pocket and unfolded it on the conference table. "Probably no prints other than mine, since there weren't any on the last one."

"Envelope?" Mallory asked.

He pulled that out of a different pocket. "I figured it'd be worthless for prints, too, considering how many people handled it. The postmark is Hastings. Mailed Saturday."

Hollis leaned a bit sideways to read the note, brows lifting. "Well, well."

Mallory joined them at the table to study the message. Like the previous note to Alan, it was block-printed yet virtually scrawled in a bold, dark hand on the unlined paper.

THEY WERE GOING TO TELL.
HE KNEW THEY WERE GOING TO TELL.
THEY WEREN'T WORTHY OF OUR TRUST.
NEITHER IS SHE.
NEITHER IS ISABEL.

18

DUSTIN FOUND IT," T.J. reported. "He knows cars better than I do. Since it's a guy thing and all."

Rafe said, "So the cruise control was engaged. McBrayer was drunk; he could have done it accidentally."

"Dustin says he couldn't have. Something about the way the cruise button is on the wheel. Of course, the wheel is mangled as hell right now, but he swears it's a safety issue or something."

Isabel straightened after looking into what was left of Hank McBrayer's car, and said, "Dustin thinks somebody else set the cruise control?"

T.J. shrugged. "I admit I thought it was pretty far out. But we checked the rear end of the car, which is mostly intact, and found signs of a jack. Lift the rear wheels off the ground, put it in gear and push the accelerate button on the wheel, set the cruise control, and, when you're ready, shove the car off the jack. The marks on the car are consistent."

"There would have been tread marks on the road at the point it came off the jack," Rafe said.

"Dustin's out now, backtracking from the scene of the so-called accident. We also found a bit of rope on the front floorboard. I'm thinking it was used to tie off the steering wheel to keep the car going in a straight line. And if that's not enough, I'm pretty sure the headlights were off." She shook her head. "A nice, neat little way to kill somebody. With McBrayer reeking of alcohol and enough in his blood to knock out a squad of marines, who would suspect it was anything but an accident?"

"Good work," Rafe told her. "You and Dustin."

"Thanks. I'll tell him you said so. And I'll send up the report when he gets back and I finish up with the car."

As they left the basement garage of the police station and headed upstairs to the offices, Isabel said, "A diversion. That *accident* happened only a couple of miles from the Brower house; the patrol on watch outside would have been the closest squad car."

"I wonder if he aimed McBrayer's car at one he could see coming or just trusted to luck he'd hit something or someone eventually?"

"I don't think our boy trusts much to luck," she said. "Finds a dark, straight stretch of road in a little-frequented area, sets up the car with McBrayer passed out inside. And waits until he sees headlights. By the time the other driver even saw the car coming at her, it was too late."

"The pay phone he called Emily from was only a few blocks from the scene of the—accident. He probably waited for the patrol car to pass him, then called her."

"I have the feeling that killing two more people just so he

could lure Emily out was another of his taunts: *Look at me, look how clever I am.*"

"You don't think it was a personal grudge against McBrayer?"

"No, I think he was convenient. From what I got talking to Ginny last night, her father's Sunday-night binges were hardly a secret around here. The killer found McBrayer, maybe even followed him to one of those basement bars you talked about. Then all he had to do was wait for his mark to pass out or be thrown out."

"And use him as a tool to get what he wanted. Emily." Rafe grasped her arm to stop her as they entered the hallway leading to the conference room. "Tell me something. Truthfully."

"Sure, if I can."

"He'll come after you next."

"Maybe. Probably. Especially if the news breaks that I'm psychic. He'd view that as an increased threat, I think."

"Will he wait a week?"

Isabel hesitated, then shook her head. "I'd be surprised if he did. Emily was damage control; she knew something he didn't want her to tell. Or at least he believed she did. I'm guessing something about that box of photographs."

"But you he wants."

"Even without the psychic nudge, yeah. Me and the last blonde on his list, whoever she is. And he's moving faster, getting sloppy. We shouldn't have found jack marks on that car, far less a bit of rope that didn't belong in it. He's feeling pressure, a lot of it. Whatever is driving him is driving him hard."

Rafe hesitated, but they were alone, and he finally said, "Whatever happened earlier did open up the shield for you, didn't it?"

"A bit. But the voices are still distant." She looked at him steadily. "There's still a part of you I can't get at."

"I trust you," he said.

"I know. You just don't trust you."

He shook his head. "I don't get it."

Isabel had to smile. "I'm not surprised. See, I think I figured out something. We both have control issues and we both know it. The difference is, I don't trust someone else to run the show, and you don't trust yourself to."

"That's a control issue?"

"Yes. I have to learn to let go, to trust someone else without giving up who I am. And you have to learn to trust yourself in order to be who you need to be."

Somewhat cautiously, Rafe said, "Are you channeling this Bishop of yours?"

"I know how it sounds, believe me. Why do you think I've been fighting this so hard? But the truth is, neither one of us has enough faith in ourselves."

"Isabel, that sounds to me like something that will take time to get itself resolved. We don't have time."

Isabel began moving down the hallway toward the conference room. "No, we don't. Which is why we'll have to take care of our issues on the fly."

"I was afraid you were going to say that."

"Don't worry. If there's anything I've learned in the last few years it's that we can make giant leaps when we have to."

"That's the part that worries me," Rafe said. "Why we might have to."

"Alan, I don't have time for this," Mallory told him as they stood just inside the foyer of the police department.

"Make time," he insisted. "Look, Mal, I know you don't want us publicly linked, but I've been doing some digging, and there's something you need to know."

Warily, she said, "About the case? Then why tell just me?"

"Call it a good-faith gesture. I could have put it in today's paper, but I didn't."

After a moment, she said, "I'm listening."

"I know there were two other sets of murders, one five and one ten years ago, in two other states."

"How did you—"

"I have sources. Never mind that. I also know that the FBI has sent investigators back to those towns to ask more questions."

Mallory hesitated, then said grudgingly, "We don't have the reports yet."

"There hasn't been time, I know. But one of my sources had occasion to talk to an investigator from the second series of murders."

"'Had occasion'? Alan—"

"Just listen. The investigator said there was something about the first murder that bugged him. It was just a little thing, so minor he didn't even put it in any of his reports. It was an earring."

"What?"

"They'd found her body out in the open, of course, the way all the others would be found. But the investigator checked out her apartment. And when he searched her bedroom, he found an earring on her dresser. Never found a match for it."

"So? Women lose earrings all the time, Alan."

"Yeah, I know. But what bugged the investigator was that the victim didn't wear earrings. She didn't have pierced ears."

Mallory shrugged. "Then a friend must have lost it."

"None of her friends claimed it. Not one. A valuable diamond earring, and nobody claimed it. It was an unanswered question, and it bugged him, has ever since."

Patiently, she said, "Okay, he found an earring he could never explain. How do you expect that to help us?"

"It's a hunch, Mal, and I wanted to let you know I was following it up. I've already talked to a friend of the second victim in Florida, and she claims to have found a single earring among her friend's things. I have somebody checking out the Alabama murders too. I think it has something to do with how he got the women to meet him."

"Alan—"

"I'm going to check it out. I'll let you know if I find anything."

Mallory thought he said something else, but a crash of thunder made it impossible to hear whatever it was, and a moment later he was gone.

She stared after him.

4:00 PM

"It's no use," Hollis said finally. "I don't know if it's the storm or me, but I just can't concentrate. And the energy of you two is not helping. If anything, it's hurting."

"We were with you the first time you saw Jamie," Isabel reminded her. "Right here in this room."

"Yeah, but it was before you two started seriously sparking," Hollis reminded her.

"Just tell me we don't have to hold hands or light candles," Mallory begged, pulling another folder toward her and looking through it with a frown.

Hollis shook her head. "What I'm telling you is that if Jamie is hovering anywhere around a doorway, it isn't mine. Or I can't open the door. Either way, it's not going to happen today."

Rafe leaned back in his chair, saying, "Look, there has to be another way to do this. Plain, old-fashioned police work. If Jamie had a secret place, there has to be a way for us to find it."

Hollis said, "And we need to do it before the six o'clock news. But no pressure."

Mallory said, "Reports coming in from all area banks have been negative. Nobody has recognized Jamie's photo or her name, and there's no way for us to guess what alias she might have used. If she's been socking away money for years with her little S&M sideline, she's had plenty of time to construct a really solid one we may never find. And I can't find anything about stray or missing jewelry, so I think Alan's off track with that one."

"It's that note I don't like," Rafe said.

"It doesn't change anything," Isabel said. "We knew I was on his list."

She pulled the note toward her and frowned down at it. "Our trust. They weren't worthy of *our* trust."

"Maybe he really is schizophrenic," Mallory said.

"Yeah, but even so, the first note made a clear distinction. *He* wasn't killing them because they were blondes. This note links the one who wrote the note and the killer. They weren't worthy of *our* trust. If he's schizophrenic, then I'd say he's on the edge of a major identity crisis."

"He didn't have one before?" Hollis murmured.

"I don't think he knew he had one. I mean, I think there was a part of him listening to whatever it was urging him to kill, and another part of him that had no idea that was happening."

"A split personality?" Hollis asked.

"Maybe. They're a lot more rare than people realize, but it is possible that's what we have in this case. One part of his mind, the sane part, may have been in control most of the time."

"And now?" Rafe asked.

"Now," Isabel said, "I think the sane part of his mind is getting lost, submerged. I think he's losing control."

"It's all about control."

"No, it's all about relationships. It's still all about relationships. Look at this note. He believes these women have violated—or, in my case, will violate—his trust. There's a secret he's protecting, and he's convinced the women he kills threaten to expose that secret."

"So they know him."

"He thinks they do."

Rafe looked at Isabel steadily. "Then he thinks you know him."

"I think I do too."

The looming storm only fed their sense of urgency, at least in part because it seemed to surround them all day long without actually hitting Hastings. Tree limbs were blown around, power crews were kept busy repairing downed electrical lines, and thunder boomed and rolled while lightning flashed in the weird twilight.

It was as if the whole world was on the verge of something, hesitating, waiting.

By five o'clock that afternoon, they had paperwork scattered across the conference table, pinned to the bulletin boards, and stacked on two of the chairs. Forensics reports, background checks on the victims, statements from everyone involved, and postmortems complete with photographs.

And still they didn't have the answers they needed.

When Travis came in with the last batch of reports from area banks, Mallory groaned. "Christ, not more paper."

"And not even helpful," he told her as he handed the notes to Rafe, then leaned his hands on the back of an unoccupied chair. "Nobody recognized the name or photograph of Jamie Brower—except to say they'd seen her picture in the newspapers and on TV."

Isabel waited out another rumble of thunder, then said, "We need a fresh mind. Travis, if you wanted to bury a secret someplace you could be sure it wouldn't be found, where would you put it?"

"In a grave." He realized he was being stared at, and straightened self-consciously. "Well, I would. Once somebody's buried, they're not often dug back up. So why not? It'd be easy enough to strip the turf off a grave, bury whatever it was I was trying to hide between the surface and the casket—assuming it was the right size—then cover it back up and re-lay the grass. As long as I was careful, nobody'd even notice."

"Son of a bitch," Rafe said.

Isabel was shaking her head. "Why isn't he a detective?"

Travis brightened. "I was right?"

"God knows," Hollis said, "but you're sending us in a new direction, so I say good for you."

"Hey, cool." Then his smile faded. "We got lots of cemeteries in Hastings. Where do we start looking? And what're we looking for, by the way?"

"We're looking for a box of photos," Rafe said, feeling the younger cop had earned the knowledge.

Isabel added, "And it has to be connected with Jamie Brower. We need to know where any deceased family or friends are buried."

"I'll go back to my phone," Travis said with a sigh. "Start calling all the local clergy and asking them. I do *not* want to have to call the Browers directly, not today. Or tomorrow, or next week."

"Yeah, let's avoid that if possible," Rafe told him.

When he'd gone, Isabel said, "You really should promote him."

"He was on my short list," Rafe said. "The only reason I've hesitated is because he's currently sleeping with a reporter who isn't quite what she appears to be."

Hollis asked, "What is she?"

"According to my sources, she works for the governor's office, and is sent in quietly during tricky investigations to keep an eye on local law enforcement. So we don't do anything to embarrass ourselves. Or the state attorney general. They're keeping a very close eye on this investigation."

"That shows a distressing lack of faith," Isabel said, but without surprise.

Mallory was looking at Rafe with lifted brows. "You know that for a fact."

"Yes," he replied with a faint smile. "I keep a fairly close eye on my people."

Mallory stared at him, then said, "Oh, don't tell me."

"You and Isabel have something in common. Neither one of you is as subtle as you think you are."

"I resent that," Isabel said.

"Besides," Hollis said, "Alan Moore is the one who isn't subtle. Even I picked up on it."

Mallory got to her feet with great dignity. "Being outnumbered by psychics is hardly fair. I'm going to use the computer in the other room. Excuse me."

"I think we pissed her off," Hollis said absently as she opened the local phone book to begin making a list of churches and cemeteries.

"She'll get over it." Rafe shook his head. "Although I don't know if Alan will. Never seen him fall so hard before."

Isabel pursed her lips thoughtfully. "Mallory doesn't strike me as the settling-down type."

"I don't think she is. I also don't think Alan has realized that yet."

"It's always about relationships," Hollis murmured, with a sidelong glance at Isabel.

Ignoring the glance, Isabel said, "We need to go back through every piece of paper associated in any way with Jamie's life and death and check out the names of all family and friends."

"Chicken," Hollis said.

"We have more imperative things to think about," Isabel told her. "Like finding that grave."

Rafe said, "You think it's there, don't you? You think Jamie buried that box in somebody's grave?"

"I think it makes sense. She was burying a part of her life, so why not put it in a grave? And I'm betting it won't be a family grave, but the grave of someone else who was important to her. A teacher, a mentor, a friend. Maybe her first lover."

"Male or female?"

"At a guess, female."

"That does help narrow the field."

"Let's hope it narrows it enough."

Of all the family and friends who had died during Jamie's life, Isabel considered three women the most likely candidates for Jamie's burial of her secrets. One was a former teacher that friends reported Jamie had seemed especially close to, one was a close friend from high school who had been killed in a highway accident, and the third was a woman who had worked in Jamie's office, dying young of cancer.

Three women, three cemeteries.

"I think we should check these out before the storm breaks," Isabel told Rafe.

Rafe wanted to argue, but he was reluctant to put off doing anything that could help them catch the killer before he took aim at his next target. Isabel.

And before the press took aim at her.

"It'll be faster if we split up," she was saying. Since she had already told him privately that she wanted to stick close to Hollis because her partner seemed to be so affected by the tension of the storm, Rafe didn't object when she added, "Hollis and I will take Rosemont."

"You'll also take Dean Emery," he added. "There's only one entrance to Rosemont, and it's fenced; he can stand by at the entrance while you two find the grave. Mallory can take Travis along to Sunset."

"And who will you take to Grogan's Creek?" Isabel asked politely.

"I might take the mayor," he answered wryly. "I need to stop and see him before he blows a fuse."

Mallory said, "We're doing all this on the way home, right? Because I'm beat."

Rafe nodded. "Check out the cemeteries, phone in reports—once you're out of the storm, that is—and then head home."

"Got my vote," Isabel said.

Twenty minutes later, Hollis was saying, "You had to pick the largest cemetery, didn't you? The one with all the tall monuments and acres of graves."

"And don't forget the pretty little chapel with the stained-glass windows," Isabel reminded, raising her voice a bit as the wind tended to snatch at it.

"I just wish the place had a caretaker on duty to point out Susan Andrews's grave," Hollis said, pausing to squint at a headstone. "Because unless . . ."

"Unless what?" Isabel asked, half turning to look at her partner.

Hollis would have answered, but she was hardly aware of

Isabel in that moment. The sounds of the wind and the thunder had retreated into that peculiar hollow almost-silence. Her skin was tingling. The fine hairs on her body were stirring. And in the strobe flashes of the lightning, she could see Jamie Brower several yards away, beckoning.

"This way," Hollis said.

Isabel followed her. "How do you know?" she demanded, raising her voice again to be heard over the rising wind.

"It's Jamie." Hollis nearly stopped, then hurried forward. "Dammit, it *was* her. But I don't see her now."

"Where was she?"

"Somewhere in this area." Hollis jumped as thunder crashed, feeling her skin literally crawl. "Have I mentioned how much I hate storms?"

"You might have, yeah. This area? We'll find it." Isabel paused as thunder boomed, and added, "Unless we get struck by lightning, that is. I just think we need to do this now. And if you saw Jamie, that makes it even more imperative, I'd say."

Hollis didn't argue, just began checking the headstones in the area, flinching with every crack of thunder and flash of lightning. "I hate this," she called to her partner. "I really hate—"

"Here." Isabel knelt by a simple headstone with the name *Susan Andrews* engraved on it.

"It doesn't look disturbed," Hollis said, then swore under her breath as Isabel dug her fingernails into the turf and neatly lifted a perfectly square section.

"You'd think it would have rooted by now," Isabel said, folding back the turf. "It's tight, but not that difficult to pull up."

Hollis knelt on the other side of the grave to help. "A very neat section just at the headstone. Now I'm glad we brought the shovel Dean had in the cruiser's trunk."

"I'm an optimist," Isabel said, unfolding the small emergency shovel.

Hollis sat back on her heels suddenly. "You knew we'd find it, didn't you?"

"I had a hunch."

"You heard a voice."

"A whisper. Help me dig."

"We should call Dean," Hollis said, but it was only a minute or two before the shovel scraped across something metallic and they were able to drag a small box about twelve inches square and five or six inches deep from its resting place at Susan Andrews's headstone.

"I think we'd better take this back to the station to open it," Isabel said, the reluctance in her tone clear despite the gusty wind and rumbles of thunder.

"You just forgot to bring your lock-pick tools," Hollis said, a little amused. "Need help carrying that?"

"No, I've got it. You get the shovel, will you, please?"

As they started back across the cemetery, Isabel carrying the box and Hollis the shovel, the latter stopped suddenly.

"Shit."

Isabel stopped as well, following her partner's gaze. "What? I don't see anything."

"Jamie. She's—"

At first Isabel thought the rumble of thunder had drowned out whatever Hollis had been saying, but then she felt a sharp tug at the small of her back and whirled, instinctively dropping the metal box, filled with the sudden cold certainty that she had been blindsided again.

A flash of lightning brilliantly lit the scene before her. Hollis falling on the ground with blood blossoming on the back of her pale blouse. Mallory standing hardly more than an arm's length from Isabel, a big, bloodstained knife in one black-gloved hand and Isabel's gun in the other.

"You know," she said, "I'm really surprised you didn't pick up on it. All those vaunted psychic abilities, yours and hers. And Rafe's, I suppose. It was so clear, and none of you saw it. None of you saw me."

Rafe was able to soothe the mayor's worries, but just barely enough to allow his own escape. He headed toward Grogan's Creek church and the cemetery behind it, a name neatly printed on a piece of paper tucked in his pocket.

But when he reached a stop sign, he found himself hesitating, looking not east toward Grogan's Creek, but west toward Rosemont.

There was no reason to worry, of course. She could take care of herself. Besides which, she wasn't alone. Hollis was with her, and Dean.

He started to turn the wheel toward the east, then hesitated again. "She's okay," he heard himself say aloud. "She's fine."

Except that his gut said she wasn't.

His gut—and the blood on his hands.

Rafe stared at the reddish stains, shocked for an instant because it had happened so suddenly.

But then, just as suddenly, he knew the truth. He understood what it meant.

And he knew Isabel was in deadly danger.

He turned the wheel hard, heading west, and reached for his phone to call Dean.

19

MALLORY—"

"You still don't get it, do you? Mallory doesn't live here anymore."

Gazing into eyes that looked dead and empty even when the lightning flashed in them, Isabel fought to keep her voice calm. "So who are you?"

With an amused little chuckle, Mallory said, "This isn't some split-personality deal, you know. That's a bunch of bullshit, what you read in the books. I was always the stronger one. Always the one who had to take care of Mallory, clean the messes after she screwed up. Always. We were just twelve when it happened the first time."

"When what happened?" Was Hollis alive? Isabel couldn't tell. And what had happened to Dean?

"When I had to kill them. Those bitches. All six of them."

"You were— Why? Why did you have to kill them?"

"Are you stalling?" Mallory asked, interested. "Because Rafe isn't coming, you know. Nobody is coming."

"Well, then," Isabel said, her mind racing, "it's just you and me. Come on, impress me. Show me all the signs I should have seen along the way."

"The only thing you and that Bishop of yours got right was gender. Male."

"Trapped in a female's body?" Isabel was deliberately flippant. "I think that's been done."

"Oh, no, I was male first. Always. I kept telling Mallory, but in the beginning she wouldn't listen. And when she did listen, she got confused. She thought she was a lesbian."

Recalling the riot of emotions and hormones of adolescence, Isabel said, "When she was twelve?"

"Those girls at camp. In her cabin. There were six of them, all giggly and girly. The one who slept with Mallory started touching her one night. And Mallory liked it. It made me sick, but Mallory liked it."

"So what happened?"

"I heard them the next day. All six of them, giggling and looking at Mallory. They knew. All of them knew. The one who'd touched her had told the others, and they were going to tell too. I knew they would. They'd tell, and everybody would know Mallory wasn't normal."

"What did you do to stop that?"

"I killed them." Her voice was eerily Mallory's and yet . . . not. Deeper, rougher, harder.

Isabel told herself what she smelled was the lightning, not brimstone. But she knew the truth.

Nothing this side of hell smelled quite like brimstone.

Except for evil.

"See, they weren't supposed to take the boats out onto the

lake, not without one of the counselors. But I made Mallory talk them into it. So they took a boat out, way out, and I made sure there were no life jackets. And then I turned the boat over. None of them made it to the shore, but I got Mallory there, of course. So sad, those other girls drowning like that. Mallory was never the same afterward."

Rafe found Dean Emery slumped over the wheel of his cruiser. He knew nothing could be done for him, but he called for backup and an ambulance, then hurried through the gates of the cemetery, gun drawn, reaching out desperately with every sense he possessed, old and new.

To hell with the goddamned shield.

Mallory shrugged. "That was when her parents moved here to Hastings. So nobody would know what had happened and she could get over it."

"But she didn't." Isabel was dimly aware of the voices, whispering louder, but the thunder and her own fixed concentration on Mallory kept them distant.

"No, not really. She was afraid to have girl friends after that, so all her friends were boys. She played sports, got tough, learned to take care of herself. So I didn't have to worry about her."

"When did that change?"

"You know when it changed, Isabel. It changed in Florida. Mallory was in college in Georgia, but she transferred to a college in Florida to take a few courses one semester."

"There was a redhead," Isabel said. "She was attracted to a redhead, wasn't she? A woman. Were they lovers?"

In the eerie twilight, Mallory's mouth tightened. "That bitch.

She got Mallory drunk and slept with her. And in the morning, she acted like it was nothing. But I knew. I knew she'd tell. I knew she'd tell her redheaded friends. So I had to take care of them, of course. All six of them, just like before."

Isabel didn't waste her breath with any reasoned argument. Instead, she said, "We wondered why the women were going with . . . him. Why they didn't feel threatened. It was because Mallory was a woman."

"It's not my fault if people don't look beneath the surface." She—or he—laughed.

"Mallory didn't know what you were doing, did she?"

"Of course not. She wouldn't have been able to hide our secret. I had to do that. And I had to protect her. When she got abnormal that way."

"What about the women in Alabama?" Isabel asked, only vaguely aware that the wind was gusting wildly now. "The brunettes? Mallory got involved with a brunette woman?"

"She was staying with a cousin over there. Just for a couple of weeks. But that was long enough. Long enough to start mooning over that dark-haired bitch. I didn't even wait for that to get started. I just took care of it. I got rid of her. And the rest of them. The other five."

"The ones who would have told?"

"Of course."

"How did you know they would have?"

"Oh, don't be stupid, Isabel. I always knew who'd tell. As soon as I saw you, I knew you would."

"But Jamie was first, wasn't she?" Isabel asked. "Jamie was the one who caught Mallory's eye."

"I thought she was over it," the thing inside Mallory said. "She was involved with Alan, she was—was *normal*. But then she talked to Jamie about buying a house. And she felt . . . that . . .

again. That longing. That desperation to be touched like that. By her."

"They became lovers."

"*Lovers?* What they were doing had nothing to do with love. Mallory thought she deserved to be punished, because she'd lived when the other girls had died. So she let Jamie punish her. And take pictures of it. But I made her stop. I made her go back to Alan."

Realizing, Isabel said, "And you made her forget. Always. You made sure that her attraction to other women was ... like a fantasy to her. Didn't you?"

"It was an aberration. She didn't need to remember that."

Isabel nodded slowly. "That's why Mallory never reacted to anything we found out about Jamie. As far as she knew, as far as she could remember, they'd never been involved."

"I protected her. I always have."

"So you sent her back to Alan. Then you watched Jamie for a while, didn't you?"

"So sick. Ugly. And she was mad at Mallory for not wanting to do those things anymore. That's why she got too rough with her next *lover* and killed her."

"Hope Tessneer."

"I decided to scare Jamie before I got rid of her. Besides, I was curious. So I took that one's body and hid it. It was fun to watch Jamie panic. Of course, she was thrilled when Mallory called her. Thrilled to meet her. And, you know, she didn't struggle at all. Isn't that interesting? Supposedly all dominant and powerful, and she died with hardly a whimper."

"But you killed her too quickly," Isabel pointed out, glancing toward the box she had flung aside. "You didn't know where she'd hidden the photos. The proof of what she and Mallory had done together."

"I thought they'd be in her apartment. But they weren't, of course. I didn't know where they were."

Isabel swallowed. "Until Emily?"

"Well, you told me to put her on the list, Isabel, didn't you?"

The sick sensation in Isabel's stomach churned even more. "I did?"

"Sure. You told me she might have seen something. Might know something about her sister's killer. And she'd seen the photographs, of course; I knew that as soon as she handed over the ones with Jamie and that other bitch. I didn't think she'd seen Mallory's, but I couldn't be sure. So I had to get rid of her."

"Blood on my hands," Isabel murmured.

"You and Rafe, both so guilty. I think part of him knew all along. I could feel it, even though Mallory never did. I think that's what made him psychic. You said the trigger had to be a traumatic shock, didn't you?"

"Yes. Yes, I did."

"Poor Rafe. He couldn't consciously believe Mallory could do anything like that. Not his friend and fellow cop Mallory. But I think he noticed something there where Jamie died. I'm not sure what; I'm very good at cleaning up after myself. Whatever it was, it told him Mallory had been there. So he knew. Deep down, he knew."

"And woke up with blood on his hands." Isabel drew a breath. "He'll know for sure now. Both Hollis and me dead, probably Dean, too, and you—Mallory—still alive. He'll know."

"No, see, you still don't get it. The change is finally complete. I got tired of only coming out sometimes, of being asleep inside Mallory so much of the time. So I've been taking over. More and more. Mallory's gone now. She's never coming back. And after I've taken care of you, I'll leave."

It was true, Isabel realized. She looked at the shell that had once held the personality, the soul, of a woman she had liked very much, and knew without doubt that Mallory Beck was gone. She had started going away when six little girls had died on a lake, and over the years more and more of her had fallen away.

Until now. There was only this. This evil thing that had lived deep inside.

Isabel knew.

This was the evil that had killed Julie. The evil Isabel had sworn to destroy. Crouching in the darkness. Waiting to sprint.

Wearing the face of a friend.

He/she glanced down at Hollis, faintly dissatisfied. "She's not blonde. Neither was that stupid, nosy reporter."

"Cheryl Bayne. She's dead?"

"Of course she's dead. Little twit hadn't even realized, but I think she'd seen me slipping into the gas station a couple of days before your partner and I *found* the body. It bugged her enough to send her snooping around the place, but I don't think she even knew what she was looking for. Until she found it, of course."

"What did you do with her body?"

"A cop to the last, aren't you?" The thing inside Mallory laughed. "They'll find her, eventually, at the bottom of a well. I didn't have time to play with her, you see. I had to get busy. Because she wasn't a blonde. But you are, and you'll make five."

Isabel knew she didn't have a hope of getting to her calf holster and second gun. Not without a distraction. But even as she thought of that, her mind was suddenly clear and calm, and she was aware of a strength and utter certainty she had never felt in her life.

She wasn't alone.

She would never be alone again.

"Mallory." Rafe was there, stepping from behind a tall monument at a right angle to the women, his gun extended in two steady hands.

"Didn't you hear me, Chief?" The black-gloved hand cocked Isabel's pistol and held it aimed at her heart. "Mallory's gone. And I'll kill Isabel if you so much as twitch."

"You'll kill her anyway," Rafe said.

"Go away like a good chief and I might let her live."

"Evil," Isabel said, "always deceives. That's what it's best at. That's why it wore the face of a friend this time. And that's why we can't let it walk away alive."

The thing wearing Mallory's skin opened its mouth to say something, but the wind that had been steadily gaining strength abruptly sent a gust of hot air through the cemetery, and the birch tree beside the chapel flung one of its broken branches through a stained-glass window.

The crash was loud and sudden, and Isabel instinctively took advantage of it, throwing herself sideways to the ground even as she reached for the gun strapped to her calf.

The black-gloved hand started to follow Isabel's path, finger tightening on the trigger, but the evil inside was just a split second slower than Rafe's training and instincts.

His shot spun Mallory around so that his/her gun was pointing toward Rafe.

Isabel's shot finished it.

The storm, uncaring of both human living and evil dying in its path, roared louder and louder as it finally made up its mind to hit Hastings.

EPILOGUE

"YOU'RE A HARD WOMAN to kill," Isabel said.

Hollis raised both eyebrows at her.

"I'm not saying it like it's a bad thing."

Looking at Rafe, Hollis said, "You realize what you're letting yourself in for? She can't *not* be flippant."

"I know. It's a character flaw."

"I resent that," Isabel said.

"You shouldn't. It happens to be a flaw I enjoy."

"Oh, well, in that case."

Hollis shifted slightly in the hospital bed to get more comfortable. Or try to. "I'm just lucky you two managed to stop Mallory's evil twin before he could finish me off."

They all found it less painful to refer to the creature they had destroyed there at the end as Mallory's evil twin—a phrase

341

naturally coined by Isabel. Not that it could be anything but painful, especially for Rafe.

Or Alan, who was still bewildered and in shock.

"What I can't figure out," Isabel said, "is what he planned to do once he left Hastings. He really was trapped in a woman's body—and had been since the male personality split off from Mallory when she was twelve."

"A sex-change operation?" Hollis suggested.

Rafe said, "I don't think so. I think *he* saw a male when he saw himself."

"A very confused male," Isabel pointed out. "He wanted Mallory to be involved with men, not women. But I'm willing to bet he would have been angry and insulted to be called homosexual."

"Didn't Bishop offer a theory?" Hollis asked. "I seem to recall a discussion going on over my mostly unconscious self a couple of days ago."

"We had to talk about something," Isabel told her. "The doctors said you were pretty out of it."

"I was. Mostly. But I remember Bishop and Miranda being here. And talking, like I said. What was the theory?"

"That Mallory's evil twin was delusional. We haven't really gotten past that part."

"It's complicated," Hollis agreed.

"She—he—was right about me, anyway," Rafe said. "I had seen something unconsciously when we were at the first murder scene. From the corner of my eye, I suppose. I'd seen Mallory touch Jamie's hair. Something about it, about the way she did it, was like a red flag."

"And a subconscious shock," Isabel said. "The hardest thing to accept about evil is that it can wear a familiar face. He was very good at hiding."

"Until Mallory did something he couldn't accept," Rafe said.

He sighed. "Just . . . thinking of her dying inside all those years, bit by bit. I keep thinking I should have known. Should have been able to help her."

"Nobody could help her," Isabel told him quietly. "Nobody was there when that boat overturned and six little girls drowned. Nobody but him. Mallory was doomed from that moment."

"And too many other women along with her," Hollis said. "Plus Ginny's father, and that poor older lady, and Dean Emery. And God knows how many others would have died if you two hadn't stopped it."

"It doesn't feel very heroic, what we did," Rafe said.

Isabel smiled at him. "It seldom does. Evil leaves so much destruction behind it that it's like a train wreck. You don't think about what was saved ahead on the tracks, just the devastation of the crash."

"And yet you're inviting me to jump on the train with you."

"Well, I'm sort of committed. To the journey, I mean. It's not something where you can just get off at the next station."

"Excuse me," Hollis said, "but are you two still speaking in metaphors?"

"You noticed that?" Isabel said earnestly.

"It amuses her," Rafe said.

Hollis shook her head. "One for the books, you two. I bet Bishop can hardly wait to get you up to Quantico."

"There was an invitation," Rafe admitted. "He didn't mention trains, though."

"So, did you accept?" Hollis asked.

"What do you think?"

"I think . . . that the SCU just took on a whole new dimension."

"How about that?" Isabel said. "And she's not even precognitive."